Vaginal Operations

Surgical Anatomy and Technique

Second Edition

Vaginal Operations
Surgical Anatomy and Technique
Second Edition

Günther Reiffenstuhl, MD
Professor Emeritus and Director Emeritus, University of Münster, Westphalen, Germany
Emeritus Chief, Salzburg Women's Clinic
Baden, Austria

Werner Platzer, MD
Professor and Chief, Anatomy Institute, University of Innsbruck
Innsbruck, Austria

Paul-Georg Knapstein, MD
Professor and Director, Clinic and Polyclinic for Obstetrics and Gynecology
Johannes-Gutenberg University
Mainz, Germany

English-Language Editor
John R. Imig, MD
Department of Obstetrics and Gynecology
The Boulder Medical Center
Boulder, Colorado

Translated by
Julika Bond
Academy of Languages
Baltimore, Maryland

SANS TACHE
Williams & Wilkins
A WAVERLY COMPANY
BALTIMORE • PHILADELPHIA • LONDON • PARIS • BANGKOK
BUENOS AIRES • HONG KONG • MUNICH • SYDNEY • TOKYO • WROCLAW

Editor: Charles W. Mitchell
Managing Editor: Grace E. Miller
Production Coordinator: Linda Carlson
Copy Editor: Therese J. Grundl
Designer: Wilma E. Rosenberger
Illustration Planner: Lorraine C. Wrzosek
Typesetter: University Graphics, Inc.
Manufacturing: Everbest

351 West Camden Street
Baltimore, Maryland 21202-2436 USA

Rose Tree Corporate Center
1400 North Providence Road
Building II, Suite 5025
Media, Pennsylvania 19063-2043 USA

Printed in Hong Kong

First Edition, in German, © 1974, Urban & Schwarzenberg

This is a translation of Reiffenstuhl G, Platzer W, Knapstein P-G. *Die vaginalen Operationen: Chirurgische Anatomie und Operationslehre*, 2nd edition. Copyright Urban & Schwarzenberg, München-Wien-Baltimore, 1994.

Library of Congress Cataloging-in-Publication Data

Reiffenstuhl, Günther.
[Vaginalen Operationen. English]
Vaginal operations : surgical anatomy and technique / Günther Reiffenstuhl, Werner Platzer, Paul-Georg Knapstein ; English -language editor, John R. Imig ; translated by Julika Bond.—2nd ed.
p. cm.
Rev. ed. of: Atlas of vaginal surgery / Günther Reiffenstuhl and Werner Platzer. 1975.
Includes index.
ISBN 0-683-07285-4
1. Vagina—Surgery—Atlases. 2. Cervix uteri—Surgery—Atlases.
3. Generative organs, Female—Anatomy—Atlases. I. Platzer. Warner. II. Knapstein, Paul Georg. III. Imig, John R. IV. Reiffenstuhl, Günther. Vaginalen Operationen. V. Title.
[DNLM: 1. Vagina—surgery—atlases. 2. Vaginal Diseases—surgery—atlases. 3. Cervix Diseases—surgery. 4. Genitalia, Female—anatomy & histology. WP 17 R361v 1996a]
RG104.R4213 1996
618.1′5059—dc20
DNLM/DLC
for Library of Congress 95-39425
CIP

96 97 98 99 00
1 2 3 4 5 6 7 8 9 10

Preface to the English Edition

It has been a privilege to edit the translation of this edition of Reiffenstuhl's text from German to English. The translation was accomplished in a superb manner by Julika Bond with the assistance of Robert Slawson, MD. My task was to edit this work into terminology in common usage by the English-speaking gynecologic surgeon. My perspective is that of a practicing gynecologist for the past 18 years at the Boulder Medical Center. Vaginal surgery remains almost exclusively within the specialty of gynecology, and in the era of "managed care," this approach often results in significant cost savings compared with abdominal surgery.

Reiffenstuhl's work is a magnificent compendium of vaginal surgery with unparalleled quality and clarity. The step-by-step illustrations and descriptions will make it possible for the gynecologist in training to quickly grasp proper surgical techniques for each procedure. The practicing gynecologist will find this text invaluable for reviewing infrequently done procedures or to prepare for newer operations. The gynecologic oncologist will appreciate the comprehensive presentation of the Schauta procedure and the coverage of fistula repair. This work will be a welcome addition to the professional library of any gynecologist.

It will be quickly evident to American readers that there are significant differences presented by the European authors regarding preoperative and postoperative care, choice of prep solutions, and choice of suture materials from those in common usage in the United States. No attempt was made to edit or change these details during the translation. Hopefully, the North American reader will note and appreciate these differences and accept that there will always be variations in practice among countries and healthcare delivery systems.

John R. Imig, MD
Boulder Medical Center

Preface to the Second Edition

In choosing the title ''Vaginal Operations,'' we do not expect to offer a comprehensive discussion of *all* vaginal operations. Rather, we intend to cover only those operations that we know from our own experience and about which we teach.

This new edition permitted a sweeping revision and broadening of the work. We slightly expanded the base of topographic-anatomical knowledge from a vaginal perspective. The chapters ''Curettage,'' ''Colpotomy,'' ''Conization,'' ''Surgical Treatment for Perineal Rupture,'' ''Surgical Treatment for Vesicovaginal Fistula,'' and ''Surgical Treatment for Vaginal Aplasia'' were further developed and clarified. We also added the chapter ''Surgical Treatment for Rectovaginal Fistula,'' which led to some new illustrations. We found that very few of the first edition's illustrations were expendable. Each discussion of a vaginal operation begins with the customary indications and ends by discussing possible technical problems. This may provide the student useful advice to avoid complications—remember that the term ''Technical Problems'' should by no means be interpreted as professional errors. Vaginal operations are in most cases a task for a group: the surgeon, two assistants, the anesthesiologist, the surgical nurse, and an assistant nurse. We once again went to great lengths to define specific tasks for the assistants during particular phases of the vaginal surgical procedures. These instructions, if followed meticulously, will create ample space for the surgeon at the operating station. Experienced assistance during vaginal surgery can be particularly crucial when difficulties must be surmounted. We paid meticulous attention to the illustrations, because they represent the most valuable aspect of the surgical text. Figure legends are used in lieu of text and should always be read conscientiously.

In discussing carcinoma of uterine cervix stage 1b, the comparison between a vaginal and abdominal radical operation caused us to expand the text of the indication statement in favor of the Schauta-Amreich operation. According to the most recent results (summer 1994) the 5-year cure rate is the same for both methods, but the radical vaginal operation has considerably fewer postoperative complications than the Wertheim procedure. Consequently, the vaginal approach is once again gaining significance. Techniques for cervical carcinoma surgery must be communicated, because this will enable the gynecological surgeon, having understood and grasped the individual phases of the Schauta-Amreich operation (especially in preventing ureteral injury), to easily stay in control of any situation during an operation.

Gynecologic minimally invasive surgery currently is synonymous with endoscopic operations. There have been numerous new developments in this genre. The German and Austrian Societies for Gynecological and Obstetric Endoscopy, both representing sections of professional societies of their countries, are engaged in developing a specific definition of indications, in standardizing techniques for operations, in legitimizing training facilities, and in including surgical methods and training standards into future professional training regulations for our field.

For decades transvaginal operations have been an essential, minimally invasive component of surgical gynecology. Particular advantages are clearly defined indications, a reliable and well-described access path for the well-trained and practiced surgeon, a small operational area producing minimal trauma for the patient, invisible scar tissue, and low perioperative morbidity with short hospitalization. Cost and time factors must also be considered. Whereas vaginal surgery uses relatively few and cost effective sutures and standard instruments, the endoscopic procedure uses expensive staplers or specialized materials as well as a high tech instrument set that carries a high acquisition price. A vaginal hysterectomy can be completed in 30 minutes; an additonal vaginal or pelvic plastic procedure might need 60 minutes, but the average scheduling time for an endoscopic supracervical uterine extirpation, even for the proficient surgeon, must be between 2 and 3 hours. A randomized psychosexual study should be performed to determine if it is truly in the patient's best interest to preserve the punched-out cervical canal, as would be the case if one used the laparoscopic technique.

Sonja Klebe created the illustrations for the additonal chapters with a great deal of sensitivity for the genius of the academic artist *Franz Batke.* We owe her considerable thanks for her commitment and diligence. We also thank *B. Scheele*, MD, the Urban & Schwarzenberg editor, who had contributed much time, care, and tremendous enthusiasm to our effort. *P. Mazzetti* must be thanked for the excellent production of the book. As production manager, he successfully expedited its production with great competence. We extend special thanks to our publisher, *M. Urban*, PhD, honorary doctor, who promoted the publication of the new edition. Amenable to all our wishes, he has given us free rein with respect to the illustrations. This made it possible to publish a high-quality product.

We hope that the new edition of our work will again contribute to the preservation of the art of vaginal surgery and serve to inspire a new generation in the medical community. We feel indebted to the outstanding performance of the Austrian and German surgical school and their pioneers, i.e., *Stoeckel, G.A. Wagner, Schauta, Amreich, Navratil.* We hope to pass their legacy to future generations. In specific cases, vaginal and endoscopic surgical techniques may in the future complement one another in a meaningful fashion.

This atlas, which is based on personal experience, is meant to be used as an instructional textbook for performing vaginal surgery. For that reason we seldom use bibliographical references and statistical data.

August 1994
G. Reiffenstuhl, Baden bei Wien
W. Platzer, Innbruck
P.-G.Knapstein, Mainz

Preface to the First Edition

The prerequisites for a successful surgical practice are talent and education. One is born with the first. Technical details can be learned but must first be developed by conscientious training. Intimate knowledge of anatomy and the experience garnered from association with and exposure to a teacher who operates whenever possible in a typical fashion are indispensable for independent execution of surgical procedures.

The German literature contains exemplary instructional material in gynecological surgery based on the collective wealth of experience of its authors. Such material warrants a prominent place in the libraries of every practicing gynecologist. This notwithstanding, we decided to create a new work on this subject in 1965. Our objective was not directed toward providing something better than previously available, but rather it originated with our thought and desire to elucidate the anatomic surgical principles that we have developed and tested in the course of evolving our extensive experience. Our aim was to coordinate this material in a uniform and comprehensively detailed manner.

In scope, this book is meant to serve in providing technical advice for performing vaginal surgical procedures. The exclusive preference for the vaginal approach in our discussion is based on the philosophy that gynecologists in particular must become proficient in these vaginal techniques, which typify the idea of gynecology, and that they should practice and nurture them.

For each gynecological disorder, there are several competing procedures available. Had we concerned ourselves with all in the same detail, the scope of this volume would have expanded excessively. We concur with *Frisch*, who stated in the preface to his atlas of surgical gynecology, ''A textbook must not become a history of gynecological operations. It is better to learn one good method than to recapitulate all methods that have been recommended over the course of the decade.'' For the same reason, we have avoided any critical mention of the relevant literature so as not to disturb the uniformity and flow of the total picture. Vaginal operations were consciously preselected for presentation on the basis of preferences engendered by their origin in the Austrian school and the fact that they have kept their place there to date. If this volume is slanted subjectively by a systematic representation of surgical procedures, some of which have been personally developed by the authors, then our purpose has been realized in helping to disseminate knowledge concerning those vaginal surgical procedures that have been and still are practiced extensively at the clinic of one of the authors. They are meant to be a reflection of the art of surgery as currently practiced by Austrian gynecologists.

Even though we must admit that we have not defended the views of our teachers of anatomy and gynecology in all matters, we believe it is the duty of respectful students toward their teachers to mention them in gratitude: *Von Hayek, Pernkopf, Antoine,* and *Navratil.* In dividing our material, we portrayed first the anatomical conditions and then built upon this information to describe the various surgical methods.

In our descriptions of operations, details were presented that were thought to be necessary to reduce the hazards of each procedure. Additionally, the activities of both assisting physicians were discussed in great detail because experience has taught us that cooperative contributions by assistants are essential for the success of vaginal surgery. The surgeon must not only have full command of the operative details of the procedure itself, but he or she must be able to instruct the assistants systematically. Only in this way can the interplay of all three operating physicians be achieved and transmit to the observer the feeling of facility and smoothness. If well orchestrated, the procedure can be shortened considerably. Furthermore, we have set out to show the hazards of the operations that proved to be problematic to both the beginner and the more advanced surgeon. Anxiety alone, while producing pearls of sweat on the surgeon's brow, is not a good advisor. It is therefore far better to explain as frankly as possible what we and others have observed as errors and dangers in performing vaginal surgery. Every surgeon who is dedicated to the surgical approach has suffered some technical setbacks, but not everyone is prepared to acknowledge them.

At the beginning, an anatomical introduction is presented. It consists of a summation based on presentations dealing with individual regions as viewed from the surgeon's vantage. We chose this approach rather than the more orthodox anatomical compartmentalization, which is not applicable to surgical practice, because it seemed to be a requisite for the surgical section that follows.

Along similar lines, we found it necessary to present sketches of the different surgical steps to indicate specific, important anatomical details. Special care has been devoted to these illustrations because the value of a surgical textbook depends to a large extent on them.

All anatomical illustrations were produced from specimens prepared at the Anatomical Institute of the University of Innsbruck through the invaluable aid of Dr. *Maurer* and others. With heartfelt thanks we acknowledge them here. In particular, we note that all semischematic and schematic illustrations were drawn from original specimens. Illustrations of the clinical aspects were based on observations made during actual procedures performed on live patients. To achieve the special characteristics of naturalness in these figures, thousands of color slides in stereoscopic photography were taken during the operations. These then served as models for the illustrations. Not one was made from memory or reproduced from previously published pictures. The stereo photography and a superior technique in drawing have permitted the artist to grasp the correct depth of the particular operative field and to represent it accurately.

All drawings were created by the academic artist, *Franz Batke*, with whom the authors have worked in collaboration for several books for more than 25 years. Franz Batke is an artist recognized by American medical illustrators as one of the best illustrators of anatomical atlases and surgical textbooks. He has brought to this book not only decades of experience but also his personal relationship and friendship with both authors. He has worked on this volume with exemplary enthusiasm. For the artistically refined illustrations contained herein, which represent 10 years of carefully detailed work, we owe considerable thanks to Franz Batke.

Significant aid in providing the slides during surgery was given by the surgical nurse, *Erasta Jagerhofer*, who applied considerable knowledge to this endeavor in an always friendly and cooperative fashion and who was willing to sacrifice much time and effort in our behalf. For all this, we express our gratitude.

For reading and correcting the anatomical section, we thank the assistants, Dr. *R. Putz* and Dr. *S. Poisel* of the Anatomical Institute of the Univeristy of Innsbruck. In editorially correcting the clinical part, Dr. *Staudach*, of the Frauenklinik Salzburg, has provided a great deal of support for which we are particularly grateful.

To our publishers, *M. Urban* of Munich and his father, Dr. *Heinz Urban*, who edited and produced the German edition of this book, we offer special thanks. Dr. *Müller*, the publisher's scientific consultant who always demonstrated a deep insight and understanding of this work, and Mr. *Gullath*, who managed the production, were both instrumental in ensuring that the book would appear in its present form.

Spring 1974
G. Reiffenstuhl and W. Platzer

Contents

SECTION I. ANATOMICAL DESCRIPTION

W. Platzer

SECTION II. SURGICAL TECHNIQUE

G. Reiffenstuhl and P.-G. Knapstein

SECTION I
ANATOMICAL DESCRIPTION

W. Platzer

EXTERNAL GENITALIA

The external female genitalia (Fig. A.1), the vulva, consists of the labia majora, labia minora, clitoris, vaginal vestibule, and mons pubis. The labia majora lie in close apposition in nulliparas, which border on the pudendal aperture. The vaginal vestibule is exposed only when the labia are parted.

The *labia majora* are separated from the genitofemoral sulci by lateral depressions and the interconnecting gluteoperineal tissues. The genitofemoral sulcus borders the interfemineum (vulva, perineum, and anus) posterolaterally toward the upper thigh and continues anteriorly into the gluteal sulcus. Medially to the genitofemoral sulcus, an accessory groove is sometimes found, beginning in the urogenital region (laterally to the labia majora) and ending in the gluteal region. The two labia come together in the midline at the anterior labial commissure that borders the mons pubis inferiorly. Toward the perineum, the posterior labial commissure is found; it appears to separate the vaginal vestibule from the sharp-edged labial frenulum (frenulum labiorum pudendi). On their outer surface, the labia majora are covered with pigmented skin that contains numerous sebaceous and sweat glands, as well as genital nerve endings and hair follicles. Hair growth covers the area after puberty. Subcutaneously within the labia majora are sheets of connective tissue that collectively form the corpus fibrosum. Adipose tissue may penetrate between these connective tissue layers from the mons pubis as well as from the perineum. Muscle fibers with a more or less smooth consistency may also be found. The connective tissue layer radiates into the perineal body at one end and into the abdominal subcutaneous tissue at the other. The deep clitoral ligament arises approximately in the middle of the mons pubis. The uterine round ligaments (ligamenta teretes, ligamenta rotunda uteri) radiate subcutaneously upward bilaterally from each inguinal canal.

The *labia minora* border medially on the vaginal vestibule and are separated laterally from the labia majora by the nympholabial sulci. They separate cranially into medial and lateral components. The medial part is the clitoral frenulum that extends to the underside of the glans clitoridis, whereas the more laterally located preputial frenulum forms the clitoral prepuce. The labia minora become smaller in their caudal extension and become apposed to each other immediately in front of the posterior labial commissure above the pudendal frenulum, a diagonal skinfold. This frenulum is sometimes inaccurately attributed to the labia majora.

The labia minora are free of hair and are covered only by a thin layer of cornified squamous epithelium. They contain mostly elastic fibers, blood vessels, and nerves as well as coarse connective tissue. In addition, they possess "free sebaceous glands" but no sweat glands. They develop to different sizes but are usually hidden by the labia majora. They can, however, protrude from between the labia majora and may actually even extend a considerable distance (as in the so-called Hottentot apron).

The vaginal introitus and the urethral meatus open into the vaginal vestibule between the labia minora. On the other side of the introitus are the openings of the ducts of Bartholin's vestibular glands. At the posterior edge of the vestibule is the fossa navicularis, whereas anteriorly, between the glans clitoridis and the urethral opening, the urethral sulcus is located. The urethral meatus opens on the urethral papilla. Anterolateral to the papilla,

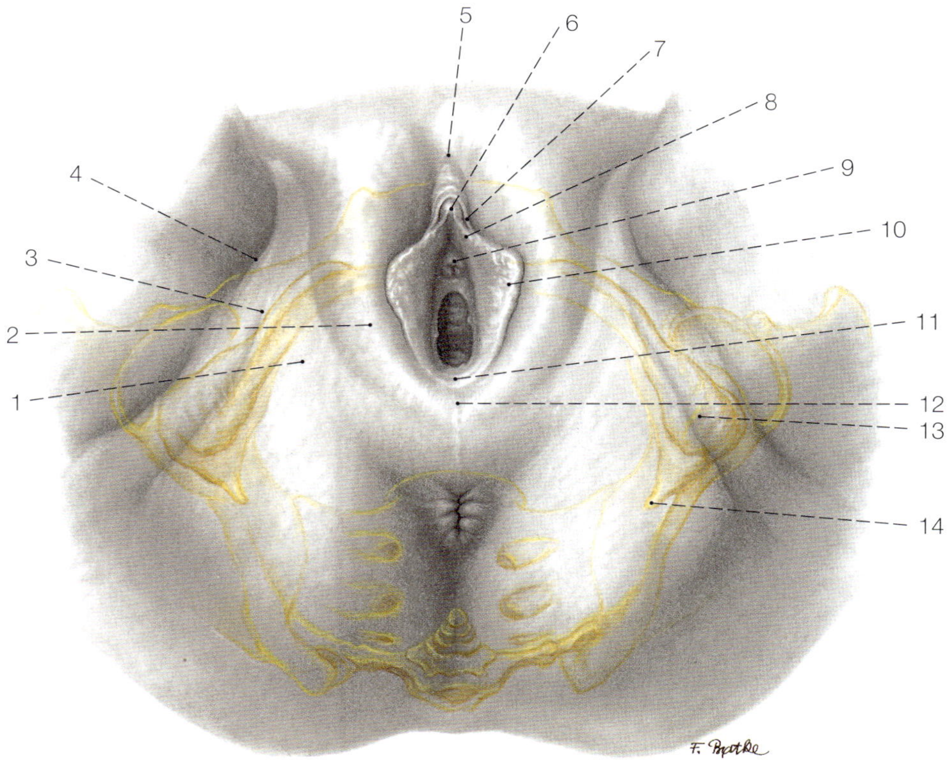

Figure A.1. External genitalia. Contours of the underlying bony pelvis are illustrated.
1 gluteoperineal area
2 labium majus
3 accessory sulcus
4 genitofemoral sulcus
5 anterior labial commissure
6 glans clitoridis
7 preputial frenulum
8 clitoral frenulum
9 urethral papilla and orifice of external urethra
10 labium minus
11 fourchette
12 posterior labial commissure
13 ischial tuberosity (palpable bony prominence)
14 ischial spine, contoured

the ostia of the paraurethral ducts can be seen leading from the periurethral glands.

The width of the introitus depends on the development of the vulva and the presence or absence of a hymen. Laterally at the edge of the introitus in multiparas are the hymeneal caruncles that constitute the remains of the hymen.

The *clitoris* is formed by the two crura that originate at the inferior pubic rami in the region of the interfascial perineal space. Both clitoral crura join to become the corpus clitoridis that ends in the rounded glans. The corpus clitoridis consists of an ascending and a descending part, forming the angle at which the clitoris is joined to the symphysis pubis by means of the suspensory ligament. Each crus clitoridis is composed of a corpus cavernosum, although it is often attenuated (in the corpus region) and incompletely divided internally by a membrane, the septum of the corpus cavernosum. The surface of this corpus cavernosum is composed of a tight, inelastic tunica albuginea. In addition, the crus clitoridis is covered by the ischiocavernosus muscle that originates on the ischial tuberosity.

At the base of the labia majora lie the vascular vestibular bulbs, the *bulbi vestibuli* (Fig. A.2). They are situated very close to the urogenital diaphragm. Their posterior ends are distended, whereas they become thinner toward the symphysis. They are interconnected between the clitoris and the urethra. The two corpora cavernosa are covered by the *bulbocavernosus muscles* (bulbospongiosus muscle, constrictor vaginae muscle) that originate from the perineal body. These muscles radiate in contiguity with the *ischiocavernous muscles* into the fascia that invests the body of the clitoris. The bulbocavernosus muscle is a relatively flat muscle covering both the vestibular bulb and Bartholin's gland. Its weakly constrictive components are strengthened by the levator sling.

The two pea-sized *Bartholin's glands* (Fig. A.2) contain mucous glandular elements and lie behind the deep transverse perineal muscles. In part they are covered superficially by the thickened posterior ends of the vestibular bulbs. Each gland complex has a duct of about 2 cm long that flows laterally from the vaginal introitus into the vestibule.

Blood supply. Blood supply of the external genital organs derives from both the internal and the external pudendal arteries. The external pudendal artery, which originates from the femoral artery in the saphenous hiatus (or fossa ovalis), supplies the anterior labial arteries. These vessels in turn reach the anterior part of the labia majora. The posterior labial arteries arise from the internal pudendal artery, usually within Alcock's canal and penetrating its wall. They supply the posterior portion of the labia minora and majora.

The clitoris is supplied with blood by the deep clitoral artery (leading to the crura) and by the dorsal clitoral artery (to the glans). The latter is the terminal branch of the internal pudendal artery. The vestibular bulb gets its blood from the internal pudendal artery bilaterally via the vestibular bulbar arteries.

Blood drainage. Blood drainage from the labia proceeds by way of the anterior and posterior labial veins to both the internal and external pudendal veins. The unpaired subfascial dorsal clitoral vein and the paired deep clitoral veins as well as the subcutaneous dorsal clitoral veins all originate from the clitoris. These veins are closely related to the pudendovesical plexus en

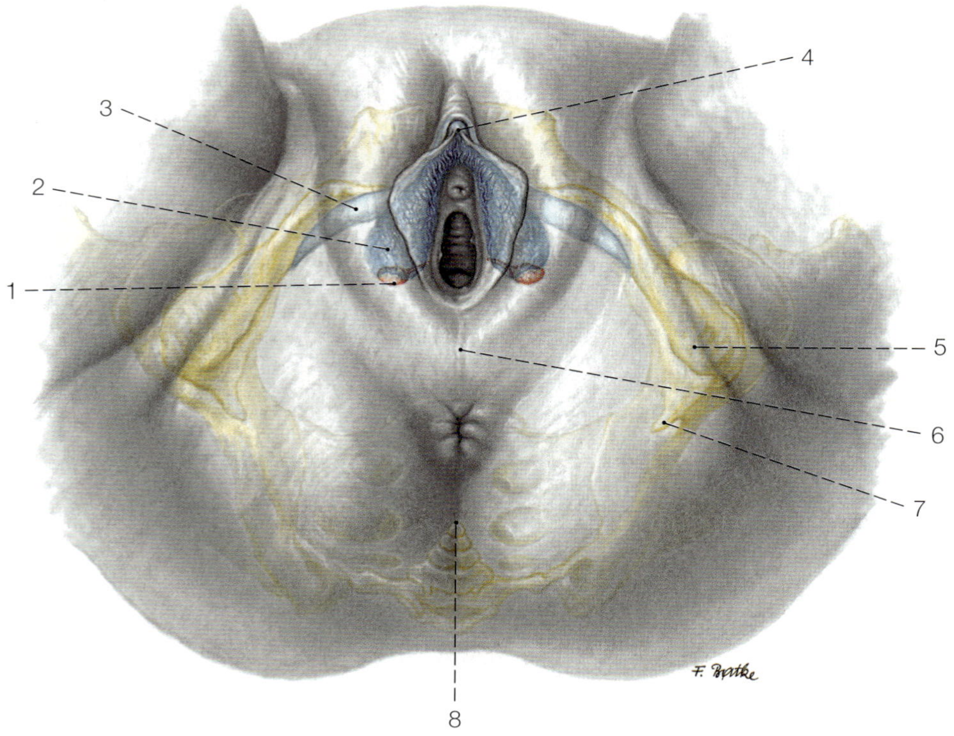

Figure A.2. External genitalia superimposed on contoured skeletal structures, illustrating clitoris and vestibular bulb.
1 Bartholin's gland
2 vestibular bulb
3 crus clitoridis
4 glans clitoridis
5 ischial tuberosity (palpable)
6 perineal raphe
7 ischial spine
8 tip of coccyx (palpable)

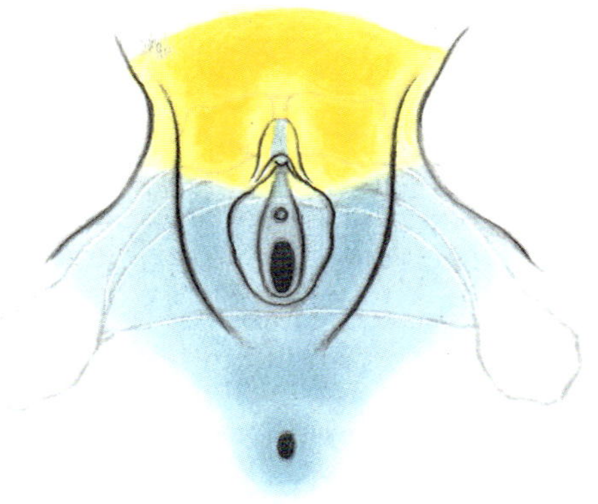

Figure A.3. Sensory innervation of vulva. *Yellow,* ilioinguinal nerve and genital branch of genitofemoral nerve; *blue,* branches of pudendal nerve.

route to the internal and the external pudendal veins into which they can also flow by a more direct pathway. Moreover, some blood from the vestibular bulb enters the pudendovesical plexus. Another portion flows directly by way of the vestibular bulbar vein into the internal pudendal vein.

Lymph drainage. Lymph drainage from the external genitalia occurs through several lymphatic collecting channels to the superficial inguinal lymph nodes. Lymphatics from the corpus cavernosum travel along the internal pudendal vein to the interiliac node groups.

Innervation. The innervation of the skin of the posterior aspects of the external genitalia (Fig. A.3) consists of the posterior labial nerves that are branches of the internal pudendal nerve. The terminal branch of the pudendal nerve, the dorsal clitoral nerve, serves the skin in the area of the clitoris. The ilioinguinal nerve coursing through the inguinal canal extends to the anterior portion of the labia in conjunction with the anterior labial nerve. The genital branch of the genitofemoral nerve also participates in the innervation of the external genitalia.

PERINEUM

The anatomy of this area is particularly relevant, because it applies to the operative treatment of Bartholin's gland cyst (Chapter 10) and to surgical procedures involving the Schuchart incision (Chapter 22).

The perineum (Fig. A.1), situated between the vulva and the anus, is about 2.5 cm long. Laterally toward the upper thigh, the perineum is bordered by the genitofemoral sulcus. The perineal raphe is a midline structure sometimes manifest as a skin fold that stretches between the pudendal aperture and the anus. The perineal body (*centrum tendineum perinei*) is the foundation of the perineum (Fig. A.4). The concept that it is composed entirely

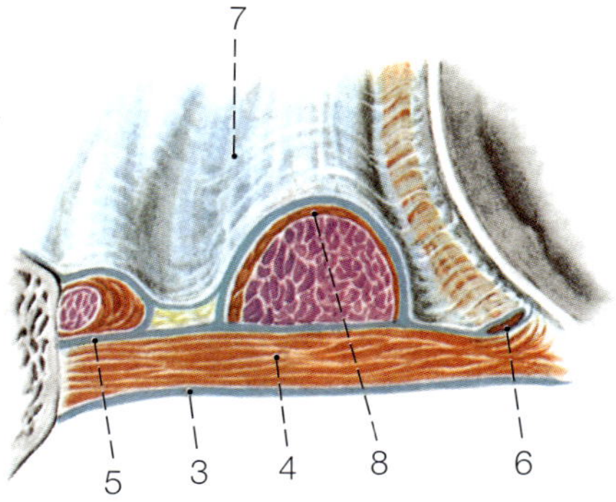

Figure A.4. Architecture of perineum. *Brown,* diagonally striated muscles; *red,* smooth muscle; *blue,* connective tissue; *yellow,* adipose tissue.

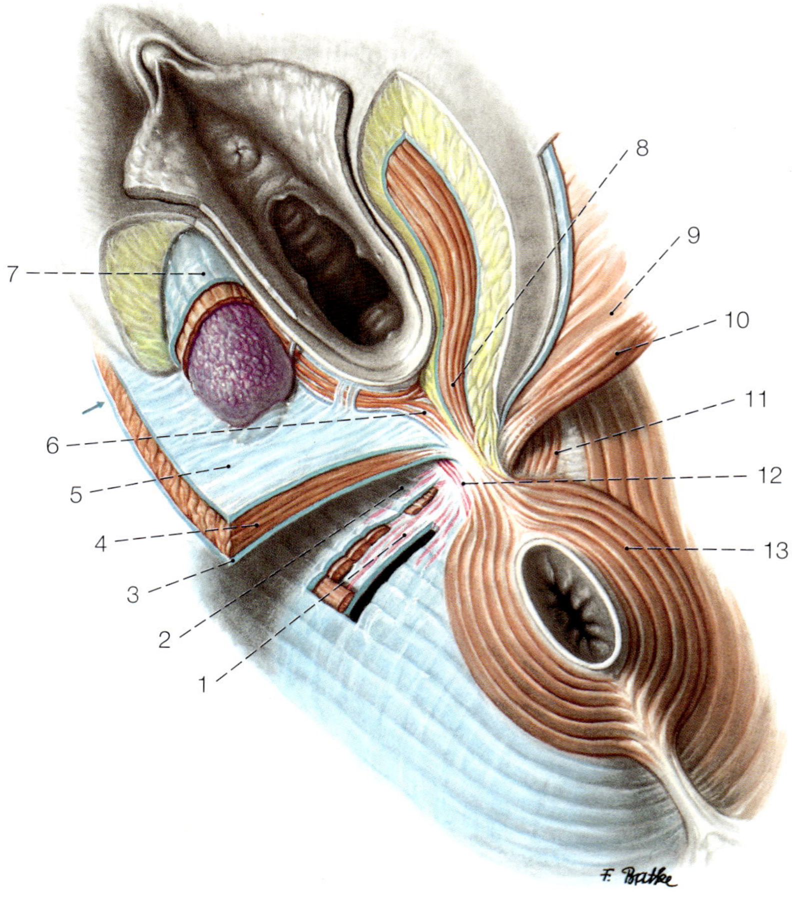

Detail. Section through urogenital diaphragm at level of *arrow* in Figure A.4.

1 superior fascia of pelvic diaphragm with smooth muscle fibers
2 inferior fascia of pelvic diaphragm with smooth muscle fibers
3 superior urogenital fascia
4 deep transverse perineal muscle
5 inferior urogenital fascia
6 urethrovaginal muscle
7 perineal fascia (superficial)
8 bulbocavernosus muscle
9 deep transverse perineal muscle
10 superficial transverse perineal muscle
11 prerectal fibers of levator ani muscle
12 rectovaginal muscle
13 external anal sphincter muscle

of connective tissue is actually incorrect, because both smooth muscle and striated muscle bundles radiate into the coarse fibrous connective tissue that it contains.

In addition to the prerectal fibers of the levator ani muscle and smooth muscle fibers of the levator vaginae muscle, muscle bundles reach the perineal body from the deep and superficial transverse perineal muscles and the superficial portion of the external sphincter ani (Fig. A.5) as well. Likewise, the medial muscle fibers of the deep transverse perineal muscle that forms the urethrovaginal muscle (vaginal sphincter muscle) also enter the perineal body. The bulbocavernosus muscle originates on either side of the perineal body. Some smooth muscle bundles stretch from the longitudinal muscle fibers of the rectum to the posterior wall of the vagina, participating as a rectovaginal muscle in the formation of the perineal body. Smooth muscle fibers of the rectococcygeus muscle that are connected to the levator fascia are similarly attached. In addition to the smooth muscle fibers arising from the inferior levator fascia (fascia diaphragmatis pelvis inferior), smooth muscle bundles reach the perineal body from the superior levator fascia (fascia diaphragmatis pelvis superior) as well as from both the superior and inferior fasciae of the urogenital diaphragm. Finally, the connective tissue membranes that form the base of the labia majora and the superficial perineal fascia take part in the construction of the perineal body.

The perineal body thus appears as a large connective tissue structure permeated with a multitude of muscle fibers. However, all the elements listed become nonfunctional if the perineum is destroyed and has to be restored by mass suturing that incorporates the levator pillar.

Blood and lymph supply. Blood supply (Fig. A.6) of the perineum is derived from the internal pudendal artery. It takes its origin at the internal iliac artery, piercing through the infrapiriform foramen and coursing around the ischial spine to reach the lateral wall of the ischiorectal fossa by way of the lesser sciatic foramen, where it enters Alcock's canal. There it gives

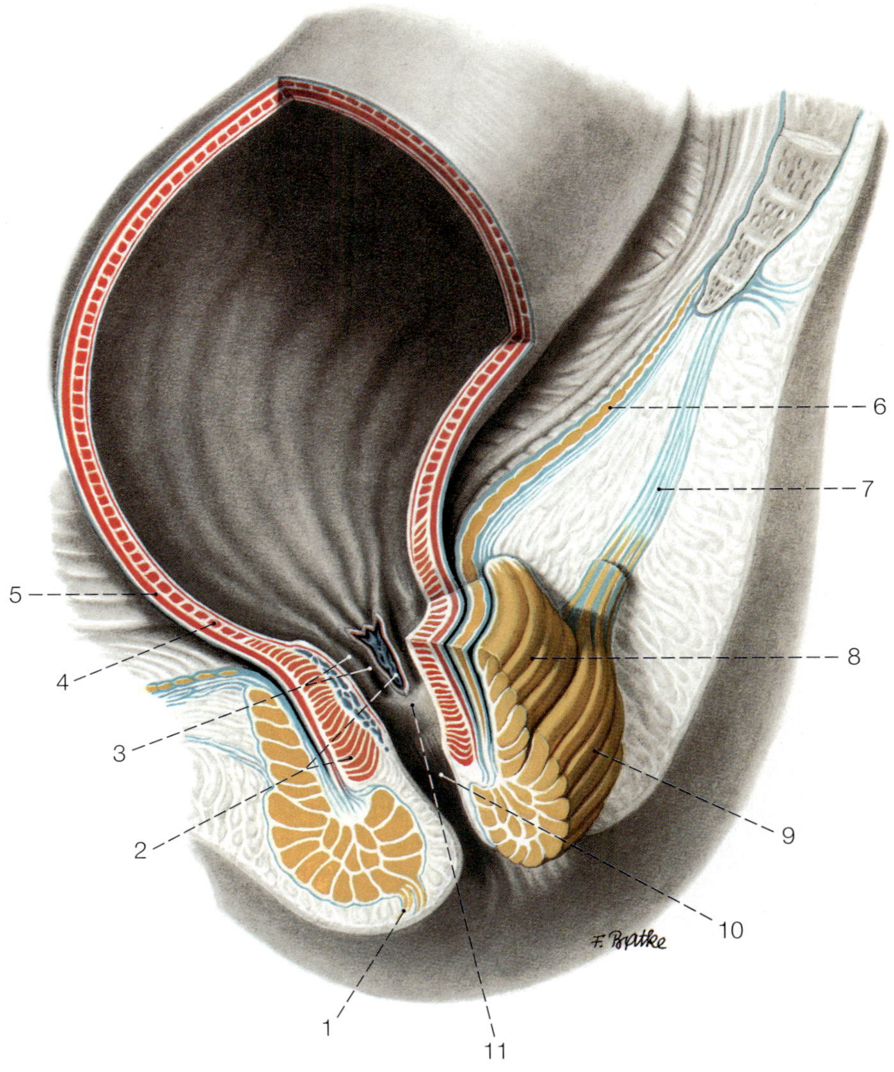

Figure A.5. Anus and external sphincter muscle (semischematic).

1 subcutaneous part of external anal sphincter
2 internal anal sphincter muscle and venous plexus in an anal column
3 anal column and anal sinus
4 annular muscle of rectum
5 longitudinal muscle of rectum
6 levator ani muscle and its fascia
7 anococcygeal ligament
8 deep part of external sphincter
9 superficial part of external sphincter
10 cutaneous zone
11 intermediate zone

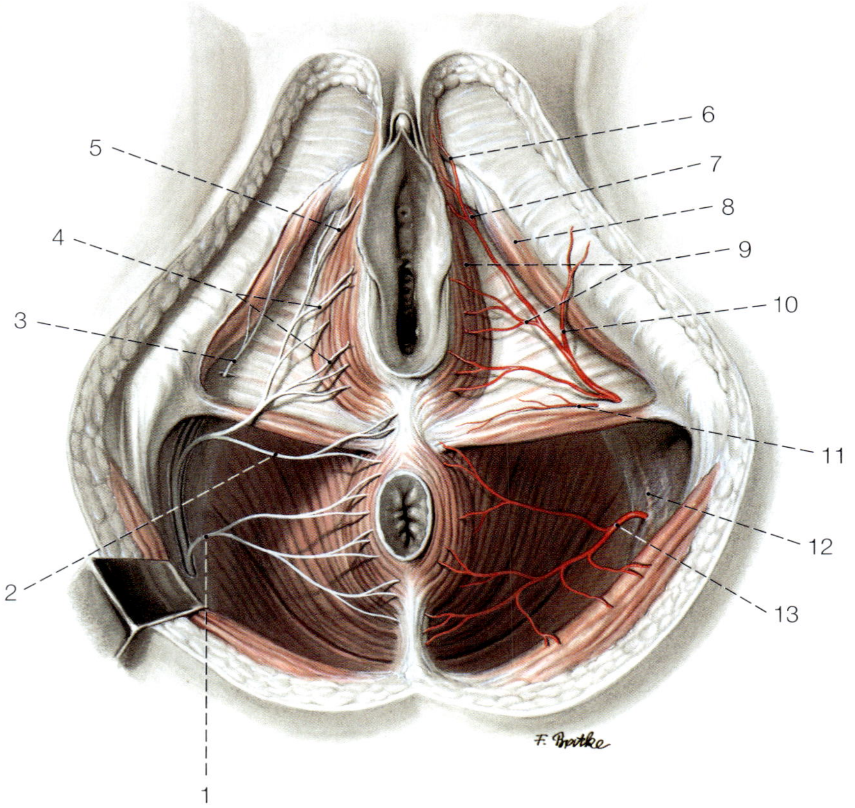

Figure A.6. Arteries and nerves of pelvic floor as seen from below. Branching of internal pudendal artery and of pudendal nerve.

1 anal nerve
2 perineal nerve
3 branch of pudendal nerve innervating ischiocavernosus muscle
4 posterior labial nerves
5 dorsal clitoral nerve
6 dorsal clitoral artery
7 deep clitoral artery
8 ischiocavernosus muscle
9 bulbocavernosus muscle and artery of vestibular bulb
10 posterior labial artery
11 perineal artery
12 internal pudendal artery in Alcock's canal
13 inferior rectal artery

rise to one or more perineal arteries. Veins with identical names accompany the arteries described above to take care of return blood flow.

Lymph drains from the perineum to the superficial inguinal nodes and from there to the deep inguinal lymph nodes.

Innervation. The skin of the perineum is innervated by one or more perineal nerves (Fig. A.6) that are branches of the pudendal nerves. Pathways of these nerves follow the similarly named arteries.

Application. The anatomy of the perineum is important with regard to episiotomies (Chapter 7), colpoperineoplastic procedures (Chapter 13), and repair of perineal lacerations (Chapter 17).

ANUS AND ANORECTAL CANAL

The anal orifice is situated in the gluteal cleft and borders the perineum posteriorly. Laterally, the anus is bordered by levator fibers as well as by the external anal sphincter into which the puborectal fibers of the levator ani muscle radiate. The anus and the perineal part of the anal canal are fixed anteriorly by the perineal body and posteriorly by means of the anococcygeal ligament (Fig. A.7).

The *anus* constitutes the opening of the anal canal (pars perinealis) and shows all transitions in its structure from the rectal wall to the skin. We will detail this area as much as is deemed necessary for those surgical procedures discussed in this book.

The *anal canal* begins with six to ten anal columns. These columns form longitudinal folds (the hemorrhoidal zone) and are supplied by venous plexuses. Outwardly, they are shut by the anal valves. Between them are the niche-shaped cavities of the anal sinuses. Nonkeratinized squamous epithelium covers the anal columns, but cylindrical epithelium can be found overlying the intervening sinuses. This is an intermediate transitional zone that reaches up to the anocutaneous line. At this point the nonkeratinized squamous epithelium becomes cornified (zona cutanea) (Fig. A.5).

The intestinal smooth muscle, which becomes intensified in the area of the intermediate zone, here abuts the internal anal sphincter muscle. A few bundles from this muscle section reach the coccyx as the rectococcygeus muscles.

The intermediate zone is also designated the pectineal line and is of interest to the surgeon from various perspectives. Besides the epithelial interface, there is a borderline of innervation. Moreover, a ''watershed'' exists here for lymph drainage, with collecting lymphatics leading to the superficial inguinal lymph nodes.

The skin layer, zona cutanea, in the anal region is thickened and invested with fatty tissue as well as circumanal sebaceous glands.

The anus is invested with the *external anal sphincter* where it passes through the pelvic diaphragm. Three sections of the

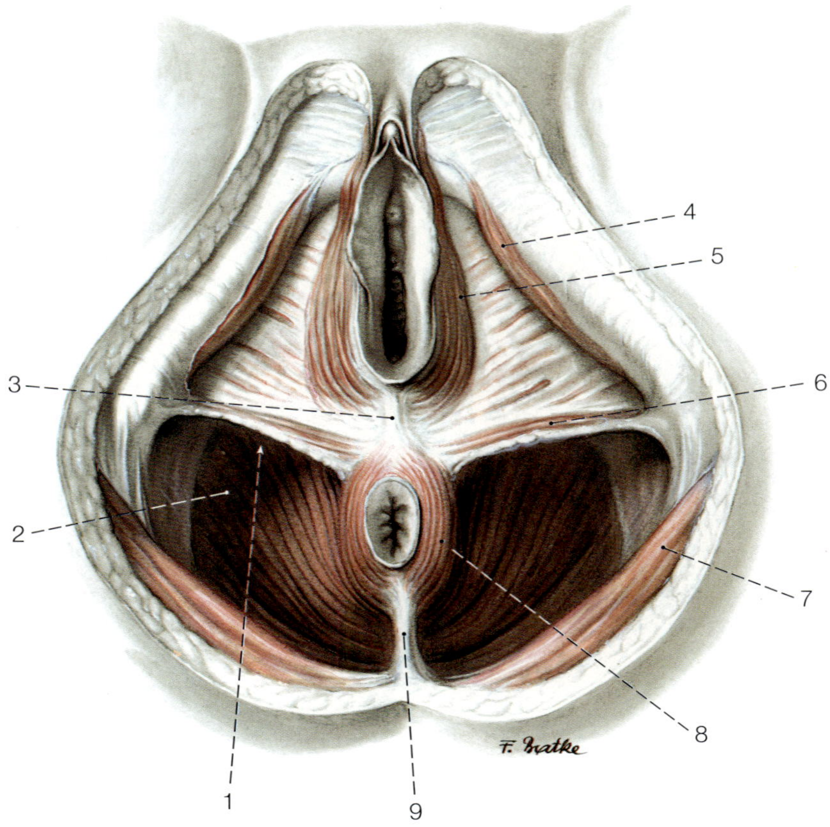

Figure A.7. Pelvic floor as seen from below. Urogenital diaphragm and pelvic diaphragm in situ.
1 ischiorectal fossa
2 levator ani muscle
3 perineum
4 ischiocavernosus muscle
5 bulbocavernosus muscle
6 superficial transverse perineal muscle
7 gluteus maximus muscle
8 external sphincter ani muscle
9 anococcygeal ligament

sphincter can be distinguished (Fig. A.5). A superficial portion, the pars subcutanea, radiates around the anus in the corium, whereas the pars superfiliales surrounds the anus in clamp-like fashion from the perineal body to the anococcygeal ligament. Only the innermost layer, the pars profundum, rings the anus over a breadth of 3–4 cm.

Blood supply. Blood supply of the rectum flows by way of the inferior rectal arteries (Fig. A.6) that leave Alcock's canal where they originate from the internal pudendal arteries to penetrate the obturator fascia. Anastomoses with the medial rectal arteries (which arise from the internal iliac arteries) and the superior rectal artery (derived from the inferior mesenteric artery) guarantee adequate circulation even if the inferior rectal arteries are interrupted.

Blood drainage. Drainage of blood occurs via veins bearing similar names that course in parallel with their corresponding arteries. A dense venous network in the hemorrhoidal zone represents the interconnection between inferior rectal, medial rectal, and superior rectal veins. The superior rectal vein also provides a communication to the portal system.

Lymph supply. Lymph drains to the superficial inguinal nodes as well as along the inferior rectal veins to the internal iliac lymph nodes. Lymphatic pathways also carry lymph to the presacral and perirectal lymph glands.

Innervation. The skin in the anal region is innervated by the anal nerve branches of the pudendal nerves (Figs. A.3 and A.6).

Application. Knowledge of this region is important in the procedures involving repair of third degree perineal lacerations (Chapter 17).

PELVIS

The bony pelvis is composed of the two innominate bones together with the sacrum and the coccyx. The pelvic bones will be discussed only as much as is relevant to surgical procedures described in this book. It is important to distinguish between the false and the true pelves. They are separated by the linea terminales that runs from the pubic bone over the arcuate line to the sacral promontory. The true pelvis is closed off caudally and dorsally by the pelvis floor.

Both innominate bones are attached anteriorly by the symphysis and posteriorly to the sacrum by means of the sacroiliac joint. Additionally, the sacrum is connected to the innominate bone bilaterally by way of the sacrotuberous and sacrospinous ligaments (Fig. A.8). Check ligaments of lesser importance are the anterior, interosseous, and posterior sacroiliac ligaments. These three ligamentous groups lie near the sacroiliac joint.

The *false pelvis* is formed principally by the two ilia and is completed anteriorly in a band-like projection from the anterior superior iliac spine and the pubic tubercle through the inguinal ligament (Fig. A.8). Two portals to the upper thigh are formed

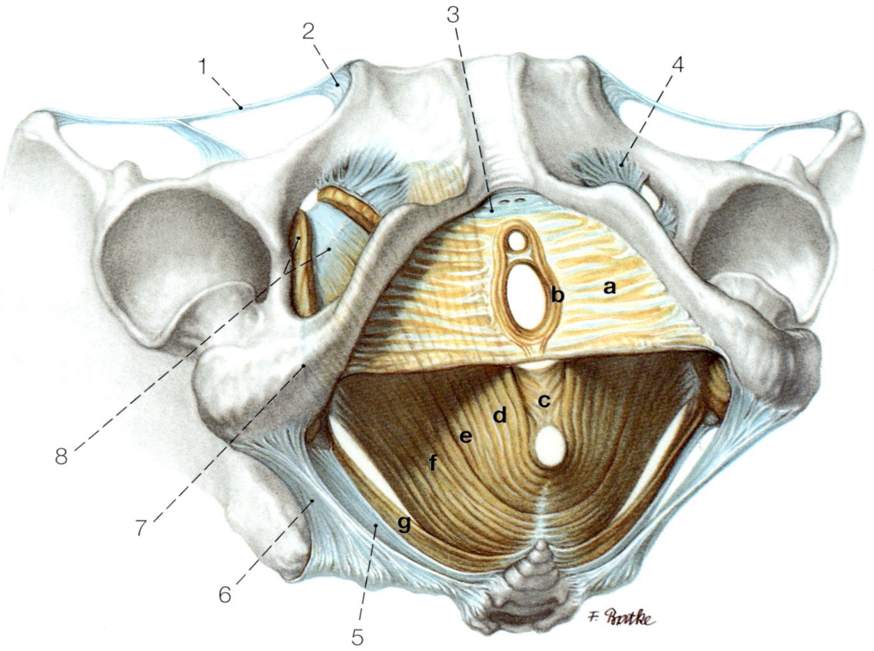

Figure A.8. Ligaments of pelvis and urogenital and pelvic diaphragms.
1 inguinal ligament
2 lacunar ligament
3 transverse perineal ligament
4 obturator membrane
5 sacrospinous ligament
6 sacrotuberous ligament
7 arcus tendineus of obturator fascia drawn translucently
8 *brown,* obturator internus muscle (cross section); *blue,* arcus tendineus obturator fascia (levator ani) drawn translucently
a deep transverse perineal muscle
b urethrovaginal muscle
c prerectal fibers
d puborectal muscle
e pubococcygeus muscle
f iliococcygeus muscle
g coccygeus muscle

between this band and the space formed by the iliac and pubic bones, subdivided by the iliopectineal line. These portals are the lacuna musculorum laterally and the lacuna vasorum medially.

The *true pelvis* is surrounded by bony structures on all sides. The obturator foramina can be found at the anterior lower wall of the pelvis. Anteriorly in the pelvis outlet, the pubic bone is palpable through the skin; posteriorly, one can palpate the ischial tuberosities and ischial spines as well. With the patient in lithotomy position, the ischial tuberosity is felt at the level of the perineum laterally at a distance of about 5–6 cm. The sacrospinous ligament stretches between the sacrum and the ischial spine and forms the minor ischial foramen (Fig. A.8) in conjunction with the sacrotuberous ligament that is attached to the ischial tuberosity.

The sacrospinous ligament arises near the sacrococcygeal transition and continues, tapering off, toward the ischial spine. The considerably wider and stronger sacrotuberous ligament originates broadly alongside the edge of the entire length of the sacrum and stretches, running laterally and dorsally to the sacrospinous ligament, toward the ischial tuberosity. Determined by their beginning, both bands cross over to form the sciatic foramina.

The true pelvis contains the following organs: urinary bladder, urethra and ureters, vagina, uterus and adnexa, and the rectum (Fig. A.9).

Musculature and Fascia

The osseous wall of the true pelvis is invested muscularly by the piriformis and obturator internus muscles. The *piriformis muscle* originates at the anterior surface of S2–S4 vertebrae laterally to the sacral foramina. It exits from the true pelvis by way of the greater sciatic foramen and reaches the greater trochanter.

The *obturator internus muscle* takes its origin at the bony edge of the obturator foramen and from the obturator membrane. It courses through the lesser sciatic foramen, using the lesser sciatic notch as a buttress to insert into the greater trochanter as well. At its origin, it completes the *obturator canal* located at the upper edge of the obturator foramen.

There are four openings in the sidewall of the true pelvis. The dorsally situated *greater sciatic foramen* is bordered by the greater sciatic notch on one side, by the sacrospinal ligament caudally, and by the anterior portion of the sacrotuberal ligament dorsally. Passing through, the piriformis muscle creates two slitted openings of different sizes—the suprapiriformis foramen and the infrapiriformis foramen.

The *lesser sciatic foramen* lies more caudally. It is bordered anteriorly by the lesser sciatic notch, cranially by the sacrospinal ligament, and caudally as well as dorsally by the anterior portion of the sacrotuberal ligament.

The *obturator canal*, always somewhat larger in women, is bordered cranially by the obturator groove, which is located at the lower edge of the superior ramus of the pubis. This groove is bordered anteriorly by the anterior obturator tubercle and posteriorly by the posterior obturator tubercle, which, however, is sometimes absent. The groove is completed into a canal by the obturator membranes caudally. It courses obliquely toward the median and downward. It is approximately 2.5–3 cm long.

Relationship of Vessel and Nerve Location of True Pelvis to Openings of Lateral Pelvic Wall

All four openings serve as passages for vessels and nerves (Figs. A.10–A.13).

The *supra piriformis foramen* serves as a passage to the outside for the superior gluteal vessels and the superior gluteus

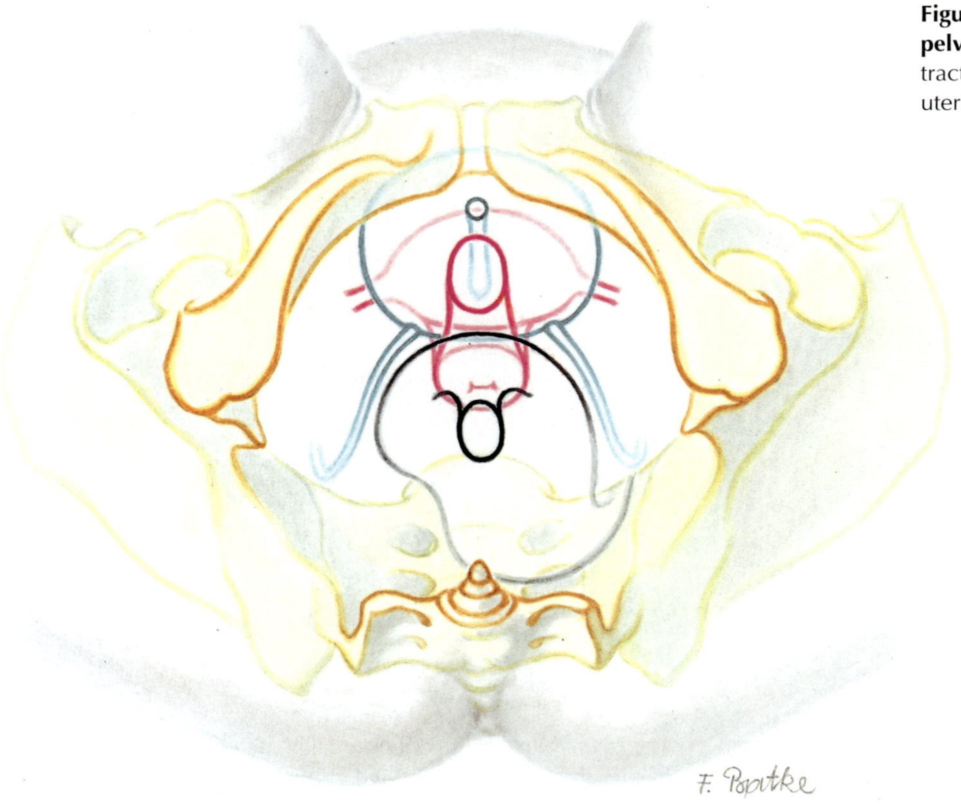

Figure A.9. Projection of bony pelvis and pelvic viscus on external surface. *Blue,* urinary tract (ureters, urinary bladder, and urethra); *red,* uterus and vagina; *black,* rectum.

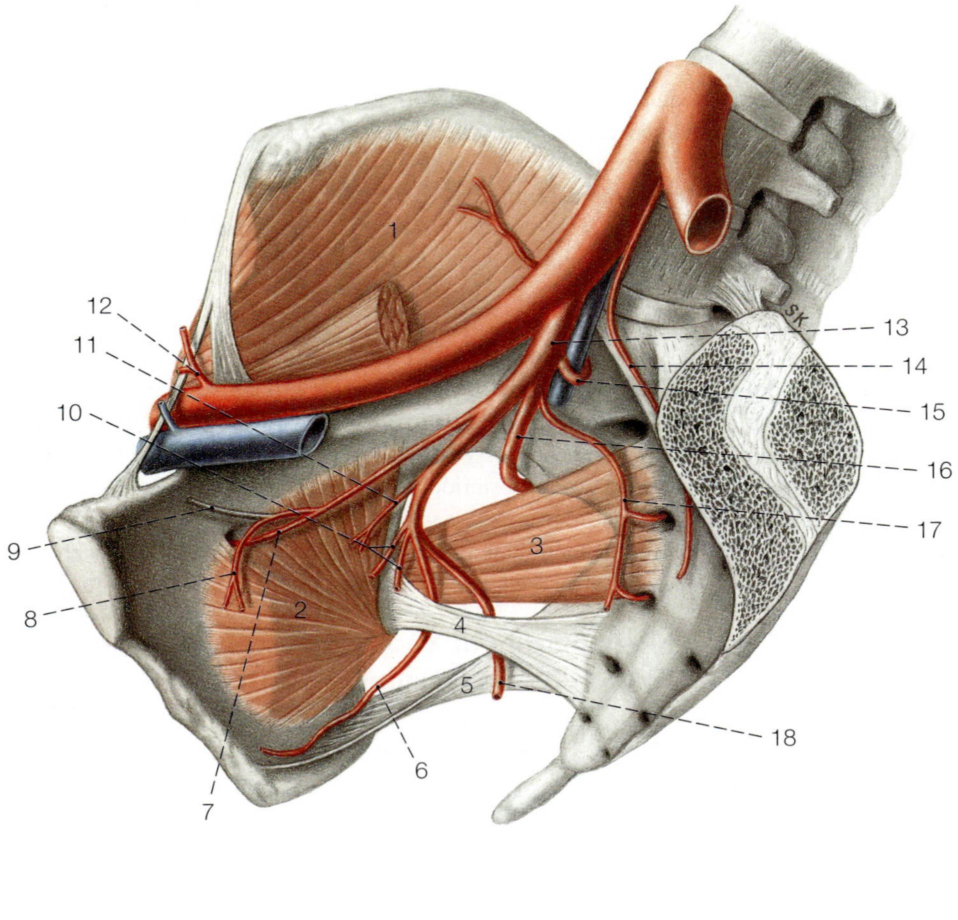

Figure A.10. Medial view of arteries of pelvic wall (somewhat schematized).

1 iliac muscle
2 internal obturator muscle
3 piriformis muscle
4 sacrospinal ligament
5 sacrotuberal ligament
6 internal pudendal artery
7 obturator artery
8 superior vesical artery
9 lateral umbilical ligament
10 inferior vesical artery (here double)
11 uterine artery
12 inferior epigastric artery
13 internal iliac artery
14 middle sacral artery
15 iliolumbar artery
16 superior gluteal artery
17 lateral sacral artery
18 inferior gluteal artery

Figure A.11. Medial view of nerves of pelvic wall (somewhat schematized).

A internal obturator muscle
B iliac muscle
S_1–S_5 ventral nerve roots from sacral segments
1 sacrospinous ligament
2 sacrotuberous ligament
3 ischial spine
4 obturator nerve
5 lacunar ligament
6 inguinal ligament
7 superior gluteal nerve
8 lumbosacral trunk (from L4 and L5)
9 coccygeus plexus
10 pudendal nerve
11 inferior gluteal nerve
12 posterior femoral cutaneous nerve

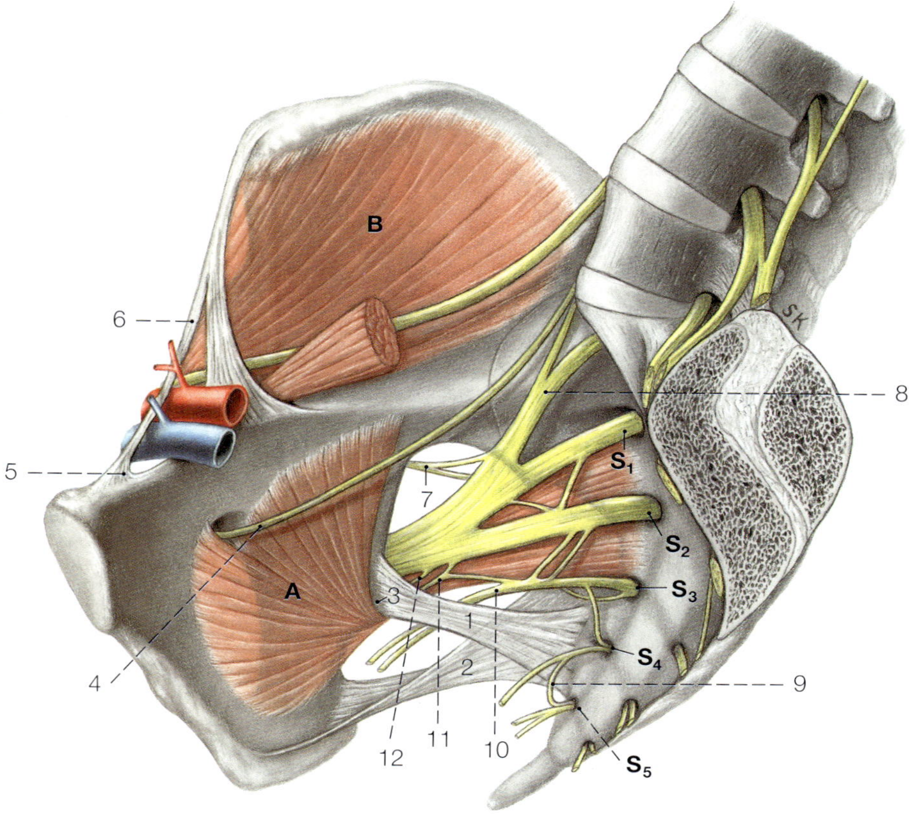

Figure A.12. Medial view of vessels and nerves of the right side; rectum is displaced toward the left (paramedial incision).

1 inferior vesical artery
2 superior vesical artery
3 urinary bladder
4 fallopian tubes
5 right ovary, lateral umbilical ligament
6 external iliac artery
7 obturator artery, obturator nerve
8 ovarian artery
9 ureter
10 superior hypogastric plexus
11 internal iliac artery
12 superior rectal artery
13 superior gluteal artery
14 inferior gluteal artery
15 internal pudendal artery
16 left hypogastric nerve
17 uterine artery

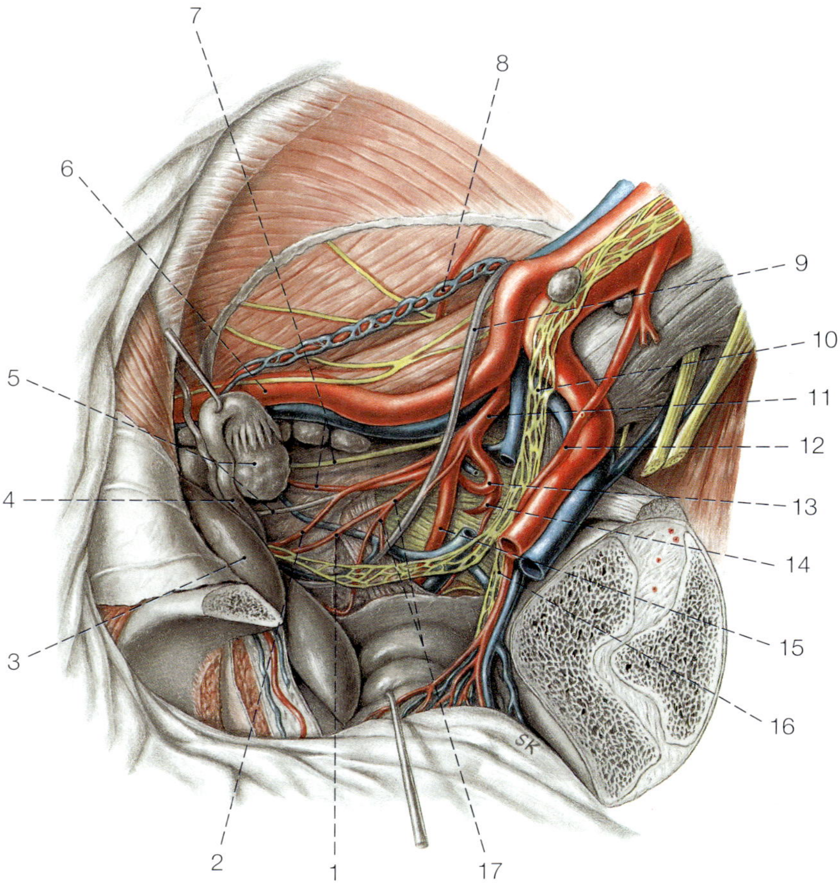

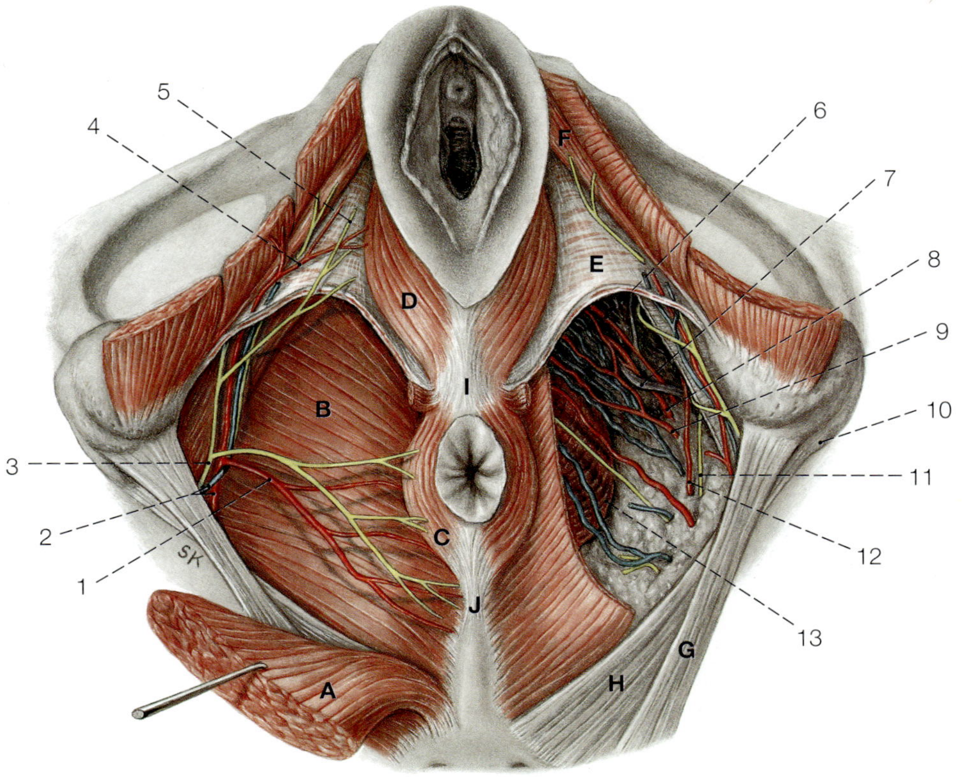

Figure A.13. Vessels and nerves of pelvis on the left side, seen from below. Pelvic diaphragm is partially removed.

A gluteus maximus muscle
B levator ani muscle
C external sphincter ani muscle
D bulbocavernosus muscle
E deep transverse perineal muscle
F ischiocavernosus muscle
G sacrotuberal ligament
H sacrospinal ligament
I central tendinous point
J anococcygeal ligament
1 inferior rectal artery
2 internal pudendal artery and vein
3 pudendal nerve
4 vestibular bulb artery
5 dorsal clitoral nerve
6 superior vesical artery
7 ureter
8 uterine artery
9 inferior vesical artery
10 ischial spine
11 obturator nerve
12 obturator artery
13 rectum

nerve. The *infrapiriformis foramen* is traversed by the following: superior gluteal vessel and nerves, sciatic nerve, posterior femoral cutaneous nerve, internal pudendal vessels, and pudendal nerve. The sciatic nerve may change, because it may exit either completely or partially between the sharp obtrusions of the piriformis muscle.

The *lesser sciatic foramen* opens into the ischiorectal fossa. The internal pudendal vessels and the pudendal nerve wind under and around the ischial spine and the supraspinal ligament. The obturator internus muscle uses the lesser sciatic notch as a passage to reach the greater trochanter. Vessels and nerves enter the pudendal canal immediately after passing through the foramen.

The *obturator canal* leads to the upper thigh and contains the obturator vessel and nerve. The often rather delicate anastomosis sometimes causes the epigastric artery to replace the obturator artery.

Internally in the true pelvis a close relationship exists between the iliac artery and its branches (which may arise in variable sequence) and the supra- and infrapiriformis foramen as well as the lesser sciatic foramen. That also holds true for the corresponding nerves.

Of special interest is the positional relationship of the nerves, in particular the sacral plexus. The root of the sacral plexus (which lies alongside the piriform muscle and also the coccygeus muscle) originates from S_1 at the cranial and from S_4 at the caudal edge of the muscle. Likewise, the pudendal plexus also lies alongside the coccygeus muscle, which in turn accompanies the sacrospinal ligament. The pudendal plexus and the root of the sacral plexus from S_2 release the pelvic nerves, which reach toward the pelvic ganglion. These nerves contain parasympathetic fibers for innervation of the pelvic organs, in particular for the ureter, vagina, and rectum.

Pelvic Floor (Muscular Foundation)

The pelvic floor is formed by two fibromuscular layers, the pelvic diaphragm and the urogenital diaphragm. Neither alone closes the pelvis completely, but closure is functionally effective, nevertheless, because the superimposed layers are arranged so that the open portions are not aligned.

The funnel-shaped *pelvic diaphragm* (Figs. A.6–A.8) consists of the *levator ani muscle* and the *coccygeus muscle*. The levator ani takes its origin at the pubic bone near the symphysis and reaches over the arcus tendineus musculus levatoris ani to the ischial spine. The three segments of the levator ani muscle are discernible and correspond to the course of its muscle fibers.

The puborectalis muscle encompasses mainly those fibers that form the so-called levator pillar, which laterally intertwines with the external anal sphincter muscle and posteriorly forms a sling for contralateral traction of the rectum.

The prerectal fibers course toward the perineum in association with the puborectalis muscle to form the levator pillar. Together with the perineal body they border the levator portal, the urogenital hiatus, beginning at the anal hiatus. Smooth muscle fibers radiate alongside these striated muscles from the levator to the perineal body, looping around the vagina in the form of the levator vaginal muscle.

The remaining levator fibers comprise the pubococcygeus and the iliococcygeus aponeurosis in conjunction with the smooth muscle bundles of the rectococcygeus. Parts of the pubococcygeus and puborectalis muscles radiate into the vaginal wall as the pubovaginalis muscle.

The levator portal is very important insofar as it is impossible to avoid intestinal descensus if the levator pillar is pulled apart (Figs. A.14 and A.15). During construction of an artificial perineum (Chapter 17), one must take care with the puborectalis muscle, because both the right and left puborectalis muscles (Figs. A.16 and A.17) have to be drawn together to ensure a secure pelvic floor to support the bowel.

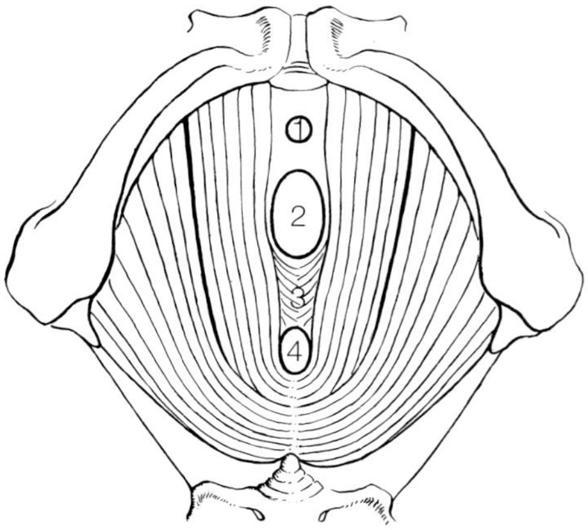

Figure A.14. Pelvic diaphragm (levator ani muscle) with a normal-sized levator portal, as seen from below.
1 urethra
2 vagina
3 prerectal levator fibers
4 anus

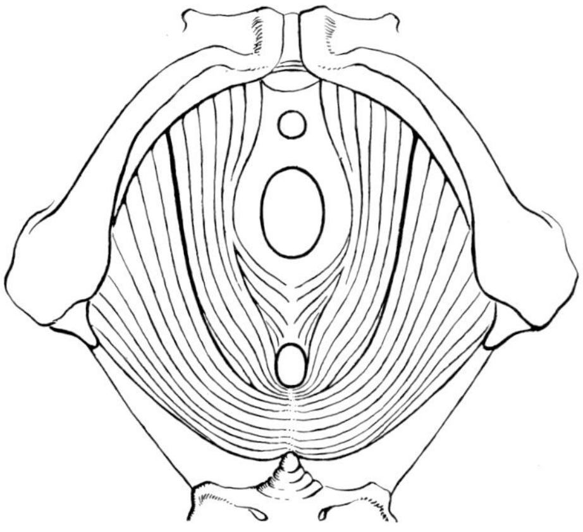

Figure A.15. Pelvic diaphragm (levator ani muscle) with an enlarged levator portal, as seen from below.

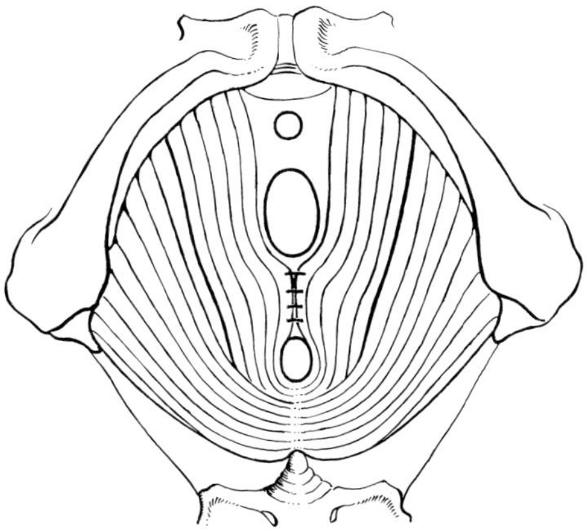

Figure A.16. Artificial construction of perineum by suturing both levator pillars between vagina and anus, as seen from below.

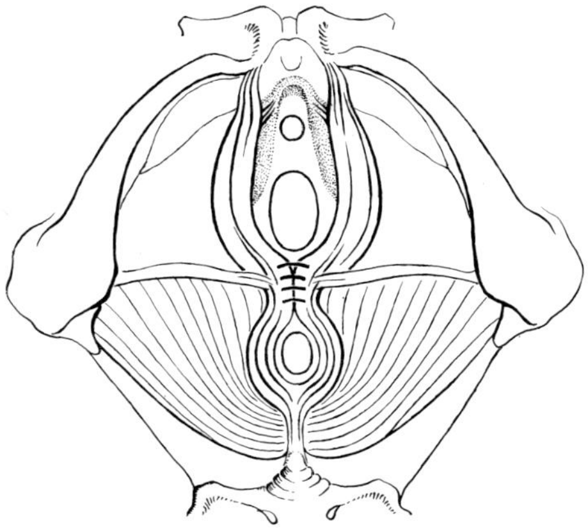

Figure A.17. Artificially reconstructed perineum is further strengthened by suturing both bulbocavernosus muscles together between vagina and anus, as seen from below.

The pelvic diaphragm is completed posteriorly by the coccygeus muscle that courses from the ischial spine to the coccyx and sacrum.

The urogenital diaphragm is of particular importance here, because it provides needed support for the levator portal, which is naturally larger in women. The *urogenital diaphragm* is mainly formed by *the deep transverse perineal muscle* that terminates in the perineal body. The diaphragm, permeated with connective tissue, originates from the lower ischium and the inferior ramus of the pubis and courses to the urogenital hiatus that it encircles to yield a urogenital sphincter (urethrovaginalis muscle, sphincter vaginae muscle). Anteriorly, its muscular layer changes into the transverse perineal ligament (preurethral ligament), which forms the anterior part of the urogenital diaphragm in conjunction with the arcuate pubic ligament. The free posterior edge of the diaphragm is strengthened by the superficial transverse perineal muscle that arises from the ischial tuberosity and inserts into the perineal body as well. Branches of the pudendal nerve serve to innervate the urogenital diaphragm. The bulbocavernosus and ischiocavernosus muscles are located superficially on the urogenital diaphragm.

Innervation. As a rule, the pelvic diaphragm is innervated by a long branch from the sacral plexus. This branch is especially endangered if a spinosacral fixation of the vagina is performed.

Application. The anatomy of this region is important in colpoperineorraphies (Chapter 13), procedures for vaginal atresia (Chapter 16), repairs of perineal laceration (Chapter 17), construction of artificial vaginae (Chapter 20), and radical vaginal operations (Chapter 22).

Fascial Base (Fasciae of Pelvic Floor)

The muscular pelvic diaphragm is covered by a fascia on both its superior and inferior surfaces. The *superior fascia* extends from the arcus tendineus of the obturator fascia (arcus tendineus musculus levatoris ani) to reach the lateral pelvic fascia (obturator fascia). Posteriorly, it attaches over the sacrum as well as to that portion of the fascia located above the piriformis muscle. At the levator pillars it meets the *inferior fascia*. Both superior and inferior levator fasciae, as derivatives of the pelvic parietal fascia, are connected to the fasciae of the rectum, vagina, and urethra, which are all portions of the pelvic visceral fascia.

Because the pelvic and the urogenital diaphragms are arranged in strata, the inferior fascia of the pelvic diaphragm also passes over the *superior fascia* (triangular ligament of Colles or middle perineal fascia). The superior urogenital fascia proceeds anteriorly under the transverse perineal ligament (preurethral ligament of Waldeyer, perineal ligament of Carcassone, Krause's ligament, interosseous pubic ligament of Winslow) and posteriorly on the free edge of the urogenital diaphragm to the *inferior urogenital fascia*.

Near the levator portal, the fasciae of the pelvic diaphragm fuse with those of the urogenital diaphragm so that the genital hiatus between them appears to be closed. Posteriorly open grooves, the ischiorectal fossae (ischioanales), are formed where the pelvic parietal fascia approaches the lateral pelvic sidewall. The pelvic parietal fascia in this area corresponds to the subdiaphragmatic portion of the obturator fascia. It possesses a duplication (sometimes designated lunar fascia) that creates an interfascial canal, the Alcock's canal (pudendal canal), between its two leaves to accommodate the internal pudendal vessels and pudendal nerve.

Closer to the skin than the inferior fascia of the urogenital diaphragm (deep layer of the perineal fascia, Colles' fascia, perineal membrane) lies the *perineal fascia* (Cruveilhier's fascia or superficial perineal fascia), which is fused with the inferior urogenital fascia at its posterior edge. Thus, an interfascial space, the perineal interfascial space, is formed between the pubic arch and the posterior edge of the urogenital diaphragm. The nomenclature applied to the fasciae in the literature differs widely, so different descriptions of individual layers are often found. The superficial perineal fascia proceeds into the superficial connective tissue membranes (Camper's fascia) of the pubic area and also into those of the thigh.

Pelvic Contents

The true pelvis (Fig. A.9) contains the vagina, uterus and adnexal structures (uterine tubes and ovaries), all constituents of the internal female genital apparatus, as well as the pelvic portions of the ureters, urinary bladder, urethra, and rectum. These structures are connected with each other and with the parietal wall by means of a connective tissue membrane that has special significance as a pelvic support and as a pathway to guide the course of vessels and nerves.

Vagina

In its relaxed, nondistended state the vagina is flattened anteroposteriorly from the the introitus to the posterior fornix. Because the vaginal portion (portio) of the uterus inserts into the upper vagina, the vaginal vault is formed around the portio as the *vaginal fornix*. The posterior lower wall is longer (about 11 cm) than the relatively shorter overlying anterior wall (about 8 cm). The fornix forms an irregularly deep groove that circles the portio and characteristically protrudes more deeply into the posterior fornix and more shallowly into the two lateral fornices and the anterior fornix.

Layers of the Wall

The wall of the vagina consists of a mucous membrane, a muscular coat, and an adventitial layer called the vaginal fascia. In surgical dissection of the vaginal wall, the mucosal and muscular strata are usually represented as a common layer separate from the vaginal fascia (Figs. A.18 and A.19). Care must be taken to ensure that the vaginal fascia maintains a close relationship with the vesicle fascia.

The epithelial layer contains greyish-red *mucosa*, which is covered by a squamous epithelium that ordinarily does not undergo cornification but can keratinize in association with prolapse. The submucosa contains much elastic tissue as well as a latticework of collagen fibers. Diagonal folds (columns of the vagina) are seen in the undistended mucosa of the adult vagina. These form the anterior and posterior vaginal columns on the respective longitudinal vaginal wall borders. The anterior border is bounded by a band of vertical muscle fibers from the tunica muscularis. The muscular layer is in close relationship with the mucosa, and, as already mentioned, tends to be surgically dissected in conjunction with the mucosa. The submucosal layer is not well defined in the vagina. In the distal continuation of the anterior vaginal column, there is a slight forward arch, the urethral carina, caused by the close relationship between vagina and urethra.

The mucosa is subject to menstrual cycle changes in that it is thicker and looser during the secretory or premenstrual phase than in the proliferate or postmenstrual phase.

Figure A.18. Layers of anterior vaginal wall. *Yellow,* mucosa of anterior vaginal wall; *pink,* muscles of anterior vaginal wall; *blue,* vaginal fascia (muscle layer of bladder can be seen through window in vaginal fascia); *orange,* mucosa and muscle of vagina (both layers together comprise the "vaginal wall").

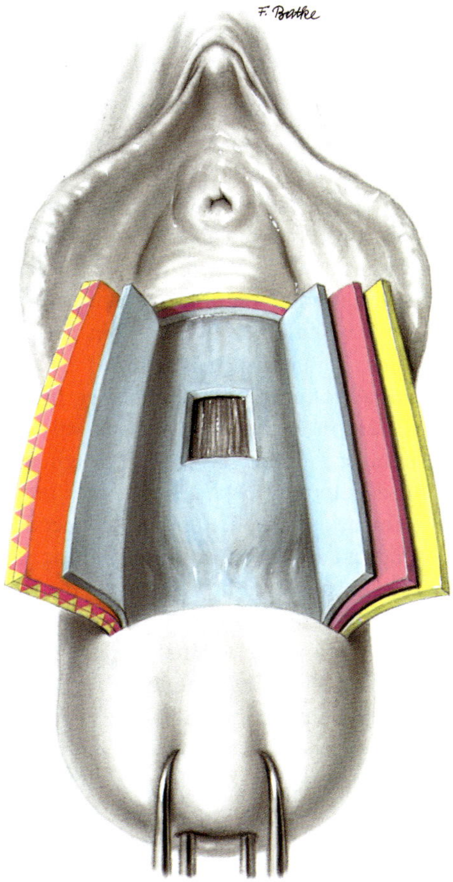

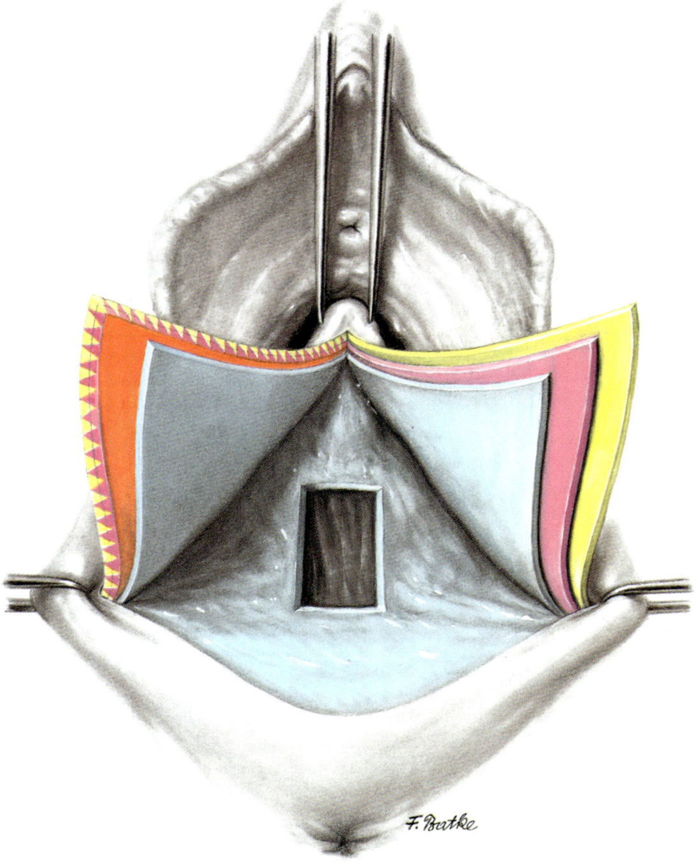

Figure A.19. Layers of posterior vaginal wall. *Yellow,* mucosa of posterior vaginal wall; *pink,* muscles of posterior vaginal wall; *blue,* vaginal fascia (folded back) and rectal fascia (below rectal muscles) (in situ); *orange,* posterior vaginal wall (mucosa and vaginal muscles, dissected together).

The mucous portion of the vaginal secretions is not generated in the few isolated glands found in the upper vagina (and which participate in the cyclic changes that the cervical glands undergo) but rather from glands in the endocervical canal.

The *muscular coat* comprises smooth musculature and a network of elastic fibers. Muscle fibers are in a fencelike arrangement in rhomboid shapes such that the vertical axis of the rhombus is perpendicular to the vertical axis of the vagina. The muscle is thicker in the anterior wall, where many muscle fibers bend vertically to form the foundation of the anterior vaginal column. There are numerous vascular plexuses within the muscle layer. These plexuses are, in turn, well developed in the region of the posterior vaginal column, here resembling the corpus cavernosum. The muscle in the upper vagina is only loosely connected with the *tunica adventitia* (fascia vaginalis), in contrast to the close interrelationship near the introitus. Here there is also intimate connective tissue connection between the vaginal fascia and the fascia of neighboring organs, designated rectovaginal and urethrovaginal septa, respectively (Fig. A.20).

In the posterior fornix, the vaginal fascia is missing, and a portion of vagina is covered by peritoneum for a distance of 1–2 cm. This constitutes the shortest distance from the posterior vaginal vault to the peritoneal cavity via the cul-de-sac of Douglas (excavatio rectouterina).

Relationship to Adjacent Organs

As already stated, a close relationship exists at the anterior wall near the introitus to the urethra through the *urethrovaginal septum*. In the upper vagina, the anterior wall is loosely connected to the base of the bladder, whereas laterally the two ureters approach the vagina. Dorsally, in the posterior fornix, the vagina is very close to the peritoneal cavity and the rectum. More distally there are connective fibers that form a relationship near the introitus in the *rectovaginal septum* that is analogous to that seen anteriorly.

Laterally, the vagina is surrounded by fibers of the deep transverse perineal muscle in the form of the urogenital sphincter. A few of its muscle bundles can encircle the vagina and the urethra as a urethrovaginal sphincter. In the intact pelvic diaphragm, the levator pillars can be felt laterally through the vagina. A few fibers of pubococcygeus and puborectalis muscles radiate as the pubovaginal muscle into the vaginal wall. These fibers are sometimes called constrictor (or compressor) vaginal muscles. The bundle of connective tissue that runs from the vagina to the lateral pelvic wall and contains blood vessels, lymphatics, and nerves can be considered collectively as the *paracolpium*.

Blood supply. The vaginal artery, a branch of the uterine artery, and smaller branches of the inferior vesical artery, the

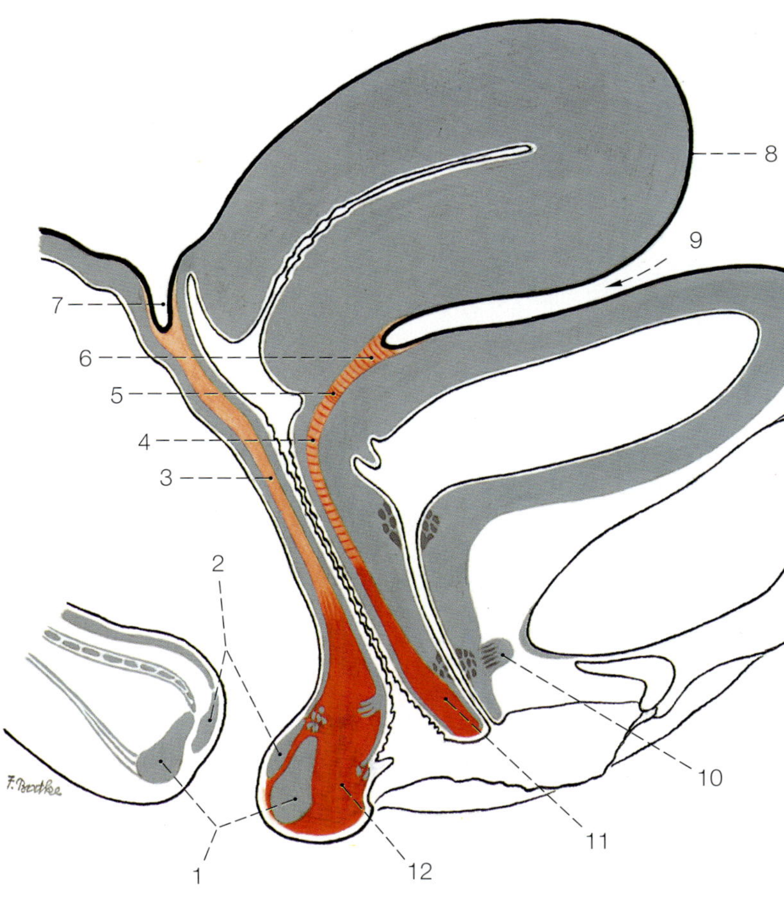

Figure A.20. Midline section of perivaginal connective tissue.
1 external sphincter ani muscle
2 internal sphincter ani muscle
3 areolar connective tissue between vaginal and rectal fasciae in rectovaginal space
4 areolar connective tissue between vaginal and vesical or urethral fasciae in vesicovaginal or urethrovaginal spaces
5 supravaginal septum
6 vesicouterine space
7 cul-de-sac of Douglas
8 peritoneum
9 vesicouterine space
10 transverse perineal ligament
11 urethrovaginal septum
12 rectovaginal septum

inferior rectal artery (see Figs. A.30 and A.31) and internal pudendal artery, reach the vagina laterally by way of the paracolpium to supply it with blood. Sometimes these branches anastomose at the posterior wall of the vagina to form a vertical anastomotic network, a vaginal azygos artery.

Vascular drainage. Vascular drainage occurs bilaterally to the hypogastric (internal iliac) veins via the uterovaginal plexus that is located in the paracolpium and the parametrium. There are anatomic connections with the internal pudendal vein and with veins of the external genitalia as well.

Lymph drainage. Lymph is drained (see Fig. A.24) from the upper half of the vagina by way of the lymphatics that also serve to collect lymph from the cervix uteri through the cardinal ligament to reach the internal iliac nodes. A few lymph vessels, after crossing the ureter (near its confluence with the bladder), also reach the internal iliac lymph nodes, especially those located most caudally. From the lower vagina, the lymph vessels (see Fig. A.24) accompany the vaginal artery laterally to the ureter to terminate in the internal iliac nodes also. Other lymphatics course through the paravesical space to the inferior gluteal nodes. Additional lymphatics reach the superior gluteal nodes in association with the vaginal artery. Finally, the afferent lymphatics of the lower vagina (see Fig. A.24) also drain into the inguinal lymph nodes. A few lymph vessels from the posterior vaginal wall (see Fig. A.24) reach the perirectal nodes by way of the rectovaginal septum.

Innervation. Near the introitus, the vagina is supplied by sensory branches of the pudendal nerve, whereas the remaining sensory and autonomic fibers originate in the pelvic plexus of Frankenhäuser, reaching the vaginal wall in association with arterial branches.

Application. Knowledge of this region is a prerequisite for all vaginal operations.

Uterus

The pear-shaped uterus has an anterior surface, a posterior surface, and laterally rounded aspects. It consists of the corpus and the cervix (collum). The latter can be distinguished by a slight constriction at the isthmus uteri. The uppermost portion of the corpus (above the mouths of the uterine tubes) is called the fundus uteri. The cervix, the collum uteri, is divisible into a portio supravaginalis (occupying two-thirds of the structure) and a portio vaginalis (one-third). In older women, the portio vaginales becomes flattened and foreshortened. The portio is that portion of the uterus that is admitted into the vagina, bearing the external os at the distal extremity between its anterior and posterior lips. The orifice represents the external opening of the cervical canal. The other end of the canal enters into the flattened, triangular endometrial cavity. The uterine tubes open into the upper lateral corners of the cavity. The internal os is the site of the junction of the cervical canal and the endometrium (canalis isthmi).

Physiologically, the uterus is in a median axial position, anteverted (with the vertical axis of the uterus perpendicular to the axis of the vagina) and anteflexed (with a forward inclination of the corpus with regard to the cervix).

Architecture of the Uterine Wall

The uterus consists of three layers: its mucosa, the endometrium; its muscle layer, the myometrium; and a serosal layer, the perimetrium, which covers it almost completely. There is no serosal perimetrium in the anterior aspect of the cervix.

The reddish *endometrium* at rest is approximately 1 mm. thick; it is covered with cylindrical epithelium and forms fine folds in the cervical canal on both anterior and posterior walls. Periodically, these small folds transform into one median vertical fold. They are called plicae palmatae by virtue of the palm-like appearance. Inside the endometrial cavity, the mucosal surface is flat and softer than in the area of the cervix. The corium is relatively thick, firm, and immovably fixed to the myometrium. Within the corium in the corpus region are the uterine glands, whereas its cervical region contains many blood vessels and cervical glands. The transition from the cervix to the corpus occurs in the isthmus. For further details on the mucosa, the reader is referred to the relevant publications on histology.

The *myometrium* consists of smooth musculature. It is in contiguity with the muscle of the uterine tube and, in the area of the cervix, with the vesicouterine and rectouterine muscle. Three layers can be distinguished on the basis of blood vessel content. Muscle fibers radiate into the broad ligament from the superficial muscle layer.

The *serosa* covers almost all of the uterus, except that it does not reach the cervix anteriorly. Laterally, the serosa becomes the two leaves of the broad ligament (plica lata). The shallow pouch of the vesicouterine excavation is formed anteriorly, whereas the deep retrouterine excavation appears posteriorly as the cul-de-sac of Douglas.

Uterine Connective Tissue

The uterus possesses two lateral mesenteries (mesometria), the broad ligaments (ligamenta lata uteri). At the free edge of the broad ligament is the round ligament or Hunter's ligament (ligamentum teres uteri, ligamentum rotunda, chorda uteroinguinalis) that courses anteriorly toward the inguinal canal. The utero-ovarian ligament travels from this site laterally toward the ovary. The fallopian tube is also found here with its mesentery (the mesosalpinx) (Fig. A.21). The parametrial connective tissue is contiguous laterally with that of the paracolpium and is interspersed with blood and lymph vessels and nerves. It contains loose as well as dense fibrous components that are interwoven with smooth muscle fibers. At the level of the cervix uteri the connective tissue becomes augmented and more compactly organized (Fig. A.22) into the cardinal ligaments (i.e., cardinal ligament of Kocks, transverse cervical ligament of Mackenrodt, retinaculum colli, lateral cervical ligament, cervical pillar). They reach the upper fascia of the levator ani muscle close to the ischial spine. Lateral to the cervix two fibromuscular bands are found

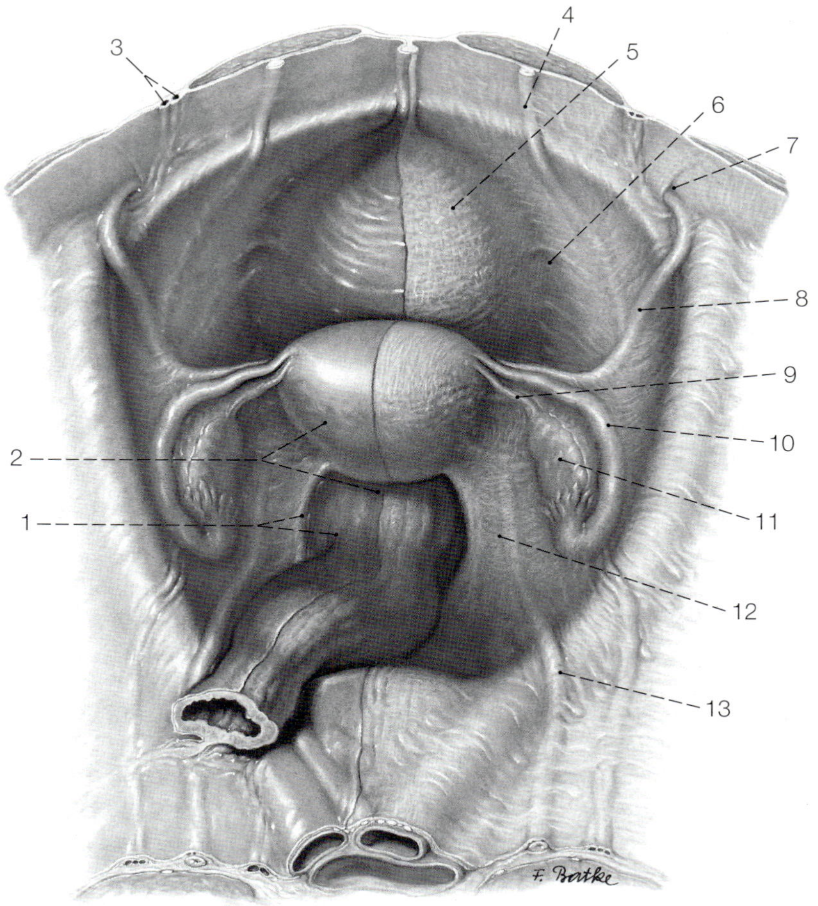

Figure A.21. True pelvis as seen from above. Peritoneum is removed on right side.

1 uterosacral fold (left), rectum (right)
2 uterus (upper), cul-de-sac of Douglas (lower)
3 inferior epigastric artery (left) and vein (right)
4 lateral umbilical fold with obliterated umbilical artery
5 urinary bladder
6 paracystium
7 deep inguinal ring
8 round ligament
9 utero-ovarian ligament
10 fallopian tube
11 ovary
12 paraproctium
13 ureter

Figure A.22. Section through bladder, uterus, vagina, and rectum with connective tissue pillars (somewhat schematized). *Blue*, connective tissue pillars; *green*, cut edge of peritoneum.

a cardinal ligament
b lateral portion of bladder pillar (with vessels and nerves)
c medial part of bladder pillar (vesicouterine ligament, sometimes contains a vesical artery)
d lateral portion of rectal pillar (with vessels and nerves)
e medial part of rectal pillar (uterosacral ligament)
f ureter in loose connective tissue (not shown) of bladder pillar
g loose connective tissue between vagina and bladder
h areolar tissue in bladder pillar
i loose fibrous tissue in rectal pillar
k lateral umbilical cord

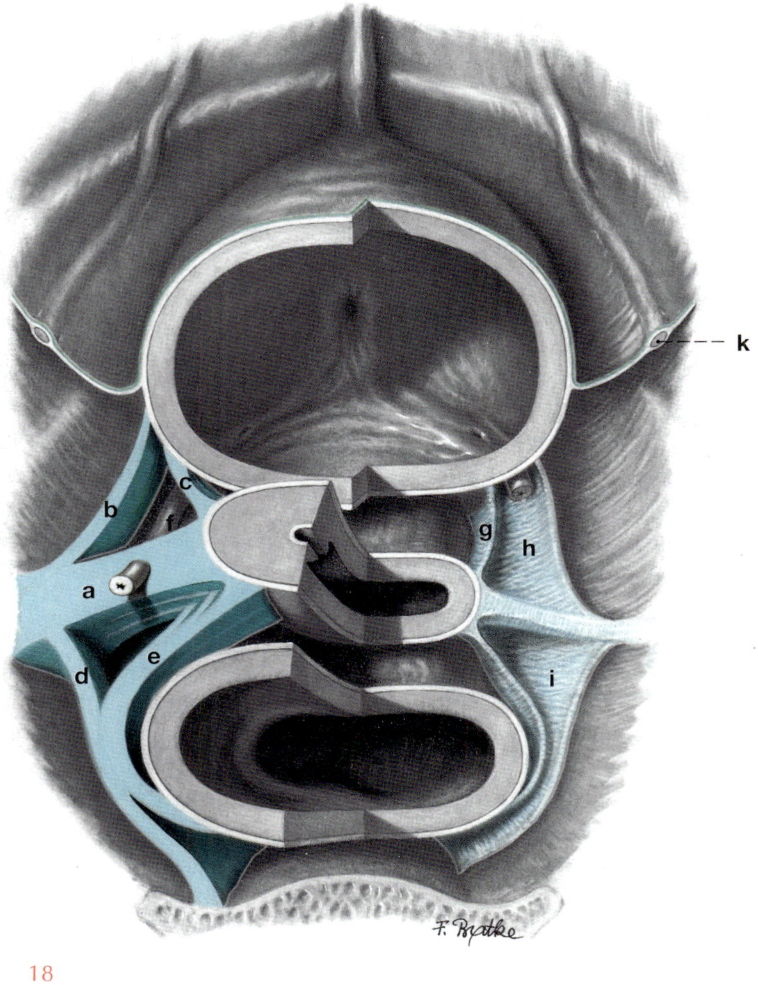

that pull the cervix forward toward the bladder as well as backward to the rectum. The vesicouterine ligament (or vesicouterine muscle) that represents the medial portion of the bladder pillar pulls toward the bladder. It reaches the lateral connective tissue of the bladder (paracystium) in the region of the bladder base. The rectouterine ligaments (sacrouterine ligament, Petit's ligament) follow the rectouterine folds (ligament of Douglas) at the lateral aspects of the cul-de-sac of Douglas, turning up on either side to reach the rectum. They constitute the medial components of the rectal crura reaching to the rectal fascia, the retrorectal connective tissue, and to the sacrum at the level of S2–S4.

Among the three fibromuscular structures described here, the cardinal ligament is of greatest practical importance because it is a principal pathway for vessels and nerves. At its upper edge, it is crossed by the ureter. Anteriorly, in the midline, another taut connective bundle that is important to the gynecologist is found: the *septum (ligamentum supravaginale)* (Fig. A.20), which courses from the cervix to the posterior wall of the bladder.

Blood supply. The principal uterine blood supply (Fig. A.23, see also Figs. A.30 and A.31) comes via the uterine artery, a major branch of the internal iliac artery. It flows in the parametrium above the cardinal ligament, crossing the ureters en route to the cervix. The ureteral crossing occurs about 2 cm from the uterus. Adjacent to the cervix, the uterine artery turns upward and reaches the tubal angle in a tortuous coiling manner. There it separates into its terminal branches, a tubal and an ovarian branch. It sends out short subserosal branches to the uterine wall along its route at the lateral margin of the uterus. These enter the anterior and posterior surfaces of the uterus and anastomose with those of the opposite side. The uterine artery may give off a vaginal artery branch either before or after it crosses the ureter. Sometimes it can divide near the uterus into an ascending branch, which is a continuation of the main vessel, and a descending branch, the cervicovaginal branch. Where it crosses the ureter, the uterine artery also gives rise to a ureteric branch. The final branches, the ovarian and tubal branches, anastomose with branches of the ovarian artery (which originates from the abdominal aorta) and transport blood to the uterus.

Venous drainage. Veins also leave the uterus at its lateral margins and course through the broad ligaments. They can be divided into three groups. These three groups, which drain blood from the fundus, corpus, and cervix, respectively, are interconnected to each other by anastomoses. Veins from the corpus and cervix form the uterine venous plexus that envelops the uterine artery. Veins from the area of the fundus drain blood mainly via the ovarian veins to the inferior vena cava. The uterine venous plexus flows into the uterine veins, one of which proceeds cranially over the ureter and the other caudally under the ureter. Blood from the cervical and vaginal veins flows from the vaginal venous plexus into the lower uterine veins. A rare pathway for drainage from the uterine fundus courses with the round ligament to the subcutaneous veins in the region of the external inguinal ring.

Lymph drainage. The lymphatics (Fig. A.24) of the uterus form mucosal, muscular, and subserosal plexuses that anastomose with each other. Lymph is collected into two groups of collecting channels bilaterally.

The first group drains the fundus and corpus into lymph vessels that course

(*a*) along the ovarian branch of the uterine artery to reach the aortic nodes,

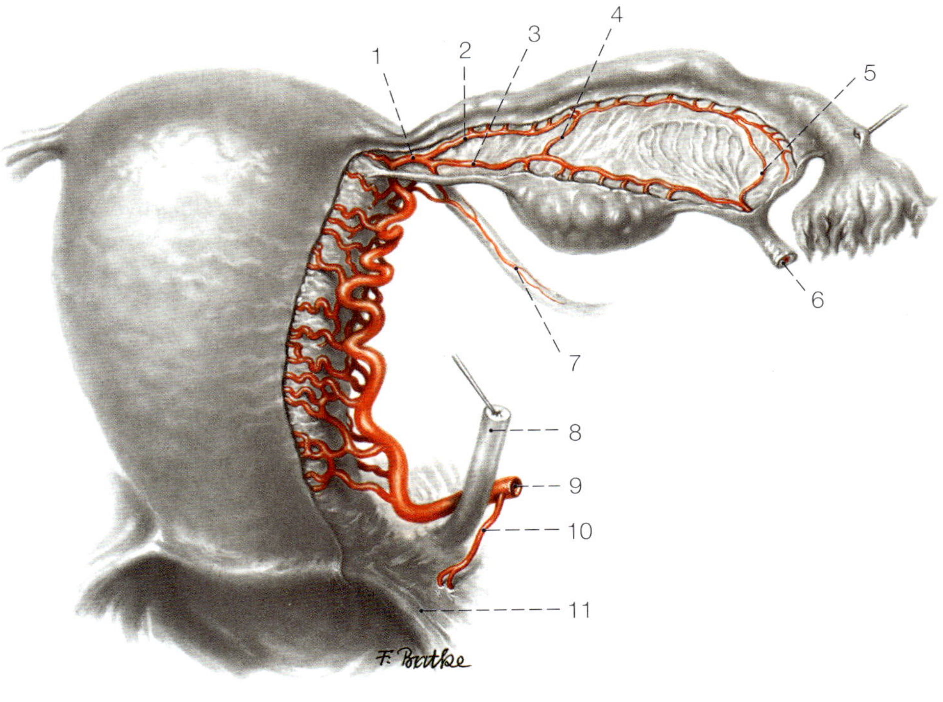

Figure A.23. Arteries of uterus and adnexa.
1 uterine artery
2 tubal branch of uterine artery
3 ovarian branch of uterine artery
4 anastomotic branch
5 tubal branch of ovarian artery
6 ovarian artery
7 round ligament with its artery
8 ureter (raised up)
9 uterine artery
10 vaginal artery
11 uterosacral fold

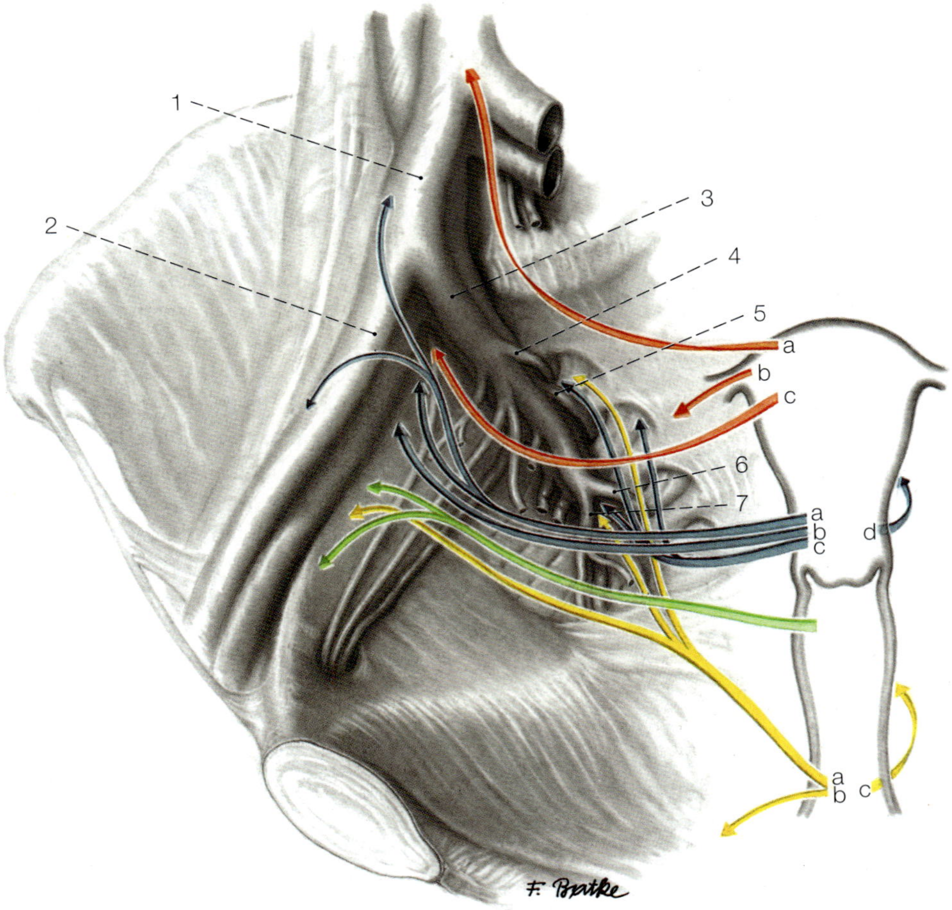

Figure A.24. Lymphatic drainage from the uterus and vagina, shown schematically. *Red,* lymph pathway from fundus and corpus uteri; *blue,* pathway from cervix; *green,* pathway from upper portion of vagina; *yellow,* pathway from lower portion of vagina. See text.

1 common iliac artery
2 external iliac artery
3 internal iliac artery
4 superior gluteal artery
5 superior gluteal vein
6 inferior gluteal artery
7 internal pudendal artery

(*b*) along the round ligament to the superficial inguinal nodes,
(*c*) within the midportion of the broad ligament to the superior internal iliac lymph nodes.

The second group of collecting lymph channels (n = 8–11 according to Reiffenstuhl) arise from the cervix uteri. There are three pathways in the region of the cardinal ligament that merit special attention:

(*a*) Lymphatics that run along the upper edge of the cardinal ligament to reach the internal iliac, lateral common iliac, and lateral external iliac lymph node groups;
(*b*) Lymph vessels that pass through the midportion of cardinal ligament (Mackenrodt's ligament) and also drain into the interiliac nodes;
(*c*) Lymphatics that course along the lower part of the cardinal ligament to the superior and inferior gluteal nodes as well as the presacral nodes;
(*d*) Additional lymphatic pathways that lead to the perirectal, para-aortic, and subaortic nodes.

Innervation. The innervation (Fig. A.25) of the uterus derives from the branches of the uterine plexus that accompany the uterine artery. The uterine plexus and the uterine nerves originate from the laterally situated pelvic plexus and its ganglia. The pelvic plexus lying near the lateral wall at the base of the broad ligament is also called Frankenhäuser's plexus (cervical ganglion of the uterus). The parasympathetic nerves arise from the sacral part of the cord (pelvic nerves) whereas the sympathetics stem from the lumbar cord (hypogastric plexus).

Application. Knowledge of the anatomy of the uterus is important for all uterine surgical procedures, including the vaginal hysterectomy (Chapter 11), cervical amputation (Chapter 14), Manchester procedure (Chapter 15), and radical operation (Chapter 22).

Uterine Tube

The fallopian tube (salpinx, uterine tube) is about 12 cm long and connects the uterine cavity to the peritoneal cavity (Fig. A.21). Its abdominal opening, the abdominal ostium, is surrounded with fimbriae. One fimbriae, the ovarian fimbria, reaches the ovary and forms an attachment. The infundibulum is reached via the abdominal ostium. It continues to the ampulla, which reaches the uterus by way of the isthmus and enters its wall with the intramural part (pars uterina). The uterine ostium opens into the endometrial cavity. The salpinx is located in the upper free

Figure A.25. Innervation of uterus, bladder, and vagina as seen from front and below.

1 pelvic nerves (parasympathetic)
2 sacral plexus (pelvic ganglion, inferior hypogastric plexus)
3 uterine plexus (uterovaginal)
4 uterine artery
5 superior vesical nerves
6 inferior vesical nerves
7 ureter
8 urinary bladder
9 uterus
10 vagina
11 uterine nerves
12 vaginal branch
13 superior hypogastric plexus
14 hypogastric right nerve

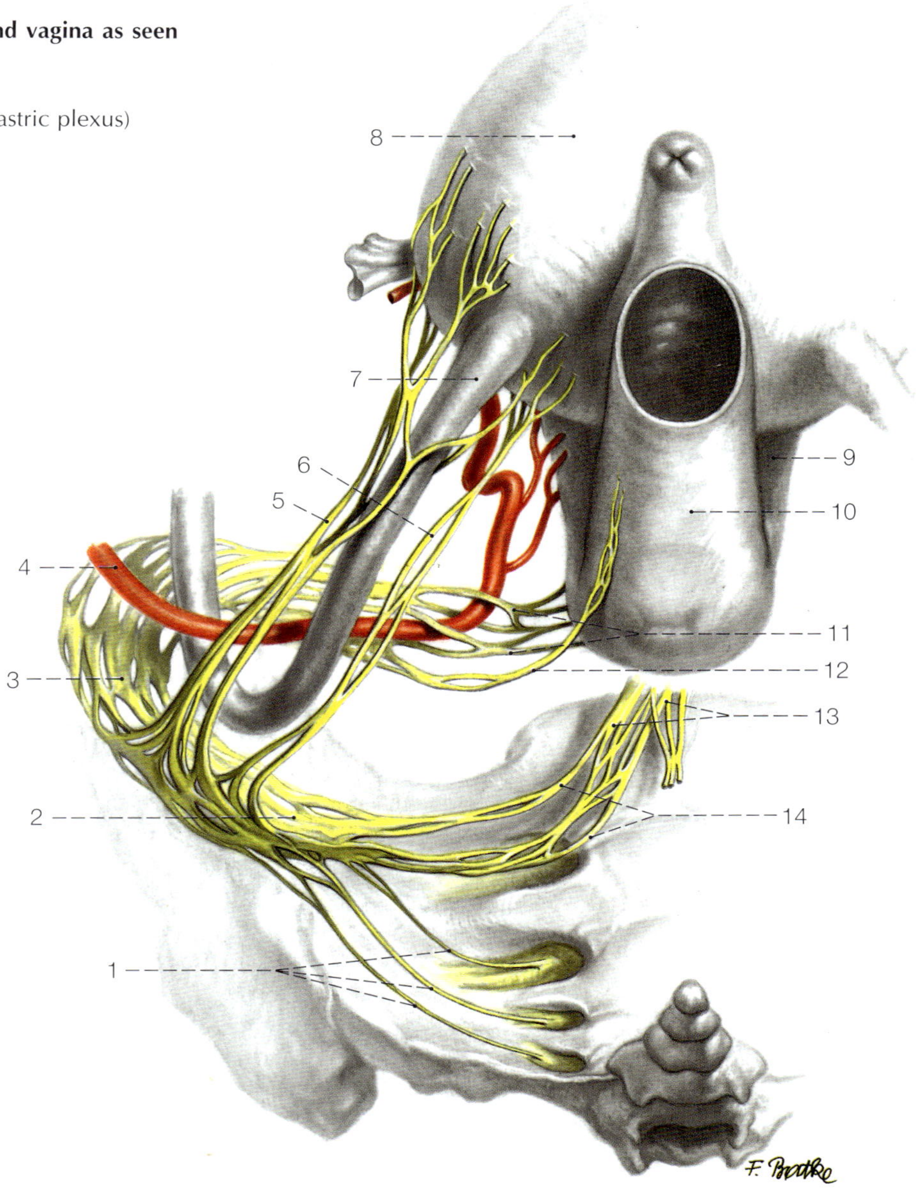

edge of the broad ligament between the round ligament and the utero-ovarian ligament. The tubal mesentery, the mesosalpinx, is short near the uterus, with only about 3–4 cm of potential elasticity in the relatively immobile isthmic portion. The ampullary part of the mesosalpinx is longer, about 7–8 cm long, and bow-shaped, and mobile. In the mesosalpinx smooth muscle fibers are found, and with them occasionally the vestigial remnants of the genitourinary system, the epoöphoron. These remnants may join to form a longitudinal duct (from the Wolffian duct), which runs parallel to the tube, and a transverse duct (derived from Wolffian body remnants). Less often, one can observe a pedunculated structure, the appendix vesiculosa, comprised of remnants from the Wolffian body.

Layers of the Wall

The tubal wall thickness narrows from the abdominal ostium (2 mm) to the uterine ostium (0.5 mm). The innermost layer, the *mucous coat*, forms many folds that disappear toward the uterus. The epithelial layer consists of ciliated, secretory, and, during the second part of the cycle, small peg cells. The cyclic development of all lining cells is dependent on the menstrual phases.

The *muscular coat* is attached to the mucosa without a submucosa and consists of an outer longitudinal and an inner annular muscle fiber layer. In addition, there are perivascular and subperitoneal muscular bundles to be found. The former direct the bloodflow; the latter serve the movement of the fimbriae. A loose *subserosal layer* (tela subserosa), containing vessels, separates the muscular coat from the *serosa*. The serosal epithelium abuts the luminal mucosa in the area of the fimbriae.

Relationship to Adjacent Organs

Bilaterally, the tube has several different areas of contact with neighboring organs. Thus, the anterior surface of both tubes touches the posterior bladder wall when the bladder is distended. The right tube is in contact posteriorly with the rectum and, in some circumstances, with the vermiform appendix. As a consequence, where the appendix is particularly long, secondary adhesions can develop. The posterior surface of the left tube is in close relationship with the sigmoid and its mesentery.

Blood supply and drainage. Blood reaches the tube distally from the branches of the ovarian artery (Fig. A.23) and proximally by way of the tubal anastomotic branches of the uterine artery.

Lymph drainage. The subserous lymphatics of the isthmus interconnect with those of the corpus uteri, whereas lymphatics stemming from the muscularis join those of the ovary (see below).

Innervation. The innervation is derived from the ovarian plexus and the uterine plexus.

Application. The anatomy of the uterine tube is significant in colpotomy (Chapters 5 and 6), vaginal hysterectomy (Chapter 11), and radical vaginal surgery (Chapter 22).

Ovary

In the adult female, the ovaries are situated bilaterally in the ovarian fossa (Fig. A.21), which is the peritoneal indentation cavity formed by the angle of the common iliac artery at its bifurcation. At the base of the ovarian fossa runs the obturator nerve, whereas the ureter traverses its posterior edge. In multiparity the ovary may be somewhat displaced dorsocaudally.

The ovary of an adult, sexually mature woman may be up to 5 cm long, 3 cm wide, and up to 2 cm thick. The pole in contact with the tube, the tubal extremity, can be distinguished from the pole directed toward the uterus, the uterine extremity. The ovarian surface facing the uterus is the facies lateralis, and the surface directed inward is the lateral surface. The dorsal edge is the free border, whereas the edge bordering the mesentery is called the mesovarian border. The mesovarium is a short mesentery that arises from the posterior surface of the broad ligament.

Superficially, the ovary is covered by the so-called germinal epithelium that becomes the peritoneal epithelium at the Farré-Waldeyer line at the mesovarian border. Immediately beneath the epithelium lies a tunica albuginea formed by condensation of the ovarian stroma. The medullary substance must be distinguished from the cortical layer. The connective tissue of the ovarian medulla blends into that of the mesentery at the hilus (which marks the beginning of the mesovarium). The vessels and nerves are also contained here. Regarding details of the cortex development etc., we suggest that relevant histological sources be consulted.

The uterine tube lies above the ovary and is in direct contact with it by way of the fimbria ovarica. A peritoneal fold, containing connective tissue, runs from the tubal extremity of the ovary; this is the suspensory ligament of the ovary (infundibulopelvic ligament), which reaches to the lateral pelvic wall in the region of the external iliac vein. In addition to connective tissue, this structure contains the ovarian vessels, nerves, and lymphatics. The utero-ovarian ligament (utero-ovarian chord) courses from the uterine extremity of the ovary as a thickened fold on the posterior surface of the broad ligament to reach the uterus, where it disappears in the angle of the tube.

Blood supply and drainage. The blood supply (Fig. A.23) to the ovary on the distal side comes via the ovarian artery from the abdominal aorta through the infundibulopelvic ligament. On the proximal side, the ovarian anastomotic branch of the uterine artery reaches the ovary by way of the utero-ovarian ligament. Both arteries anastomose in the mesovarium. From this anastomosis they send out small branches into the ovary. Blood drainage occurs through similarly named veins. In the hilar region, these veins form a plexus, the ovarian bulb, that can distend with blood and reach nearly the size of the ovary.

Lymph drainage. Lymph drainage occurs by way of channels that course in the infundibulopelvic ligament along the ovarian vessels up to the para-aortic lymph nodes. Because they are interconnected with lymphatics from the tube as well as with those from the uterine fundus, the possibility exists that lymph from the ovary follows a common pathway with lymph from the uterine fundus to reach the corresponding lymph nodes.

Nerve supply. The ovarian nervous plexus (derived from the aortic plexus) runs along the ovarian artery to the ovary. It contains both autonomic and sensory fibers supplying the ovarian surface.

Application. Anatomical knowledge of the ovary is important for radical vaginal surgery (Chapter 22).

Pelvic Ureter

The pelvic portion ot the ureter, about 15 cm long (Fig. A.26), extends from the linea terminalis to the confluence of the bladder. In practical terms, one can distinguish three parts of the pelvic ureter. First, a *descending portion* describes a curve that is convex outwardly, changing into the *ascending retrovesical part* at the so-called *ureteral knee*. The ascending segment, together with the intramural part, enters obliquely into the bladder wall and opens into the bladder cavity at the ureteral orifice.

Layers of the Wall

The wall of the ureter is three-layered. The innermost layer, the *mucosa*, is formed into folds during contractions (resulting in a star-shaped lumen) and carries a transitional epithelium. There is no submucosa, so the *muscularis*, consisting of a loose

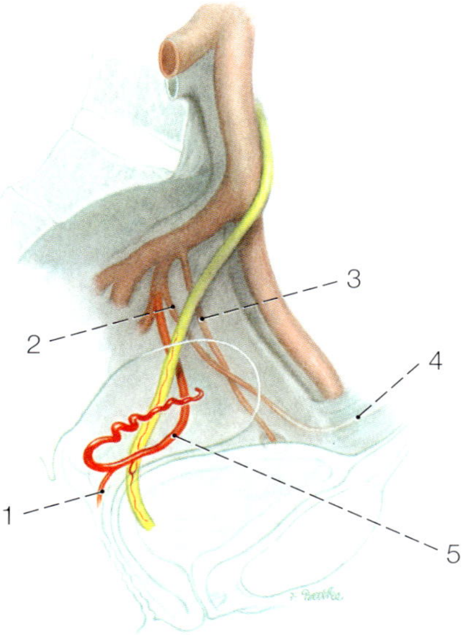

Figure A.26. Course of ureter and uterine artery (parasagittal section). Ureteral branch is given off from uterine artery where it crosses ureter. Medially, a cervicovaginal branch is sometimes encountered.

1 cervicovaginal branch
2 umbilical artery
3 obturator artery
4 lateral umbilical cord
5 uterine artery

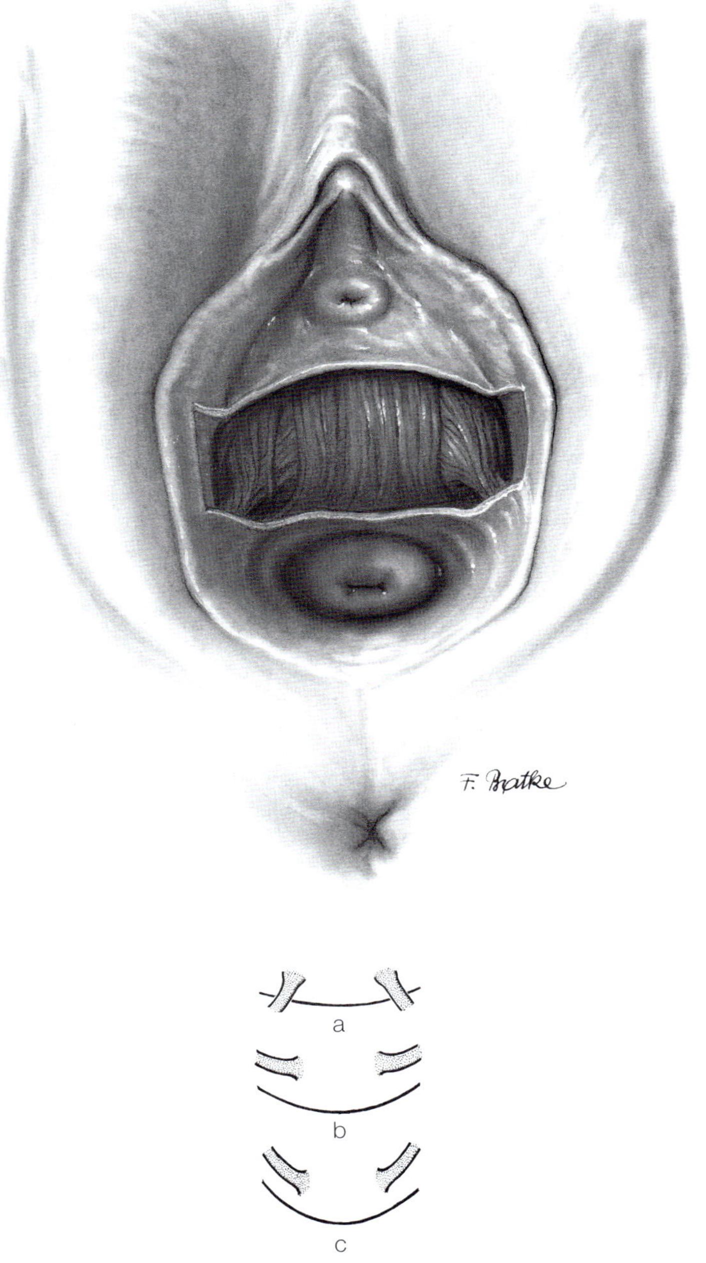

Figure A.27. Bladder base as seen from below. Connective tissue (vaginal and vesical fasciae) has been completely removed.

Detail a: direction of ureteral segment near bladder in normal position.
Detail b: ureteral course in association with descensus uteri.
Detail c: ureteral course in association with uterine prolapse.

inner longitudinal muscle layer and a dense outer circular layer, connects directly with the mucosa. In the anterior part of the intramural segment, longitudinal fibers are also present outside the circular muscle layer. In the region of the intramural portion, the ureteral musculature changes into the bladder musculature (Fig. A.27; see also Fig. A.32). The outermost layer is a connective tissue covering, the *adventitia*, which contains the blood vessels that supply the ureter. This adventitia can enter into a closer, more intimate relationship with the surrounding connective tissue.

Relationship to Adjacent Organs

On entering the true pelvis, the ureter crosses the common iliac artery near its bifurcation (Fig. A.26; Figs. A.35 and A.36). Sometimes it lies somewhat more laterally and instead crosses the external iliac artery. The crossing point corresponds to the approximate location of the sacroiliac articulation. The ureter describes a descending laterally convex curve in the first part of the pelvic portion. Laterally lie the ovarian vessels just before reaching the base of the suspensory ligament of the ovary (infundibulopelvic ligament). Further down, it is situated medially to the internal iliac artery (hypogastric artery) and its branches and also medially to the obturator nerve, sometimes reaching the posterior border of the ovarian fossa subperitoneally behind the ovary. Subsequently, the ureter loses its close relationship to the peritoneum and courses through the cardinal ligament above the rectal pillar. As it reaches the rectal pillar (or even afterward), the ureter possesses a connective tissue sheath originating from its adventitia (ureteral lamina) that is connected to the rectal

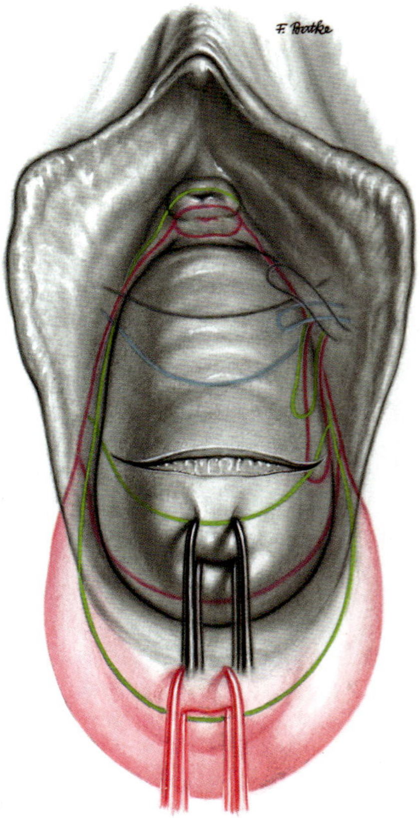

Figure A.28. Position of ureters and bladder in uterine prolapse. Ascending ureter in its normal state (*grey*) becomes almost horizontal (*blue*) when bladder sinks anteriorly (*blue edge*). In more extensive cases (*green*, bladder edge; *pink*, portio edge), the ureter will descend moderately (*green*), whereas it descends vertically in most severe cases (*green*, bladder edge; *pink*, portio fully depicted).

pillar. Presupposing normal locations of the pelvic viscera, the ureter describes a convex descending curve here and then passes through the bladder pillar to the base of the bladder. As mentioned before, this transition is also described by the surgeon as the *ureteral knee* (Figs. A.27 and A.28).

In its passage through the cardinal ligament, the ureter is crossed by the uterine artery (Figs. A.26, A.30, and A.31) and lies about 1.5–2 cm from the cervix. However, in isolated cases it can be as close as 1 cm to or as far as 4 cm from the cervix. Before the ureter reaches the base of the bladder, it is still in fairly close contact with the anterior vaginal fornix.

The ascending portion of the ureter can alter its direction as a consequence of a change in the position of the genital organs (Fig. A.27). Thus, in the case of a cystocele, for example, the ureter approaches the bladder laterally only when the cystocele is associated with uterine prolapse; the ureter also descends (from lateral above) toward the bladder (Fig. A.28).

Blood supply. Blood supply (see Figs. A.30 and A.31) to the pelvic ureter comes from several different arteries, and a certain degree of variability is to be expected. In addition to a branch of the ovarian artery that reaches the ureter, this structure receives blood by way of branches from the common iliac artery. All these supplying vessels vary in their number and caliber as well as in their antecedent arterial sources.

The ureteral portion near the bladder is of particular interest to the gynecologist, because during surgery, damage to *all* supplying vessels at this site can lead to inadequate tissue perfusion and thus necrosis of this section. This diminished perfusion occurs even though the very delicate adventitial arterial network possesses numerous anastomoses. In a healthy ureter these anastomoses are not sufficient to provide adequate blood supply alone. Damage to the adventitia during ureteral enucleation may also interrupt the blood supply here.

Near the bladder, a branch from the uterine artery arises at the crossing with the ureter. It usually separates into an ascending and a descending branch; the descending branch anastomoses with branches from the superior and inferior vesical arteries to supply the ureter. Additionally, a branch of the vaginal artery also frequently leads into the adventitial network. Because of the numerous supplying arteries, any one branch, including the vessel from the uterine artery, can be ligated during the Schauta operation without any problem. It must be stressed, however, that the ureteral adventitia and its blood supply must be preserved intact (see above).

Blood drainage. Blood drainage occurs to the vesical plexus, to the uterine plexus, and directly to the internal iliac vein and the ovarian vein.

Lymph drainage. Lymphatics follow the blood vessels to reach the internal iliac and common iliac nodes.

Innervation. Innervation of the pelvic portion of the ureter comes by way of the pelvic plexus as well as the vesical plexus. In addition to autonomic fibers, sensory nerves also reach the ureter via the important vesicourethral ganglion located near the entrance of the ureter into the bladder.

Application. The anatomy of the pelvic ureter is important for all vaginal operations. Of particular significance is the changed anatomy when prolapse occurs (Figs. A.28 and A.29).

Urinary Bladder

The urinary bladder (Fig. A.21) lies above and behind the symphysis in the retropubic space. At its lower surface in the area of the bladder base (vesical fundus), it is connected with the urogenital diaphragm. The bladder base continues anteriorly in an upward direction into the corpus uteri, which rises to the bladder vertex (vesical vertex). At the inner surface of the bladder base is the trigone, whose posterior angles are formed by the ureteral orifices. The interureteral fold stretches between the two ureters that empty here. Anteriorly, the bladder trigone is bordered by the internal orifice of the urethra, whose lumen forms a half-moon in the closed state by virtue of a projection of the mucous membrane (uvula vesicae).

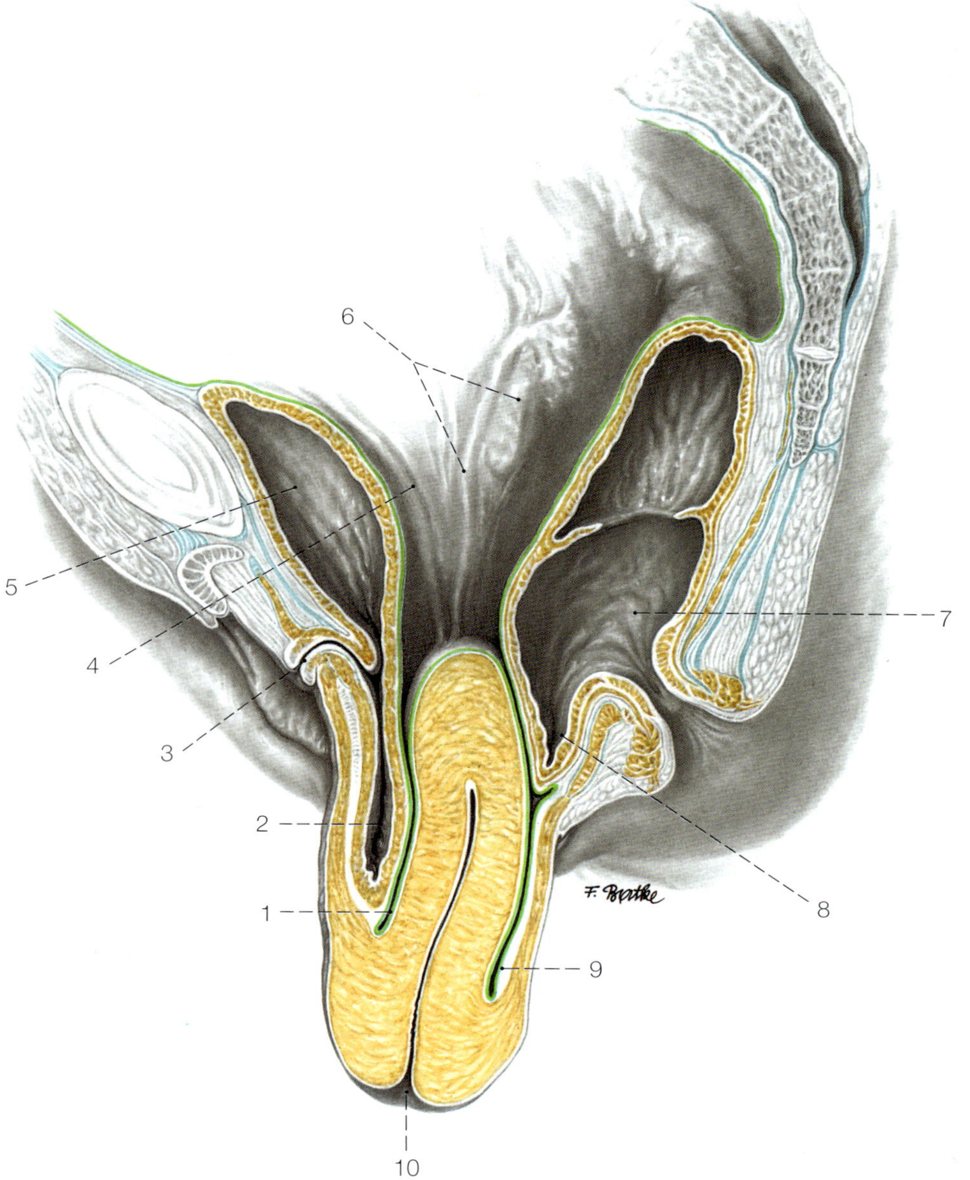

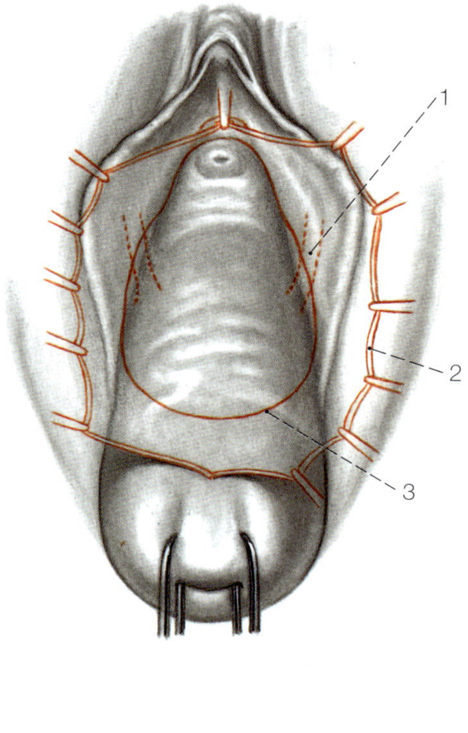

Figure A.29. Uterine prolapse with cystocele and rectocele in a median sagittal section. *Green*, peritoneal cut edge.

1 vesicouterine excavation
2 cystocele
3 urethra
4 round ligament
5 urinary bladder
6 uterine tube and ovary
7 rectum
8 rectocele
9 cul-de-sac of Douglas
10 external cervical os

Detail. Operative field in prolapse of bladder and vagina, with section of ureter near bladder, cut edge of vaginal wall, and operative margins.

1 ureteral course near bladder
2 separated vaginal wall
3 edge of operative field

Layers of the Wall

The reddish *mucosa* possesses a transitional epithelium and a loose lamina propria that is rich in blood vessels. Except in the trigone, there is an adjoining *submucosa*. The immovable mucosa of the trigone is directly juxtaposed to the subjacent *muscularis* (see Fig. A.32). A definite layer of muscle is not found; it appears more as a netlike reticular arrangement of muscle fibers. Only in isolated areas (e.g., the dorsal part) is there a three-layered architecture with outer longitudinal fibers (detrusor urinae muscle), middle annular and spiral fibers (compressor urinae muscle), and an inner reticular layer.

In the region of the trigone, the musculature is distinguished by its fine muscle bundles and its content of elastic fibers. From there, muscle fibers of the outer layer reach the anterior pelvic wall (at the symphysis) as the pubovesical muscle (pubovesical ligament); they reach the uterus as the vesicouterine muscles within the vesicouterine ligaments. Posteriorly, a diagonal muscle enlargement, the torus uretericus, is formed; the ureteral musculature continues into the torus uretericus to yield the structural base for the interureteral fold. Longitudinal muscle fibers course directly beneath the mucosa, converging toward the urethral orifice that they surround from behind like a bridle. In this way, a half sphincter is formed. From the anterior aspect, a corresponding reversed half sphincter forms around the opening made in the annular fibers and functions to close the urethral orifice. Additionally, a smooth muscle lissosphincter urethrae (*Hayek*) converges toward the urethra. The outer layer of the bladder is partially formed of *serosa* and partly by *adventitia (vesical fascia)*. The posterior bladder wall is covered by peritoneum that is only loosely adherent to the muscularis. When the bladder is empty, one or more *transverse folds* course diagonally across the posterior wall of the bladder in the form of reserve peritoneal folds. The vesical fascia is firmly attached to the vaginal fascia in some places and, especially, to the fascial adventitia of the cervix in the supravaginal septum (Fig. A.20).

Attachments of the Bladder

The base of the bladder lies approximately at the level of the lower edge of the symphysis pubis to which it is densely adherent by means of the fascia of the superior urogenital diaphragm (Figs. A.20, A.35–A.37). The bladder is anchored anteriorly over the pubovesical ligament in the area of the sym-

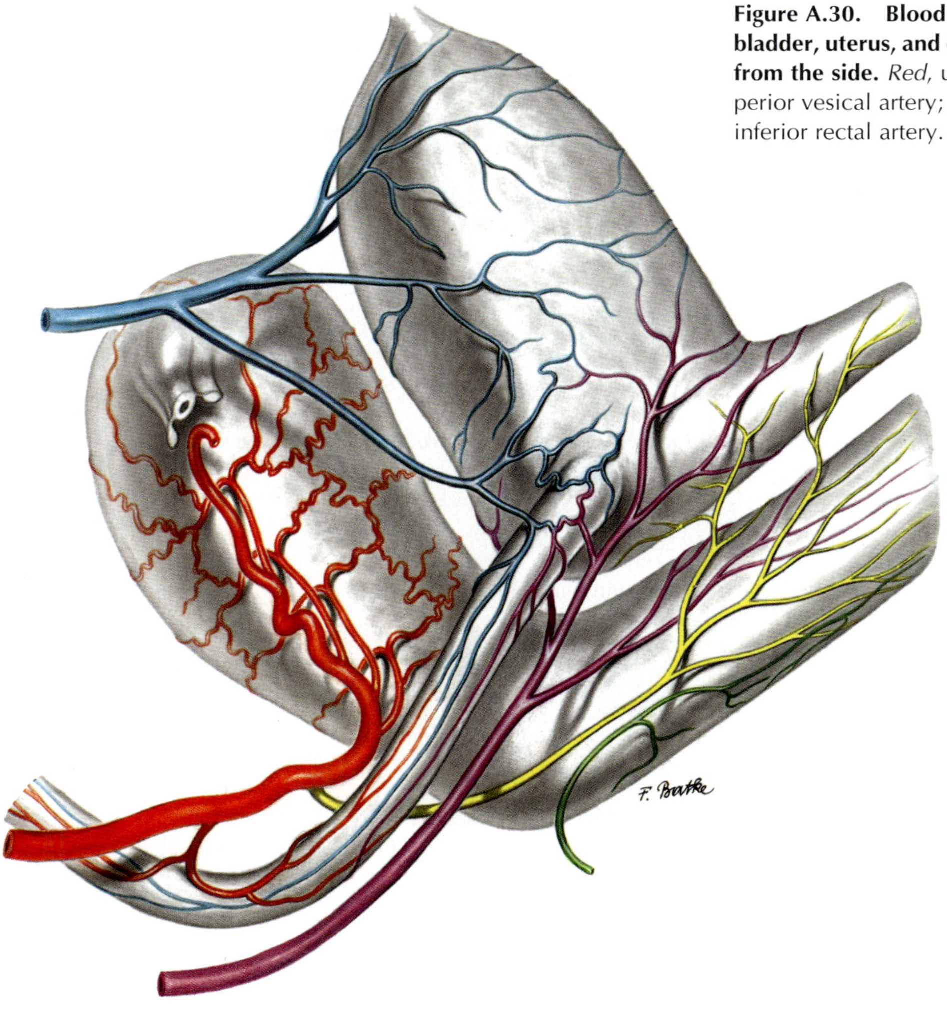

Figure A.30. Blood supply of portion of ureter near bladder, the bladder, uterus, and central parts of the urethra and vagina as seen from the side. *Red,* uterine artery; *yellow,* vaginal artery; *blue,* superior vesical artery; *violet,* inferior vesical artery; *green,* branch of inferior rectal artery.

physis. The bladder is also bound to the vagina where loose areolar connective tissue is found between the vesical fascia and the vaginal fascia. This structure is termed the vesicovaginal septum by various authors. In actuality this undoubtedly is not a real septum but rather connective tissue that can be pushed together during surgery to evoke the impression that it is a septum or a ligament. It is more correct to speak here of a vesicovaginal space that is filled with loose connective tissue (sliding tissue) and is situated between the two fascial layers. It is only between the cervix and the bladder that one encounters a true condensation of connective tissue that can be described as the *supravaginal septum* (Fig. A.20).

Laterally to the bladder is the loose areolar tissue of the *paracystium* that also possesses denser fibers. These fibers are arranged to form the *bladder pillars* that course from the anterior part of the cardinal ligament to the bladder base. The medial part of the bladder pillar originates near the cervix. It corresponds to the vesicouterine ligament (or vesicouterine muscle by virtue of its smooth muscle content) and sometimes contains a vesicovaginal branch from the uterine artery.

A wider band courses from the vertex of the bladder; this is the middle umbilical ligament (vesicoumbilical ligament) that contains the obliterated urachus (chorda urachi) reaching to the umbilicus.

Blood supply. The blood supply (Figs. A.30 and A.31) comes via a pair of vesical arteries. The superior vesical artery (often consisting of two branches) originates at the beginning of the umbilical artery and terminates in the upper lateral part of the bladder pillar. The inferior vesical artery, a direct branch of the internal iliac artery, reaches the bladder by passing through the lower lateral aspect of the bladder pillar. Numerous anastomoses exist between these two arteries. In addition, the bladder may be supplied by branches arising from the uterine and vaginal arteries.

Blood drainage. Similarly named veins form a plexus within the bladder pillar, which represents a portion of the vesical plexus. This plexus is connected to both the uterine and vaginal venous plexuses near the cardinal ligament. The anterior vesical veins course from the anterior surface of the bladder; they unite into a single trunk to join the pudendal plexus or the dorsal cli-

Figure A.31. Blood supply of portion of ureter near bladder, the bladder, uterus, and central parts of the urethra and vagina as seen from front and below. *Red,* uterine artery; *yellow,* vaginal artery; *blue,* superior vesical artery; *violet,* inferior vesical artery; *green,* branch of inferior rectal artery.

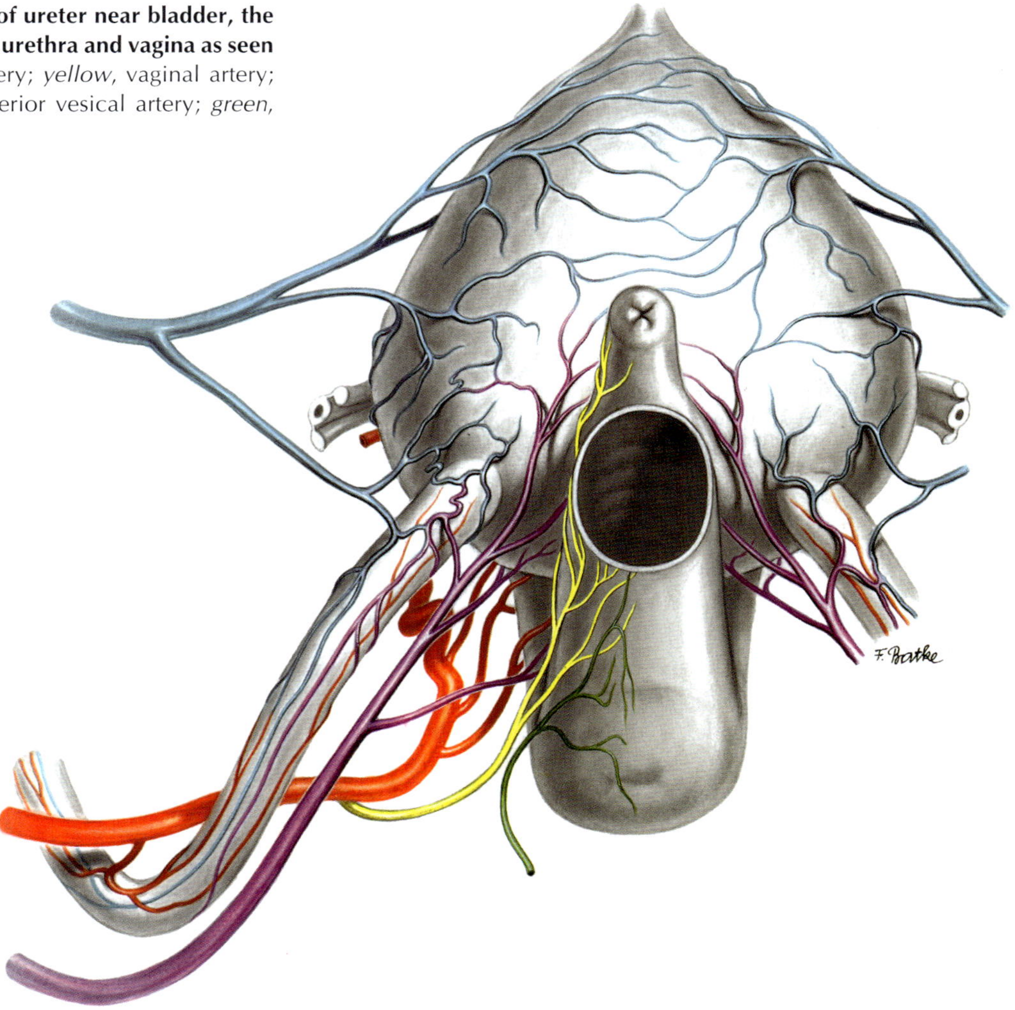

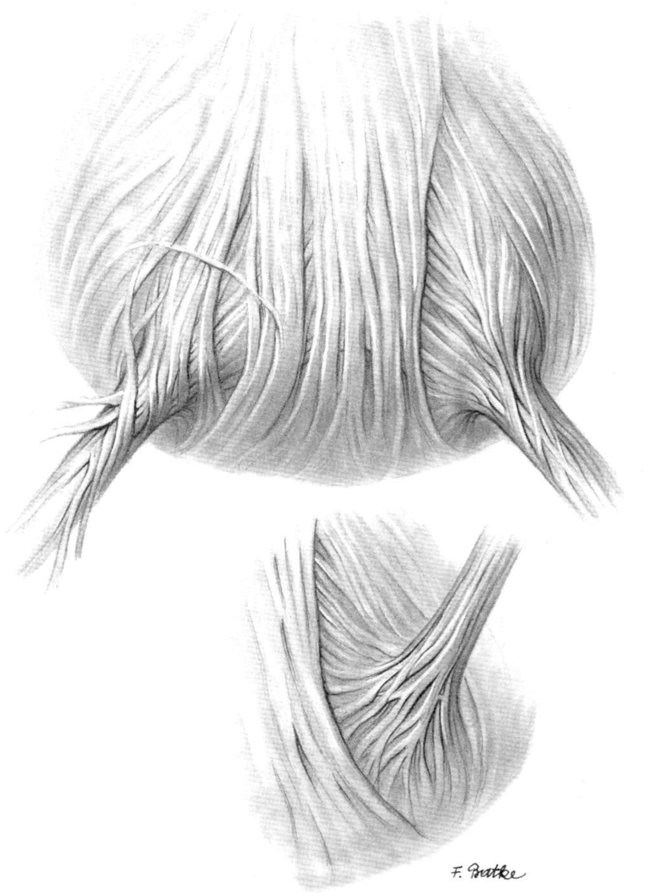

Figure A.32. *Top:* musculature of fundus of urinary bladder as seen from below. Ureteral muscle radiates into deep layer of bladder muscle. *Bottom:* muscular ureterovesical junction shown with right ureter retracted upward.

toral vein. These tributaries allow blood to drain not only to the internal iliac veins but also to the femoral veins.

Lymph drainage. The lymphatics reach from the bladder pillars to the internal iliac nodes.

Innervation. Innervation occurs by way of the vesical nerves from the vesical plexus, which is formed in turn from the pelvic plexus. The pelvic plexus derives its parasympathetic elements from the sacral cord (pelvic splanchnic nerve) and its sympathetic fibers from the lumbar portion of the spinal cord (superior hypogastric plexus). The major part of the vesical nerves innervates the lateral aspect of the bladder pillar laterally to the vesicouterine ligament. These nerves may therefore be damaged during the division of the bladder pillars and preparation of the paravesical space during surgery.

Application. It is essential to be familiar with the anatomy of the bladder during vaginal hysterectomy (Chapter 11), anterior colporrhaphy (Chapter 12), Manchester procedure (Chapter 15), surgical treatment of vesicovaginal fistula (Chapter 18), and radical vaginal surgery (Chapter 22).

Urethra

The relatively short (3–5 cm) female urethra extends from the bladder through the levator portal to empty into the vaginal vestibule at the external urethral orifice. For expediency, the gynecologist should distinguish between two parts of the urethra: (*a*) the upper portion, loosely attached to the vaginal fascia, called the *superior part* (or free part) and (*b*) the contrasting *inferior part* (or fixed part) that is fixed by the urethrovaginal septum.

The *mucosa* exhibits a variable epithelial layer, which may consist of either transitional or cuboidal epithelium or even of a squamous covering. Glands can be found in the lamina propria; their numbers increase toward the external urethral meatus. A *submucosal layer* separates the mucosa from the *muscle layer*. The latter consists of smooth muscle with superimposed layers of diagonally striated muscle. The smooth muscle is composed of an inner longitudinal and an outer annular fiber layer. Both layers are essentially continuations of the bladder musculature. The fiber bundles of the pubovesical muscle run from the os pubis to the bladder and radiate into the inner longitudinal muscle tracts anteriorly. An outer supplementary longitudinal fiber layer courses in thin layers to the preurethral ligament or to the superior fascia of the urogenital diaphragm. From the posterior aspect of the urethra, longitudinal branches radiate into the vaginal wall. These are intrinsically involved in the formation of the urethrovaginal septum. The circular fiber layer forms the smooth muscle lissosphincter urethrae (*Hayek*) in the central region of the urethra.

The diagonally striped muscle fibers originate from the deep transverse perineal muscle and form a urethrovaginal sphincter muscle and a rhabdosphincter urethrae. In the area of the urethrovaginal septum, the striated muscle bundles of the urethrovaginal sphincter radiate into the vaginal wall.

The *adventitia* is loosely applied in the upper posterior urethra, whereas it is densely adherent to the fascia vaginalis in the lower urethra within the urethrovaginal septum.

Blood supply and drainage. The arterial vessels originate from the inferior vesical arteries, the vaginal arteries, and from branches of the internal pudendal arteries. Venous drainage is directed toward the pudendal plexus and to the veins of the external genitalia.

Lymph drainage. The lymphatics reach from the lower urethra to the superficial and deep inguinal lymph nodes. From the upper urethra, they travel along the bladder pillar to the internal iliac and the subinguinal node groups.

Innervation. Innervation is from the vescical plexus as well as from the pudendal nerve. The latter carries both motor and sensory fibers.

Application. Anatomical knowledge of the urethra is vital

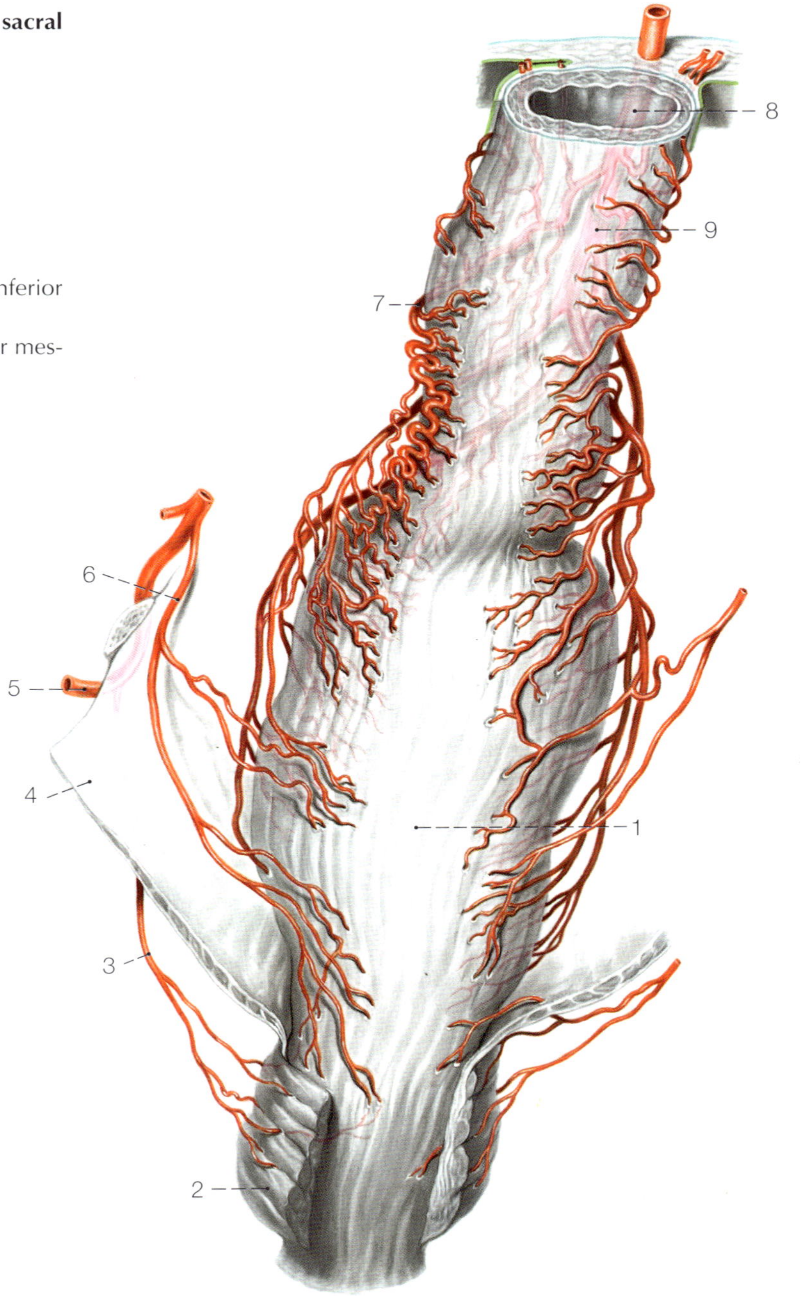

Figure A.33. Blood supply of rectum. Branches of middle sacral artery are not shown.
1 rectal ampulla
2 external ani sphincter muscle
3 inferior hemorrhoidal artery
4 pelvic diaphragm
5 internal pudendal artery
6 middle hemorrhoidal artery
7 rectosigmoid artery
8 Sudeck's point where rectosigmoid artery takes off from inferior mesenteric artery
9 superior hemorrhoidal artery (endarterial branch of inferior mesenteric artery)

in anterior colporrhaphy (Chapter 12), Manchester operation (Chapter 15), and repair of vesicovaginal fistula (Chapter 18).

Rectum

The rectum reaches approximately from S2 to the anus. However, it is more appropriate to speak of a "rectosigmoidal" transition, because its boundary may fluctuate according to the structure of the rectal wall. It curves along the sacrum (Figs. A.21 and A.33) to form the sacral flexure in the *pelvic part*; then, in its *perineal part* (canalis perinealis), it arcs anteriorly to yield the perineal flexure. In the region of the sacral flexure, the rectum is displaced to the right, whereas it occupies the midline in the perineal part. Immediately above the perineal portion is the ampulla of the rectum.

Layers of the Wall

The architecture of the rectal wall corresponds more or less to that of the large intestine in the pelvic part. Only the longitudinal musculature completely and uniformly envelops the rectum in the form of an outer muscle layer. There are but a few (at most three) diagonal folds, the transverse rectal folds, that can be found in the mucosa. The largest fold (the middle one) is named after Kohlrausch. The anal canal is discussed under "Anus and Anorectal Canal."

Relationships to Adjacent Organs

There is no peritoneum over the posterior wall of the rectum, and loose connective tissue extends from the sides. This lateral connective tissue is called the *paraproctium*. The anterior rectal wall is connected to the posterior wall of the vagina by means of the rectovaginal septum. Three peritoneal pockets are formed above this area. In the middle is the cul-de-sac of Douglas (rectouterine excavation) and laterally are the pararectal fossae.

The anal canal is fixed within the pelvic diaphragm, where it is surrounded by the levator ani muscle and the external anal sphincter muscle.

With regard to *arteries* (Fig. A.33), the rectum is supplied by the unpaired superior hemorrhoidal artery (the superior rectal artery arising from the inferior mesentery artery), the paired middle hemorrhoidal arteries (from the internal iliac artery), and the paired inferior hemorrhoidal arteries (from the internal pudendal artery). The middle hemorrhoidal arteries reach the rectum by way of the pararectal connective tissue (the lateral aspect of the rectal pillar); they anastomose with both superior and inferior hemorrhoidal arteries. The superior hemorrhoidal artery, at the dorsal side of the rectum, sends out two main branches, each of which further subdivides into a left and a right branch, respectively. Laterally to the rectum, the uppermost of these branches forms anastomoses by means of vascular arcades that originate in the rectosigmoid artery.

The point where the rectosigmoid artery takes off from the mesenteric artery is called the "critical point" (Sudeck's point), because it is the last artery that is connected with the other colonic arteries by adequate anastomoses.

Blood supply. The middle hemorrhoidal arteries anastomose with the superior hemorrhoidal arteries at the arcades where the two main branches divide. The anastomoses with the inferior hemorrhoidal arteries occur within the muscular layer. Small branches of the middle sacral artery reach the posterior wall of the rectum above the pelvic diaphragm.

Blood drainage. Blood flowing from the rectum is collected in the superior hemorrhoidal veins (superior rectal veins) that are formed from the rectal venous plexus (superior part) situated in the paraproctium. These veins reach the inferior mesenteric vein. From the rectal ampulla, veins also lead to the rectal venous plexus (which, in this location, has connections with the uterine or vaginal venous plexuses) and then, by way of the middle hemorrhoidal veins, to the internal iliac veins. In addition, other veins arise from the dorsal side of the rectum to reach the middle sacral vein and finally from the inferior hemorrhoidal veins to the internal pudendal veins. All these veins are interconnected with each other via the rectal venous plexus.

Lymph drainage. Lymph vessels follow the veins in their course and drain into the rectal, internal iliac, presacral, and inguinal lymph node groups.

Innervation. The rectum is innervated by the hypogastric plexus (Fig. A.34). The superior hypogastric plexus represents a continuation of the plexus that accompanies the inferior mesenteric artery. It supplies the portion that connects to the sigmoid with both sympathetic and parasympathetic nerves. The superior hypogastric plexus is formed from the lumbar splanchnic nerves of the sympathetic trunk and continues laterally into the hypogastric nerve. The latter develops on either side of the sympathetic root of the pelvic plexus (inferior hypogastric plexus). The parasympathetic roots of this plexus originate from the sacral region (S2–S4) and reach the plexus by way of the pelvic nerves (pelvic splanchnic nerves). The lower portion of the rectum receives both sympathetic and parasympathetic innervation from the median rectal plexus that begins in the pelvic plexus. The pelvic plexus lies within the paraproctium and is connected to the uterovaginal and the vesical plexuses. Sympathetic fibers entwining the rectal arteries also reach the rectum as the inferior rectal plexus. Finally, the external anal sphincter is innervated by means of the inferior rectal nerves that arise from the pudendal nerve.

Application. Intimate knowledge of the anatomical details of the rectum is needed in the performance of vaginal hysterectomy (Chapter 11), colpoperineorrhaphy (Chapter 13), procedure for vaginal atresia (Chapter 16), repair of perineal laceration (Chapter 17), and radical vaginal surgery (Chapter 22).

Pelvic Connective Tissue

The pelvic connective tissue invests those subperitoneal or extraperitoneal tissues that connect the viscera and the abdominal wall. In addition to loose areolar tissue, there are denser, fibrous, syndesmotic elements that are reinforced by smooth muscle.

Pelvic connective tissue surrounds the viscera in denser layers called adventitia or fascia. Laterally to the organs, the connective tissue is arranged to serve as guiding tissues for vessels and nerves in the paracolpium, parametrium, paracystium, and paraproctium leading to specific organs. The anchoring tissues are called bands, muscles, and pillars. Thus, one may distinguish between bladder pillars, cervical pillars (perhaps even uterovaginal pillars), and rectal pillars (Fig. A.22). These pillars, however, have no supporting function but rather a hardening function for the viscera, but they do check organ displacement. Support against pressure from above is only from pelvic floor musculature.

There are innumerable terms for pelvic connective tissue and its component parts, e.g., intrapelvic body, vessel-nerve-guiding tissues, connective-tissue matrix (horizontal and frontal), endopelvic fascia and similar designations. Realize, however, that different authors have used the *same* terms for *different* structures, adding confusion to an already complicated connective tissue construction. Only the most common and meaningful expressions will be used in this text.

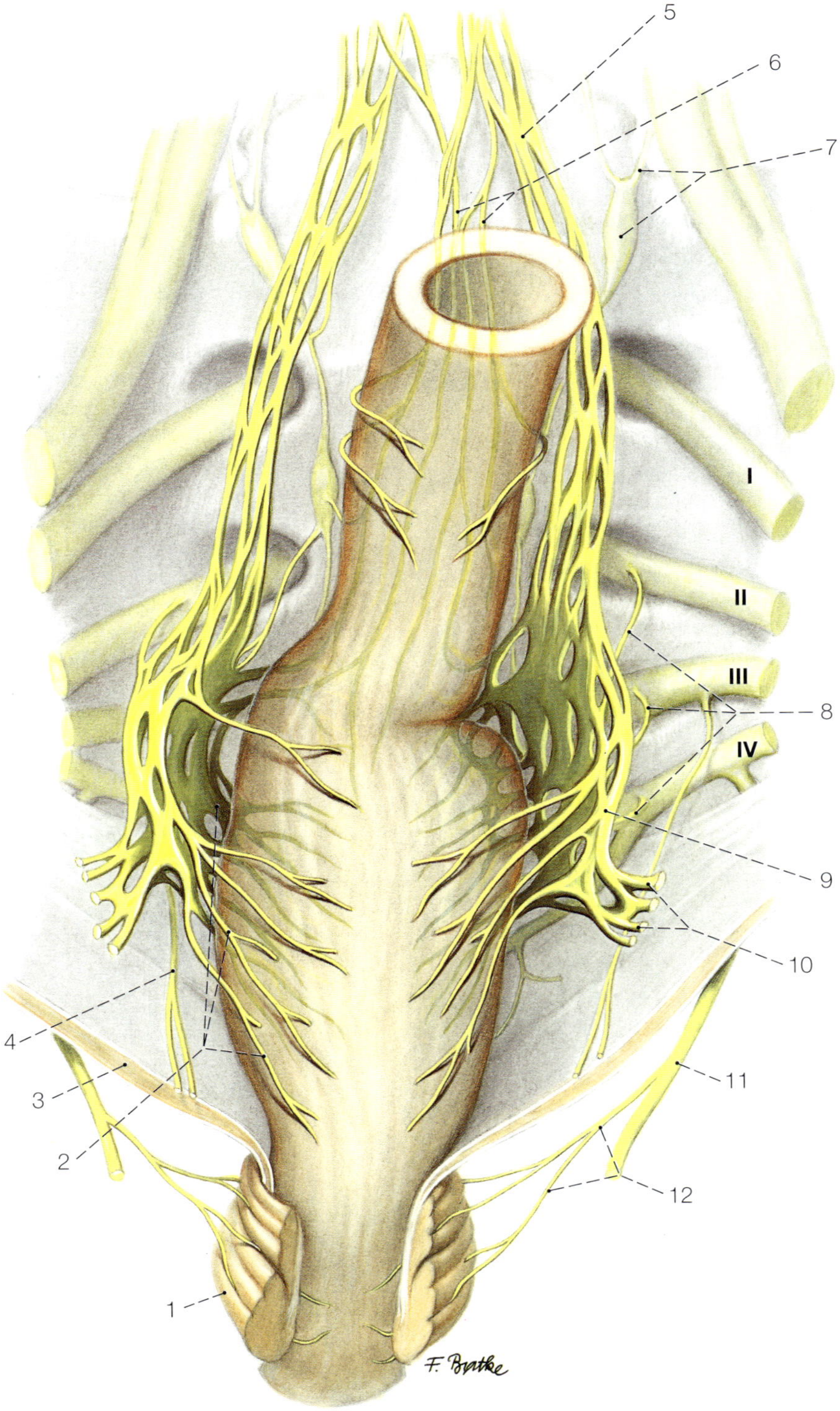

Figure A.34. Innervation of rectum. ***I–IV:*** **ventral branches of sacral nerves 1–4.**

1 external sphincter ani muscle
2 median rectal plexus derived from sacral plexus
3 levator ani muscle
4 long branch innervating levator ani muscle
5 hypogastric nerve arising from superior hypogastric plexus
6 rectal nerve branches
7 sympathetic trunk with a ganglion
8 pelvic nerves (S_2–S_4)
9 sacral plexus (inferior hypogastric plexus, pelvic ganglion)
10 communication with uterovaginal and vesical plexuses
11 pudendal nerve
12 inferior rectal rami

The loose areolar tissue interposed between denser connective tissue strands fills those cavities that can be easily seen during surgery. One differentiates the prevesical, paravesical, pararectal, retrorectal, vesicocervical, vesicovaginal, urethrovaginal, and rectovaginal spaces (Figs. A.35 and A.36).

Anteriorly, the pelvic connective tissue attaches to the pelvic wall along the arcus tendineus of the pelvic fascia. This border begins near the lower edge of the symphysis pubis and crosses the tendinous arc of the obturator fascia (levator ani muscle) close to the ischial spine to reach the pelvic fascia. The arcus tendineus of the pelvic fascia corresponds to a striped thickening of the superior levator fascia. Anteriorly, between the symphysis and the bladder, stretches the *pubovesical ligament* (also called the pubovesical muscle) permeated by smooth muscle fibers. This band represents the most anterior part of the pelvic connective tissue. The posterior part is weaker; it belongs to the rectal pillar and reaches the pelvic wall approximately in the angle of bifurcation of the common iliac artery.

The center of the intrapelvic body is that point at which the connective tissue is most powerfully developed. It is found where the visceral vessels separate from the pelvic wall. Denser strands are developed from this part within the connective tissue as guiding pathways for vessels and nerves. The strongest structure is the *uterovaginal pillar*. This pillar, also called *cardinal ligament*, participates in the formation of the parametrium and connects the lateral pelvic wall with the cervix uteri. It is attached to the pelvic floor only with loose areolar tissue. It does continue, however, into the lateral connective tissue of the vagina, i.e., into the endopelvic fascia.

With regard to the cardinal ligament, its various designations and interpretations should be discussed.

The term "cardinal ligament" was first introduced in 1880 not by *Mackenrodt* but by *Kocks*, who spoke of the pars cardinalis ligamentum lati when referring to the basal part of the broad ligament. *Mackenrodt*, in 1895, used an even narrower definition for the taut connective tissue fibers that stretch from the cervix to the pelvic wall with the term "ligamentum transversale colli or ligamentum latum colli." In 1899, *Waldeyer* introduced both expressions into the anatomy. *Halban* and *Tandler* in 1907 again used both expressions in the gynecological anatomy. *Martin* originally characterized (in 1911) all connective tissue fibers leading to the uterus as retinaculum uteri, whereby he designated the section, which corresponds to the cardinal ligament, as pars media retinaculi uteri. He changed this expression himself in 1950 when he introduced an additional new term "pars media fasciae pelvis." *Pernkopf* and *Pichler* spoke in 1945 of a "tunica vasorum uteri, id est ligamente cardinale Mackenrodt." They were the ones, in addition to *Martius* (1936), who connected the term cardinal ligament with the name Mack-

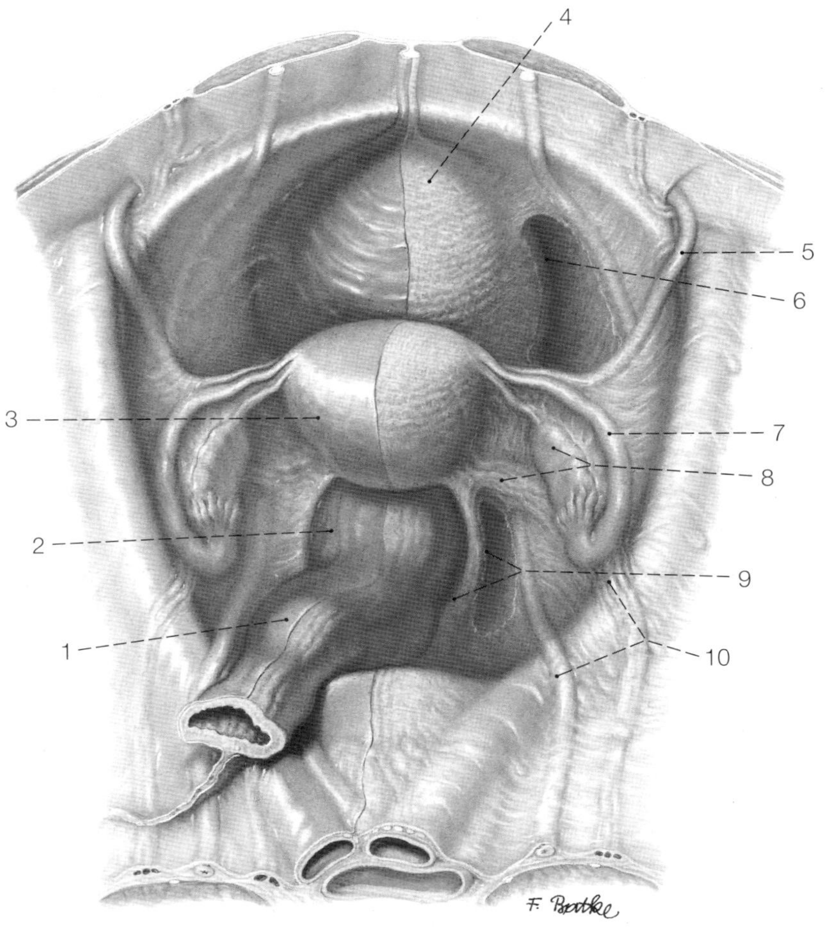

Figure A.35. Connective tissue spaces of true pelvis as seen from above. Peritoneum has been removed from left half.
1 rectum
2 cul-de-sac of Douglas
3 uterus
4 urinary bladder
5 round ligament
6 paravesical space
7 fallopian tube
8 ovary and cervical pillar
9 rectouterine ligament and artificial space created within paraproctium
10 infundibulopelvic ligament and ureter

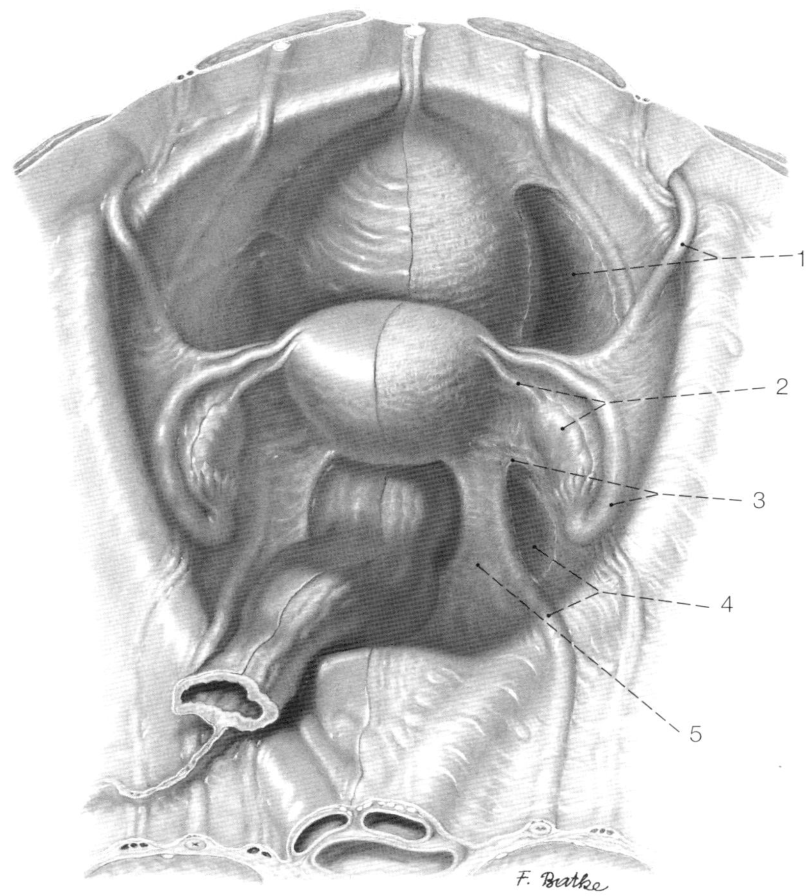

Figure A.36. Connective tissue space of true pelvis as seen from above. Peritoneum has been removed from left half.

1 paravesical space and round ligament
2 utero-ovarian ligament and ovary
3 cardinal ligament and fallopian tube
4 ureter and artificial space in lateral aspect of rectal pillar
5 medial portion of rectal pillar

enrodt. The terms "cardinal ligament of Mackenrodt," "lateral cervical ligament," and "transverse cervical ligament" are considered synonymous in the American surgical-anatomical literature (*Hollinshead 1956*).

In 1930 *Amreich* defined the term "frontal connective tissue" in his Operational Theory (*Peham-Amreich*) and made it synonymous with the term "ligament of Mackenrodt." More recently, *Artner, Holzner,* and *Schaller* (1972) tried to find a clear description—and bring about a resolution in defining these conflicting expressions.

To summarize, note that the terms cardinal ligament, transverse cervical ligament, Mackenrodt's ligament, and cervical pillar (as defined by *Amreich*) all represent the same structure. For *Amreich,* the term cervical pillar represents only the intermediate portion of Mackenrodt's ligament. This seems to be perfectly understandable, if one considers that he includes the entire frontal portion of the connective tissue foundation in the term Mackenrodt's ligament. In 1936, *Martius* used the term "retinaculum" to equate the pars media with the cardinal ligament. Based on the rules of priority, the terms under discussion may only be used for tissue connecting the pelvic wall to the cervix. Connective tissue lying above that region must be designated as parametrium connecting to the corpus uteri. It seems to make sense to use the term cervical pillar, in particular when one also speaks of bladder pillar and rectal pillar.

Augmented connective tissue fibers embedded with smooth muscle fibers are found on the anterior surface of the cardinal ligament (cervical pillar). They course laterally near the pelvic wall and medially near the uterus, extending to the vesical fascia. Collectively, these fibers represent the *bladder pillar*, whose medial fibers are also called the vesicouterine ligament (*ligamente vesicouterinum*). Most blood vessels and nerves pass through the pillar's lateral portion that reaches the pubovesical ligament (pubovesical muscle). Within the vesicouterine ligament courses an always present vesicovaginal artery, which arises from the uterine artery (variably). Between the medial and lateral parts of the bladder pillar loose areolar tissue is found. All connective tissue lying laterally to the bladder, including the loose areolar tissue, is called the *paracystium* (Fig. A.37).

Dorsally, the *rectal pillar* stretches from the cardinal ligament to the rectum. The rectal pillar curves relatively far toward lateral because the space of Douglas descends between the medial aspects. Located near the uterus, the uterosacral ligaments (*rectouterine ligament*), arising from the cervical pillar, form the medial border of the rectal pillar. These two ligaments represent the connective tissue base of the rectouterine fold. These two peritoneal folds form the lateral border of the cul-de-sac of Douglas. The lateral aspect of the rectal pillar originates form the dorsal part of the cardinal ligament and contains vessels and nerves. The ureter is found between these two ligaments embedded in its connective tissue sheath (ureteral adventitia). Loose areolar

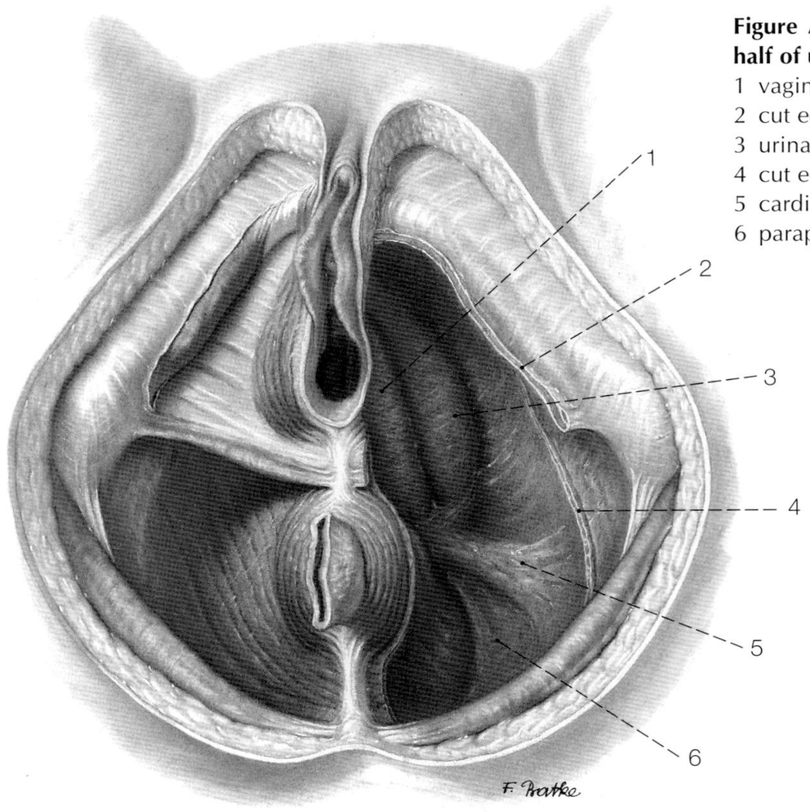

Figure A.37. Pelvic connective tissue as seen from below. Left half of urogenital and pelvic diaphragms have been removed.
1 vagina with vaginal fascia
2 cut edge of urogenital diaphragm
3 urinary bladder with vesical fascia, paracystium
4 cut edge of pelvic diaphragm
5 cardinal ligament
6 paraproctium

tissue fills the surrounding spaces. In that sense, the entire investing tissue around the rectum can be designated the *pararectal fascia* (Fig. A.37).

The urinary, genital, and digestive tracts are all interconnected in the midline by connective tissue infiltrated with smooth muscle. Included in this structure are the urethrovaginal septum, rectovaginal septum, and supravaginal septum.

Fascial Spaces

The connective tissue spaces are filled with loose areolar tissue that can easily be entered by blunt dissection during surgery. This allows individual spaces to be seen.

Paravesical and Prevesical Spaces

The paravesical space is found laterally to the bladder and the anterior aspect of the formed connective tissue that constitutes the bladder pillar (Figs. A.35, A.36, and A.38). It is bordered posteriorly by the root of the bladder pillar from the center of the intrapelvic body (the root of the cardinal ligament) and laterally by the pelvic wall. Anteriorly, the paravesical space proceeds to the prevesical space, which connects, in turn, with the paravesical space of the opposite side. The prevesical space is occluded below by the pubovesical ligaments. The paravesical and prevesical spaces represent parts of the overlying preperitoneal (retropubic) space of Retzius.

Pararectal Space

This space is bordered laterally by the pelvic wall and anterolaterally by the posterior edge of the cardinal ligament or its root, which consists of the center of the intrapelvic body. The medial border is the rectal pillar. Caudally, it reaches to the pelvic floor (Figs. A.35, A.36, and A.38).

The ureter progresses in its connective tissue sheath, the ureteral adventitia, through the rectal pillar. The medial part of the rectal pillar is formed from the uterosacral ligament; vessels and nerves course through its lateral aspect. It contains loose connective tissue. In a surgical preparation it is possible to enter *from above* between the rectal pillar borders to create spaces that are medial and lateral to the ureter and the ureteral fold (Figs. A.35 and A.36) but that do not actually represent the pararectal space. The spaces lie within the rectal pillars. If one enters between the borders of the rectal pillars, one can advance up to the rectovaginal space. Medially, the pararectal space is separated from the retrorectal space by the uterosacral ligament. The pararectal space communicates with the paravesical space beneath the cardinal ligament because, as mentioned earlier, the cardinal ligament is attached dorsally to the pelvic floor by loose areolar tissue (the horizontal pelvic fascia, according to *Amreich*).

Retrorectal Space

The retrorectal space is separated laterally from the pararectal space by the uterosacral ligaments. Its anterior wall is formed

Figure A.38. Median sagittal section of lateral connective tissue spaces, shown as artificially created. *Blue*, paravesical space; *red*, connective tissue space lateral to uterus; *green*, pararectal space.

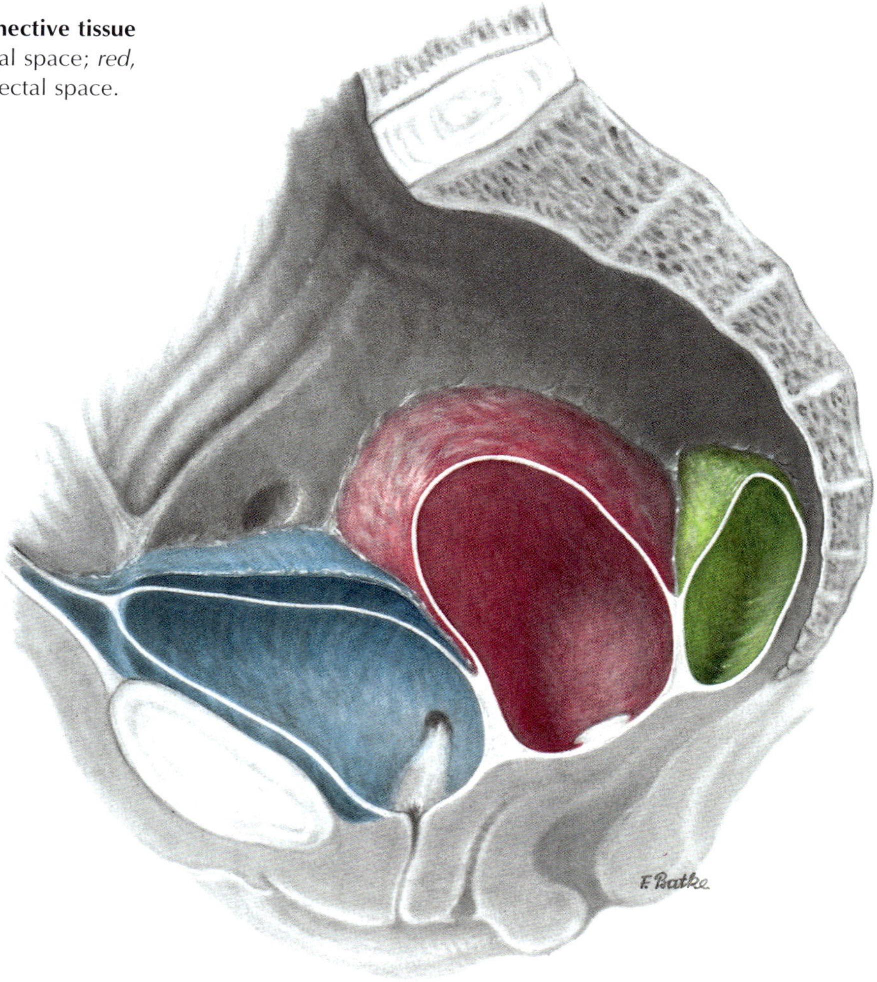

by the rectal fascia, its posterior wall by the sacral fascia, and its floor by the transition of the superior levator fascia into the sacral fascia.

Vesicocervical Space

The vesicocervical space stretches between the urinary bladder (vesical fascia) and the cervix uteri (cervical adventitia or fascia). It is separated from the vesicovaginal space below by the supravaginal septum. Cranially, this space is bounded by the lower surface of the vesicouterine cul-de-sac (vesicouterine excavation), whereas its lateral border is formed by the vesicouterine ligaments.

Vesicovaginal and Urethrovaginal Spaces

The vesicovaginal space is bordered anteriorly by the bladder (vesical fascia), posteriorly by the vagina (vaginal fascia), and superiorly by the supravaginal septum. Lateral to this space is the denser connective tissue of the endopelvic fascia and the paracystium (here the vesicouterine ligament). The vesicovaginal space continues inferiorly into the urethrovaginal space. This short cleavage space is present only at the uppermost portion of the urethra (Fig. A.20) because its fascia is securely adherent to the vaginal fascia for about three-fourths of the length of the urethra in the urethrovaginal septum.

Rectovaginal Space

This space is bounded above by the lower surface of the peritoneum abutting the cul-de-sac of Douglas. It is occluded anteriorly by the vaginal fascia and posteriorly by the rectal fascia. The space narrows below where it borders the dense rectovaginal septum. Laterally lie the lowest offshoots of the rectal pillar, i.e., their uterosacral ligaments. Thus, one can also penetrate from there into the loose connective tissue within the rectal pillar.

Intimate knowledge of the anatomy of the pelvic connective tissue and the fascial spaces is especially necessary for all vaginal surgical procedures.

INGUINAL REGION

The inguinal area is demarcated cranially by a line (the interspinous line) that bows across the abdomen between the anterior superior iliac spines, medially by the outer edge of the rectus sheath, and caudolaterally by the inguinal ligament (iliopubic ligament, Poupart's ligament, pubic ligament of Cowper, arcus inguinalis) (Fig. A.39). The inguinal ligament represents the lower edge of the aponeurosis of the external oblique abdominal muscle as well as the beginning of the fascia lata of the thigh. The subcutaneous fatty tissue is permeated with connective tissue and becomes the mons pubis medially. The subcutaneous connective tissue may be arranged in a layer, which has led to its designation in the Anglo-American literature even today as fascia or *Camper's fascia* (Fig. A.40). If one wishes to adopt this interpretation, then the actual external abdominal wall fascia, the *superficial abdominal fascia*, must be designated separately as a deep layer and called *Scarpa's fascia* (used also in Anglo-American literature). This fascial structure radiates under the inguinal ligament into the fascia lata and in the perineal region into the perineal fascia. It can be assumed, however, that neither *Camper* nor *Scarpa* ever actually described these fasciae. Moreover, the so-called superficial leaf is so permeated with fatty tissue, and the connective tissue layer so variable, that it is difficult to provide support for the concept (in the anatomical literature) that it represents a true fascia. Nevertheless, this superficial connective tissue layer can guide surgeons in their quest for subcutaneous vessels and nerves and deserves to be mentioned from a practical point of view. The subcutaneous vessels usually first course beneath this connective tissue layer.

Ascending diagonally in the subcutis, the superficial epigastric vessels course toward the umbilicus. They become subcutaneous in the saphenous hiatus (fossa ovalis). Lymphatic vessels accompany them to reach the horizontal tract of the superficial inguinal lymphatic nodes. When the subcutaneous tissue has been removed, including the external abdominal fascia (the deep leaf of Scarpa's fascia), the external inguinal ring is exposed. Immediately above this ring (*external inguinal ring*) the iliohypogastric nerve emerges. The external ring is bordered by the reinforced fiber fasciculi of the aponeurosis of the external oblique abdominal muscle. At the upper medial border is the medial crus; at the lower lateral border is the lateral crus; between them are the intercrural fibers. A thin fascial leaf that radiates into the labium majus can be considered a continuation of the aponeurosis and should be removed during surgical preparation of the inguinal ring. The lateral crus ends together with the inguinal ligament at the pubic tuberculum, whereas the medial crus forms the posterior wall of the external inguinal ring as the reflected inguinal ligament (ligamente reflexum Collesi, ligamente inguinale reflexum, triangular ligament of thigh) and attaches at the superior ramus of the pubis.

The round ligament (ligamentum teres uteri, ligamentum rotundum) exits through the inguinal canal accompanied by blood and lymph vessels and radiates into the connective tissue of the labium majus (Fig. A.39). It is associated with the ilioinguinal nerve and the genital branch of the genitofemoral nerve. The latter nerves supply the skin in the area of the labium majus and the adjoining inner surface of the thigh. Preperitoneal adipose tissue (Imlach's fat pad) becomes visible in the external inguinal ring next to the round ligament. The external inguinal ring rep-

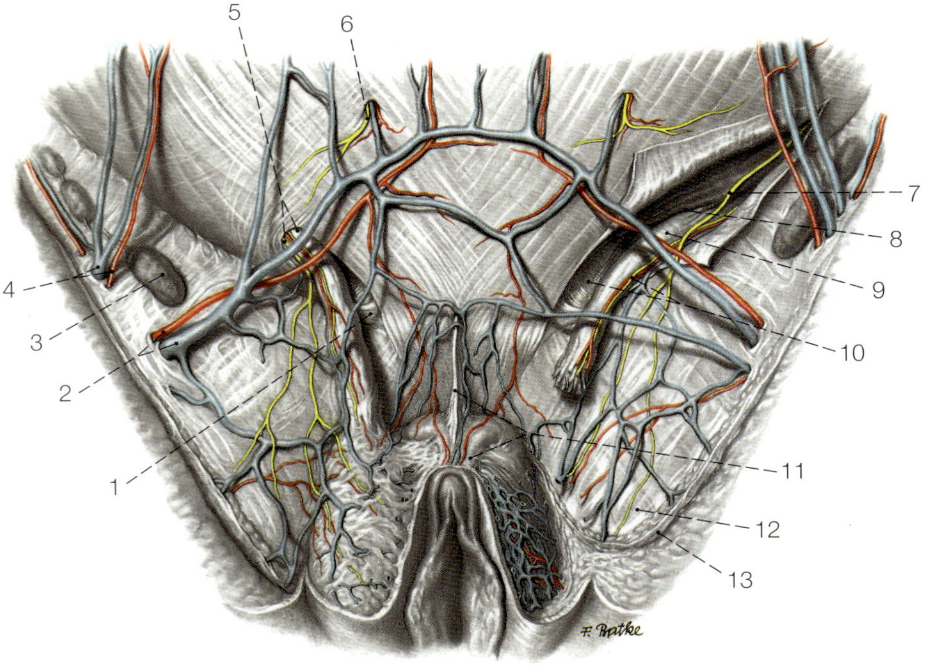

Figure A.39. Pubic and inguinal regions. Inguinal ring on right is sharply delimited; left inguinal canal has been opened and round ligament divided.

1 ligamentum inguinal reflexum
2 external pudendal artery and vein
3 superficial inguinal lymph node
4 superficial epigastric artery and vein
5 external inguinal ring and ilioinguinal nerve
6 iliohypogastric nerve (right anterior)
7 ilioinguinal nerve
8 caudal edge of internal oblique abdominal muscle
9 round ligament
10 transversalis fascia and genital branch of genitofemoral nerve
11 suspensory ligament of clitoris and corpus clitoridis
12 fascia lata
13 connective tissue layer (Camper's fascia)

resents a site of minimal resistance for the anterior abdominal wall.

The *inguinal canal* (Fig. A.39) is bounded caudally by the inguinal ligament, and cranially by the lower edge of the transverse abdominal muscle. The anterior surface is formed of the aponeurosis of the external oblique abdominal muscle; the posterior wall is the transversalis fascia, strengthened by the interfoveolar ligament (Hesselbach's ligament, inguinal ligament of Blumberg). For additional anatomical details the reader is referred to appropriate text books in the anatomy literature.

Knowledge of the anatomy of this area is especially important in the surgical treatment of vulvar carcinoma (Chapter 21).

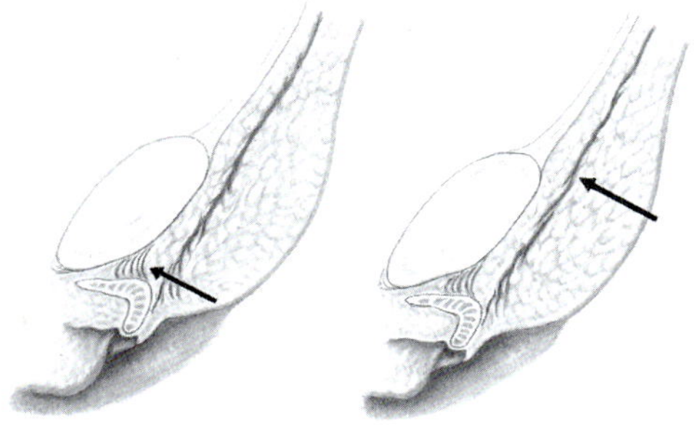

Figure A.40. Median sagittal section through anterior abdominal wall. *Left,* arrow points to suspensory ligament of clitoris; *right,* arrow points to Camper's fascia that terminates caudally in deep clitoral ligament.

PUBIC REGION

The inguinal regions of both sides are connected through the pubic area, which extends up into the mons pubis by way of the pubic sulcus. It is bordered cranially by the interspinous line. Subcutaneously, once again one finds fatty tissue that diminishes toward the labia majora, interspersed with fibrous connective tissue corresponding to Camper's fascia. The latter is also called the tunica fibrosa urogenitalis externa (*Pernkopf*). Medially, this connective tissue becomes denser toward the *deep clitoral ligament* (Fig. A.40). At the mons pubis there are branches of the external pudendal vessels.

Detailed anatomical knowledge of the pubic area is of great importance for surgical treatment of vulvar cancer (Chapter 21).

SUBINGUINAL REGION

The subinguinal region, or groin, is bordered cranially by the inguinal ligament, laterally by the sartorius muscle, and medially by the abductor longus muscle. It gains its practical significance for the gynecologist by the lymph nodes situated here. In addition, in this region below or behind the inguinal ligament, vessels and nerves, as well as the iliopsoas muscle, pass through two portals (lacuna vasorum and lacuna musculorum) to the thigh.

As a rule the subcutaneous fatty tissue is abundant here and, as in the inguinal and pubic regions, contains a coarse connective tissue layer that can divide the fatty layer into a superficial and a deep layer. These layers correspond to *Scarpa's fascia* (old designation is superficial femoral fascia). According to the literature, they unite with the fascia lata about one finger breath beneath the inguinal ligament. However, so far, I cannot verify this observation. According to my experience, these connective tissue layers stretch up to beneath the saphenous hiatus and vanish there (Fig. A.41). Only after the connective tissue layer is removed does one reach the subcutaneous vessels distal to the inguinal ligament. The significance of these "fasciae" is the same as that discussed under "Inguinal Region."

The *fascia lata*, the fascia of the thigh, is aponeurotic in construction. It covers the musculature and also separates the sartorius muscle laterally from the gracilis muscle medially. The fascia lata originates at the inguinal ligament and extends as far as the knee. It closes off the subinguinal fossa ventrally. The iliopsoas fascia and the iliopectineal fascia line this cavity in its depth, therefore dorsally. The large vessels and nerves course through the subinguinal fossa. In this area, the fascia lata is not of aponeurotic nature; rather it is more loosely constructed and reticular in character (Fig. A.42). This loose portion, the *fascia cribrosa* (or cribriform fascia), begins in the curved, laterally convex bow of the dense fascial portion. Through the cribriform fascia pass the subcutaneous vessels. The laterally convex edge, the *falciform margin* (Fig. A.43), runs medially into the *superior cornu* (ligament of Hey) (Figs. A.43 and A.44) and also into the *inferior cornu* (ligament of Burns) as shown in Fig. A.44. Both cornua fuse with the fascia of the pectineus muscle. An oval field is exposed when the cribriform fascia is removed; this is the *saphenous hiatus* (fossa ovalis).

Blood and lymph vessels and nerves. Subcutaneously, the superficial inguinal lymph nodes are found lying on the cribriform fascia (Fig. A.43). They are arranged in two groups: one node group, the horizontal tract, lies rather parallel to the inguinal ligament, whereas the other group, the vertical tract, is approximately vertical and follows the largest subcutaneous structure, the greater saphenous vein. This vein penetrates the saphenous hiatus to join the femoral vein. Ascending distally, the greater saphenous vein may be accompanied by an accessory saphenous vein that usually lies medially to it (but may sometimes be lateral). Medially, the external pudendal veins extend from the mons pubis; the superficial epigastric veins descend from above over the inguinal ligament to the cribriform fascia. Between the connective tissue bands of this fascial plate, the veins traverse to enter into the greater saphenous vein or directly into the femoral vein. From the lateral side, running parallel to the inguinal ligament, the circumflex iliac vessels reach this area.

In the depth of the hiatus, lying laterally to the femoral vein, is the femoral artery. Medially to the veins course the efferent lymphatic vessels that originate from the superficial lymph nodes or from distal regions of the leg. The lymphatics course through

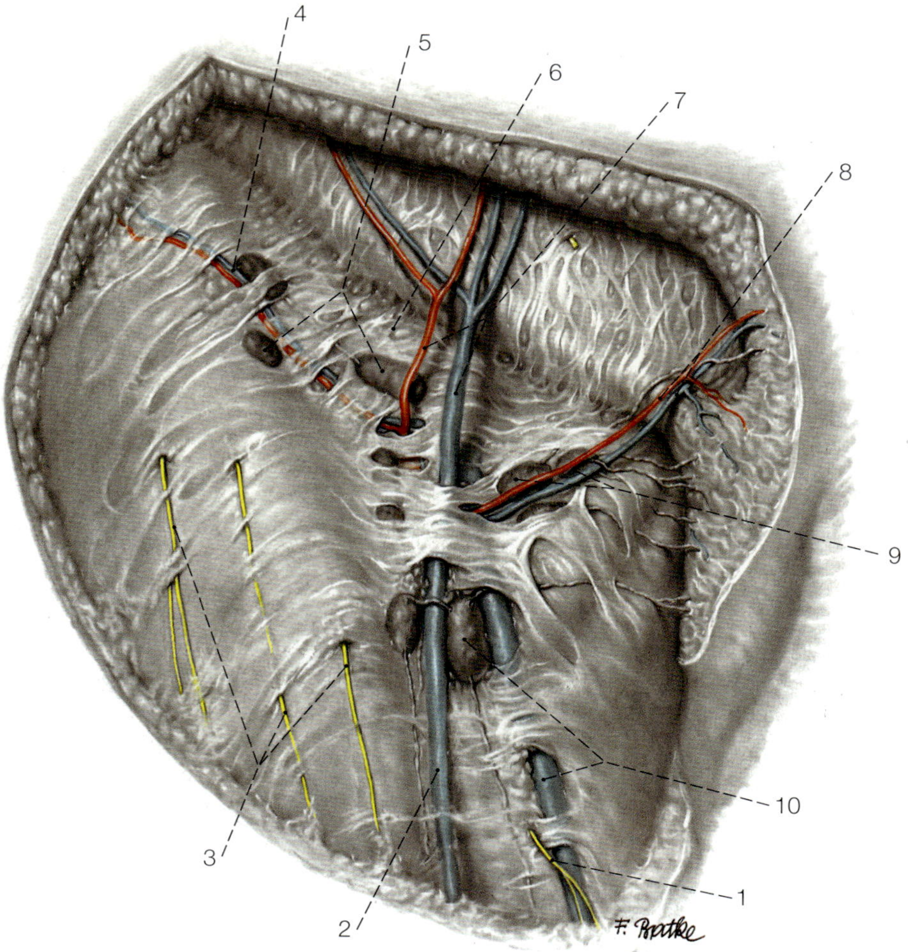

Figure A.41. Subinguinal region demonstrating subcutaneous layer with its coarse connective tissue (previously designated superficial femoral fascia).

1 anterior femoral cutaneous nerve branch
2 lateral accessory saphenous vein
3 branches of lateral femoral cutaneous nerve
4 superficial circumflex iliac artery and vein
5 superficial inguinal lymph nodes (lateral horizontal tract)
6 subcutaneous connective tissue
7 superficial epigastric artery and vein
8 external pudendal artery and vein
9 superficial inguinal lymph nodes (medial horizontal tract)
10 greater saphenous vein and superficial inguinal nodes (vertical tract)

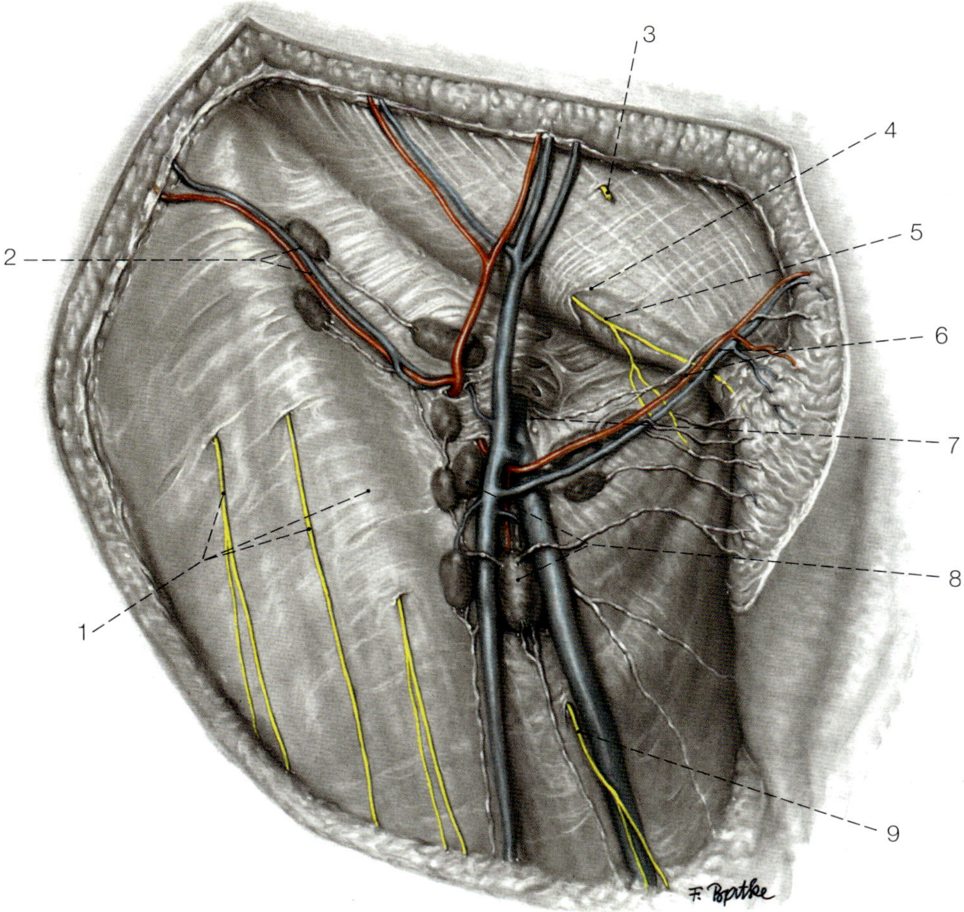

Figure A.42. Inguinal and subinguinal regions and fascia lata.

1 fascia lata, branches of lateral femoral cutaneous nerve
2 superficial circumflex iliac artery and vein
3 iliohypogastric nerve (anterior branch)
4 external inguinal ring
5 ilioinguinal nerve
6 external pudendal artery and vein
7 fascia cribrosa
8 inferior superficial inguinal lymph nodes
9 anterior femoral cutaneous branch

Figure A.43. Inguinal and subinguinal regions with cribriform fascia removed.

1 femoral artery
2 falciform margin
3 superficial circumflex iliac artery and vein
4 superior cornu
5 intercrural fibers
6 femoral vein, Rosenmüller's node
7 medial crus, ilioinguinal nerve
8 lateral crus, ilioinguinal nerve
9 external pudendal artery and vein
10 greater saphenous vein

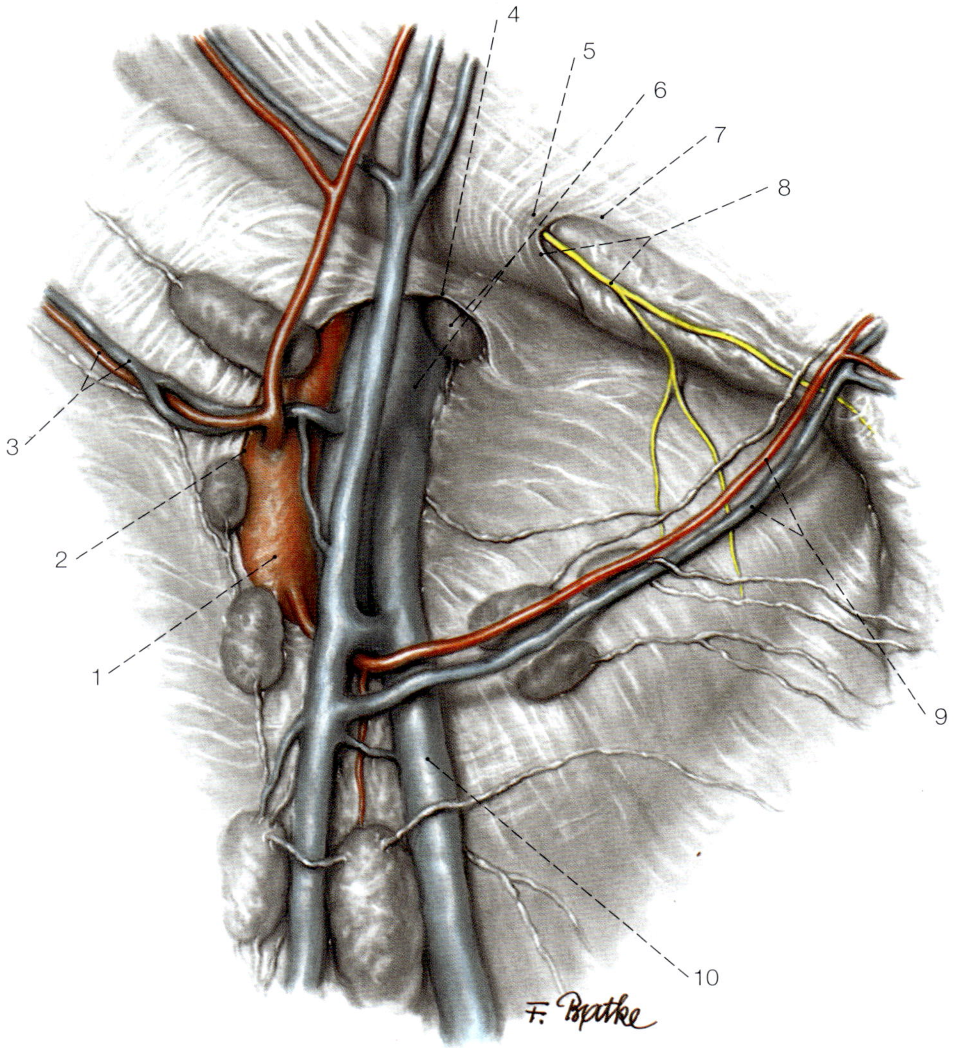

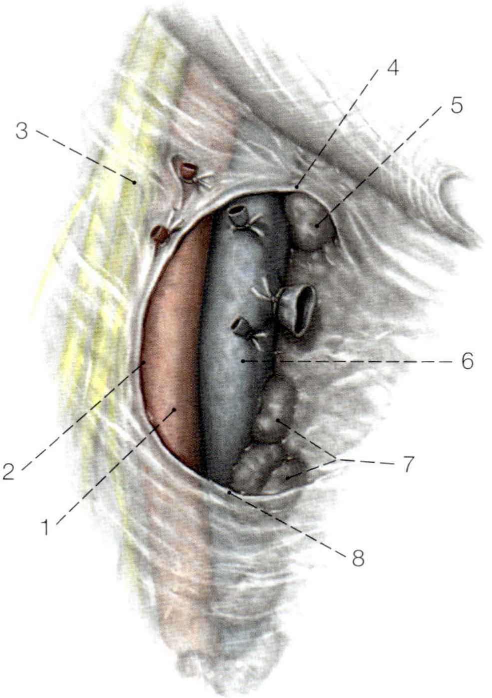

Figure A.44. Fossa ovalis.

1 femoral artery
2 falciform margin
3 fascia lata with femoral nerve (drawn translucently)
4 superior cornu
5 Rosenmüller's node
6 femoral vein
7 deep inguinal lymph nodes
8 inferior cornu

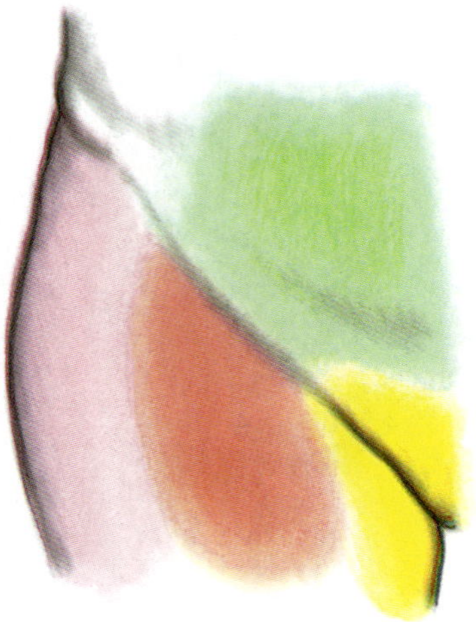

Figure A.45. Areas supplied by cutaneous nerves. *Green,* iliohypogastric nerve (anterior ramus); *yellow,* ilioinguinal nerve; *red,* femoral branch of genitofemoral nerve; *violet,* lateral femoral cutaneous nerve.

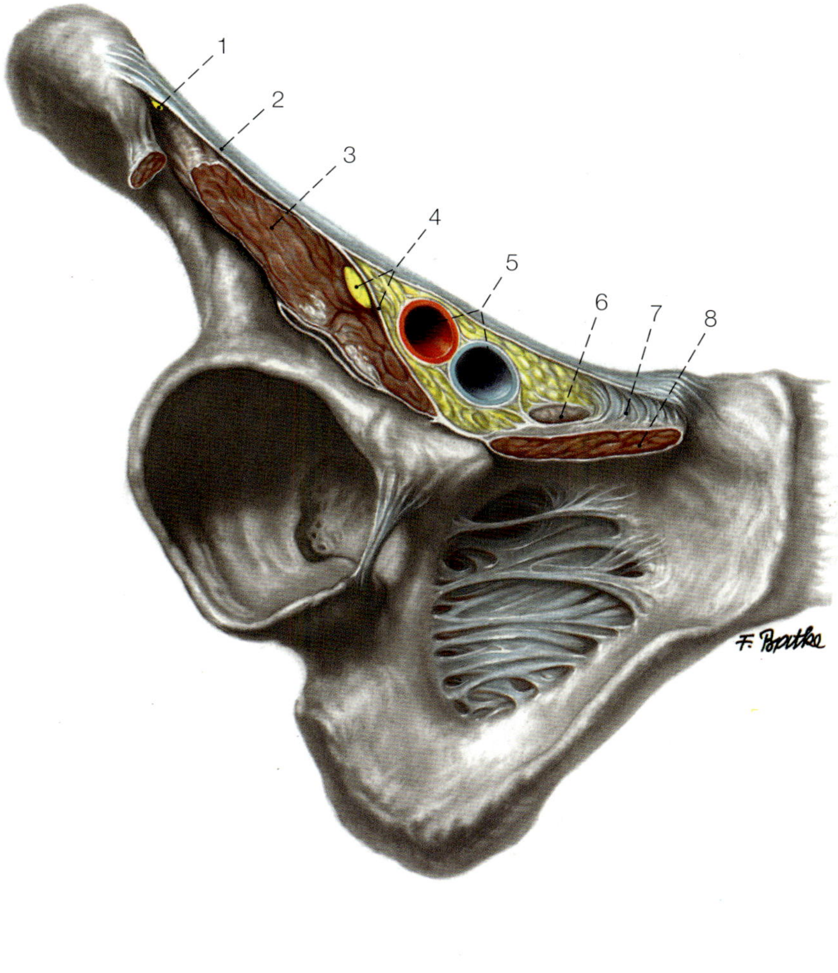

Figure A.46. Lacunae in cross-section.
1 lateral femoral cutaneous nerve
2 inguinal ligament
3 iliopsoas muscle
4 femoral nerve, arcus iliopectineus
5 femoral artery and vein
6 Rosenmüller's node in femoral canal
7 lacunar ligament
8 pectineus muscle

the *femoral canal* (see below) situated in the middle of the lacuna vasorum (for the femoral vessels). An especially large inguinal lymph node is encountered deep in the femoral canal; this is the Rosenmüller's or Cloquet's node.

The femoral artery, located laterally to the femoral vein, is often covered by the falciform margin. Here the femoral artery sends out subcutaneous arteries coursing through the cribriform fascia. It gives off the external pudendal artery medially, passing either proximally or distally to the junction of the greater saphenous vein into the femoral vein. Cranially, the superficial circumflex iliac artery and superficial epigastric artery also branch from the femoral artery.

Innervation. In the area of the cribriform fascia, the lumboinguinal nerve (femoral branch of the genitofemoral nerve) becomes subcutaneous with one or more branches supplying the skin in the region (Fig. A.45). The femoral branch reaches the thigh through the lacuna vasorum in conjunction with the femoral vessels.

Lacunae

Beneath the inguinal ligament is a vascular orifice medially and a muscular orifice laterally (Fig. A.46).

Lacuna Vasorum

The anterior border of the lacuna vasorum is the inguinal ligament; medially is the lacunar ligament (*Gimbernat*) that terminates in the fascia of the pectineus muscle. Inferomedially, the lacuna is assumed to be bounded by the pectineal ligament (posterior iliopubic ligament, pubic ligament, Cooper's ligament), which slips by the pubic bone. The lacunar and pectineal ligaments are both strengthened by the inguinal falx (Henle's band). The lateral border is formed by the arcus iliopectineus (ligamentum lacunare, iliopectineal ligament) stretching between the inguinal ligament and the iliopubic eminence (iliopectineal eminence).

The femoral artery, vein, and lymphatics pass through the lacuna vasorum in a medial direction. The medial portion of the vascular orifice corresponds to the femoral canal, the inner opening of which (the femoral ring) is closed off by a loose septum, the femoral septum (*Cloquet*).

Lacuna Musculorum

The muscular orifice is joined laterally to the lacuna vasorum and bordered in front by the inguinal ligament, medially by the arcus iliopectineus, and posterolaterally by the iliac portion of the innominate bone (coccyx). Through it pass the iliopsoas muscle with its fascial covering and the medially associated femoral nerve. Laterally, immediately adjacent to the anterior superior iliac spine, courses the lateral femoral cutaneous nerve.

Anatomical knowledge of this region is of utmost importance for the surgical treatment of vulvar carcinoma (Chapter 21).

SECTION II
SURGICAL TECHNIQUE

G. Reiffenstuhl and P.-G. Knapstein

1/ Patient Preparation

When surgery is indicated, patients must be prepared so that possible complications during surgery and convalescence can be avoided. Modern medicine with its numerous prophylactic, diagnostic, and therapeutic resources renders superfluous an exhaustive coverage of this subject in the context of this book; therefore only a few fundamental observations will be emphasized.

The more extensive the procedure, the more important the presurgical preparation becomes. Nowadays, the patient's age is no longer a limiting factor because vaginal operations, in contrast to abdominal procedures, offer a significantly lower risk. Women can undergo vaginal surgery at an advanced age provided their bodies are in reasonably good health. For example, the oldest patient undergoing a Schauta radical vaginal operation for a cervical carcinoma was 86 years old.

Because gynecological operations are generally not considered emergency procedures, optimal timing may be chosen. To allow smooth collaboration between the anesthesiologist and the internist, the patient should be admitted 1 or more days before the operation. Conscientious physical and mental preparation will favorably influence the healing process, because it places the patient in better condition for the operation.

General Preparations

The following general preparations are suggested for any operation. They become more important as the procedure becomes more severe.

1. A good case history and a doctor-patient relationship based on trust are imperative. They establish the correct procedure through dialogue. Important questions are those about prior operations, births, and delivery methods, because these may either support or impede a planned surgical procedure or may suggest other alternatives.
2. The surgeon must be aware of the patient's present gynecological and general physical condition.
3. Of critical importance is awareness of the condition of the leg veins and the connective tissue of the lower pelvic area. In contrast to standard medical practice, if varicosities are present, or if there is an elevated risk factor for thromboembolism, thromboprophylaxis will be used before surgery. An elevated risk of thromboembolism may also be caused by latent anemia resulting from hypermenorrhea, which in turn may cause intraoperative blood loss. Thromboprophylaxis includes compression of the leg veins, blood clotting retardants with heparin derivatives and acetylsalicylic acid, and early mobilization aided by passive and active movement exercises beginning a few hours after surgery. Women using hormonal contraceptives should stop using them 6 weeks before the procedure to reduce the risk of thromboembolic complications. See Chapter 3 for detailed discussion of the thromboprophylaxis procedure.
4. Clinical diagnostics include the following: daily temperature, pulse, and blood pressure monitoring; comprehensive blood work for blood group, Rh factor, HIV, erythrocyte sedimentation rate, electrolytes, kidney and liver function tests, and clotting factors; chemical and microscopic urine analyses; ECG; routine chest x-ray; and a vaginal sonography of the interior genitalia. Subsequently, the patient should be seen by an internist, who might mandate further tests and who will decide about "medical operability," which is delivered in writing.
5. Before performing an ordinary or expanded radical vaginal hysterectomy, or before correcting prolapse, we suggest a urologic analysis via cystoscopy and perhaps pyelography. For incontinence we advocate a cysto- and sphinctero-manometry. Carcinoma surgery is not the only procedure that requires knowledge of the current condition of the urinary tract to prevent intraoperative injury and also to interpret and treat postoperative urologic complications.

   Gynecological operations, which almost always occur near the bladder and which often result in injury to the bladder, may worsen a pre-existing cystitis and encourage bacterial ascension into the renal pelvis. The specific description of fistula operations is addressed in Chapter 18.
6. Two days before the procedure the patient should take a mild laxative. The morning before surgery we prescribe an enema to prevent defecation during surgery. In addition, a low residue diet (no vegetables, no potatoes, no milk, preferably a low meat diet) reduces stool volume. The evening before surgery, nurses will shave the patient's pubic hair. This is painless in most cases if plenty of shaving cream is used and the skin is properly stretched while shaving. (With particularly sensitive patients we postpone shaving to the day of surgery and wait until the patient is anesthetized.) The patient then takes a full bath, after being advised to take extra care while cleaning her navel and nails.

All patient preparation described so far occurs during the days before surgery. The following discusses preparations immediately before the onset of surgery.

Preparation Immediately before Surgery

For the vaginal procedure, the patient will be placed in lithotomy position as far as necessary above the lower edge of the operating table. The legs are bent at the hip and knee, and the feet are secured by straps in the stirrups. Articulated leg rests, which can be adjusted in length and allow circular motion, may be used instead of the leg supports. The articulated leg rests slide easily back and forth, which allows their precise calibration for different lengths and positions of the calves. The articulated leg rest is used to hold and support the calf, which is resting on a foam cushion, right above the ankle joint. The distal segments of the lower extremities will be wrapped with a wide bandage.

Vaginal surgery requires two assistants to stand between the straddled legs of the patient (one on the right side of the patient, the other on the left). They may use their backs to turn the leg supports toward the outside before they are secured. This will widen the abduction of the patient's legs, should that become necessary.

While positioning the arms, one arm will be prepared for the anesthesiologist by placing it on a hand rail. The other arm is secured parallel to the side of the body and must be cushioned by a pad on the inside of the upper arm to prevent pressure from the edge of the operating table (radial paralysis).

While the pelvis is raised, additional shoulder support is needed to prevent the patient's entire weight from hanging on the leg support, which might induce thrombosis through pressure on the veins in the hollow of the knee.

The skin of the surgical area must be disinfected carefully. A swab is used to first cleanse the external genitalia and surrounding area with soap and water, and then a disinfectant is applied. Usually we use orange or colorless Merfen. Be careful to prevent the disinfectant solution from running onto the patient's back and buttocks: severe necrosis may result if the patient is exposed to the caustic medium. We avert complications of this nature by placing compresses under the patient's back and buttocks to absorb any liquid. They are discarded after the disinfecting process is completed.

The patient is catheterized immediately before surgery begins, and the vagina is rinsed with a disinfectant solution that must correspond to the acidity level of 1% lactic acid. (The self cleansing mechanism of the vaginal flora is not affected by a pH factor of <4). All requisites for disinfection are arranged on a separate table.

A sterile cloth is used to cover the patient's abdomen and buttocks. Legs and calves are also covered with sterile cloth. The lower extremities and the lower end of the patient's body, except for the external genitalia, are closed off with sterile covering reaching up to the frame located above the patient's head.

2/ Postoperative Care

General Aspects

Various hospitals handle aftercare differently, less with regard to generally accepted guidelines than with regard to the details. Thus, personal preferences may be involved in the discussion of this subject. It seems only natural that methods, which have been tried and practiced personally, are given preferential treatment.

The type of surgery will determine how aftercare is individualized. However, an individual aftercare program will be constrained by these 18 steps that must be followed to ensure recuperation from the surgical procedure.

1. The vaginal cuff must be treated with antibiotic powder at the end of surgery.
2. With the use of a gauze strip, the vagina must be tightly tamponaded for 24 hours (use four layers, 3 cm wide, 1 m long).
3. The skin of the perineal sutures must be sprayed briefly with adhesive spray (make sure to cover the anus with a gauze pad).
4. A permanent catheter must be inserted into the bladder for at least 6 hours, and up to 3 days, to prevent postoperative urine retention (use a Foley balloon catheter or suprapubic drainage); rinse the urinary bladder once a day with lukewarm boric acid solution (100 ml); 48 hours after the permanent catheter is removed, residual urine volume must be determined. At a retention level of more than 150 ml, replace the permanent catheter for 2 or 3 more days to relieve the overstretched urinary bladder. Tenesmus requires chemical, microscopic, and bacteriological urine examinations and often daily instillation of antibiotics as well as antispasmodics. For atony of the bladder, parasympathomimetics might be useful.
5. The patient should wear support hose during surgery and during the hospital stay.
6. Do not use general antibiotic prophylaxis during the first few days after surgery; temperatures up to 38°C are within the normal absorption range. Secretions at the vaginal cuff after a hysterectomy should be drained through blunt probing.
7. After a hysterectomy or colporrhaphy a thromboprophylaxis with heparin derivatives is a routine procedure that reduces the danger for thromboembolic complications. The evening after surgery, we encourage the patient to get up and, aided by a nurse, briefly move around. This will then be repeated several times a day. The danger for hemorrhage is minimal at this stage because the tissue stumps have been ligated several times and the vaginal circumcision wound margin and the medial colpotomy have been secured with interrupted sutures, thus achieving hemostasis.

   For patients especially vulnerable to thrombosis (anemia, local stasis varicose veins, leg ulcer, adiposity, hypertonia, cardiac insufficiency, carcinoma, diabetes, hypermenorrhea), a thromboembolic prophylaxis must be conducted in three phases.

   (*a*) Preoperative: circulatory function must be improved (support hose or cardiac medication support may be used). For elective surgery, hormonal (oral) contraceptive intake should be discontinued at least 6 weeks before the date of surgery. For acute cases, women taking oral contraceptives should be given a postsurgical prophylaxis with heparin and dihydroergotamine starting on the day of surgery.

   (*b*) Intraoperative: leg support used in lithotomy position may be uncomfortable. To minimize this discomfort, inflatable leg sleeves called BOC Roberts Venous Flow Stimulators may be used. These will ensure that there is no substantial negative impact on blood circulation in the legs. Atraumatic surgery and thromboprophylaxis will prevent major vascular endothelial injury.

   (*c*) Postoperative: prophylaxis with heparin will begin the day of surgery 2 hours before the procedure and continue until complete patient mobilization is achieved. Heparin will not penetrate the placenta and may therefore be used to treat patients during pregnancy and delivery and after childbirth. It will not affect breast milk. Physical measures to consider include exercising in bed, wearing support hose, and rising from bed as soon as possible.
8. On the day of surgery, and also during the first postoperative day, fluid and nutrition must not be taken orally but rather intravenously until the bowel functions properly. The anesthesiologist will determine the exact fluid dosage; up to 2500 ml daily and more may be used should the patient be very thirsty. Nutrition intake per mouth is also restricted up to that point.
9. One day after surgery, in the evening, the patient should take 2 tablespoons sodium picosulfate (Agaffin laxative gel). Its median level of effectiveness is 10 hours, which will ensure an undisturbed rest at night and a soft stool discharge the next morning. Should bowel movement not be satisfactory, an enema (Mikroklist) may be used 48 hours after surgery after the vaginal packing has been removed.
10. The long vaginal packing must be removed from the vaginal cuff at least 48 hours after surgery. If the last portion of the strip adheres subperitoneally, causing extreme pain when pulled, it may be softened by pouring water over the portion sticking out from the vulva. The strip may then be removed painlessly after a short wait.
11. If the postoperative process proceeds normally, after the fourth day (the day of surgery is counted as the first day) the patient may take a lukewarm full shower but may not use soap on the lower portion of the body.

12. A sponge bath or a soft external shower is permitted after bowel movement, but a bidet may not be used.
13. Sanitary napkins should be changed several times a day, but tampons may not be used.
14. The perineal sutures may be removed on the sixth day (this may perhaps be done on an outpatient basis).
15. The patient may be released after sutures have been removed or on the fourth day after surgery should an early release be desired. Before the patient leaves, she will be advised to take a daily sitz bath (see step 17).
16. Postoperative vaginal secretion, which will diminish every day, is considered to be normal because the vaginal cuff has deliberately not been completely closed [330 hysterectomies in which the vaginal cuff was left wide open were compared with 215 cases in which sutures were used to completely close the end of the vagina; in those cases that had a closed vaginal end, 6% retroperitoneal cyst formation was evident; not one case using the open method demonstrated such cyst formation because even though an open wound always produces secretions, these secretions could flow toward the outside and the necrotic tissue of the tissue stumps could drain toward the exterior.

Cyst formation from secretions after primary vaginal cuff closure are relatively high, produce fever, and may become infected. In these cases, one or two sutures must be removed to allow proper drainage. If the vaginal cuff is not widened enough, the infected fluid may spread through the loose subperitoneal connective tissue cranially and may in extreme cases lead to a lymphocele abscess. To prevent such complications, we suggest leaving the vaginal cuff open after a hysterectomy to allow downward drainage of the retroperitoneal area.
17. The daily lukewarm sitz bath can be started 6 days after surgery and can be supplemented with chamomile, oak bark, or cheese poplar. Water temperature should be about 37°C; the bath should last no longer than 15 minutes. These sitz baths clean vaginal secretions from the exterior genitalia. The vulva then receives an application of absorbent powder to prevent vulvitis and to granulate the vaginal wound. The absorption process will also benefit from the warm sitz bath. In general, full baths are allowed approximately 2–3 weeks after surgery. At that time, vaginal secretions have generally stopped. A full bath promotes circulation as well as cleanliness. Taken before bedtime, it has a calming effect and induces sleep. Supplements of aromatic substances—perhaps pine oil extract—are pleasant.
18. Five weeks after surgery the patient returns for a follow-up examination that will check for possible granulated tissue, which may be found at the end of the granulated vaginal blind sack. It may be treated at the office with a lapis ointment tampon. The patient is advised to remove the tampon after 24 hours. At that time the vaginal secretion will have ceased completely, and the patient may now resume regular activities.

Special Postoperative Care

Carcinoma Patients

For postoperative care of women who have undergone carcinoma surgery, the primary care physician plays a major, if not crucial, role. He or she will be responsible for constant patient observation and will ensure that the patient misses none of the follow-up examinations. These should take place every 2 months during the first year, every 3 months during the second year, every 4 months during the third year, every 5 months during the fourth year, and twice a year beginning with the fifth year.

Today, care for tumors involves postoperative checking for tumor markers (e.g., CA125), photo-imaging procedures (e.g., computed tomography of abdomen and pelvis, magnetic resonance imaging, intravenous pyelogram, sonography), and measurement of bladder function in regular intervals. In addition, to guide the patient toward a natural lifestyle, we suggest that she "take it easy" during convalescence, spend time in fresh air, and watch distribution of meals. We also prescribe appetite inducing preparations, treatment for anemia, and, if necessary, preparations to regulate bowel movement.

Urinary Bladder and Kidneys

The urinary bladder and kidneys of patients who underwent radical surgery must be watched specifically. Maximal separation of the bladder from its foundation, isolation from its neighboring tissue, and denervation are often the cause of all postoperative bladder complications. The degree of bladder displacement and the radicalness of tissue resection normally determine the severity of bladder malfunction. Important vessels and nerves are separated, and the bladder becomes atonic and inelastic. These innervation disorders cause loss of feeling followed by problems with the evacuation mechanism and often long-lasting urinary retention. In addition, the ureters, which have been exposed for a long stretch, are hampered in their action, which might produce vesicoureteral reflux. This might lead to ascending infection.

In addition, some possible aftereffects pose a threat after gynecological carcinoma surgery: fresh infections from residual urine in the damaged bladder as well as long-term damage of the ureter (ureteral stenosis), with resulting irreversible damage to kidneys and connecting pelvic calyces. This damage may clinically manifest itself long after late convalescence has been in progress. Prophylaxis and therapy concentrate mainly on the prevention and removal of residual urine. We therefore recommend during late convalescence, and even afterward, to check frequently (every 4 weeks) for residual urine and to conduct a chemical, microscopic, and bacteriological urine analysis. In most cases, the family physician will be responsible for toning the bladder and treating already existing cystitis. Readmission to the hospital may become necessary should urinary retention and urinary tract infection persist, because such cases warrant short-term insertion of an indwelling bladder catheter.

For already entrenched pyelitis, in addition to antibiotics, some old, well-tried measures such as warm compresses, diuretic teas, and intestinal cleansing with the help of a strong enema are still justified. However, for a patient recuperating from radical surgery it is often not only recommended but also imperative to admit her to the hospital if she suffers from pyelitis because the chance for ureteral stricture exists. This may be detected with ultrasound of the urinary tract.

Having said all this, we emphasize that it is just as important to pay as much attention to the kidneys as to the prevention of a possible relapse after radical surgery.

Hormonal Syndromes

Hormonal syndromes—which may occur after an oophorectomy or after postoperative radiation—must be treated with appropriate substitution. The primary care physician will try to prevent skin damage on radical surgery patients undergoing postoperative radiation therapy. He or she will advise that a brassiere may rub the skin and that warm, moist compresses and intense exposure to a thermophore, a sunlamp, or the sun are not recommended. Use of a brush, strong soaps, and/or irritating substances must be avoided. During the first 4 weeks after radiation, the exposed skin may be washed only with lukewarm water or, better yet, with olive oil. Vaseline, lanolin, or a zinc preparation may be used to lubricate the skin of the abdomen.

Social Interaction

We highly recommend social workers to aid patients in need of social programs. Improvement of economic and living conditions will expedite the healing process. Full cooperation between the primary care physician and the hospital, as is already practiced in most large treatment centers, will prove beneficial for the patient.

3/ Curettage

Indications

Curettage is performed for diagnostic and therapeutic purposes. This procedure is indicated when irregular bleeding occurs, in particular perimenopausally, and to identify endometrial carcinoma. In many cases, either a hyperplastic mucosa or polyps are the cause of irregular bleeding. The decision for curettage is also made in cases of endocrine disorders to detect the functional structure of the mucosa.

Nowadays for patients at very high risk of surgical complications, persistent uterine bleeding after removal of a carcinoma may be stopped via hysteroscopic ablation of the endometrium.

For pregnant women curettage is performed to remove the remains of an incomplete abortion or postpartum if persistent bleeding occurs in case placental fragments were left behind (differential diagnosis: endometritis postpartum vs. placental polyp).

A sharp curette is used to perform a curettage indicated for gynecological reasons. In contrast, a blunt curette should be used for an abortion so that the uterine mucosa, already softened through pregnancy, will be scraped only in the area of the endometrium. When a sharp curette is used in this case, the softened uterine mucosa (including the basal layer) is removed all the way to the muscularis. This might cause traumatic amenorrhea.

Contraindications

Here, inflammatory adnexal illnesses, adnexal tumors, and endometritis must be cited because a curettage quite often causes the severity of these illnesses to worsen.

If heavy uterine bleeding persists beyond 2 weeks postpartum, the placental polyp can be differentiated from endometritis in the following manner: 5 days Metherin i.m., antibiotics, bed rest. Should this conservative treatment not stop the bleeding, i.e., there is no considerable improvement, one is dealing most likely with a placental polyp rather than endometritis. Curettage is then recommended. (There are known cases involving postpartum bleeding where curettage was performed up to ten times because a placental polyp was thought to be present. This treatment did not stop the genital bleeding, because the cause was really endometritis, which occurs much more frequently and which worsened from one curettage to the other.)

Patient preparation. In most cases patient preparation for curettage is the same as that for vaginal surgery. The patient is placed on the operating table in lithotomy position, anesthetized, and catheterized. The vagina and exterior genitalia are thoroughly disinfected, and the vulva is covered with sterile pads.

Size and position of the uterus are determined once more through combined bimanual palpation. Exact knowledge of uterine position and size is imperative for safe instrument insertion.

Technique

Curettage of the uterus occurs in three steps:

1. Sounding the uterus and measuring the length of the endometrial cavity;
2. Dilation of cervix;
3. Curettage of endometrial cavity.

Postoperative care. Postoperative care is simple: at the end of surgery, inject a dose of Metherin i.v. to aid contractions. Perform an additional Metherin prophylaxis during the next 5 days (20 drops t.i.d. or one tablet t.i.d.). Regeneration of uterine mucosa after a dilation and curettage is completed 5 days after surgery; it is regulated by glands that have not been touched during curettage. The interior plane of the uterus is now lined by a contiguous cover of epithelium.

In abortion cases with Rh-negative women who have Rh-positive partners, immune prophylaxis with anti-D-globulin is performed after the procedure.

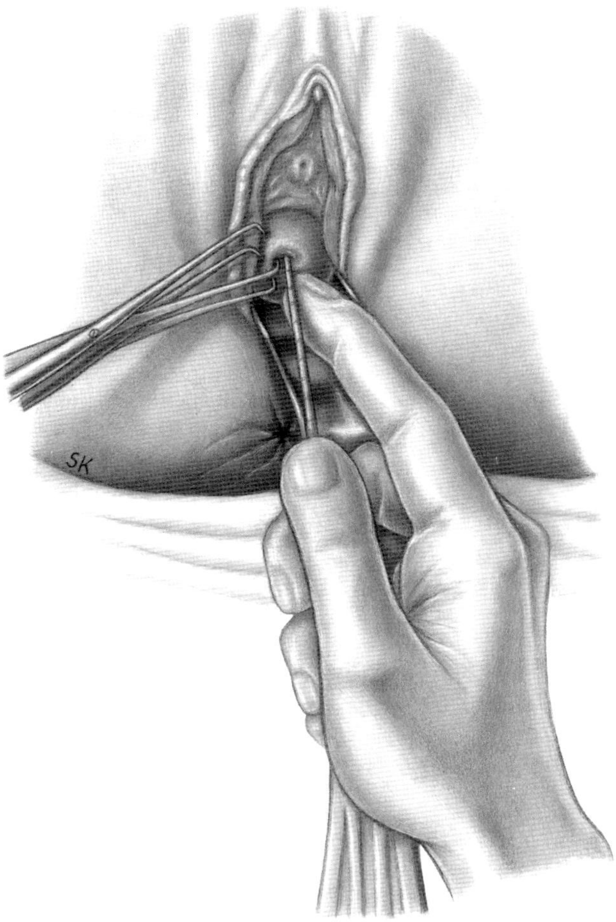

Figure 3.1. Curettage. Sounding the uterus.

The vagina is exposed with a self-retaining anterior retractor. The anterior cervical lip is grasped with two single-toothed tenacula, and the uterus is stretched downward forcefully.

The sound is extended to the fundus uteri; the index finger is used to fixate the exterior cervix; and the length of the uterus marked on the sound. Uterine length is normally 7–8 cm.

The uterine sound is seldom used now to determine the length of the uterine cavity; recently perfected ultrasound diagnosis is preferred. Sounding of the uterus is contraindicated if the slightest suspicion of an abortion exists because the sound might easily perforate an already softened uterus.

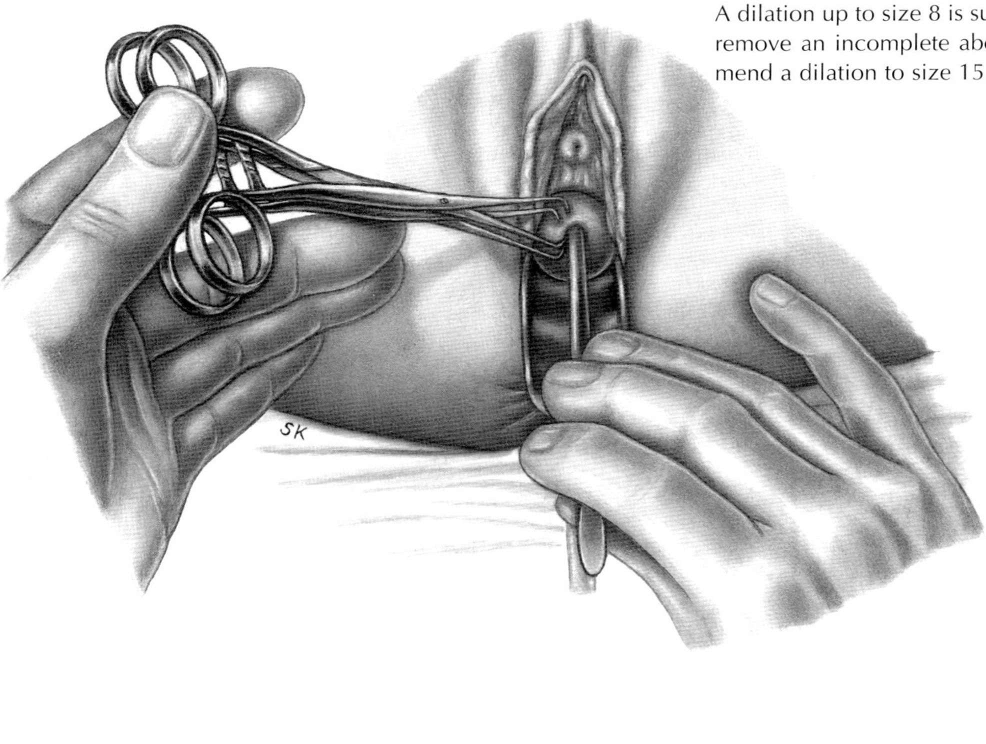

Figure 3.2. Curettage. Dilating the cervical canal.

The tenacula are attached at the anterior cervical lip. The surgeon pulls the tenacula downward and inserts a metal dilator through the external os into the uterus, using the small finger to brace against the perineum.

A metal dilator is used for insertion into the uterus. One begins with the smallest instrument (that which may just barely pass through the opening) and advances slowly, size by size, depending on the elasticity of the cervical canal. Each dilator remains in place for a short time and is then withdrawn rapidly, and the next larger dilator is slowly and carefully inserted through the internal os.

A dilation up to size 8 is sufficient for a gynecological curettage; to remove an incomplete abortion (abortus incompletus) we recommend a dilation to size 15.

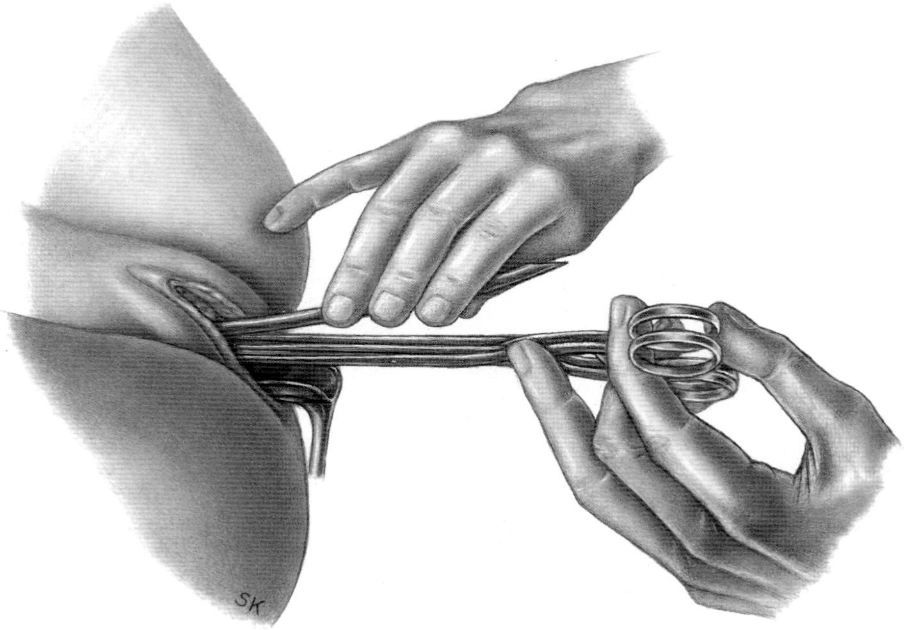

Figure 3.3. Curettage. Dilating the cervical canal (lateral view).

The anterior cervical lip is pulled downward forcefully by the attached tenacula, which stretches the uterus.

The surgeon holds the dilator using the first, second, third, and fourth fingers and inserts its tip gently (without force) into the cervical canal. If the cervix is rigid, strong resistance must be overcome at the level of the internal os.

After pushing past the resistance at the internal os, the surgeon must ensure that the dilator will not advance uncontrollably into the uterine cavity and perhaps perforate through the fundus. He or she will therefore support the small finger of the controlling hand against the perineum while the dilator is pushed forward.

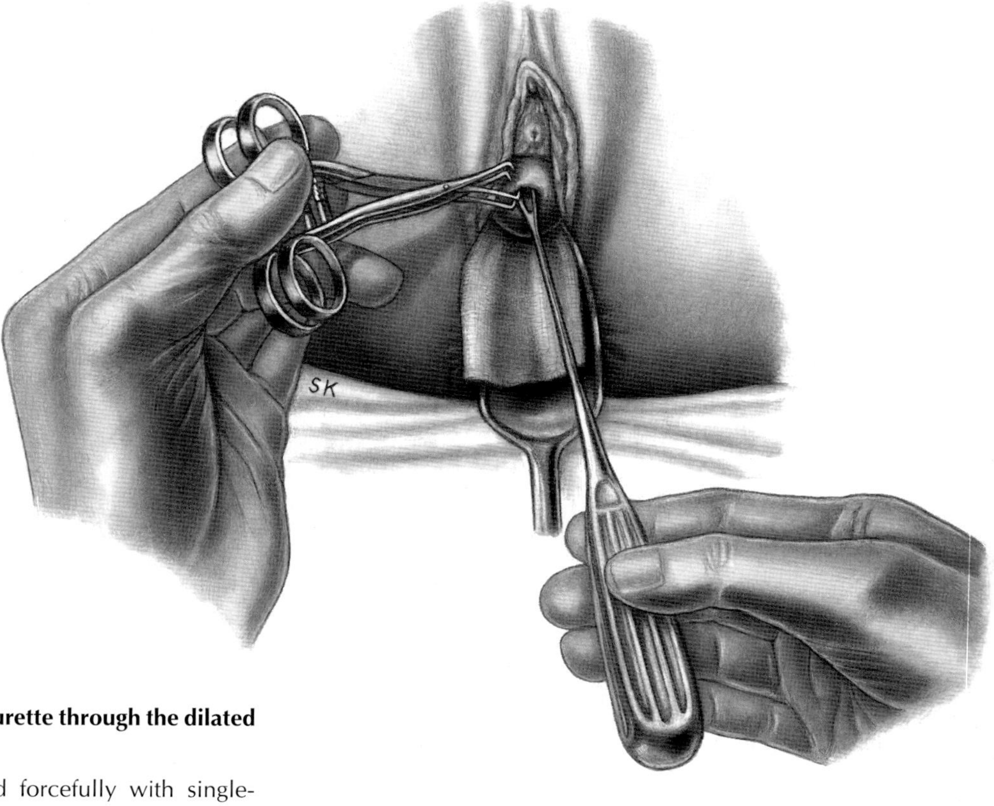

Figure 3.4. Curettage. Insertion of the curette through the dilated cervical canal.

The surgeon pulls the uterus downward forcefully with single-toothed tenacula.

The curette handle is placed on the second, third, and fourth fingertips and then gently secured with the opposing thumb. In this position, the curette is slowly inserted into the uterine cavity through the now sufficiently widened cervical canal.

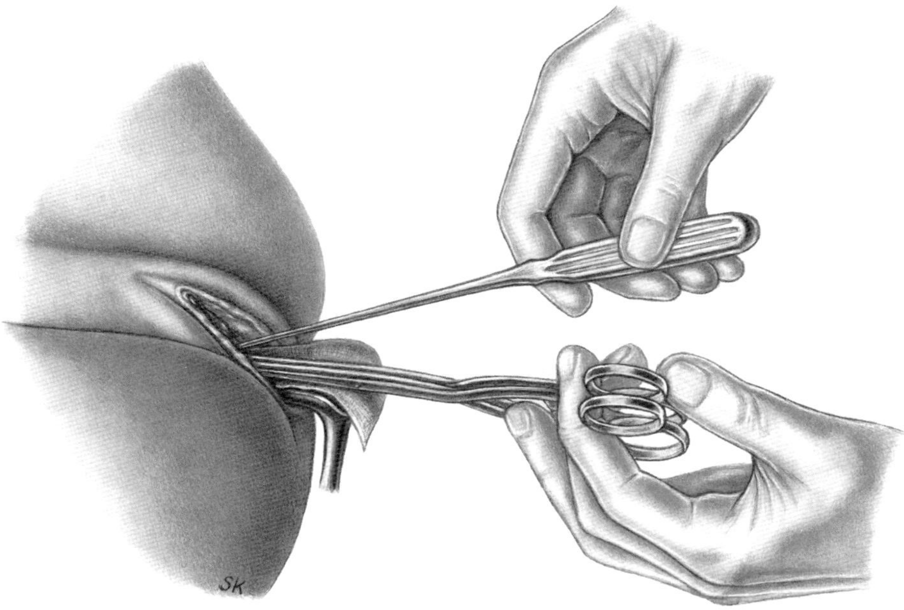

Figure 3.5. Curettage. Insertion of the curette (lateral view).

The curette, held delicately in place by the fingertips, is pushed forward slowly until it meets the fundus. To accommodate uterine anteflexion, the handle must be lowered somewhat as the instrument is advanced.

For a diagnostic curettage of the uterus, a "fractional curettage" is generally performed. This is done by curetting the cervical canal first and then the corpus uteri.

Figure 3.6. Curettage. Scraping the uterus.

The curette has been carefully inserted to the fundus uteri. The surgeon now grasps the curette handle firmly and pulls it back as far as the internal os at the uterine wall. In this process, the curette loop is turned toward the mucosa and is used to scrape off the loose mucous membrane.

The curette is then pushed carefully back to the fundus, turned slightly along its longitudinal axis, and pulled back once more. This stroking procedure is repeated several times, gradually turning the curette 360°. The procedure is repeated as long as there is any mucous membrane or product of conception remaining.

A sharpened sense of hearing and feeling control the effect of this procedure. The mucosa is completely removed and the uterine cavity is empty when one feels the curette gliding over a coarse foundation and when a scraping sound ("muscular tone") can be occasionally heard.

The curette is removed through the cervix after the circular procedure is completed. The scraped tissue must be placed on a gauze strip and sent to the lab for microscopic testing.

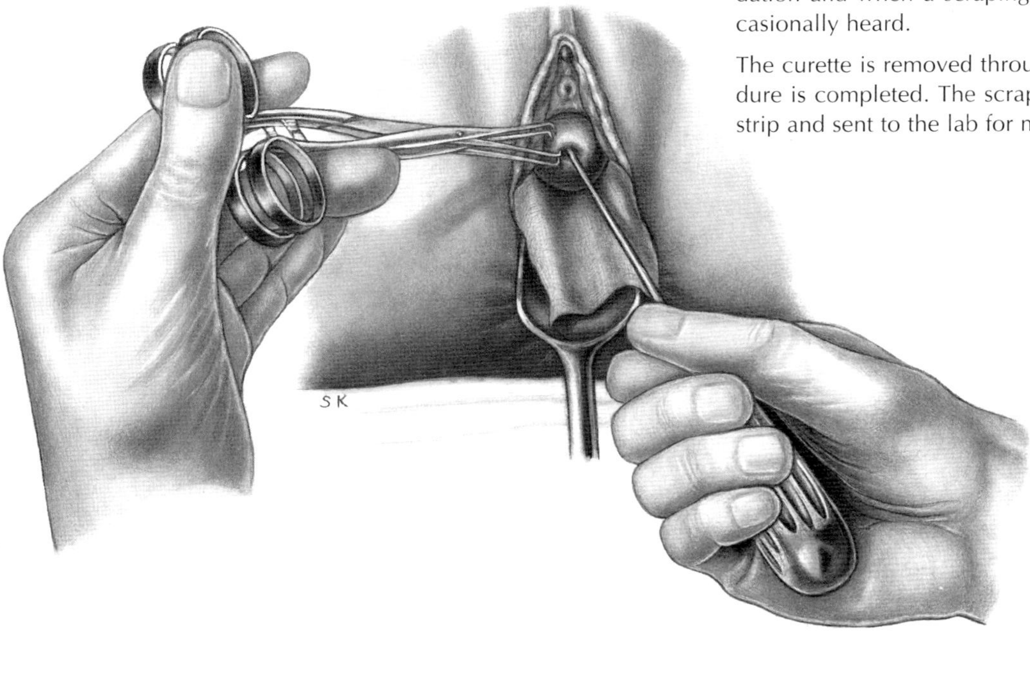

Technical Problems

1. Most perforations of the uterus do not occur with the curette during scraping of the uterus; they occur when *too much force is used* while the cervical canal is dilated. The uterine wall can also be damaged when jerky movements are used to push against resistance in the regions of the internal cervical os.
2. Capillary tears may happen if the cervical canal is *dilated too forcefully and too rapidly*. These serve as pathways for infectious agents. Even with a rigid cervix there is danger that the muscular wall will be deeply lacerated if suddenly dilated, sometimes extending into the parametrium. Such ruptures can lead to heavier bleeding and even to severe parametritis.
3. If *retroflexion of the uterus* exists and if dilation in the direction of the anteflected uterus occurs, the anterior portion of the uterine wall may be penetrated and vice versa. This may be prevented by using bullet forceps to pull the cervix down forcefully. This allows the uterus to stretch and remain in that position during the entire surgery.
4. Any penetration with an *instrument that goes too deep*, regardless whether a sound, a dilator, or a curette, must be equated with a perforation. It is imperative, the moment the surgeon recognizes his or her mistake, that the instrument be immediately withdrawn, without exerting any force, along the same pathway in which it was inserted and the operation aborted—regardless of what was planned, whether the operation was completed, or whether anything was left in the uterus. Depending on the degree and position of the injury one can wait, but a laparotomy may need to be performed. More extensive perforations require a hysterectomy.
5. It is especially easy to *perforate* the senile uterus, the puerperal uterus, or the uterus with an advanced corpus carcinoma. Uterine perforations can occur in the hands of the most practiced and careful surgeon. He or she will, however, immediately recognize the event and proceed accordingly.

4/ Culdocentesis

Indications

With the development of the laparoscopic diagnostic, the cul-de-sac of Douglas puncture has been pushed into the background. Nevertheless, even today culdocentesis retains its value for differential diagnosis of tubal pregnancy, ovarian cysts, and adnexal tumors. In addition, it is feasible to puncture cul-de-sac abscesses, pyosalpinges, endometrial tumors, and ovarian cysts. The patient scheduled for this procedure should be prepared as if for a laparotomy; she is completely anesthetized and relaxed before being placed in lithotomy position.

Technique

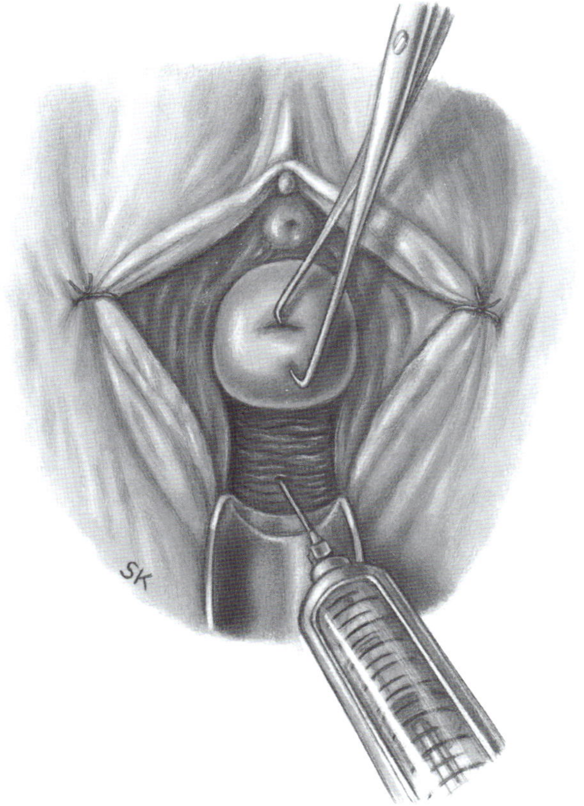

Figure 4.1. Cul-de-sac puncture.

The vagina is exposed with a self-retaining retractor, and the anterior cervical lip is grasped with tenacula and forcefully pulled straight upward.

If the posterior fornix is ballooned (as with a space of Douglas abscess or with retrouterine hematocele), a 2-mm thick, 15-cm long *straight* needle (which is securely affixed to a 20-ml syringe) is used for puncture. The needle is inserted through the vaginal wall in the midline of the posterior fornix. It is then advanced 3 cm into the cul-de-sac of Douglas, while one continuously aspirates with the attached syringe. If no liquid can be aspirated, the needle is withdrawn somewhat and then advanced once more 3 cm to the right and then to the left.

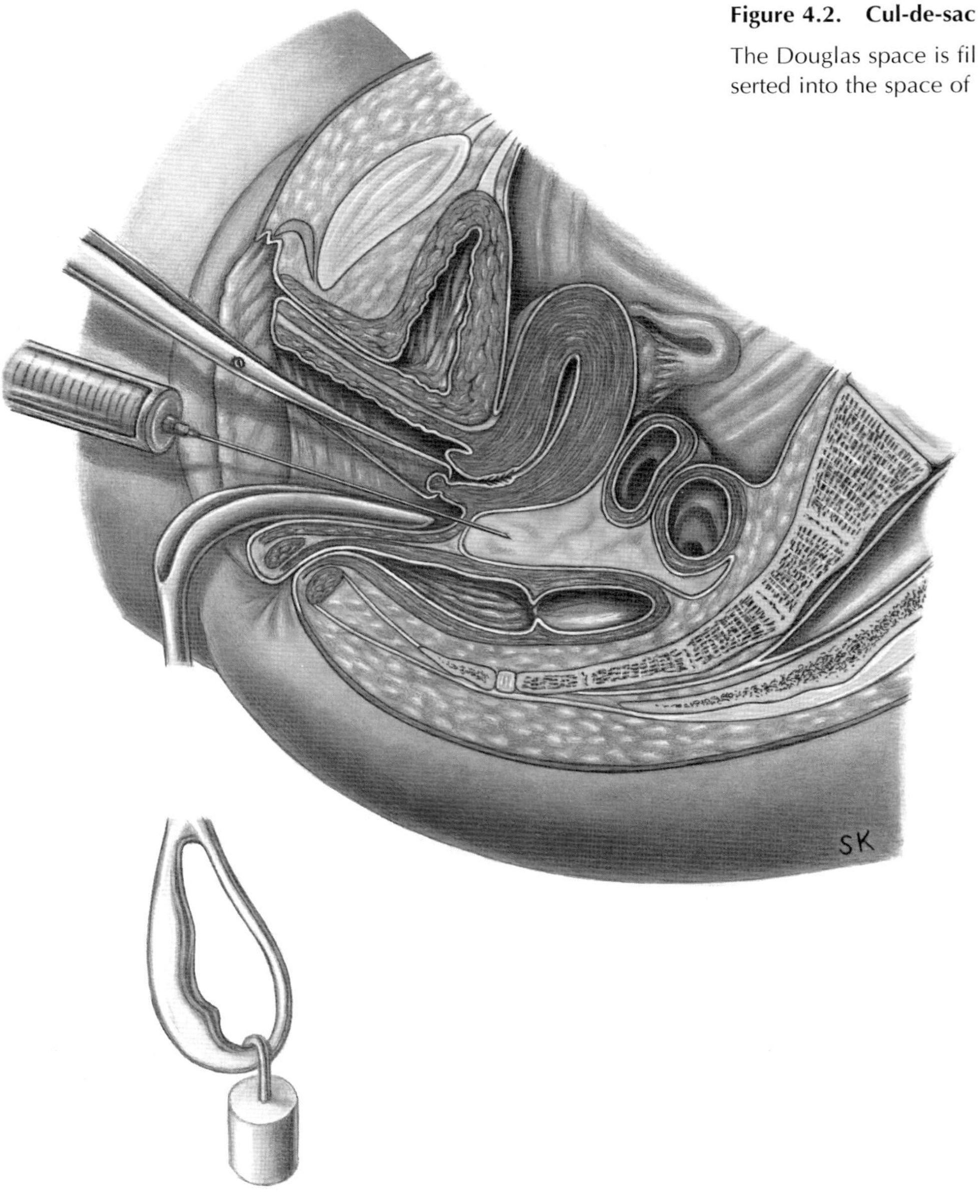

Figure 4.2. Cul-de-sac puncture. Lateral view.

The Douglas space is filled with liquid. The puncture needle is inserted into the space of Douglas through the posterior fornix.

Figure 4.3. Cul-de-sac puncture. Adnexal puncture. Lateral view.

Douglas space is free of liquid accumulation; the ovary is enlarged.

For puncture of the adnexa (ovarian cysts, pyosalpinges, endometrial tumors), a long curved needle is used. The needle punctures the cul-de-sac of Douglas through the posterior fornix and is advanced with the attached syringe safely up to 6–8 cm into the abdominal cavity. The syringe must be depressed maximally to ensure that the needle tip is turned upward.

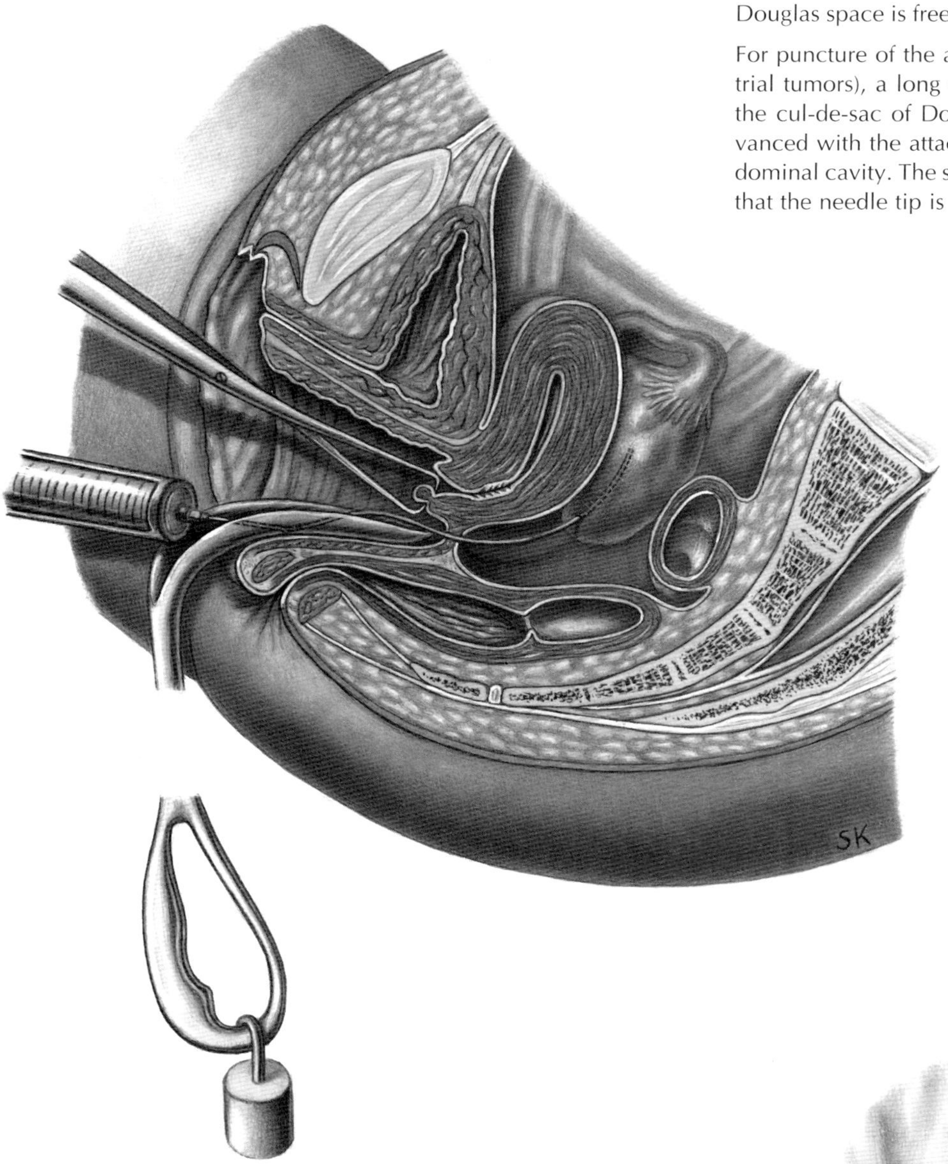

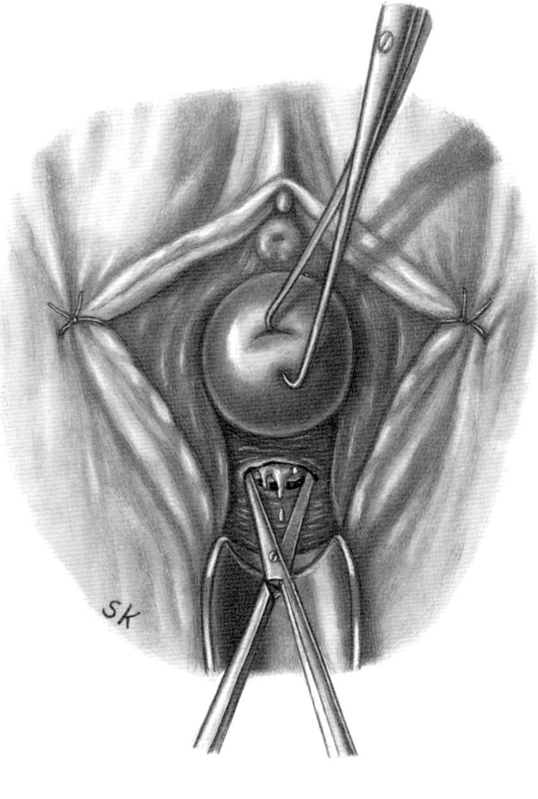

Figure 4.4. Pouch of Douglas abscess. Opening.

To drain the pus collected in the cul-de-sac of Douglas, the ballooning vaginal wall and Douglas pouch peritoneum are incised transversally with a scalpel immediately posterior to the cervix. Dressing forceps are used to dilate the opening; the pus then drains.

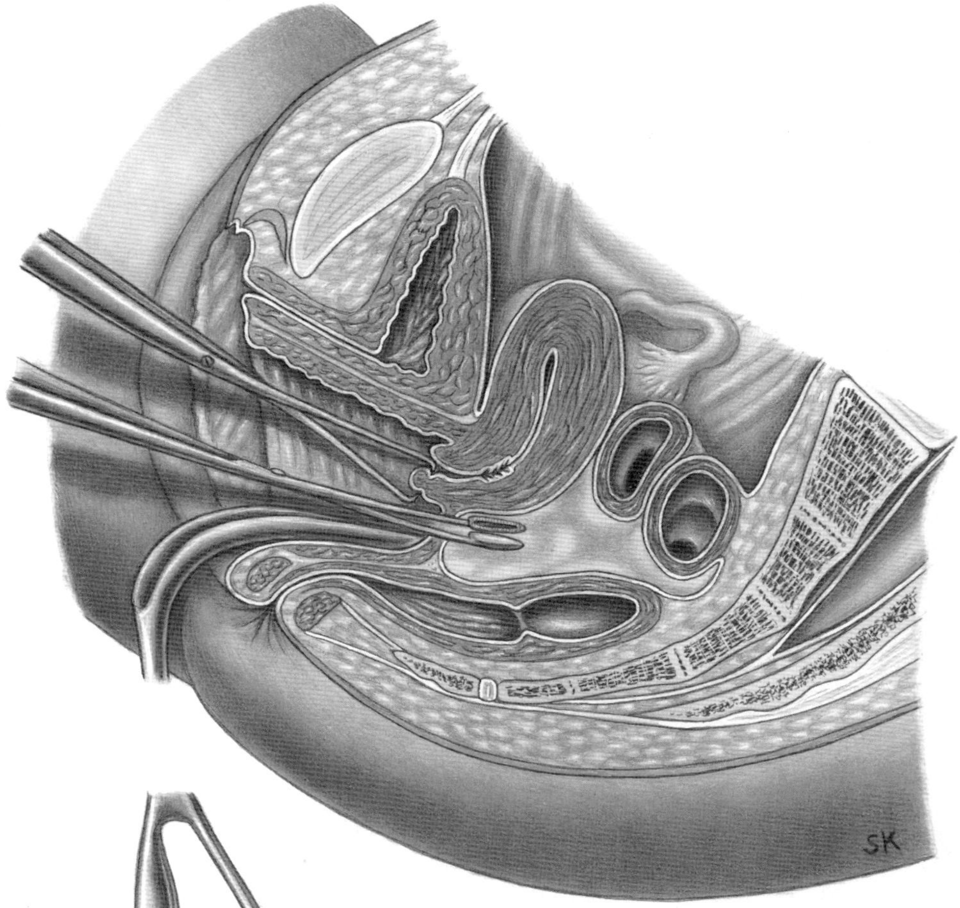

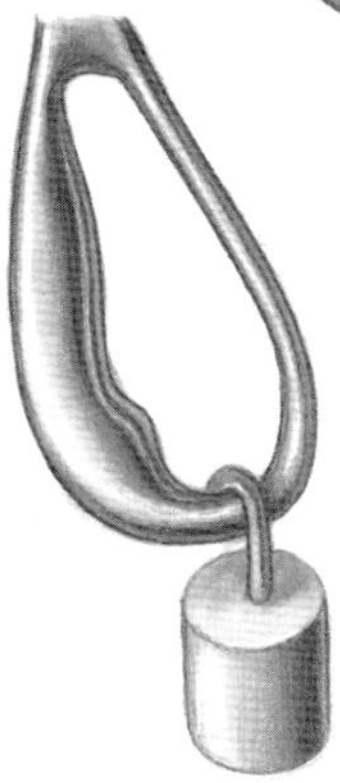

Figure 4.5. Pouch of Douglas abscess. Drainage. Lateral view.

The space of Douglas contains pus that is encapsulated cranially toward the abdominal cavity.

To dilate the incision in the posterior fornix, forceps are inserted and then spread.

We do not recommend palpation of the abscess cavity, because the cranial border of the encapsulated abscess might be punctured accidentally; this could result in diffuse peritonitis.

Instead, a rubber T-drain (*left detail*) is inserted into the abscess cavity. This T-drain is grasped with forceps (*right detail*) so that the horizontal bar of the T lies parallel to the longitudinal axis of the drain, which allows easy insertion into the Douglas pouch.

A sample of pus is sent for bacteriological culture and sensitivity. The drain is used to thoroughly rinse the abscess cavity with an antibiotic solution.

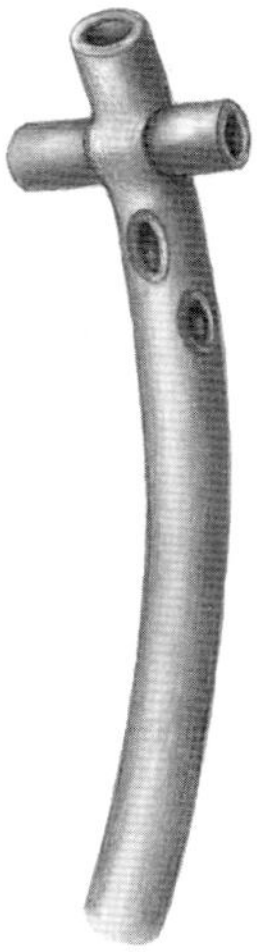

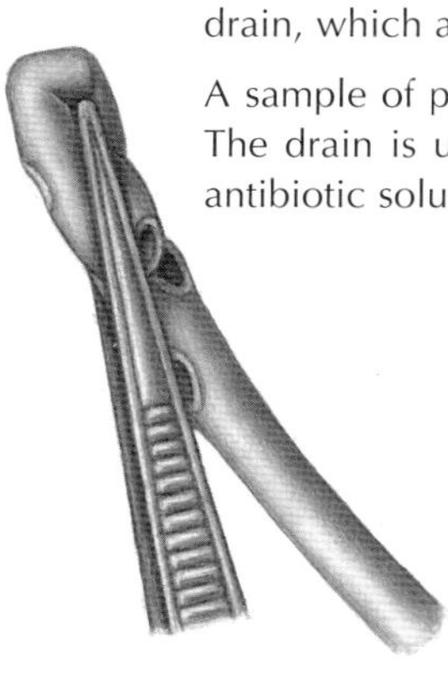

Technical Problems

1. For fear of puncturing the rectum, the curved needle might be *inserted too close to the posterior wall of the cervix*. In this case, the needle tip will not enter the cul-de-sac of Douglas but will burrow into the cervical tissue instead. This is easily noticed by increased resistance as the needle is advanced.
2. Even though the curved needle is inserted medially, if the syringe is depressed too soon after the needle is advanced, the tip of the needle might *puncture the posterior cervical or uterine wall*.
3. The needle might be *inserted laterally in the posterior fornix* rather than in the midline. As the needle is advanced, the parametrium is entered, and the vessels located there are punctured.
4. The needle may be *advanced too far into the abdomen*. Loops of bowel can be punctured, especially when they are fixed to the adnexa by adhesions. Such complications arise occasionally during puncture of adnexal cyst tumors when the tumor is punctured. Secondary infection of such cysts may result from bacterial contamination of the cyst from the adherent bowel via the needle channel. This can be avoided if one aspirates continually as the needle is being advanced and stops advancing as soon as fluid is obtained.
5. The *rectum may be punctured* as the needle is advanced toward the sacrum. Although this complication occurs occasionally, in our experience it has had no further serious consequences.
6. One should not persist and *make numerous attempts to obtain fluids* if preliminary puncture fails. This is not only senseless but dangerous.
7. Should a Douglas abscess be *mistaken for a pyosalpinx*, and drainage occur into the vagina, a fistula may develop because the drainage canal of the pyosalpinx epithelializes quickly. Tubo-ovarian abscesses should never be incised and drained via the cul-de-sac of Douglas; they may be aspirated only. In contrast, a Douglas abscess must be opened and drained vaginally.

In most cases, tubal vaginal fistulae may be removed surgically with tubal extirpation only; a spontaneous healing of the fistula cannot be expected because it may constantly be reinfected by vaginal bacteria and by steady secretion of the tubal epithelium.

5/ Posterior Colpotomy

Indications

Posterior colpotomy is indicated for smaller surgical procedures of the uterus and adnexa—specifically for vaginal sterilization—and to drain a cul-de-sac abscess.

Three methods of vaginal sterilization are discussed: vaginal fimbriectomy, Irving technique, and Pomeroy technique.

Technique

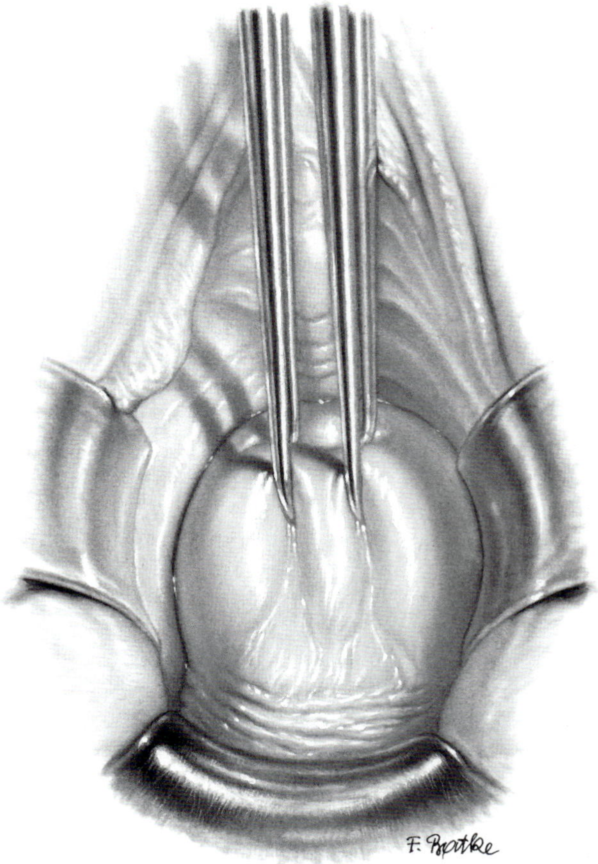

Figure 5.1. Posterior colpotomy.

The vagina is extended with three retractors. Two tenacula are applied to the posterior cervical lip. Moving the tenacula on the cervix up and down will reveal the border between the smooth cervical mucosa and the wrinkled vaginal mucosa.

To open the cul-de-sac of Douglas, a transverse incision is performed in the wrinkled vaginal mucosa of the posterior fornix. The portio is pulled upward to stretch the posterior fornix wall. In this area the transverse incision is performed.

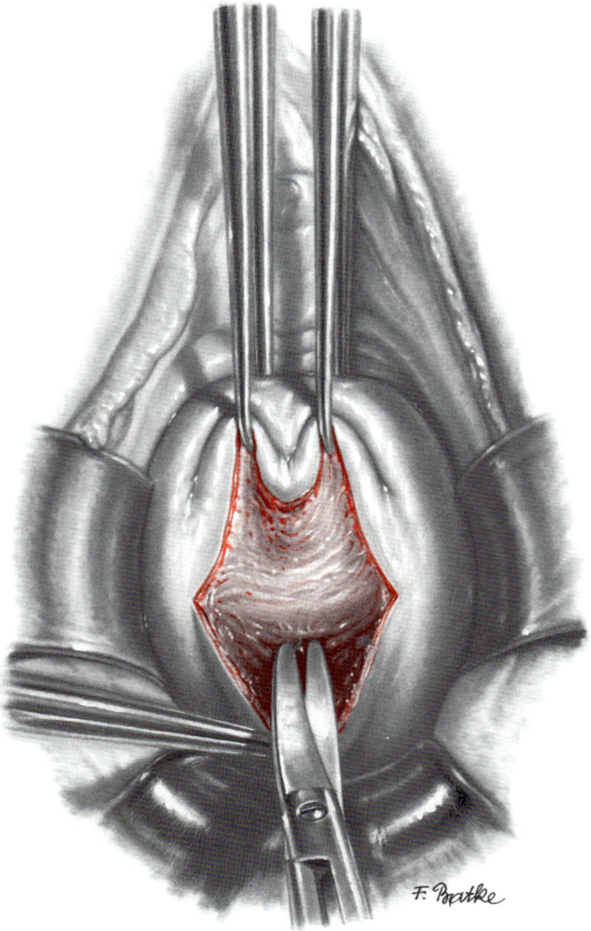

Figure 5.2. Posterior colpotomy. Dissecting the rectum.

The vaginal wall has been transversely incised with a scalpel in the posterior fornix. The anterior vaginal wound edge is held together with the portio by the tenacula and pulled upward. This causes the wound to gape widely.

The surgeon grasps the posterior vaginal wound edge with tissue forceps and pulls it downward. At the same time, curved, slightly opened scissors are used to dissect the rectum free caudally.

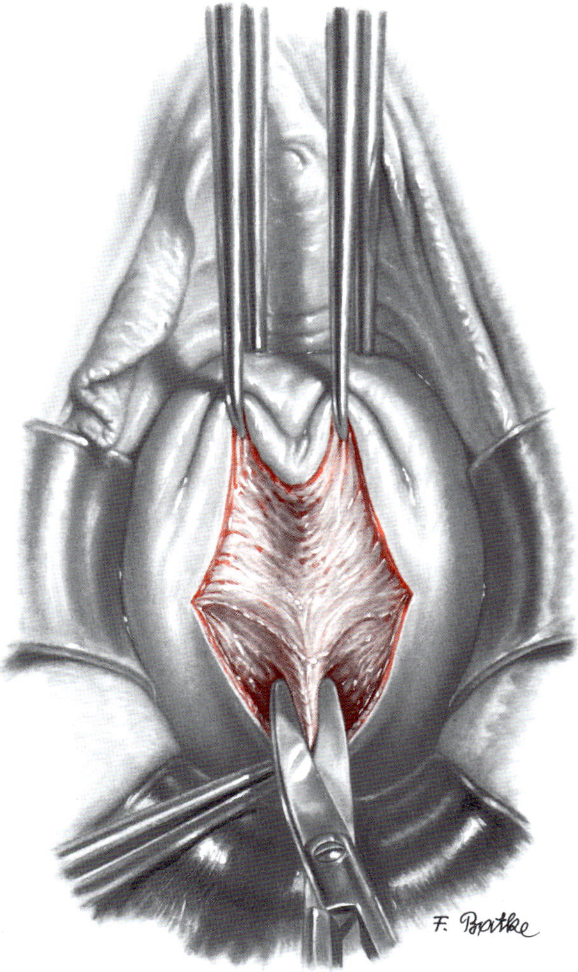

Figure 5.3. Posterior colpotomy. Opening the cul-de-sac of Douglas.

The rectum has been pushed caudally.

The surgeon grasps the peritoneal reflection with toothed forceps and pulls it slightly outward. The peritoneum is opened with one incision of the scissors. One should expect that loops of bowel might be fixed in the cul-de-sac, especially in association with adnexal tumors or endometriosis. It is therefore advised to open the space of Douglas carefully in a step-by-step fashion.

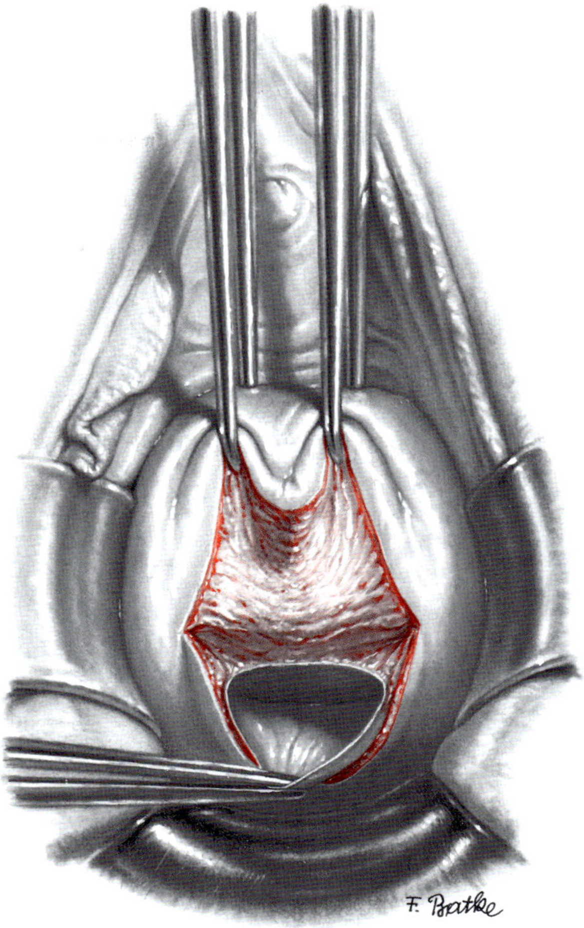

Figure 5.4. Posterior colpotomy. Extending peritoneal wound edge.

The pouch of Douglas has been opened.

For a better view, and for easier intraperitoneal retractor insertion, the posterior wound edge is pulled downward with forceps. To expose the adnexa, the intestinal loops are pushed away with long retractors. Tubes are grasped with forceps and pulled forward so that they are exposed in their entirety (from their extension from the uterus), provided that there are no inflammatory adnexal changes or that the adnexa are easily mobilized.

In some cases it may be difficult to gain access to the adnexa. The following procedure is then advisable.

1. Extreme pelvic elevation.
2. Deep anesthesia and good relaxation.
3. Bowel and omentum are packed back with a large gauze tampon strip.
4. Tenacula are removed from the posterior lip of the cervix.
5. Two long, narrow spatula retractors are inserted laterally into the space of Douglas, and a wide posterior spatula is used to hold the rectum back. Lateral spatula retractors are used to push packed bowel upward; they should not be applied against uterus.
6. A blunt hook is introduced into the cul-de-sac to help retroflex the corpus uteri and pull the posterior wall of the fundus into the colpotomy wound. This makes it possible to bring both uterotubal junctions into view.

Minor ovarian or tubal surgical procedures can now be performed, or a tubal pregnancy may be removed vaginally. Tubal sterilization via the vagina is also possible by this approach.

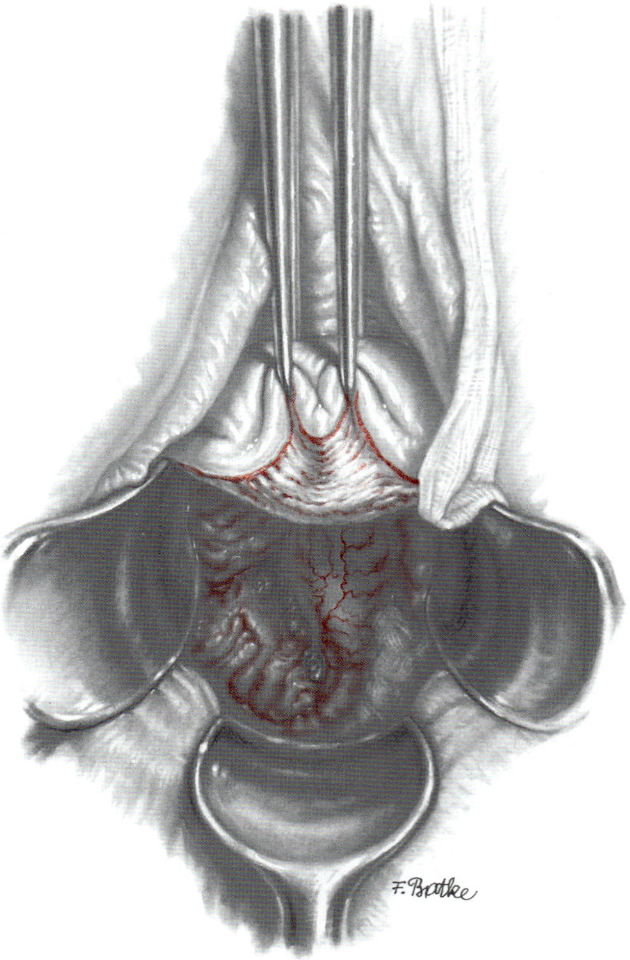

Figure 5.5. Posterior colpotomy. Removal of a tubal abortion. The pouch of Douglas is exposed with two lateral and one long posterior retractor, all inserted intraperitoneally. The loops of the bowel are packed back with a gauze strip.

The distended ampullary end of the tube, whose wall is heavily vascularized, can be seen.

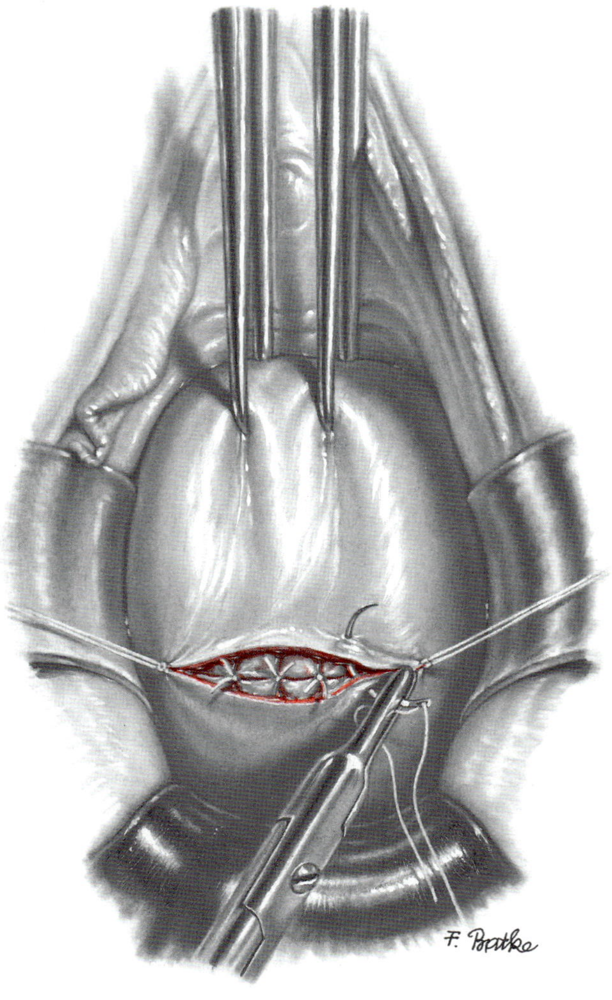

Figure 5.6. Posterior colpotomy. Closing the wound in layers.

The anterior and posterior peritoneal wound edges are united with interrupted sutures. In the second layer, the horizontal colpotomy wound is closed with interrupted catgut sutures, beginning with the angle sutures that are used for traction.

Vaginal Fimbriectomy

Indications

Resection of the entire fimbria funnel with the distal portion of the tube is the safest and thereby the easiest method of sterilization. The patient must be informed, however, that this procedure is irreversible. However, modern microsurgical techniques using the Irving or Pomeroy method allow tubes to be recanalized with an 80% success rate.

Technique

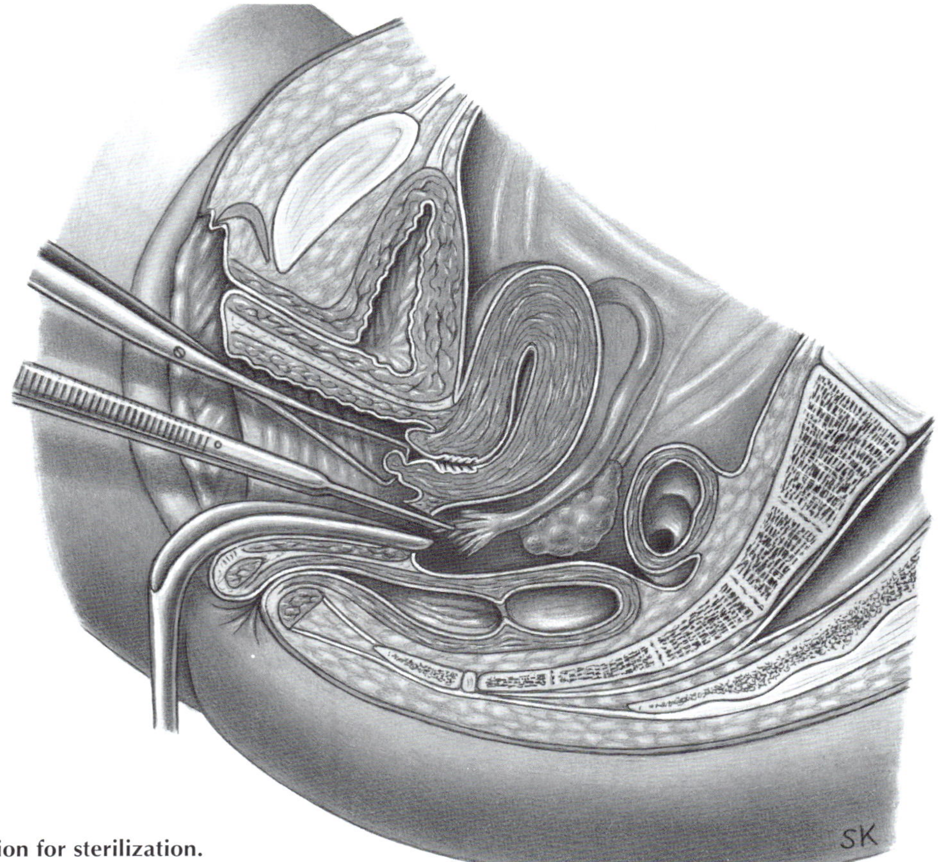

Figure 5.7. Posterior colpotomy. Tubal ligation for sterilization.

A wide, posterior band retractor dilates the space of Douglas dorsally; a wide bladder retractor pushes the uterus ventrally, and forceps are placed on the posterior cervical lip to deflect it. A blunt tenaculum grasps the fimbria.

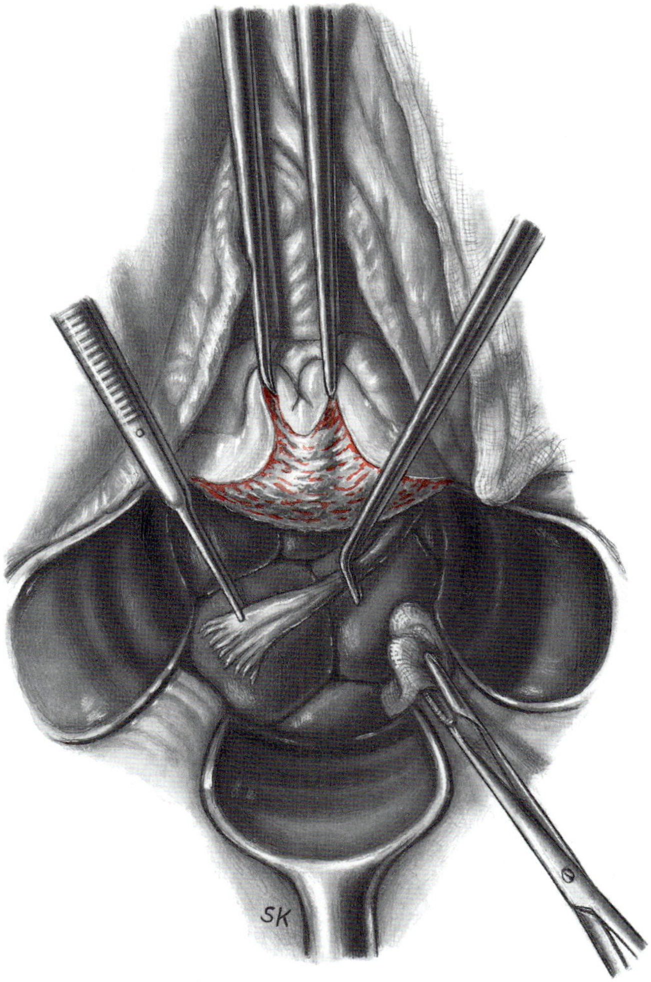

Figure 5.8. Posterior colpotomy. Fimbriectomy.

A pediculated gauze swab is used to slide the loops of bowel from the pelvic wall; this makes it easier to find the tube. It will be dislocated downward and severed above a long Overholt clamp. The stump is carefully ligated (use 00 absorbable suture).

Technical Problems—Figures 5.7 and 5.8

It is generally easy to find and mobilize the tubes at the pelvic wall. However, a prior case of pelvic inflammatory disease may cause difficulty. This procedure is made easier by elevating the operating table until the space of Douglas is at eye level with the surgeon. Long instruments should be used. The gauze swab must be firmly held by the forceps to ensure that it will not be lost between the bowel loops. A laparotomy and an arduous search might be the consequence.

Irving Technique

The isthmic segments of the uterine tubes are resected in a tubal sterilization using the Irving technique. One cut end of the tube is buried in a mesosalpinx pocket, and the other is sutured subperitoneally at the posterior surface of the uterus.

The tube is ligated with two sutures and then incised between them. At the same site, the peritoneum of the mesosalpinx is incised so that the distal stump of the tube can be buried in the mesosalpingeal pocket thus created to relocate it extraperitoneally.

The proximal tubal stump (on which the suture end was left long for traction) is then dissected free from the mesosalpinx up to the uterotubal junction and mobilized. A small transverse incision is made (with a scalpel) in the uterine serosa near the cornu on the posterior wall. A small pocket is formed in the myometrium with curved dissecting scissors, and the proximal stump of the tube is buried here. Each suture is provided with a needle that is used to pierce the myometrium within the newly formed pocket. The needle emerges in 1-cm intervals on the posterior uterine wall.

After all those sutures are tied together, the tubal stump is pulled into the musculature of the posterior uterine wall and buried there. The uterine wound is closed with one or two catgut sutures, and the peritoneal wound in the mesosalpinx is also closed with catgut button sutures.

Pomeroy Technique

Tubal sterilization by the Pomeroy technique entails lifting the exposed tube with a Babcock clamp to form a loop that is tied with a transfixed ligature. The proximal pillar of the loop is ligated, and then the distal pillar is sutured into the same ligature. Each pillar should be 2 cm long; they will be shortened to 1.5 cm at the conclusion of the procedure.

6/ Anterior Colpotomy

Indications

Cervical myomata, deep-seated myomata of the anterior wall corpus, and large uterine polyps may be removed conservatively with an anterior colpotomy. In addition, with intrauterine benign tumors (submucosal or pedunculated myomata) the uterine neck may be split and the tumors enucleated (gynecological indication for anterior vaginal hysterotomy). Colpotomy may also be considered for gaining access to the adnexa. However, this vaginal procedure has lost its significance because we now have the option of laparoscopic myomectomy.

Technique

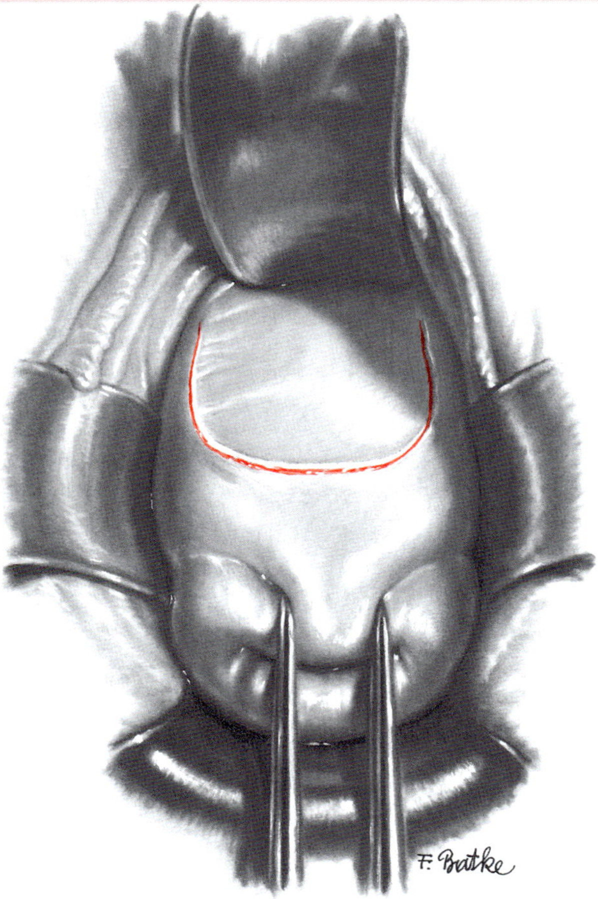

Figure 6.1. Anterior colpotomy. Incision.

The vagina is exposed with one anterior, two lateral, and one posterior self-retaining retractor. The anterior cervical lip is grasped with two single-toothed tenacula, and the portio is pulled forward.

In the region of the inverted anterior vaginal wall a caudally convex curved incision is made with the lower pole reaching into the anterior fornix, i.e., above the smooth vaginal mucosa covering of the portio. The lateral ends of the incision reach approximately up to the level of the internal cervical os.

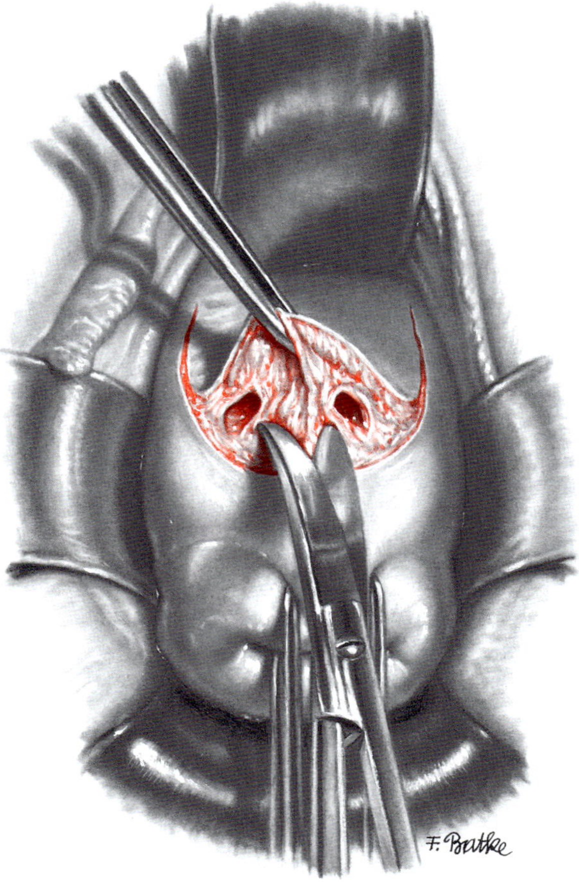

Figure 6.2. Anterior colpotomy. Dividing the supravaginal septum.

By lifting the flap of the vaginal mucosa, fibers of the supravaginal septum are stretched medially. They are severed with curved scissors, with tips pointing toward the cervix.

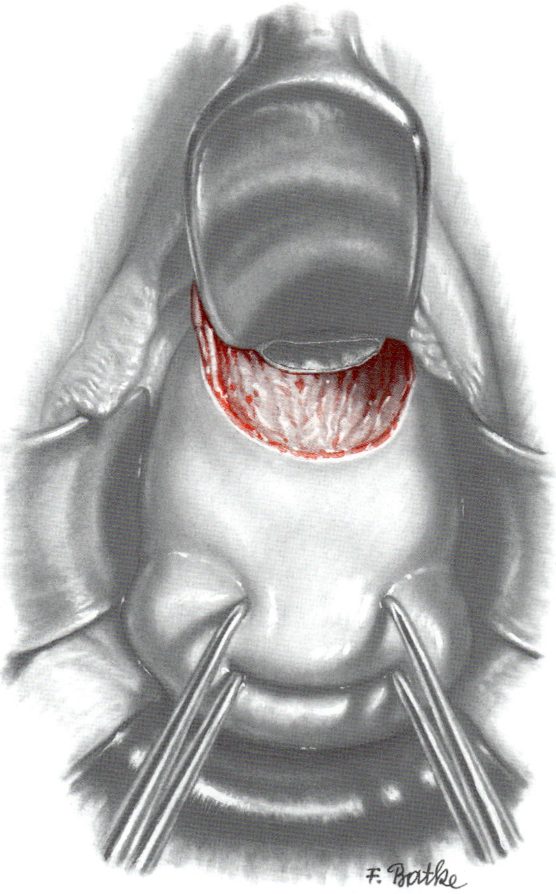

Figure 6.3. Anterior colpotomy. Opening the vesicouterine fold.

The bladder is dissected and is held upward by a retractor; fibers of the lateral bladder pillar were not severed.

The anterior peritoneal fold, which is just barely visible anteriorly, is exposed with a scissors incision after the bladder has been pushed back.

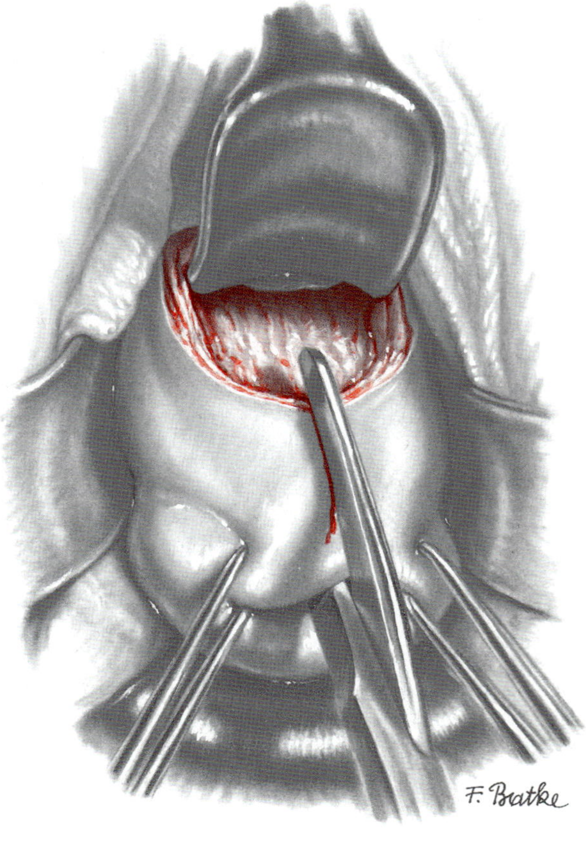

Figure 6.4. Anterior vaginal hysterotomy. Splitting the anterior wall of the cervix.

The peritoneal cavity has been exposed. The bladder is forcibly retracted upward with an anterior intraperitoneal retractor. The anterior cervical wall is split in the midline with strong straight scissors up to the ureteral isthmus.

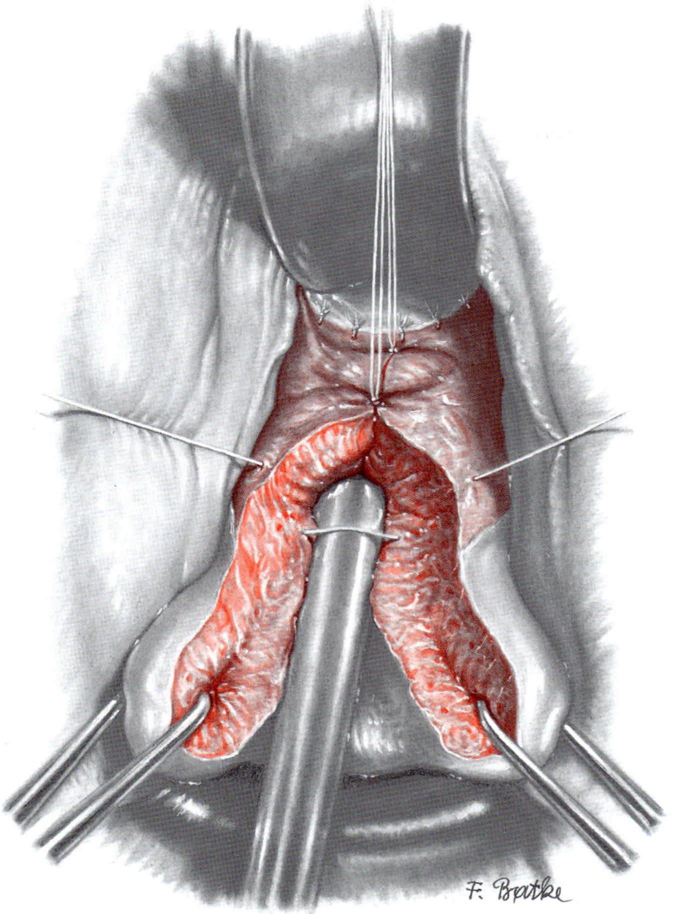

Figure 6.5. Vaginal hysterotomy. Suturing the cervical canal.

The peritoneal cavity is closed with button sutures.

A Hegar dilator (no. 8) is inserted into the cervical canal; above it the anterior cervical wall is closed with interrupted button sutures.

Note that only the muscle, not the mucosa, is sutured.

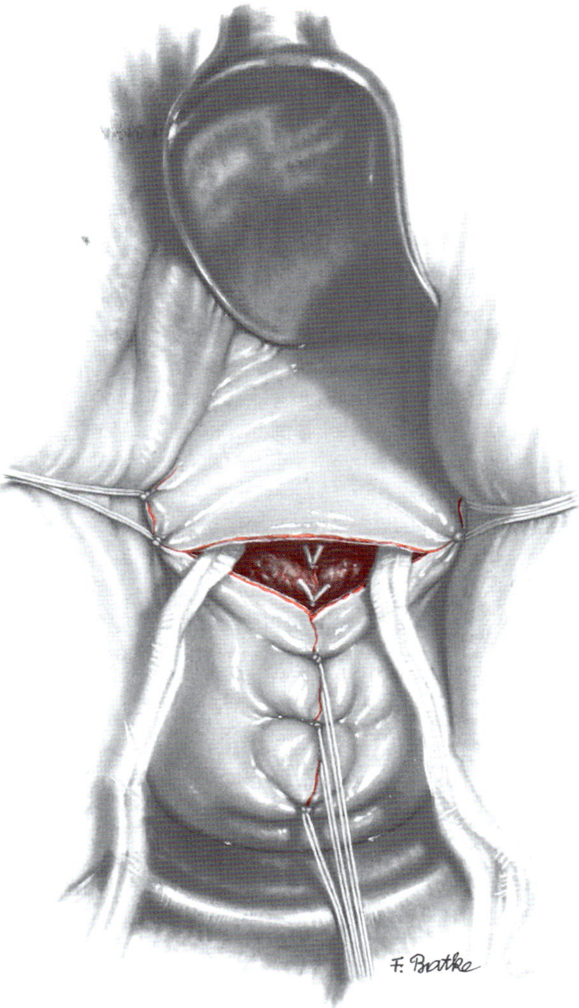

Figure 6.6. Anterior vaginal hysterotomy. Suturing the colpotomy wound.

The anterior cervical wall and the portio are united with interrupted sutures.

Two thin gauze strips are inserted into the vesicocervical space for drainage and left for 48 hours.

Edges of the bow-shaped colpotomy wound are closed with button sutures.

Technical Problems

The tongue-like incision in the anterior vaginal wall might *not reach far enough upward laterally*. As a result, the lower, mobilized bladder pole and its overlying adherent anterior vaginal flap cannot be advanced sufficiently cephalad; the anterior cervical wall is therefore not exposed enough to gain sufficient access to the vesicouterine fold.

7/ Episiotomy

Indications

An episiotomy is done at parturition whenever the perineum is inflexible and tense, the pubic arch is narrow, and the fetal head is large or deflexed. It is especially useful in forceps deliveries, vacuum extractions, manual manipulations, and breech procedures when the integrity of the pelvic floor musculature is endangered. To avoid injury under these circumstances, an episiotomy should be performed as a general rule.

A timely episiotomy of appropriate depth may prevent an imminent tear of the perineal mucosa, as well as overstretching and laceration of the pelvic floor musculature. When performed at the right time, an episiotomy will also serve to shorten the birth process by diminishing the resistance of the perineum and the pelvic floor, by widening the birth passage, and by shortening the birth canal. Finally, the widened birth passage will diminish the pressures that are applied to the cranium of the premature infant who is at increased risk during vaginal delivery.

There are two types of episiotomy: mediolateral and median. The mediolateral episiotomy, if sufficiently deep, protects the levator pillars from being overstretched and torn. In contrast to the median episiotomy, there is no danger of a further tear, which yields a third degree perineal laceration. Suturing the mediolateral episiotomy requires more practice and skill than closing the median episiotomy because the wound edges are distorted by muscle pull. However, the mediolateral episiotomy will heal just as well as the median procedure—without offering any of its disadvantages—provided one observes exact apposition of the levator pillars and of the urogenital diaphragm during the reconstruction.

Technique

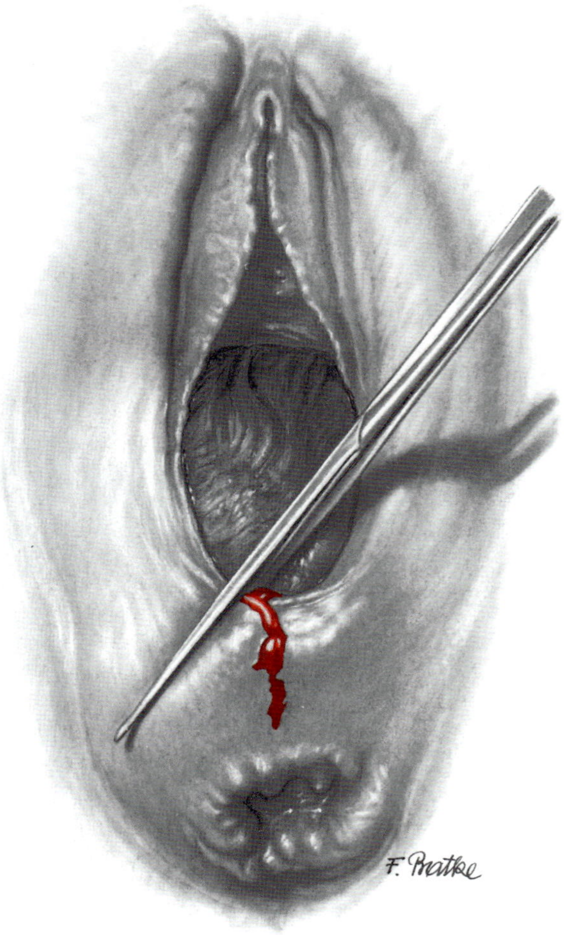

Figure 7.1. Mediolateral episiotomy. Making the incision.

The advancing fetal cranium crowns over the perineum and begins to tear into the vulva. At the height of a uterine contraction, the perineum is stretched and becomes pale. There is some bleeding from the vagina. The anus is gaping in response to the pressure of the fetal head. With long straight scissors, the obstetrician makes a radial incision into the right side of the perineum at 7 o'clock: one scissor blade is inserted approximately 1 cm from the midline at the posterior commissure. The incision is performed under slight pressure in the direction of the ischial tuberosity. The flat sides of the scissor blades are always held at right angle to the tissue being severed to ensure a transverse division of perineal tissue.

The incision should extend at least 3–4 cm onto the perineum. If the levator muscles have been overstretched, the puborectal muscle (median part of the levator) is also indented.

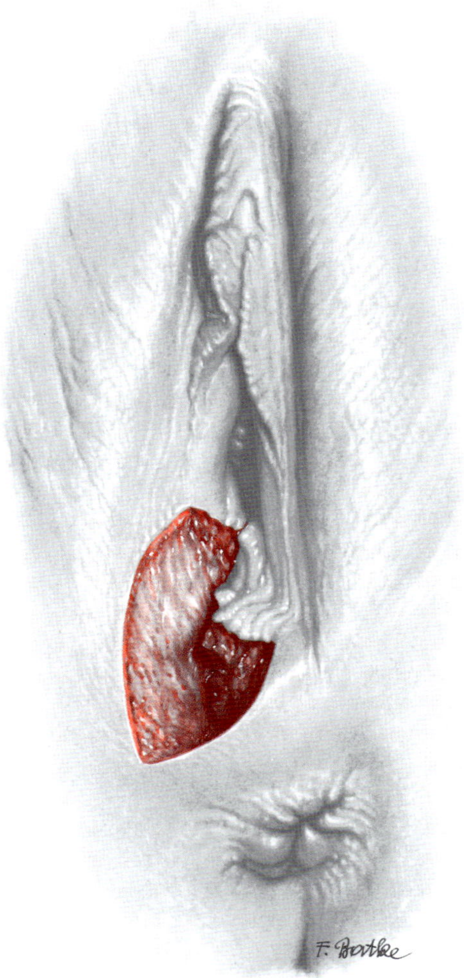

Figure 7.2. Mediolateral episiotomy. After delivery.

The mediolateral wound edge of the perineal incision has retracted into the vagina somewhat as a consequence of contraction of the bulbocavernous muscle (musculus bulbospongiosus).

Before the episiotomy wound is sutured, the birth canal is exposed with large vaginal retractors and closely inspected to find possible cervical or vaginal lacerations. These are then repaired before suturing begins.

A large gauze tampon (with a string attached) is then packed in front of the cervix to hold back uterine bleeding temporarily. This will allow an undisturbed view of the episiotomy wound surface, which can now be presented clearly.

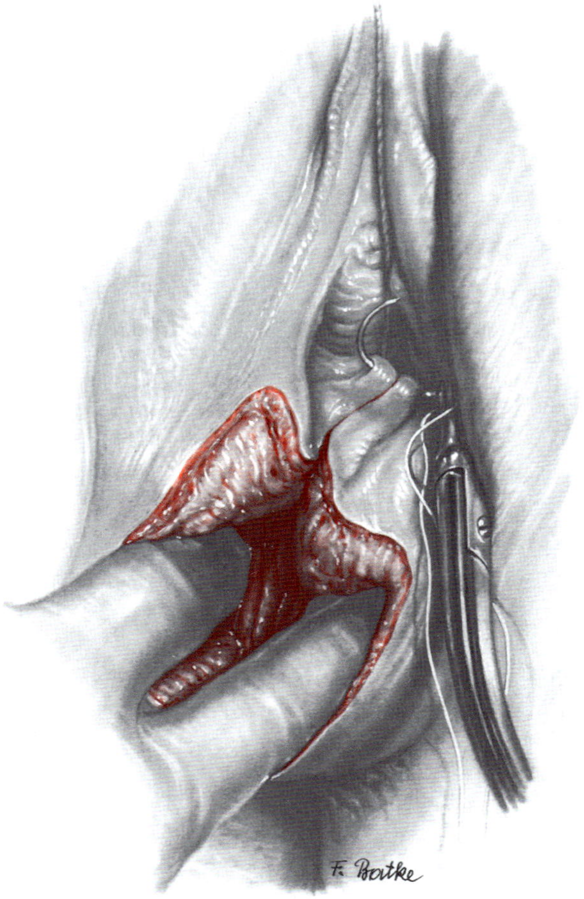

Figure 7.3. Mediolateral episiotomy. Suturing the perineal incision.

A large tampon is packed into the vagina; its distal marker is placed on the mother's abdomen.

Because repair of a vaginal perineal incision is performed in most cases without assistance, the surgeon spreads the perineal tissue with the second and third fingers of the left hand into the vagina, pushing it lightly in a caudal direction. This will provide access to the uppermost vaginal wound angle, which is closed with the first catgut suture.

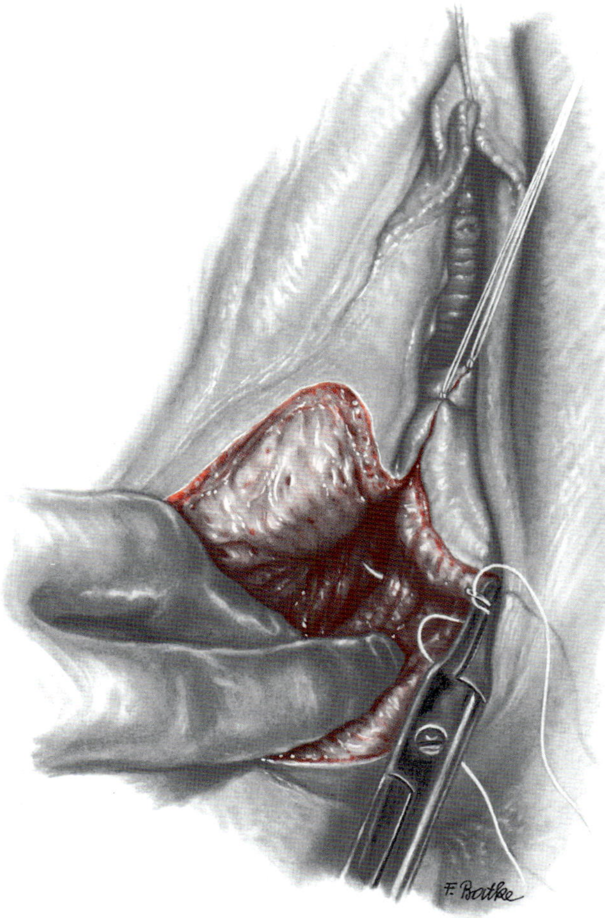

Figure 7.4. Mediolateral episiotomy. Suturing the perineal tissue.

The vaginal wound is closed not quite up to the posterior commissure.

The surgeon spreads the perineal wound widely and unites the deep perineal tissue to avoid leaving dead space. Medially, relatively little tissue is taken on the needle to ensure that the rectum will not be punctured.

Note that to unite corresponding wound surfaces, the needle is not inserted horizontally but at an angle, with the medial side lower than the lateral.

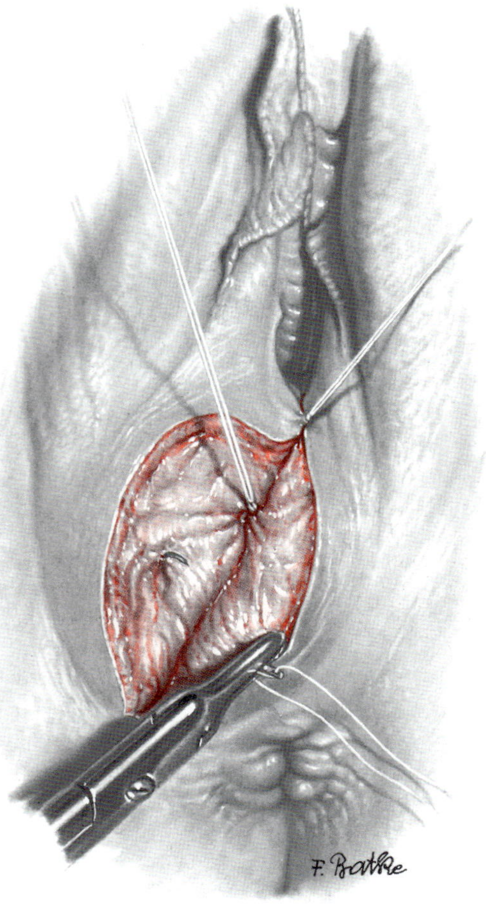

Figure 7.5. Mediolateral episiotomy. Reconstructing the perineum.

The vaginal wound has been closed almost as far as the posterior commissure; the deep perineal tissues have been joined with a suture.

Additional deep sutures are applied; note again that the needle is pushed from lower medial to higher lateral direction.

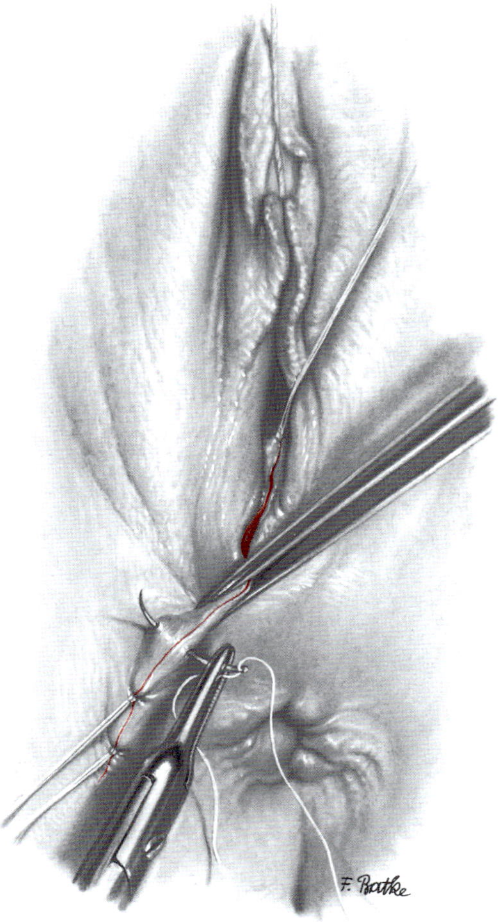

Figure 7.6. Mediolateral episiotomy. Suturing the perineal skin.

A series of catgut sutures has brought the vaginal wound edges together down to about 2 cm from the posterior commissure.

As the skin at the perineal wound edges is sutured, one begins at the caudal angle of the wound and proceeds from caudal to cranial. The surgeon holds the skin edges together with tissue forceps while the third suture is placed. The perineal skin is sutured with fine silk (or a subcuticular suture is used); compare with Figure 17.11.

Technical Problems

1. When the episiotomy is *too small,* it will not be sufficient to relieve the tensions on the perineum, and, if stressed further, there is danger of uncontrolled lacerations. We use large straight scissors for a mediolateral episiotomy. They should have enough leverage to incise the tissue at the height of a contraction with a single cut. At that point the patient, if possible, is briefly anesthetized with inhalation anesthesia.
2. If the episiotomy has been placed *too far laterally,* it will not provide the desired relaxation of the median portion of the levator.
3. An episiotomy can be made with *several successive cuts.* This is disadvantageous because the wound edges become distorted by the pull of the muscle after the first incision into the stretched perineum has been made; any additional perineal cuts will yield a zigzag incision line.
4. *Deep sutures* can be required high in the vagina. If the vaginal wall was cut too high or has torn further upward into the lateral fornix or beyond, a wide gaping wound will result. In the upper reaches of such a wound one can occasionally see the exposed urethra (which always remains uninjured). Under these circumstances, only the vaginal wound edges need be brought together with fine (size 0) catgut sutures. Placing submucosal sutures to occlude dead space is inappropriate here. We are dealing in this case only with reapposing the posterior vaginal wall to the rectum—not with a deep wound. After uniting the vaginal wound edges, the posterior wall will adhere to the anterior wall of the rectum, and no dead space will remain between them. Deep sutures are required only near the vaginal introitus.
5. The large, gaping wound described under point 4 seldom bleeds actively and should therefore *never be drained.* Rather hemostasis should be performed whenever it is indicated. A drain in the paravaginal wound space serves as a conducting pathway for lochial secretions; its presence will usually lead to infection of the wound cavity. It is preferable to close the large vaginal wound primarily.
6. During reconstruction of the pelvic floor and the perineum, the *sutures might have been limited only to the superficial layers of tissue.* This may produce dead spaces deep in the wound, and blood will tend to collect there. Deep approximating sutures are needed here.
7. With *deep perineal sutures*, it is possible *to grasp too much tissue medially* on the needle and puncture the rectum. This is a common error committed by beginners.
8. The severed muscles of the *urogenital diaphragm or levator ani* are *incorrectly approximated* (i.e., deep sutures have been placed incorrectly in a horizontal direction). The perineum will now have a "slanted look"; it will heal in slantwise fashion, and vaginal descensus may develop later.

8/ Surgical Treatment of Cervical Incompetence

Indications

Indication depends on the following three criteria:

- Past history of two or more midtrimester abortions (specifically excluding habitual abortions occurring in the first trimester);
- Dilation of external and internal cervix; the amniotic membranes are ballooning forward to the external os;
- Demonstration in the nongravid state that the cervical canal will accommodate an 8-mm Hegar dilator without discomfort.

Three different methods of surgical procedures are used to close the prematurely dilating cervix: Shirodkar cerclage, McDonald cerclage, and Wurm-Hefner closure.

If possible, the procedure is performed at the end of the fourth lunar month of pregnancy. If cervical incompetence is discovered later, the procedure can still be performed up to the 28th week of gestational age, provided the portio is still preserved, the amniotic sac is still intact, and there is no bleeding.

The cervix is encircled with a band of synthetic material (Mersilene band). Use of heavy silk suture is not advisable. It can result in severe strangulation of the cervical tissue and even complete amputation of the cervix.

Shirodkar Cerclage

In general, the Shirodkar technique is preferred today.

Technique

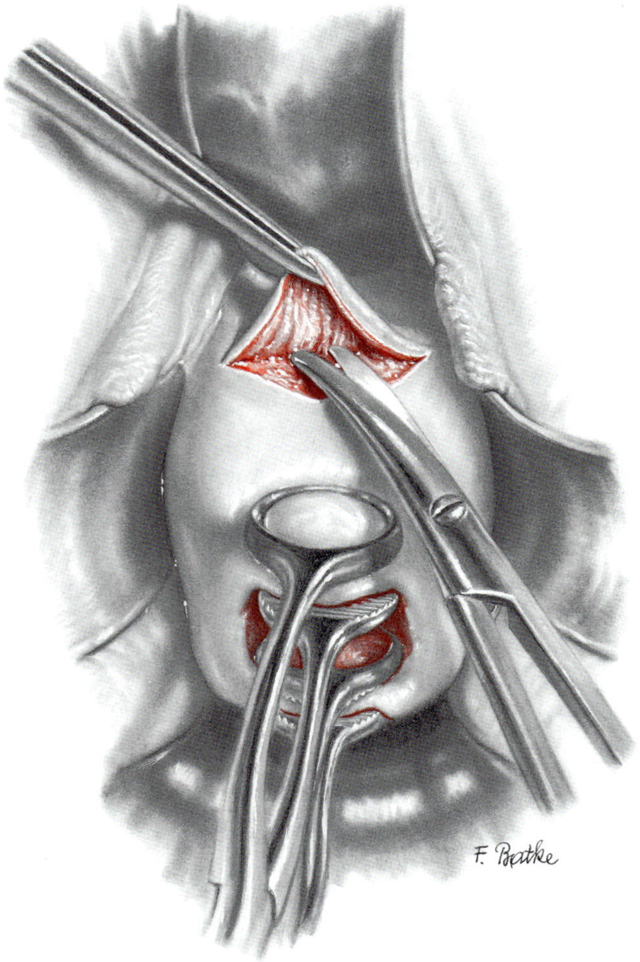

Figure 8.1. Shirodkar cerclage. Dissecting the bladder.

Both the anterior and posterior cervical lips are gently grasped with ring forceps; special care must be taken to avoid rupturing the lower pole of the protruding chorioamniotic membranes.

A transverse incision is made in the vaginal wall in the anterior fornix region. The lower pole of the bladder is somewhat dissected.

A similar transverse incision is also performed in the posterior fornix region so that the rectum can be pushed caudally out of the way.

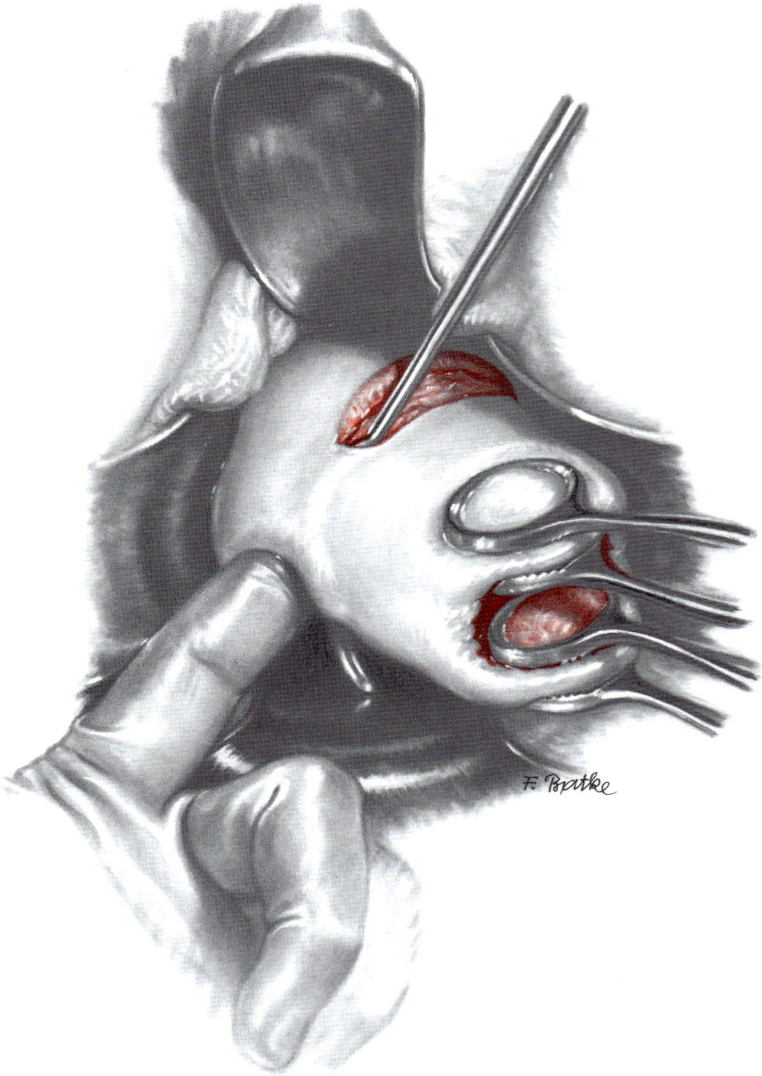

Figure 8.2. Shirodkar cerclage. Inserting the left-handed Deschamps needle subfascially.

The vaginal wall is transversally incised in the anterior and posterior fornices; bladder and rectum are somewhat advanced.

On the right side, an empty left-handed Deschamps needle is inserted into the anterior fornix and pushed forward under the fascia of the vaginal wall until its tip exits at the posterior fornix. At the same time the surgeon exerts counterpressure with the left index finger.

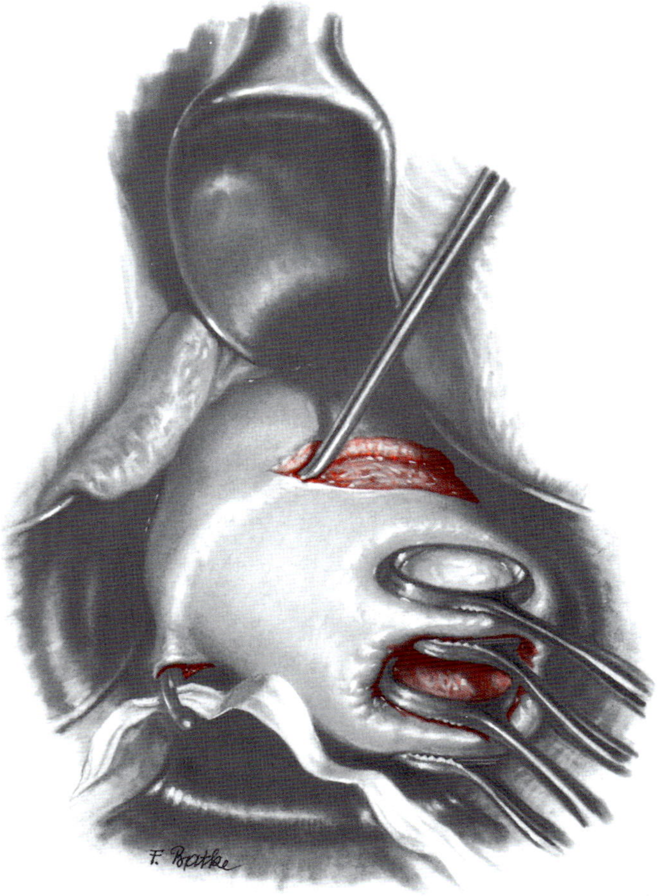

Figure 8.3. Shirodkar cerclage. Threading a Mersilene band.

The end of a Mersilene band is inserted into the eye of the needle that protrudes through the posterior incision. When the Deschamps needle is withdrawn, the band is led out at the anterior fornix incision.

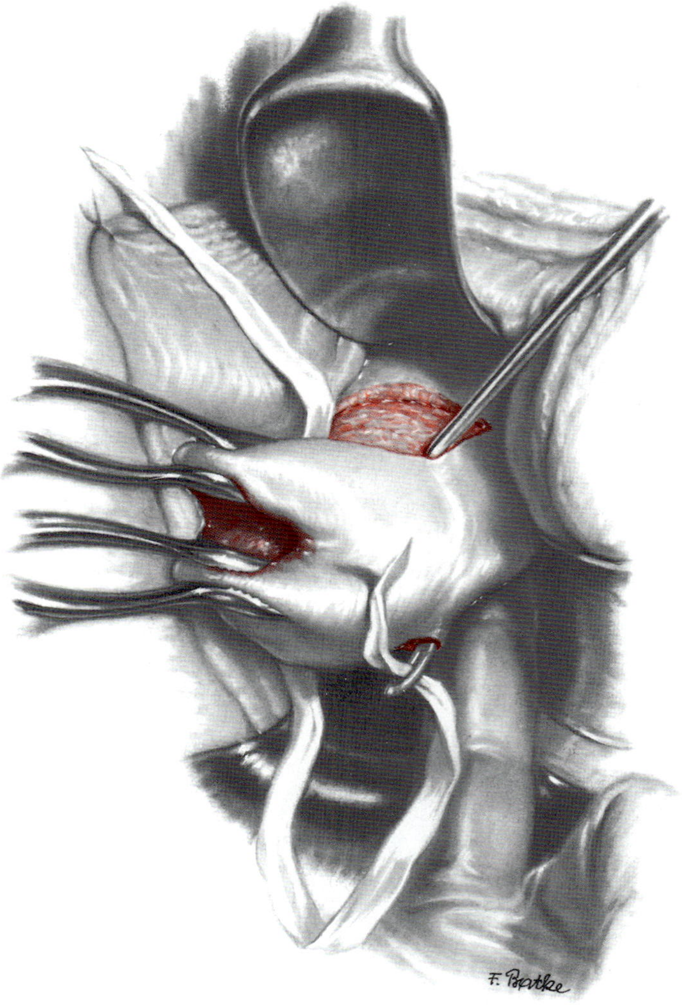

Figure 8.4. Shirodkar cerclage. Applying the right-handed Deschamps needle subfascially.

On the right side, the end of the cerclage band is guided through the anterior wound opening, where it exits.

On the left side, using counterpressure of the left index finger at the posterior incision, the surgeon has inserted a right-handed Deschamps needle subfascially from the anterior fornix around to the posterior fornix. The other end of the cerclage band is then threaded into the protruding tip of the needle.

By pulling the Deschamps needle back, this second cerclage band end is pulled out through the anterior fornix.

Instead of using Deschamps needles, a Mersilene band with a large, round needle already attached to it may be used. The cerclage band is also slung subfascially around the cervix at the level of the internal cervical os and tied anteriorly.

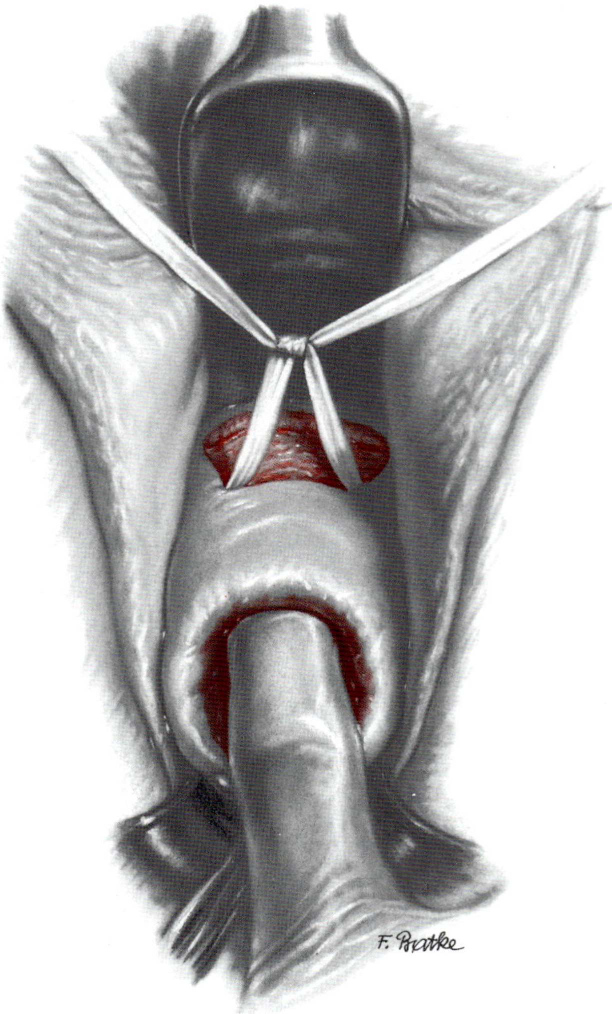

Figure 8.5. Shirodkar cerclage. Tying the cerclage band.

The ring forceps on the anterior lip of the cervix are removed.

The Mersilene band encircles the cervix subfascially at the level of the internal cervical os. It is tied anteriorly by the surgeon. Simultaneously, the assistant slightly inserts the index finger into the cervical canal to control how tightly the internal os is being closed by the band.

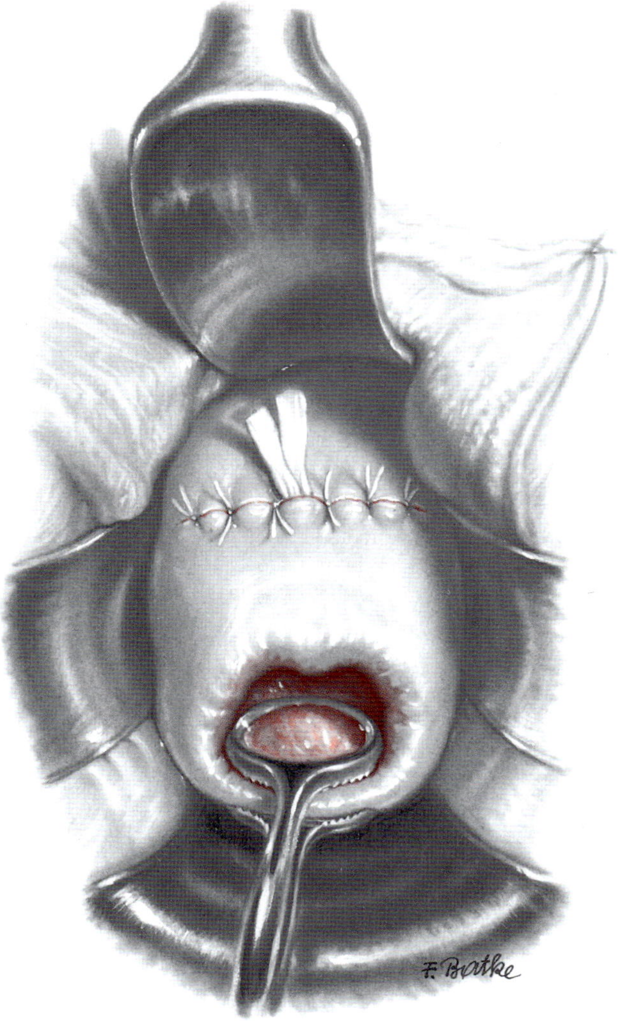

Figure 8.6. Shirodkar cerclage. Suturing the colpotomy wounds.

The band has been placed to encircle the cervix at the level of the internal os under the vaginal wall and is tied. In this way, it effectively closes the internal os. The ends of the band are guided through the anterior colpotomy wound and shortened.

The edges of the vaginal incision are joined together with interrupted catgut sutures.

Technical Problems—Figures 8.1–8.6

1. Should the cerclage band be *tied around the cervix too close to the external cervical os*, the internal os will not be closed sufficiently and be able to withstand the pressure coming from the uterine cavity, even though the cerclage is in place.
2. Occasionally, at the conclusion of pregnancy, it is *difficult to locate* the band encircling the cervix, especially in cases when it was cut too short or if it was cut into the cervical tissue because it had been pulled together too tightly. A small cervical wall incision will expose the band so that it can be removed completely.

McDonald Cerclage (Purse-String Suture)

Technique

A purse-string suture with large gauge nylon or silk suture is placed at the level of the internal cervical os but beneath the lower bladder poles. One sutures through the vaginal wall at the left side and posteriorly, then at the right side and anteriorly. The suture is slung around the portio and tied in front. (The suture is left in place until term. It is removed at the due date or when labor begins).

Wurm-Hefner Closure (Mattress Suture)

Technique

In cases when pregnancy is far along and/or cervical incompetence is recognized late (cervix is noticeably dilated and portio already effaced), one may try to delay the onset of labor by closing the external cervical os with mattress or U sutures. Prognosis is poor; this effort is only justified if contractions have not yet begun. One must be particularly cautious to avoid puncturing of the amniotic sac and/or the progressing infant's head.

9/ Conization

Scott Conization

Indications

Suspicion of the presence of a precancerous lesion of the cervix or the desire for definite histological verification warrants the performance of conization of the cervix, by the technique described by Scott, in conjunction with uterine curettage. Indications include

1. Suspicious cytology (repeated Class III Pap smears, unaltered by local treatment, as well as those of Class IV or Class V);
2. Suspicious histology (in tissues obtained by punch biopsy or curettage of the cervical canal);
3. Suspicious colposcopy.

Routinely combining a sharp conization with a follow-up curettage is entirely justified because these procedures will survey the entire cervical canal and also the uterine cavity for diagnostic purposes.

In young women, during their phase of sexual maturity, a flat conization is sufficient for histological verification because their squamocolumnar junction (most frequent point of origin for a cervical carcinoma) extends well out onto the surface of the vaginal portio. In elderly women, at least two-thirds of the cervical canal must be removed during conization because the squamocolumnar junction has receded into the cervical canal.

This procedure, if performed for diagnostic purposes, may also serve as a therapeutic measure in dysplasia or carcinoma in situ (carcinoma colli 0) that had been removed in healthy tissue (histology: overlapping step-serial sections) via conization.

Technique

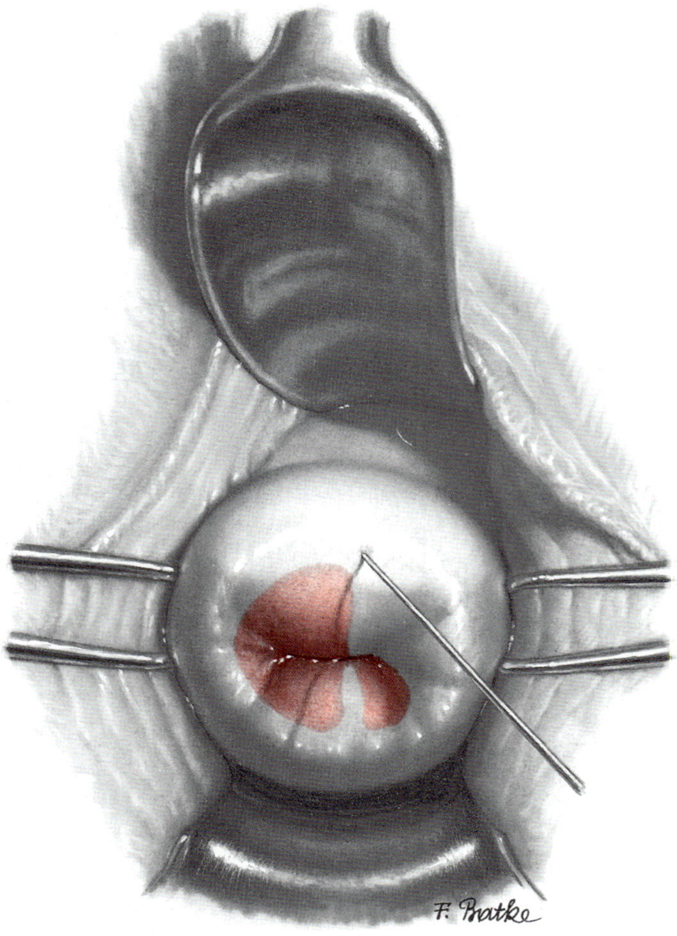

Figure 9.1. Scott conization. Infiltrating the portio.

The vagina is exposed with an anterior retractor and a self-retaining posterior retractor. The portio is grasped laterally with forceps and pulled forward.

The anterior and then the posterior lip of the cervix are each infiltrated with 4–7 ml fluid and rendered ischemic until the tissue appears pale (add 5 IU Pitressin in 100 ml physiologic saline solution).

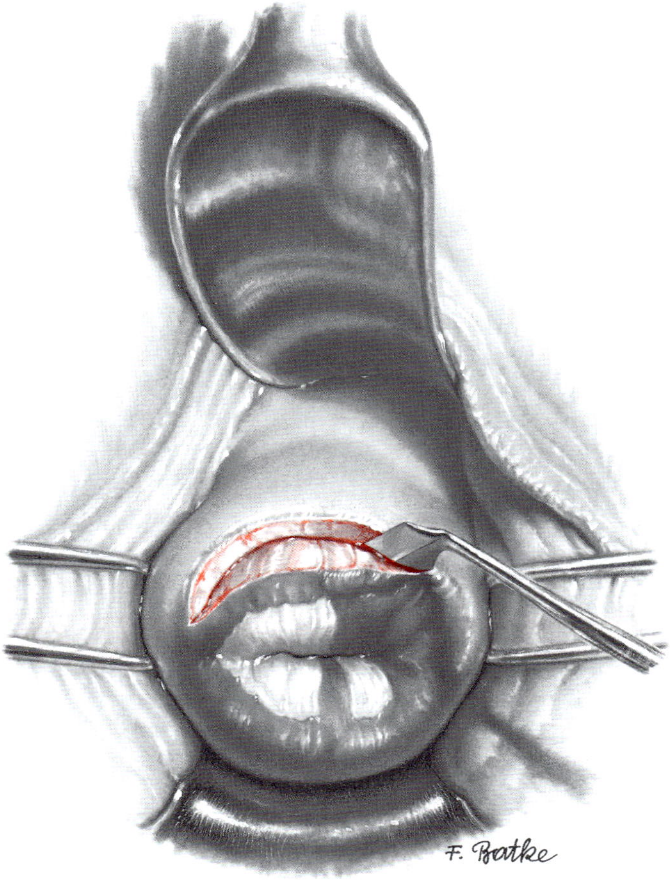

Figure 9.2. Scott conization. Incising the cone.

After staining the mucosa of the portio with Lugol's iodine solution, the sharp-edged, iodine-negative areas can be recognized on the anterior and posterior cervical lip.

Using a double-edged knife, one begins to excise the cone anteriorly in the healthy iodine-positive tissue. The knife is held with its tip directed toward the internal os of the cervix.

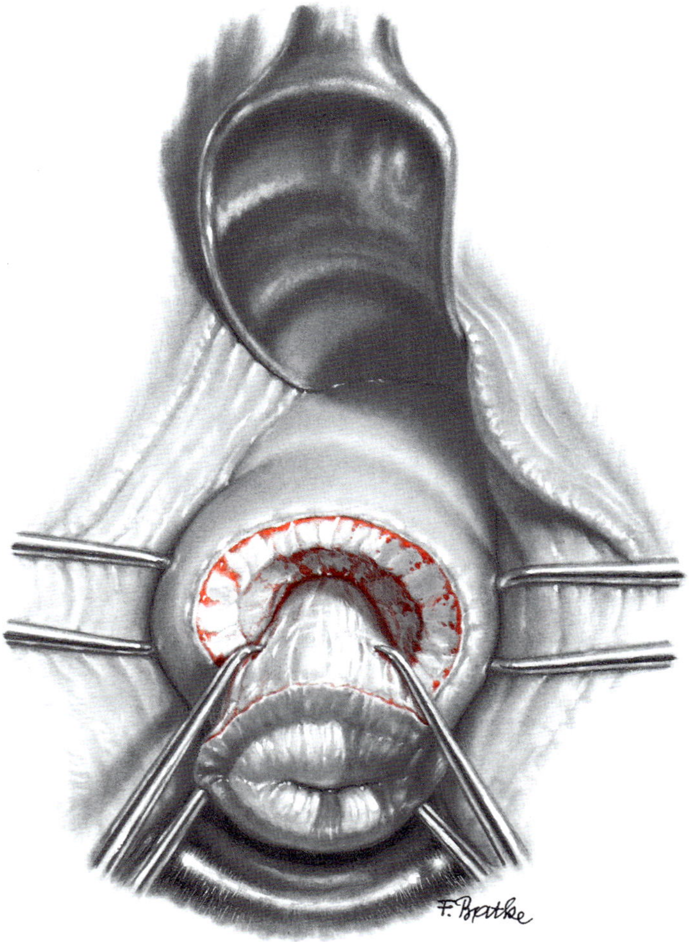

Figure 9.3. Scott conization. Dissecting the cone.

The cone and entire cervical canal are largely excised from the portio.

Precise removal of the entire cervical canal is facilitated after the circumferential portio incision is made by grasping the external wound edge of the cone with two forceps (without injuring the portio epithelium or the cervical canal) and pulling the cone downward.

Curettage of the uterine cavity follows.

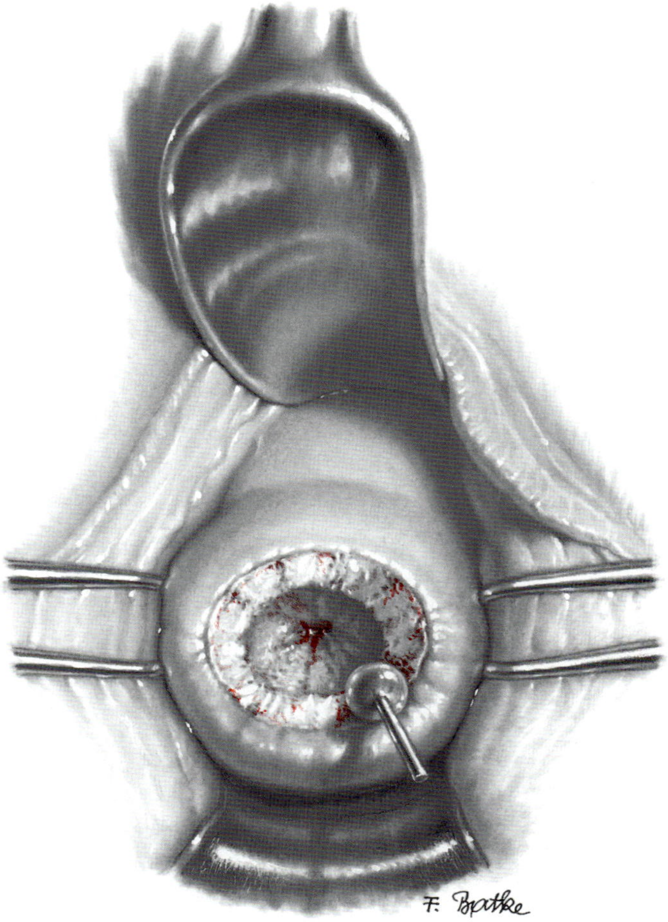

Figure 9.4. Scott conization. Care of the wound surface.

The cone has been excised from the infiltrated portio. By means of coagulation with a button tip electrode (or with a laser), hemostasis of the surface of the wound is achieved.

Technical Problems—Figures 9.1–9.4

1. Curettage is performed before conization. This will destroy the architecture of the cervical canal, and the histological diagnosis will be inexact.
2. If *strength of the current chosen* during electrocoagulation is too high, deep necrosis will develop, and the tissue will not heal for a long time. Excessive current will be manifest when the tissue begins to blacken.
3. If *bleeding continues despite coagulation*, the lateral margins of the cervix must be ligated at 3 and 9 o'clock with size 00 chromic catgut sutures.

After hemostasis has been accomplished, sulfonamide powder is instilled into the vagina, and the wound surface is tamponaded with a vaginal packing strip for 24 hours. If these measures are followed, the most unpleasant complication of this procedure, postoperative bleeding, can usually be avoided.

Laser Conization (Conization with a CO_2 Laser)

Indications

Hospitals with access to the relatively expensive CO_2 laser may use it for conization. This technology offers several advantages: infiltration of the portio with saline solution is unnecessary; a laser beam incision will immediately produce secure hemostasis; the wound surface will heal quickly and without problems (generally within 6–8 days); and postoperative infiltration of infection of the paracervical tissue is minimal. In addition, a well-focused laser beam will produce clearly defined wound edges at the cone and allow excellent diagnostic assessment with the histological examination.

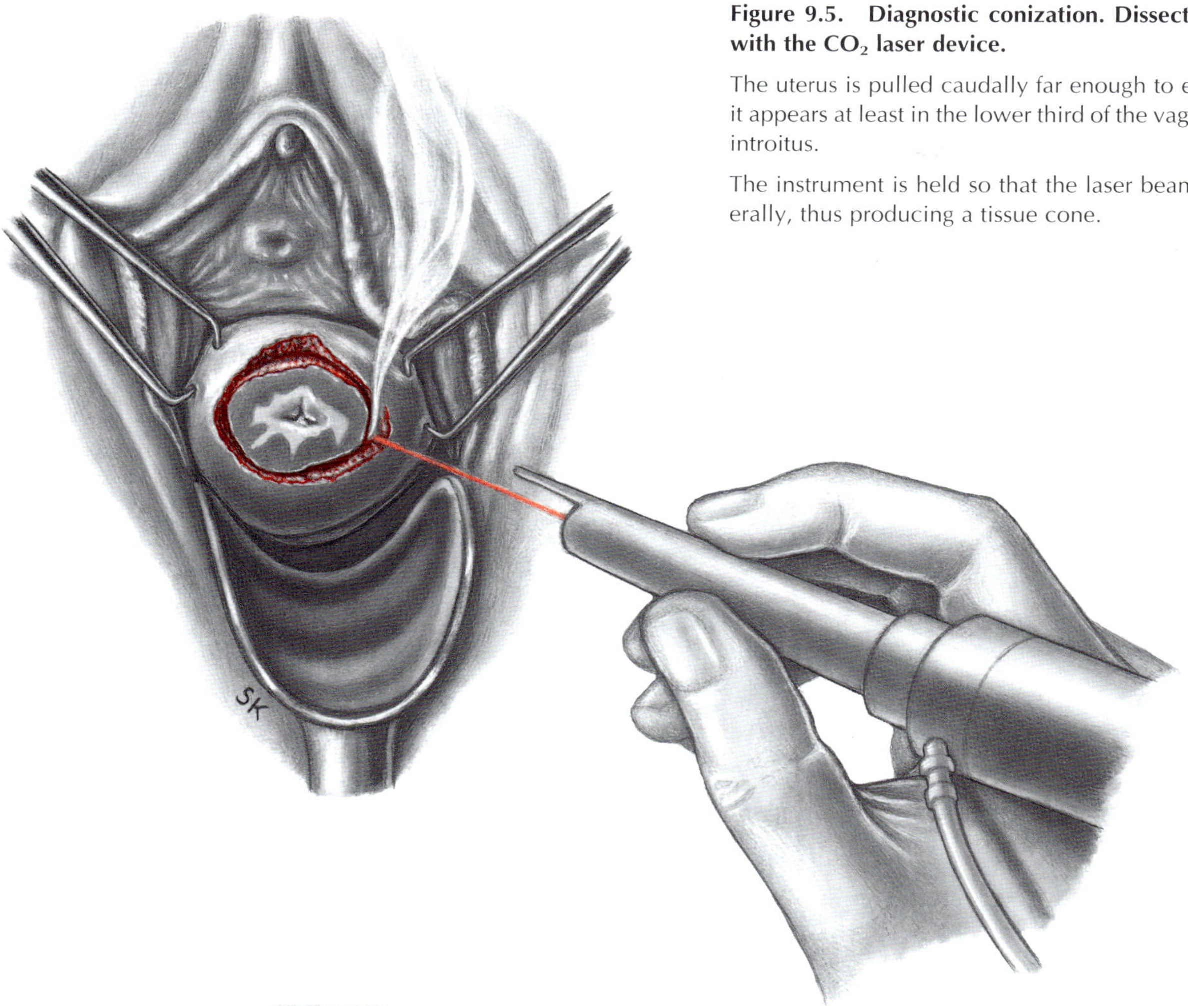

Figure 9.5. Diagnostic conization. Dissecting the cervical cone with the CO_2 laser device.

The uterus is pulled caudally far enough to expose the portio until it appears at least in the lower third of the vagina, i.e., in the vaginal introitus.

The instrument is held so that the laser beam meets the portio laterally, thus producing a tissue cone.

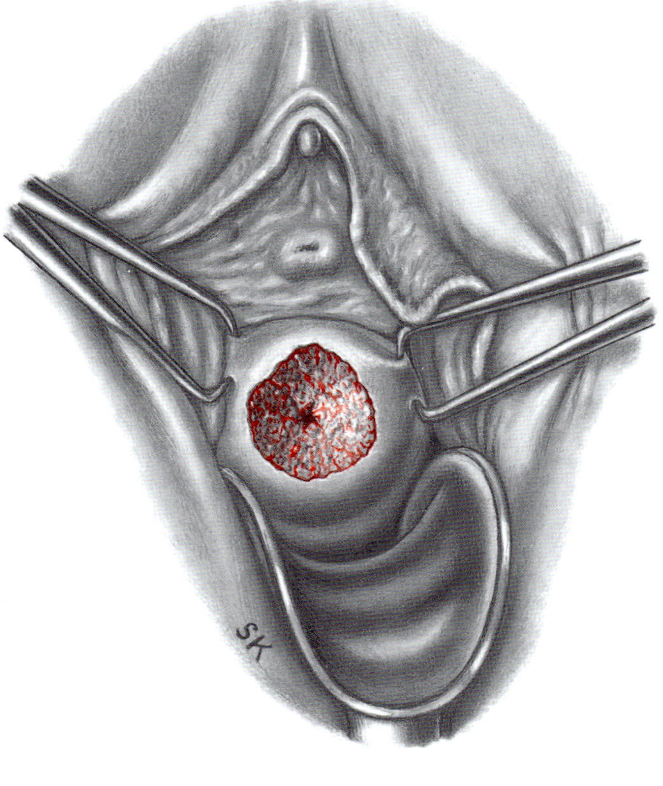

Figure 9.6. Diagnostic conization. Wound surface shows sharp edges after the laser beam was used.

The incision process has produced hemostasis simultaneously.

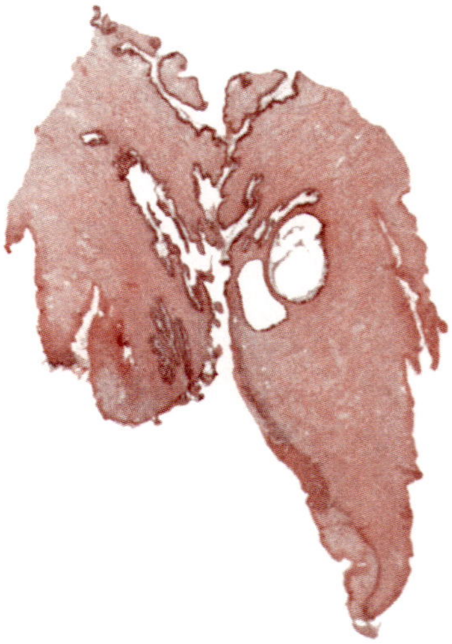

Figure 9.7. Diagnostic conization. Large surface incision through a portio cone produced with a CO_2 laser.

The squamous epithelium of the portio [a region with cervical intraepithelial neoplasia (*right*)] proceeds to the columnar epithelium of the cervix. There are smooth incision edges that are easily assessed. Hemostasis in this region may be accomplished again with the laser beam.

TECHNICAL PROBLEMS—FIGURES 9.5–9.7

A prerequisite in using the laser instrument is to pull the uterus down far enough with the laterally attached forceps for the portio to be exposed in the lower third of the vagina. The straight, nonangled beam makes a conical incision impossible. In some cases, the upper end of the cone will have to be cut with an angled scalpel or scissors.

10/ Surgical Treatment of a Bartholin Cyst (Abscess)

Marsupialization

Indications

In dealing with cysts of Bartholin's gland, one is not primarily concerned with cystic changes in the glandular parenchyma but rather with a dilation of the excretory duct whose exit into the vestibule is closed as a result of preceding inflammation. These cysts are actually retention cysts containing thick, viscid mucus and are thus more appropriately named pseudocysts. Secondary invasion by virulent organisms will cause pus to collect, converting the structure into a pseudoabscess located in the lower half of the labia majora.

Until recently, the treatment for a Bartholin cyst was extirpation and that for Bartholin abscess was incision. Both methods have the disadvantage of being associated with recurrence; extirpation will sometimes remove only the enlarged excretory duct, leaving the glandular parenchyma in situ to continue secreting and accumulating. When an abscess is incised, the wound usually heals over rapidly. Furthermore, extirpation of a cyst can be a particularly bloody and, with larger cysts, technically demanding procedure. Such cysts tend to extend posteriorly toward the rectum, and the cyst wall may be found in close proximity to the rectal wall. After an excision, the very thin labial skin must often be resected, and, as a consequence, the cosmetic results are poor. Finally, young women in particular may complain about an uncomfortable feeling of dryness after bilateral cyst extirpation, because glandular excretions no longer discharge into the vestibule.

For these reasons, it is generally preferred today to leave the glands in situ and instead to try to ensure adequate drainage by way of a widened gland exit created by marsupialization. This method demonstrates good cosmetic results, even though recurrences occur occasionally.

Marsupialization can also be done in the presence of an abscess of the excretory duct of the Bartholin's gland. However, under these circumstances, exact approximation of the cyst wall to the skin edges is not possible to achieve because sutures placed in the inflamed tissue will easily cut through.

Bed rest is maintained during the first 5 postoperative days. The abscess cavity is held open by a gauze strip soaked in an antibiotic; the packing is changed daily, with subsequent daily sitz baths recommended to ensure that the wound region is kept clean. Marsupialized abscesses are more likely to recur than comparably managed uninfected Bartholin cysts.

Technique

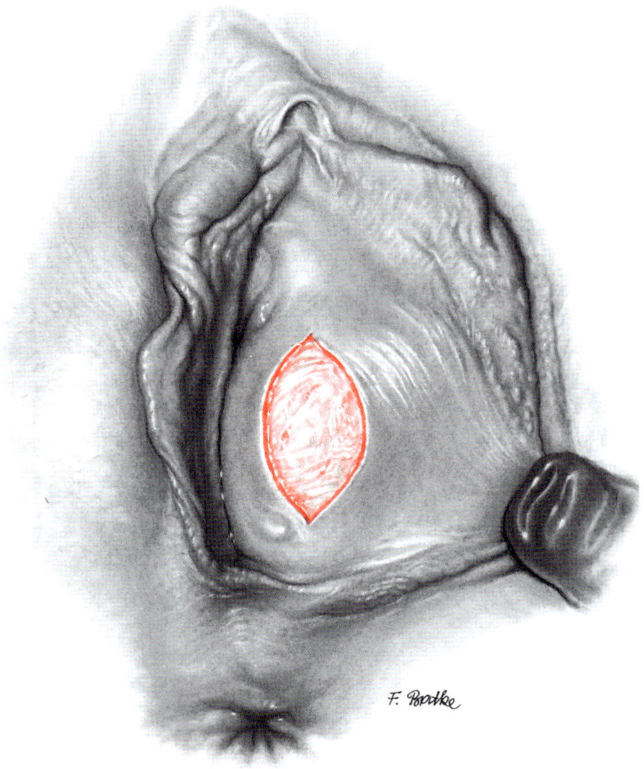

Figure 10.1. Left marsupialization. Incising the labial skin.

The assistant uses the thumb to retract the left labium minus laterally and then pushes somewhat into the genitofemoral sulcus with the index finger to clearly expose the Bartholin cyst.

The surgeon makes a 3-cm lengthwise incision in the skin of the inner aspect of the protruding labium over the convexity of the cyst, which runs approximately 0.5–1 cm laterally from the hymenal ring. First, only the labial skin is incised. This reveals the underlying cystic structure.

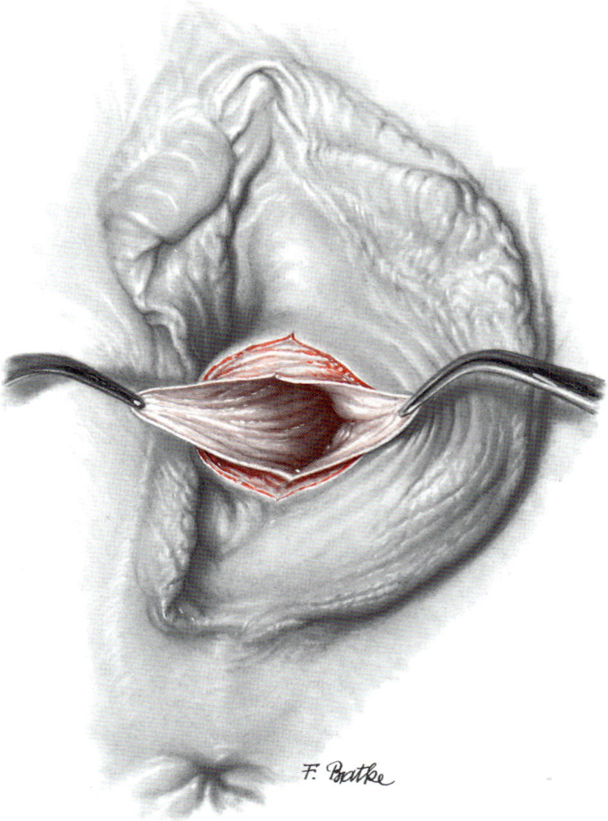

Figure 10.2. Left marsupialization. Opening the cyst cavity.

The labial skin has been incised longitudinally, and the cyst wall is also incised lengthwise, which releases contents of the cyst, mainly thick viscid mucus.

Wound edges of the cystic structure are grasped with two delicate clamps so that they will not retract.

Technical Problems—Figures 10.1–10.3

1. The longitudinal incision in the vestibular mucosa might be placed too far laterally; in such a case, the newly formed gland exit will not open onto the vestibule.
2. The opening of the retention cyst may be made too small. The cyst opening must be large enough to accommodate the insertion of a finger; if smaller, it will close off completely through the shrinkage process, and the cyst will recur.
3. If the cyst is entered with a single thrust of the scalpel, the cyst wall and skin edges will be difficult to distinguish from each other. Approximation, therefore, will be a problem. Thus, it is preferable to incise the mucosa of the labium minus first and cause the wound to gape before proceeding to open the cyst wall itself.

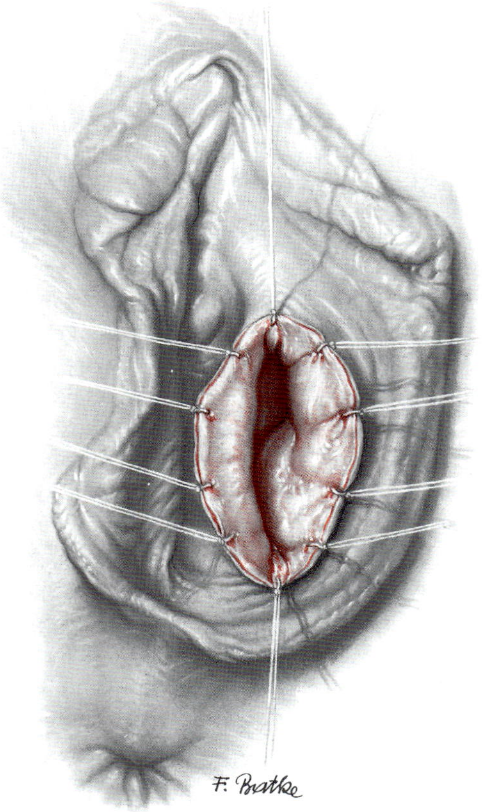

Figure 10.3. Left marsupialization. Exteriorizing the cyst wall.

Cut edges of the cyst wall are joined to wound edges of the vestibular skin with a series of delicate, interrupted catgut sutures applied radially (size 00 atraumatic needles).

The interior of the cyst cavity is sponged out with a hot gauze strip and loosely tamponaded for 24 hours with soft packing material that has been soaked in antibiotic.

The opening of the cyst, originally admitting one finger breadth, shrinks over the course of the next week to pinhead size.

In the presence of intact functioning gland parenchyma, mucus continues to be secreted; the mucus drains through the newly formed ostium. Beginning with the fourth postoperative day, daily sitz baths are indicated to clean the wound region.

Bartholinectomy

Indications

If retention cysts recur, a complete extirpation of the entire gland is indicated. Because a Bartholin cyst develops as a consequence of a preexisting inflammation, the pseudocyst body is often adherent to surrounding tissues. It can, therefore, be removed only by means of sharp dissection. Extirpation of the Bartholin cyst is technically difficult and should not be considered as an operation for a beginner, because the wall of larger cysts always seems to extend close to the rectal wall.

Technique

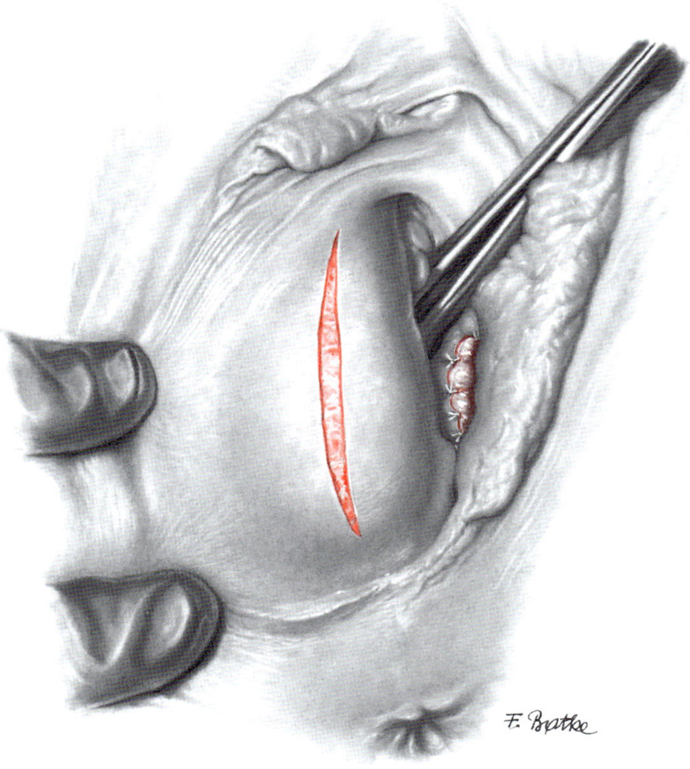

Figure 10.4. Right bartholinectomy. Incising the labial skin.

The assistant uses two fingers to retract the inner aspect of the labium minus laterally, which exposes the lower pole of the protruding cyst.

The other assistant, who is positioned opposite, inserts sponge forceps into the vagina, lifting the Bartholin cyst forward, which tightly stretches the labial skin above.

The surgeon incises the skin of the vestibule at the inner aspect of the labium minus with a longitudinal incision extending from the upper to the lower pole of the cyst.

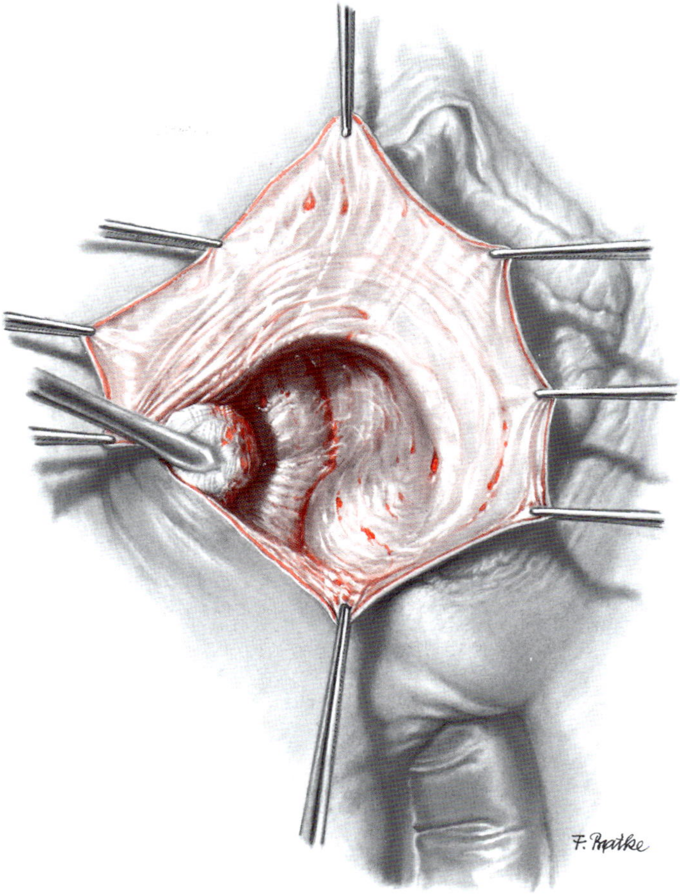

Figure 10.5. Right bartholinectomy. Mobilizing the cyst.

So far, only the labial skin has been dissected from the cyst in stepwise fashion. Labial wound edges are spread with delicate toothed clamps.

The surgeon retracts the partially dissected cyst laterally with a sponge clamp, determining how close the medial pole of the cyst reaches to the rectal wall with the index finger inserted into the rectum.

Observe how the finger in the rectum balloons its lateral wall, and note also the adherence of the cyst to the rectum.

We prefer to place the incision in the vestibule, rather than on the perineal skin outside the labium minus, because wound edges of the vestibule (thinned by the expansion of the cyst) can be resected with better cosmetic results. Additionally, the glandular loculations are easier to dissect off the lateral skin of the labium than from the medially thinned wall of the vestibule. If, however, a longitudinal incision were to be made on the outer surface of the labium minus, one could anticipate multiple perforations of the vestibular skin in the course of attempting to dissect the cyst off the thinned medial labium surface, thus creating both medial and lateral wounds. This usually necessitates extensive resection of the labium minus.

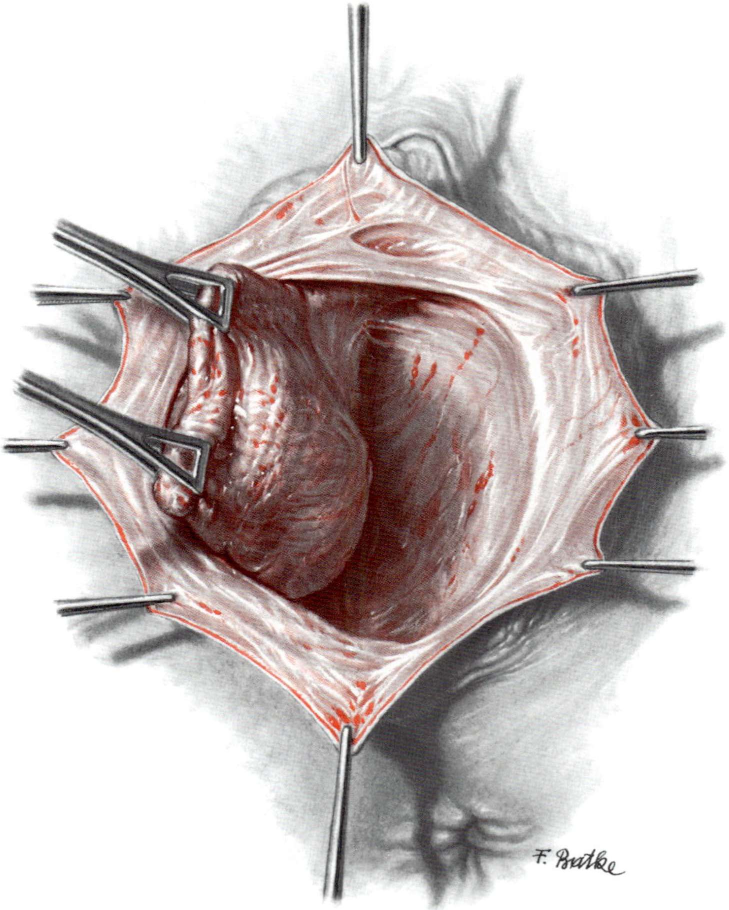

Figure 10.6. Right bartholinectomy. Mobilizing the lower cyst pole.

Wound edges are fanned out, and the wall of the partially mobilized cyst is grasped with delicate fenestrated clamps and lifted forward.

Sharp mobilization of the lower cyst pole requires staying close to the cyst wall; otherwise severe hemorrhage may result.

Large cysts tend to extend especially in a caudal direction toward the rectum. This must be considered when sharply dissecting the medial and posterior parts of the cyst. We advise a second rectal examination to check whether one is dissecting in the correct layer.

When large cysts are removed, one's close proximity to the rectal wall may be surprising.

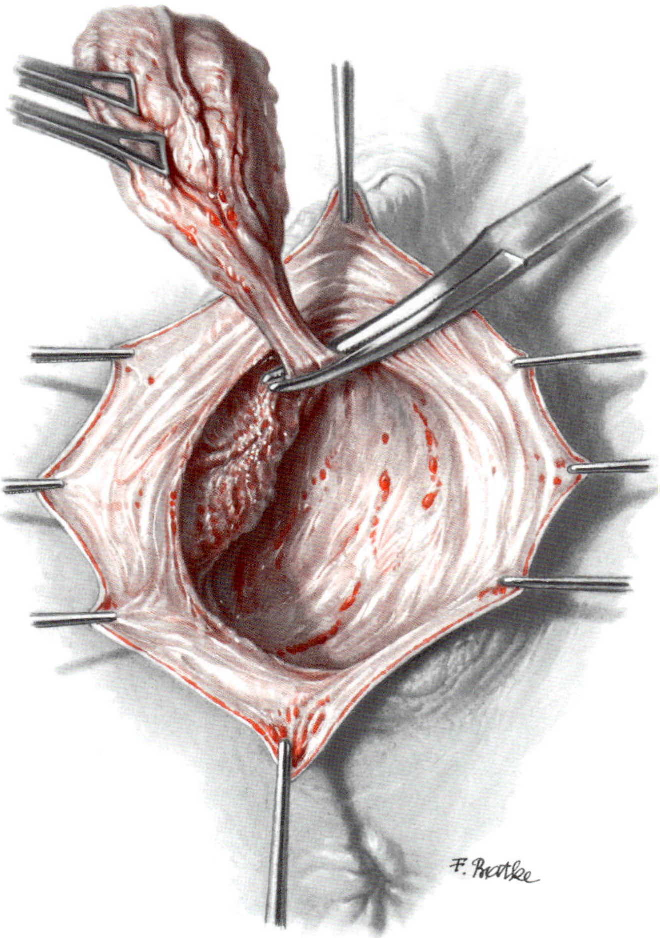

Figure 10.7. Right bartholinectomy. Extirpating the cyst.

After dissecting the cyst wall from the rectum and mobilizing the lower pole of the cyst, one frees the upper pole. This part of the dissection is technically easier, but severe hemorrhage can result from the venous plexus of the vestibular bulb.

The cyst is enucleated from its bed and pulled out with delicate forceps. The cranially arising cephalad attachment is vascular and must therefore be clamped.

Laterally in the depth of the wound cavity the bulbocavernous tissue can be seen.

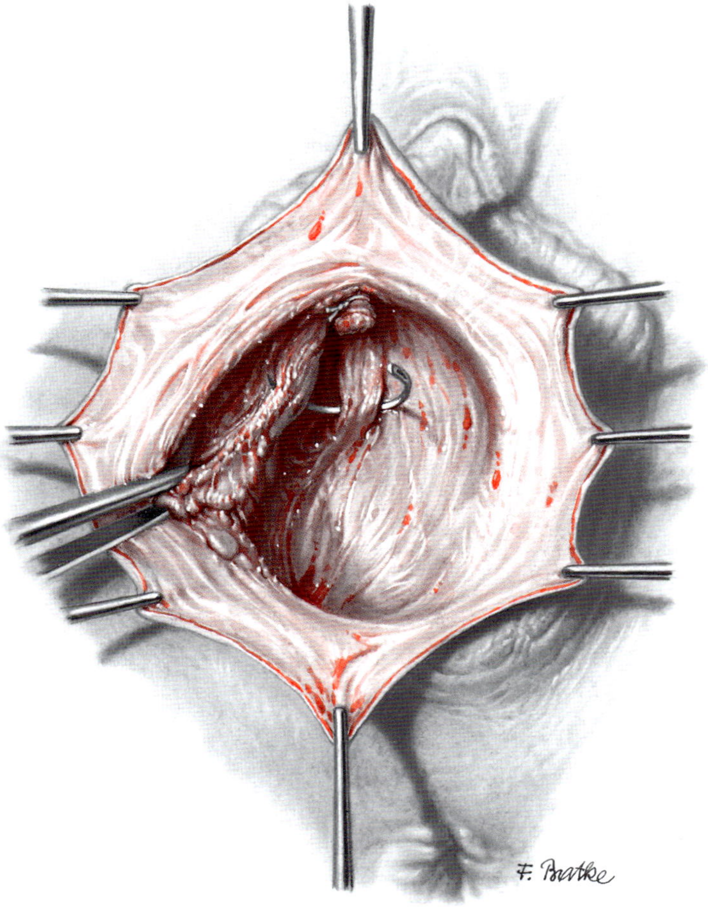

Figure 10.8. Right bartholinectomy. Closing the wound cavity.

The wound cavity is closed with multilayered interrupted catgut sutures after precise hemostasis has been performed. Note that medially relatively little tissue is taken on the needle because the rectum is here in immediate proximity.

Parts of the wound edges that are thinned are resected, if necessary, and the freshened skin edges are united with fine silk sutures.

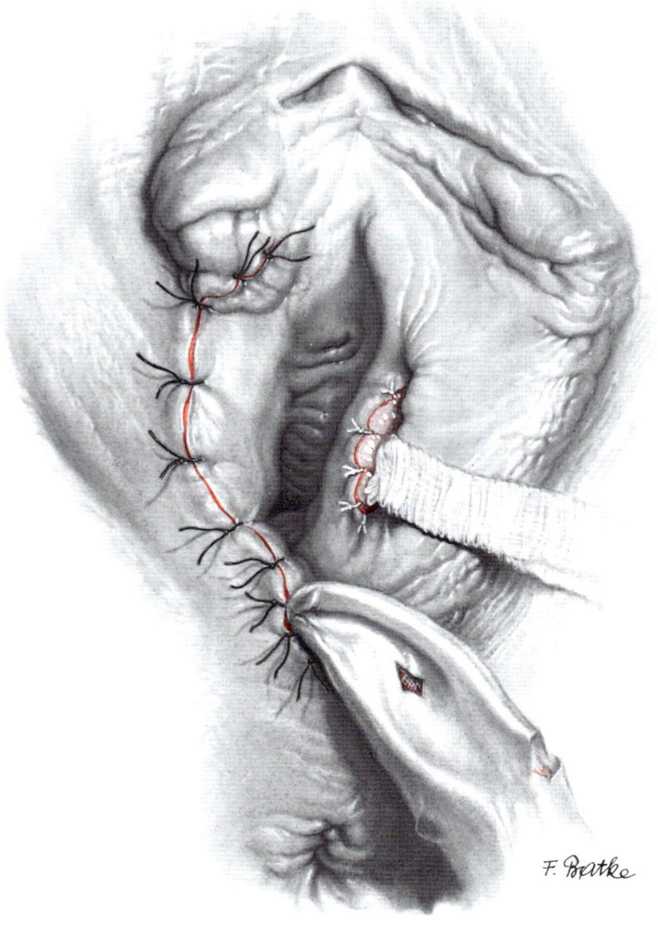

Figure 10.9. View after marsupialization (*left*) and bartholinectomy (*right*).

The cyst cavity on the marsupialization side is drained with a gauze strip.

On the bartholinectomy side, after the cyst was enucleated, most of the thinned labial skin had to be resected. This wound cavity is drained with a Penrose drain.

Observe the considerable cosmetic difference between these surgical methods.

TECHNICAL PROBLEMS—FIGURES 10.4–10.8

1. If the *cyst wall is perforated* during dissection of the cyst, the margins of the evacuated cyst will become difficult to identify; a portion of the gland is often left, and recurrence can be expected.
2. *Mobilization* of the cyst should not be started at the upper pole. This will cause severe hemorrhage from the nearby vestibular bulb. Moreover, by not first freeing up the lower pole, one no longer has the attached pedicle to aid in identifying the remaining glandular parenchyma, and an incomplete resection of the gland may result.
3. The posterior aspect of the cyst may be *dissected too closely to the rectum*, causing injury. Dissection under the guidance of a finger in the rectum will prevent such injury, although one must be careful not to perforate the thinned anterior rectal wall with the finger.
4. To avoid recurrences, the retention cyst as well as the entire glandular parenchyma must be removed. If this is not done, the remaining glands will continue to secrete mucus, which has no means for drainage into the vestibule, and a new cyst may later be formed. The noncystic portion of the Bartholin's glandular parenchyma can be delineated by palpation. In contrast to the soft surrounding tissue, it feels firm. The glandular parenchyma often reaches far upward underneath the bulbocavernous muscle. Such extensions should be clamped and then resected to ensure that bleeding will not occur.
5. Insufficient hemostasis of the large wound cavity can lead to formation of a massive hematoma postoperatively. If precise hemostasis cannot be conducted, drainage with a gauze wick or fine Penrose drain should be instituted for 24 hours.
6. If pus has been unexpectedly encountered during the incision of a *pseudo* retention cyst, one should first split open the abscess widely and perform marsupialization and drain the abscess cavity. If it recurs, it should be excised later after a quiescent interval.

11/ Vaginal Hysterectomy

Basic Operation

Indications

During the decision making that leads to recommendation for surgical removal of the uterus, there is no room for dogmatic explanation. As surgeons have gained experience in the art of vaginal surgery, it has become clear that patient recovery time after a vaginal hysterectomy is considerably better than after an abdominal hysterectomy. Furthermore, when one considers its cosmetic aspect, vaginal hysterectomy by far surpasses other methods (abdominal, laparoscopic) because there is not even a small abdominal incision. Finally, the vaginal surgical procedure offers optimal opportunity to correct already existing problems of vaginal wall and bladder prolapse.

For several years, the media has criticized the frequency of hysterectomy procedures, which to them appears to be too high. Actually, the frequency of operations fluctuates considerably among countries and regions, whereas the frequency for disease is stable. The problem lies with the indication statement itself. The real question is not whether too many hysterectomies have been performed but whether these procedures are truly indicated. However, the question about the ''right'' indication has always been under discussion and will remain so.

From a clinical viewpoint, a valid indication statement must be based on the following considerations.

1. The sum of all complaints will be improved by a hysterectomy.
2. The percentage rate of surgical complications must be so minimal and women who have undergone a hysterectomy should be so obviously content that later discussions about pros and cons need not even arise. Important contributing factors follow.
   - The quality of the surgeon must be first-rate; he or she must exhibit superior mastery of the techniques for vaginal operations.
   - The patient must be reassured before surgery that capability for orgasm is retained. This will ensure that women do not view a hysterectomy in context with a loss of femininity.

We have performed more than 2000 vaginal hysterectomies without the death of a single patient. Changes in position of the uterus (descent, prolapse: 40%), myomatous uterus (30%), and recurring climacteric bleeding (4.5%) provide the main indications. In addition, vaginal hysterectomy (*beyond the age of 40*) is gaining more importance under the following circumstances.

- A vaginal hysterectomy that retains the adnexa may be considered a *preventive measure for reducing the death rate from carcinoma*, even though the 30% rate of participation in Pap smears is relatively low and is not expected to improve (despite educational campaigns ongoing for decades). The probability for death caused by cancer of the uterus among women between age 35 and 65 is approximately 1.5%. In contrast, the primary death rate for vaginal hysterectomy is 0 to 0.05% and thus obviously below the mortality rate for uterine carcinoma. This proves that vaginal hysterectomy contributes to preventative measures taken to lower carcinoma mortality.

Endometrial hyperplasia, cervical dysplasia, and especially carcinoma-in-situ incompletely removed during conization are further indications for vaginal hysterectomy.

In addition, we offer for discussion the following argument: a vaginal hysterectomy may be used as a *final means of contraception* in women older than 40 who have chosen to limit the size of their family, because hormonal contraception measures during the next 10 years of their life means an unphysiologic reduction in production of their own hormones. After all, the treatment for adverse menopausal symptoms and prophylaxis for osteoporosis is less problematic when the uterus has been removed.

However, in cases of extended indication for ordinary vaginal hysterectomy with adnexal retention among women older than 40, one must consider on an individual basis the psychological aspects and sexual reactions that may affect women who have had their uterus removed. While giving due weight to the tendency to extend indications for uterine extirpation, we paid particular attention to the following problems.

For 35- to 40-year-old women, there was no radioimmunological increase detected in the amount of follicle-stimulating and luteinizing hormone concentration after a hysterectomy with adnexal retention.

Another study followed more than 1000 hysterectomy cases of women in childbearing years who were no older than 45 at the time of their hysterectomy and who were examined 1.5–8 years after the procedure. Comparison of these cases with a control group (350 women of childbearing age who did not have the operation) yielded the following results:

- 92% of the women who had the operation did not suffer from the absence of menstruation, and among the remaining 8%, most women had been insufficiently prepared for this consequence before their operation.
- Desire for intercourse remained almost the same or was even slightly higher among the operated women compared with those in the control group.
- Frequency of intercourse increased among women who had the operation because fear of pregnancy was no longer a factor.
- Among 10% of the operated women, dyspareunia occurred; 4% of the women regretted their choice for the operation. This may be due to poor technique while performing

a colporrhaphy, which often becomes necessary during a hysterectomy (this may result in scar formation or in a vagina that is too narrow as a consequence of a colpoperineoplasty).

- Vaginal hysterectomies have an extremely low *mortality record.*

Extended indication for sexually active women older than 40 should include especially careful patient preparation in cooperation with the internist. In addition, thorough and informative dialogue should take place before surgery—preferably in her partner's presence—during which the physiology of hormones is discussed. This is done to guard the woman against postoperative psychosexual disorders. After such an extended (although time-consuming) discussion, both partners should indicate their agreement to the operation.

The following must be regarded as *prerequisites* for a vaginal hysterectomy.

- Mobility and easy access to the uterus and good adnexal mobility.
- Concerning the size of an uterine myoma, opinions differ regarding whether to use the vaginal or abdominal approach, because the surgeon's experience and practice are the deciding factors. A general rule might be that as long as the myomatous enlarged uterus may be pulled into the false pelvis (which corresponds in uterine size to pregnancy in the fourth to fifth month) one may choose the vaginal approach in cases of primiparae as well as multiparae. Even in cases where the uterus has surpassed the size of an infant's head, the experienced and well-practiced surgeon may apply the technique of uterine bisection and morcellation and finish the operation vaginally (Fig. 11.2).
- The size of the vagina is relatively unimportant in the choice for the vaginal approach to surgery. In most cases, the vagina is easily stretched during anesthesia; if necessary, it may be widened with the aid of a Schuchardt incision. The surgeon who masters the vaginal technique will tend to operate vaginally more often, as his or her experience and practice increase. Even extensive vaginal operations are extremely well tolerated by patients.

Contraindications

Contraindications include patients with scar tissue, inflamed or endometrial changes of the adnexa, and ovarian tumors. In addition, patients with several prior laparotomies (including a perforated appendix) and those with abscesses of the cul-de-sac of Douglas in anamnesis must be excluded from a vaginal hysterectomy because adhesion formation is to be expected in such cases.

Reasons to avoid the vaginal route of hysterectomy may include patients with adhesive disease, inflammatory processes, or endometriosis of the adnexa, as well as ovarian tumors. Additionally, patients with several prior laparotomies (especially for a perforated appendix), and those with a history of cul-de-sac abscesses must be excluded from the vaginal approach because adhesions are to be expected.

Technique

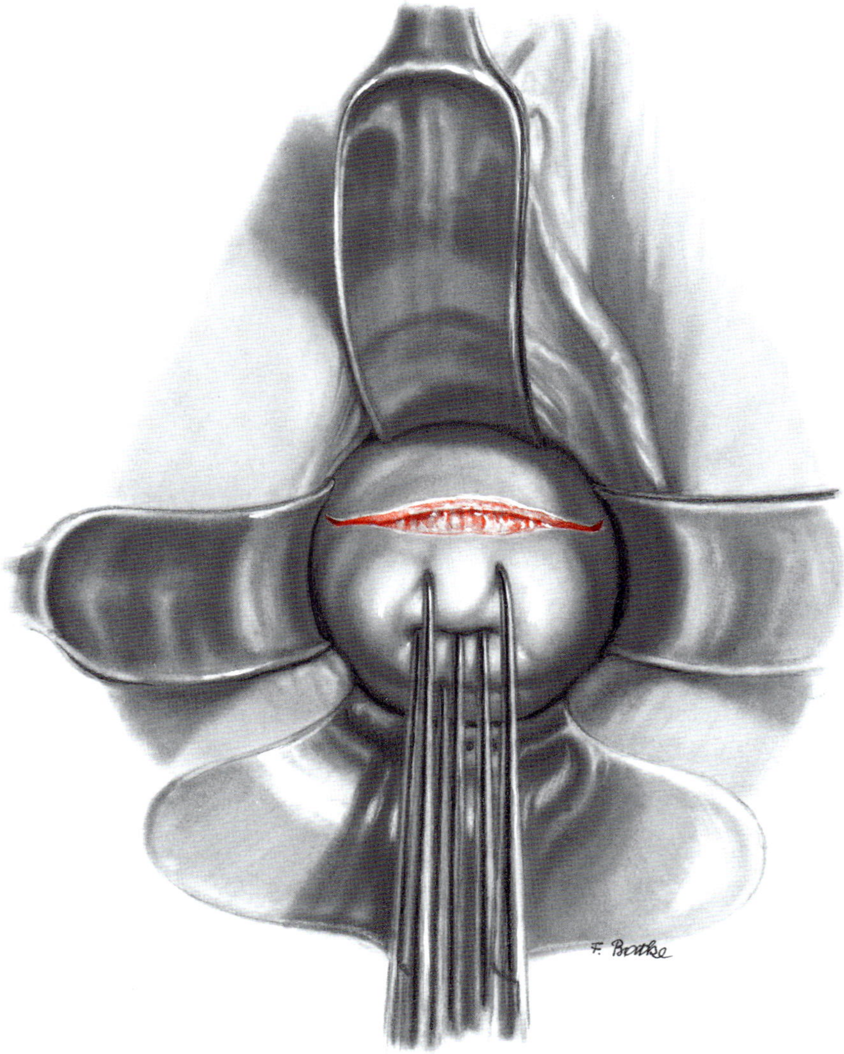

Figure 11.1. Vaginal hysterectomy. Anterior vaginal circumcision.

The vagina is spread by four retractors (anterior and right side by the right assistant, posterior and left side by the left assistant). The anterior lip of the cervix is grasped with two single-toothed tenacula and the posterior lip with one tenaculum, and the uterus is pulled down. This causes the upper part of the vagina to invert.

Vaginal circumcision provides access to the vesicovaginal space anteriorly and the rectovaginal space posteriorly.

The anterior circumcision is performed immediately above the transition of the smooth portio wall into the wrinkled vaginal wall mucosa. One identifies this border by moving the tenacula on the portio up and down. The circumcision is begun in the anterior vaginal fornix in a curved incision, its curve somewhat elongated upward on both sides.

With this curved incision, which posteriorly runs parallel to the anterior incision, the cranial opening of the vaginal canal is larger than that produced by a circular incision. This allows more space for the following surgical procedures.

At first the depth of the incision reaches only through the vaginal mucosa; it is deepened in its midsection only as the exposed vaginal fascia is severed and the vesicovaginal space is opened.

A typical sign for the surgeon to know that he or she is working in the proper anterior region is that the bladder and its covering fascia will retreat cranially up to the cervix when pressure is applied by the retractor.

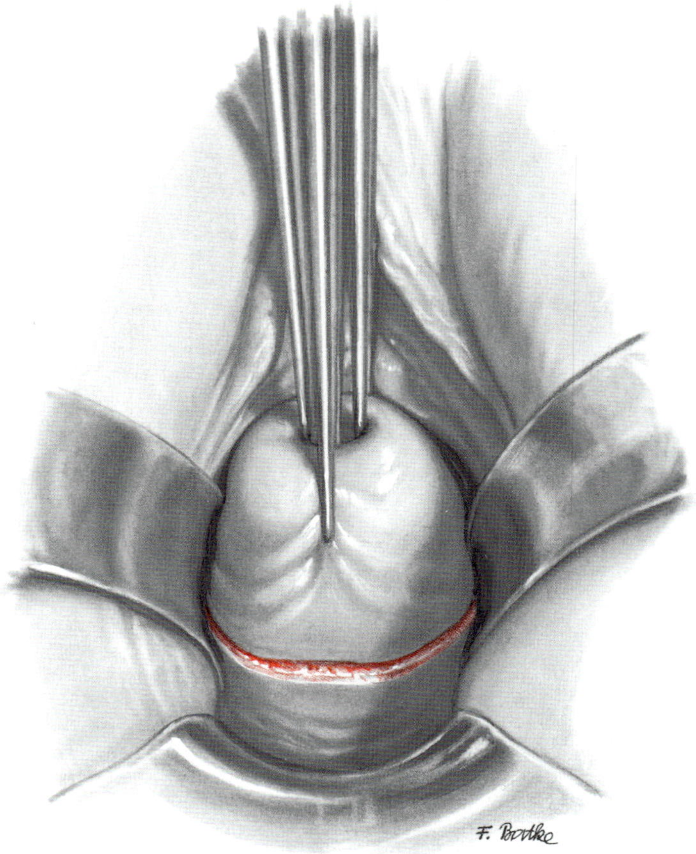

Figure 11.2. Vaginal hysterectomy. Posterior vaginal circumcision.

It begins at the right end of the anterior incision and courses in a bow shape to meet the left end of the vaginal circumcision.

Both the vaginal wall and vaginal fascia are cut in the midline (which opens the rectrovaginal space), whereas at the lateral parts of the circumcision the vaginal wall alone is incised.

These lateral parts of the circumcision serve only as a demarcation line where the parametrial sutures will be anchored later.

Technical Problems—Figure 11.2

1. If the incision is made *too far caudally* in the smooth cervical wall, rather than anteriorly in the vaginal fornix, one cannot open the vesicovaginal space nor can the supravaginal space be reached. Moreover, the lower bladder pole will be fixed to the anterior cervix in the vesicovaginal space by dense connective tissue, making it difficult to separate the bladder from the cervix later.
2. If the circumcision is *not performed deep enough* so that the vaginal fascia is not penetrated, the vesicovaginal space is not opened. As a result, the view of the tissue layers becomes obstructed, and attempts to dissect the lower bladder pole may result in damage to the bladder by virtue of the fact that one is dissecting too close to it.
3. If the circumcision is performed *too deeply laterally*, the vaginal wall and the vaginal fascia are penetrated. Unnecessary bleeding will ensue from injuries to the veins of the vaginal plexus coursing in the lateral aspects of the vaginal fascia.
4. The circumcision can be conducted *in the posterior fornix too close to the cervix* while dissecting the rectum. In such a case, one comes too close to the cervix and may be dissecting in the wrong tissue layer so that the cul-de-sac of Douglas is found only with great difficulty. One may think the problem is due to adhesions, but this is not the case; instead, one has been deluded by the original error in dissection.

Figure 11.3. Vaginal hysterectomy. The supravaginal septum is divided.

The circumcision has been completed. The tenacula were repositioned anteriorly and posteriorly; their external claws grasp the vaginal wound edge of the circumcision and make the wound gape more.

The left assistant uses a downward pulling motion with the tenacula, while counterpressure is applied upward with the anterior blade. Thus fibers of the supravaginal septum, which course medially from the anterior surface of the cervix to the lower pole of the bladder, are stretched. The supravaginal septum forms the border between the vesicovaginal and the vesicocervical space.

The surgeon lifts up the lower pole of the bladder with toothed tissue forceps and dissects the fibers stretching toward median of the supravaginal septum near the cervix. Tips of the curved scissors should point toward the cervix.

After dividing the supravaginal septum, the lower pole of the bladder can be easily pushed above the peritoneal reflection with the index finger.

Detail. Place of dissection of supravaginal septum.

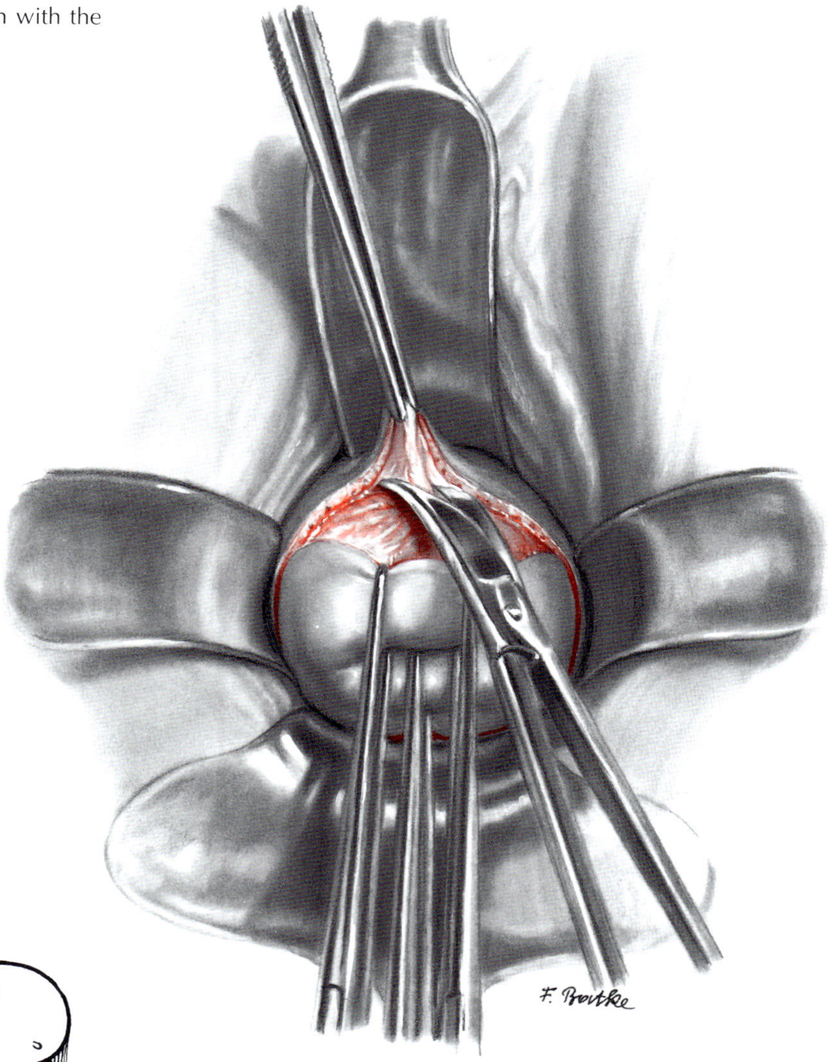

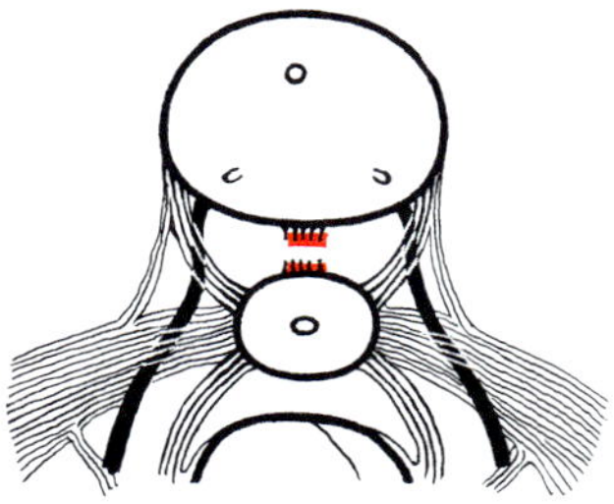

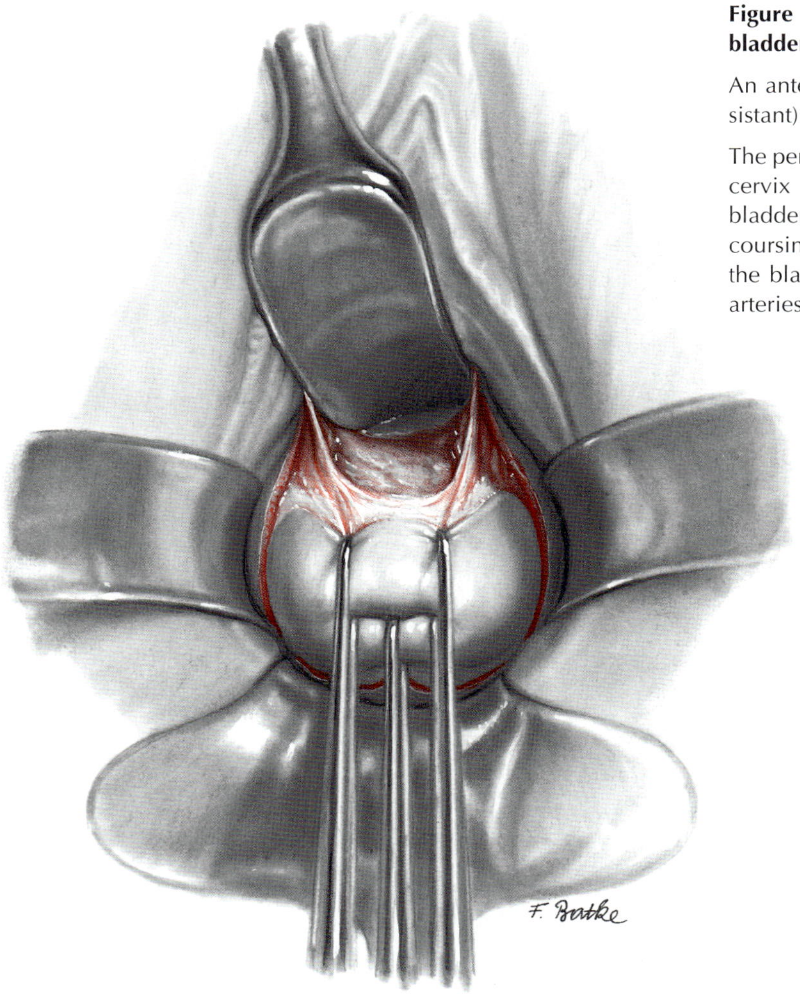

Figure 11.4. Vaginal hysterectomy. Dissection off the urinary bladder.

An anterior retractor inserted in the vesicocervical space (right assistant) advances the mobilized lower bladder pole.

The peritoneal reflection becomes visible on the anterior wall of the cervix as a tongue-shaped, shiny white membrane. Laterally, the bladder pillars (vesicouterine ligaments) are stretched; its fibers coursing from the bladder to the cervix. Portions of the ureters enter the bladder near here. Medially to the bladder pillars the uterine arteries can be seen at the edge of the cervix.

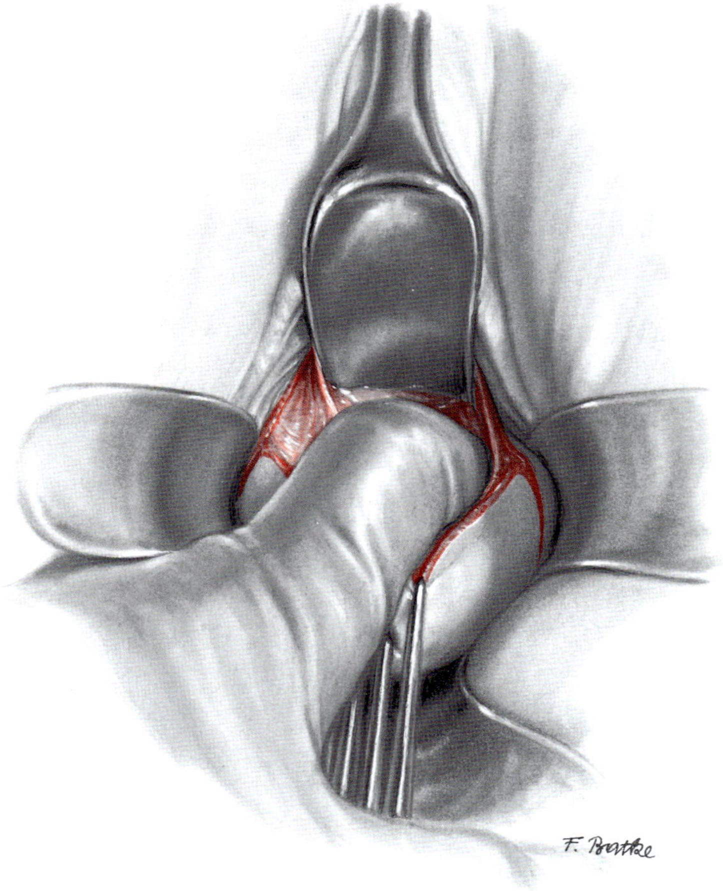

Figure 11.5. Vaginal hysterectomy. Displacing the ureter.

The bladder is held up by the right assistant with a retractor inserted in the vesicocervical space.

To avoid endangering the ureter (coursing through the bladder pillars) during later ligation and dissection of the parametria, the surgeon pushes away the bladder pillar fibers to the sides bilaterally with the index finger until the ureters are displaced well out of the operative field.

Detail. Displacement of left ureter.

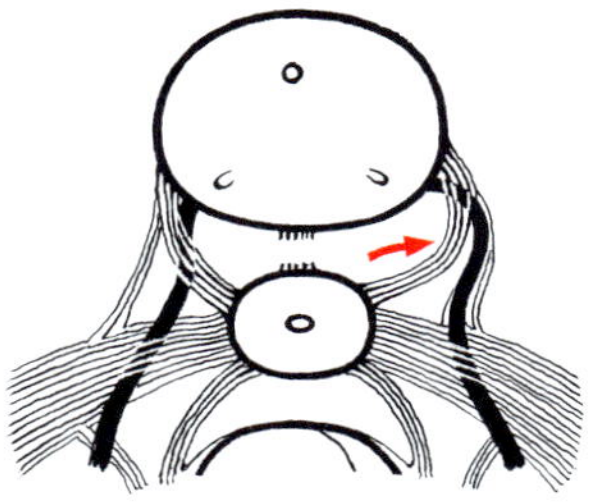

Technical Problems—Figures 11.3–11.5

1. If the assistant elevates the anterior vaginal wall *with the anterior retractor too strongly*, the surgeon cannot lift the lower pole of the bladder enough, and the fibers of the supravaginal septum are insufficiently stretched.
2. When sharply dissecting the fibers of the supravaginal septum, the *fibers may only be partially incised*. If this occurs and one disregards the remaining connective tissue fibers of the septum that fix the bladder densely to the anterior wall of the cervix, the bladder wall can be damaged by bluntly displacing the partially mobilized lower bladder pole with the finger or by increased anterior retractor pressure. Most instances of inadvertent bladder entries occur in this manner.
3. If one severs the supravaginal septum *too close to the cervix* (an error often made by the novice for fear of injuring the bladder) then the vesicocervical space will not be reached. Instead one will be probing laboriously into the cervical wall, presuming incorrectly that the faulty planes are the result of a previous infection. This is the lesser worry. To extricate oneself from this maze, one should locate the lower pole of the bladder with a blunt probe inserted into the bladder through the urethra. In this way one will determine if the dissection has come too close to the cervix. Conversely, if the supravaginal septum is dissected *too close to the bladder*, the bladder may be injured or even entered. This can happen easily and is more likely if the lower bladder pole is not pulled up sufficiently with toothed forceps so the fibers of the supravaginal septum are insufficiently stretched while one is sharply dividing the fibers of the septum.

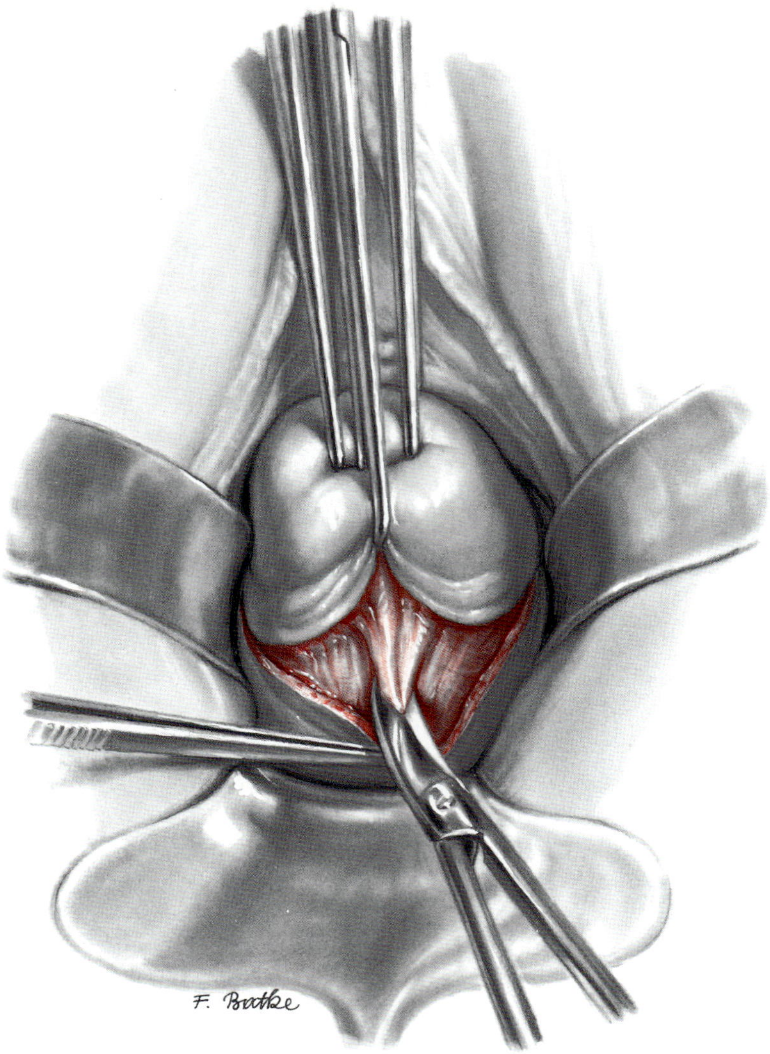

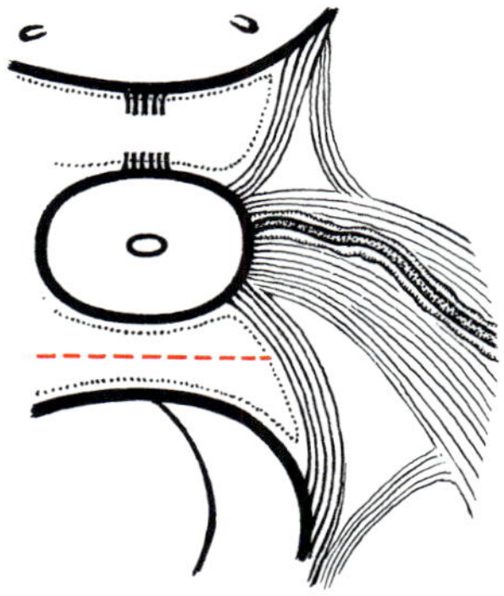

Figure 11.6. Vaginal hysterectomy. Opening the cul-de-sac of Douglas.

The uterus is pulled steeply upward on the tenacula by the right assistant; the posterior tenaculum has likewise been "repositioned" and grasps the posterior portio wound edge. The surgeon pulls the posterior vaginal wound edge outward with tissue forceps while pushing the perirectal connective tissue fibers downward with slightly opened dissecting scissors and dissects the rectum caudally. The midline portion of the posterior vaginal wound now gapes widely.

Now the rectouterine fold is pulled down medially with toothed tissue forceps. This causes the cul-de-sac peritoneum to stretch as a sagittal fold, and the space of Douglas is opened just above the forceps with a transverse scissors cut. The scissor blades point toward the cervix.

Detail. Location of cul-de-sac of Douglas opening.

TECHNICAL PROBLEMS—FIGURE 11.6

1. While dissecting the rectum from the posterior vaginal wall and from the cervix, one may approach *too closely to the uterus* with the scissors because of fear of injuring the rectum. In such a case the posterior peritoneal reflection is dissected further away from the posterior wall of the uterus so that the cul-de-sac is not opened because one is opening in the wrong layer. The situation is corrected by grasping the freed fold near the uterus with a toothed clamp, pulling it up and incising it transversally just caudally to the clamp. This will make it possible to open the space of Douglas.

2. If the *rectum* has been displaced from the median aspects of the circumcision wound and is dissected *laterally*, the vessels coursing in the fibers of the rectal pillars may be damaged.

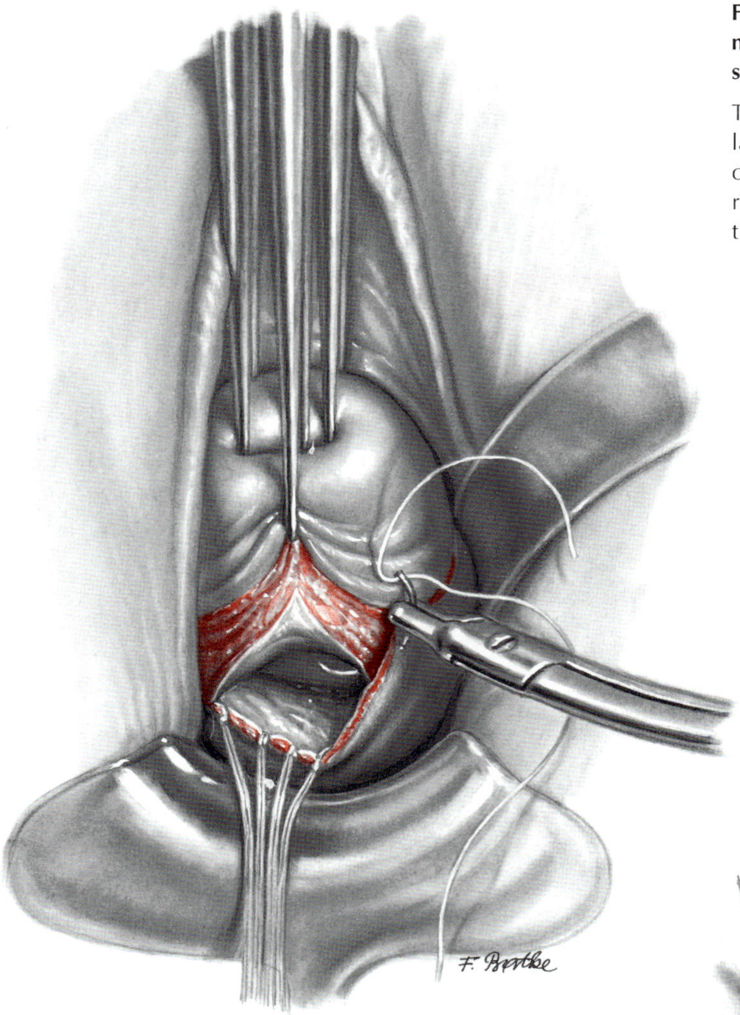

Figure 11.7. Vaginal hysterectomy. Fixing the posterior peritoneal cut edge to the posterior vaginal wound edge. Interrupted sutures.

The space of Douglas has been opened. On the right side, the Douglas peritoneum has been fixed with four sutures. This is continued on the left side. This achieves hemostasis in the vaginal wound edge region and exposes the entrance to the space of Douglas. Ends of the sutures are left long, held in a clamp, and used as a marker.

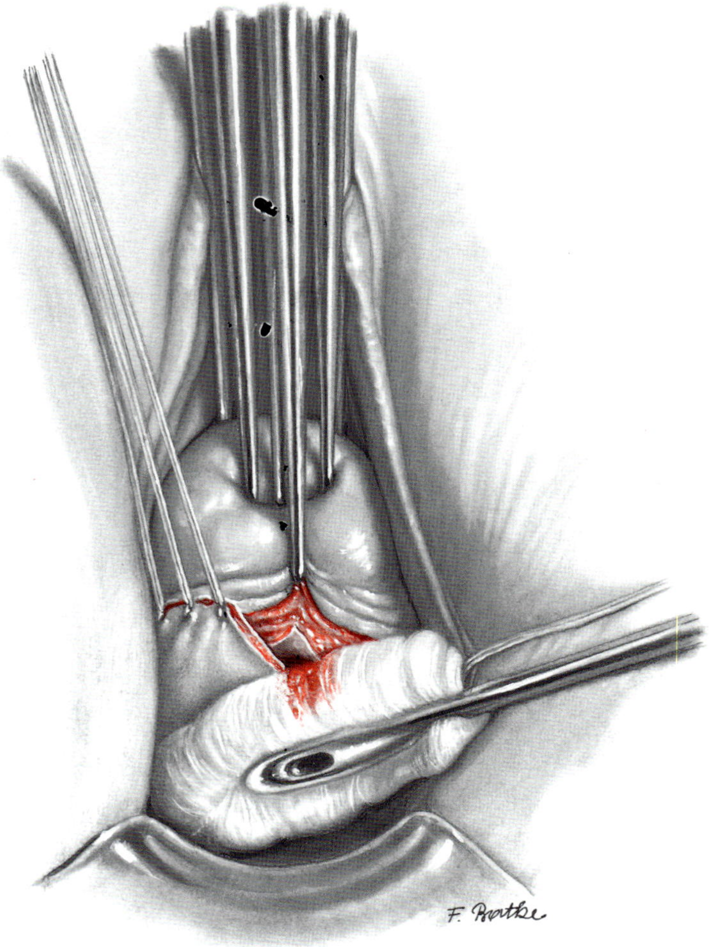

Figure 11.8. Vaginal hysterectomy. Removing blood from the peritoneal cavity.

The assistant will not insert the sponge forceps into the space of Douglas because such pressure on the delicate peritoneal leaf will tear out the posterior vaginal sutures. Instead, the posterior vaginal wall is pushed against the posterior cervix with the sponge forceps. This will express the blood collected in the peritoneal cavity.

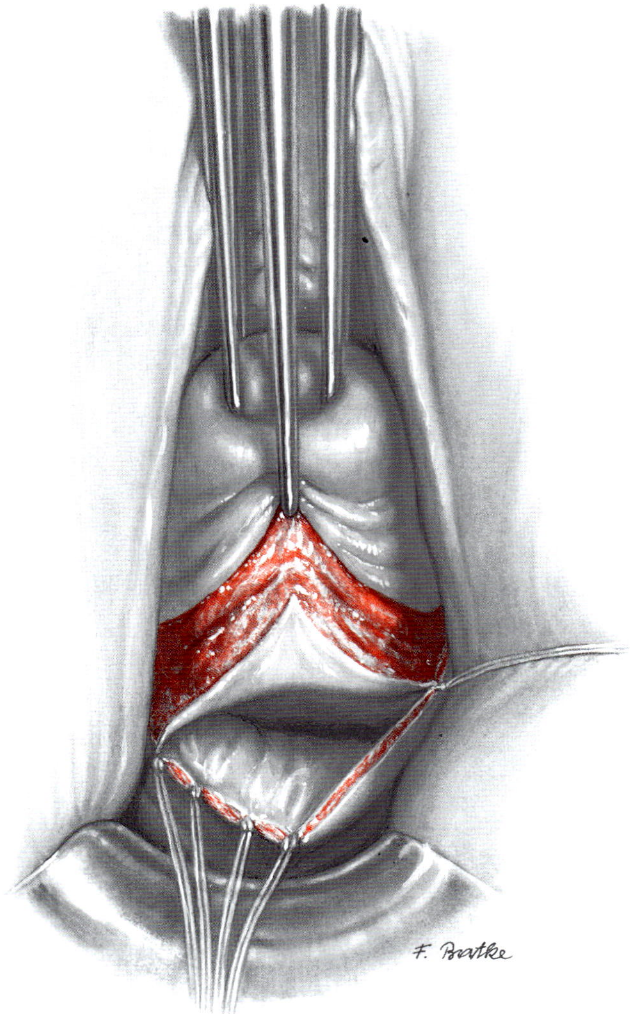

Figure 11.9. Vaginal hysterectomy. Additional interrupted sutures.

The posterior peritoneal cavity gapes to show the absence of blood: the cut edge is now fully exposed and can be fixed to the posterior vaginal wound edge.

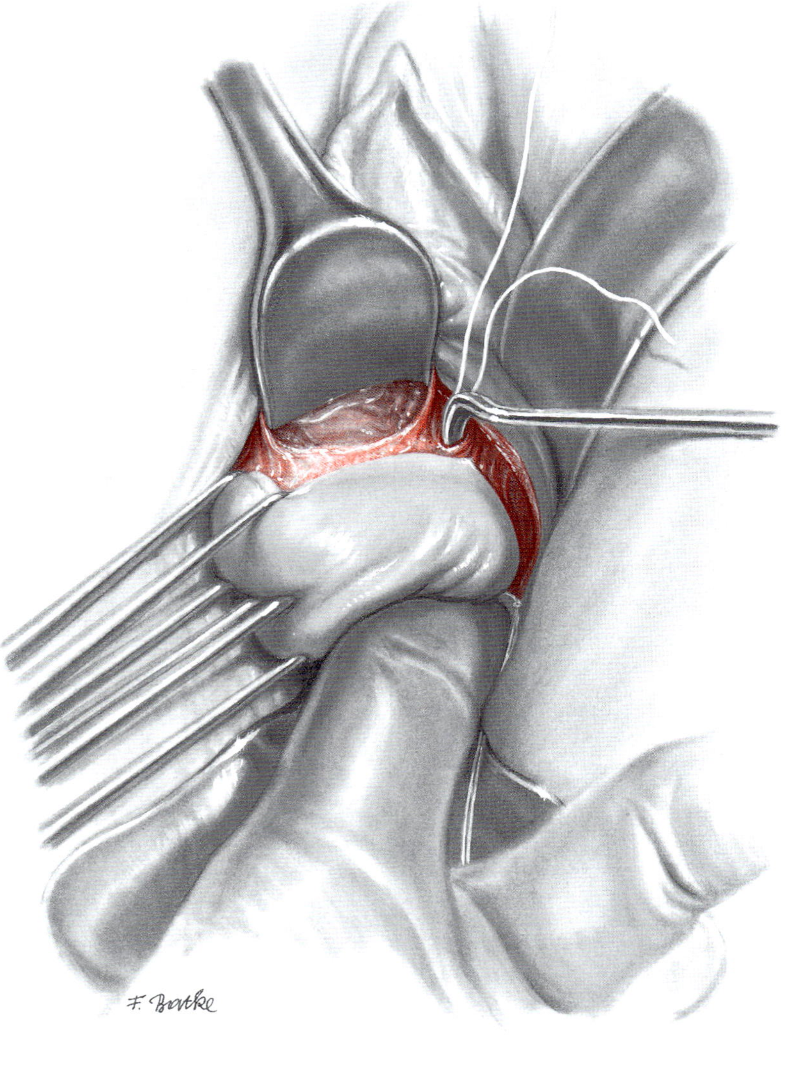

Figure 11.10. Vaginal hysterectomy. Ligation and retraction of the left parametria. First suture of the uterosacral ligament.

The portio is pulled toward the right with the single-toothed tenacula. The mobilized lower bladder pillar is advanced upward to the right with a retractor inserted into the vesicocervical space. The anterior peritoneum has not yet been opened; this avoids prolapse of the intestinal loop.

The surgeon places the left index finger (palmar surface turned upward) into the open space of Douglas and grasps the left parametrial tissue bundle so that the fingertip lies at the edge of the uterus. He or she partially ligates the posterior aspects of the parametrium using a flat curved Deschamps needle; placement is guided from above down with the finger. The right assistant slowly raises the portio with single-toothed tenacula so that the tip of the needle is visible and the suture is easily pulled through with the small thread hook.

The knot of the ligature is tied in the groove formed at the lateral vaginal circumcision.

Medial from the Deschamps needle the left uterine vascular bundle is visible, which had not been included in the first parametrial ligature.

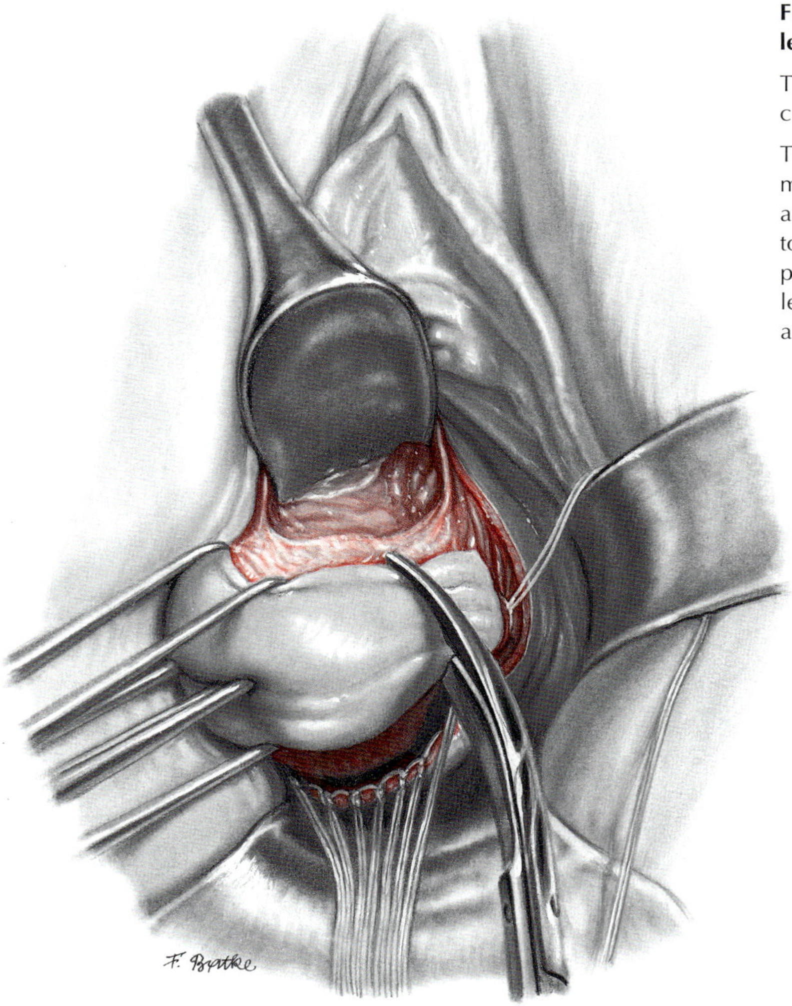

Figure 11.11. Vaginal hysterectomy. Partial division of the left parametrium.

The first parametrial suture is tied in the groove that had been created laterally during vaginal circumcision.

The posterior parametrial tissue bands are severed approximately 1 cm distally from the ligature. Sharply curved scissors are used to make the incision; scissor points should be directed toward the portio, angulated in to the border of the cervix and parallel to the ligature. A small piece of the portio mucosa is left on the stump to broaden the distal end of the stump and anchor the ligature on the stump still more securely.

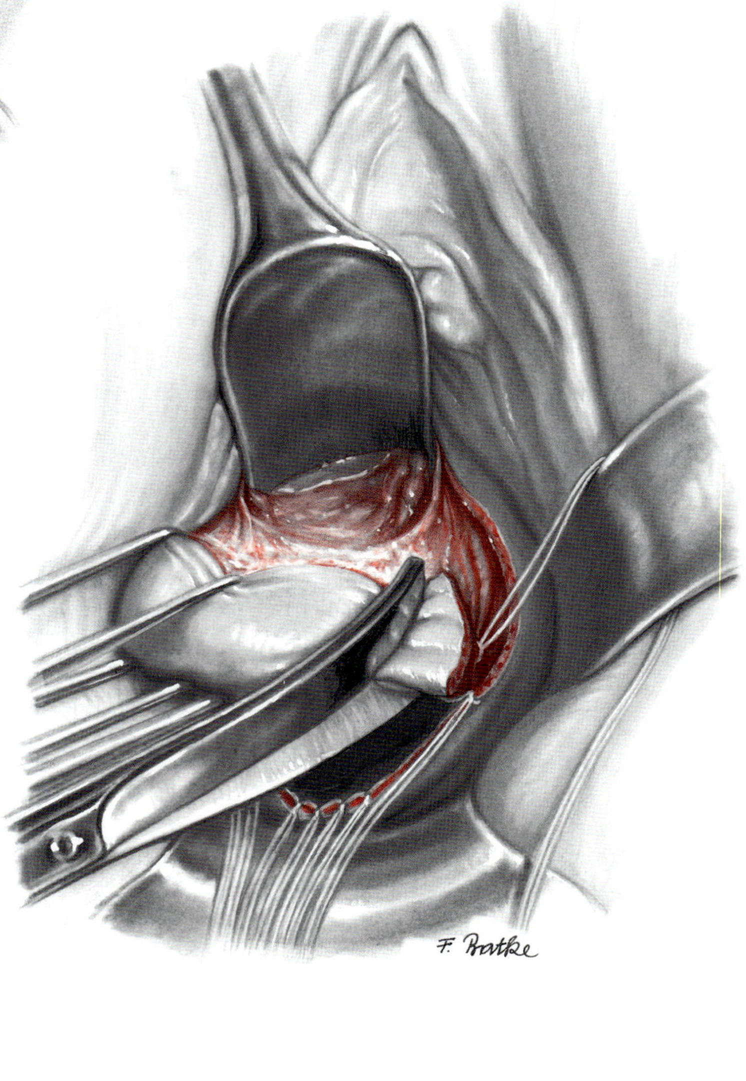

Figure 11.12. Vaginal hysterectomy. Incorrectly incising during division of the parametrium.

Blades of the scissors are not being held diagonally to the cervix but parallel to the edge; as a consequence, during division of the parametrium from the cervix, the upper fibers of the stump are cut short and may slip out of the ligature.

Figure 11.13. Vaginal hysterectomy. Ligating the left parametrium. Second suture.

The surgeon once more inserts the index finger into the space of Douglas to grasp the *entire* left lateral parametrium at the lateral edge of the cervix. By using a Deschamps needle, the uterine vascular bundle is now sutured together with the remaining unligated lateral parametrium and the previously ligated posterior parametrial connective tissue.

The anterior parametrium (vesicouterine ligament, bladder pillar) may not be included in this ligature because the ureter courses through it.

Detail. Space of Douglas is opened; cardinal ligament (lateral parametrium) is severed.

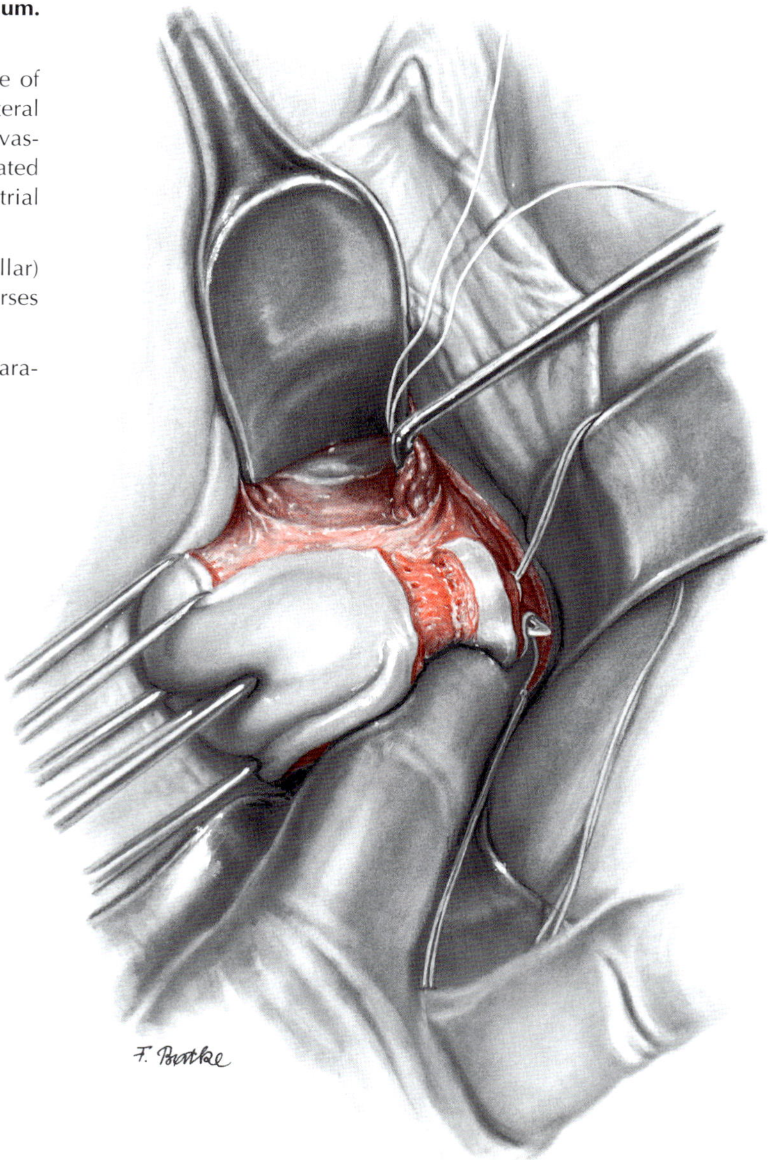

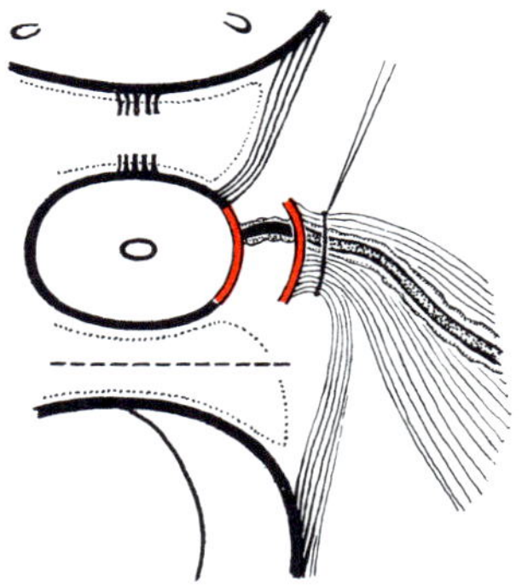

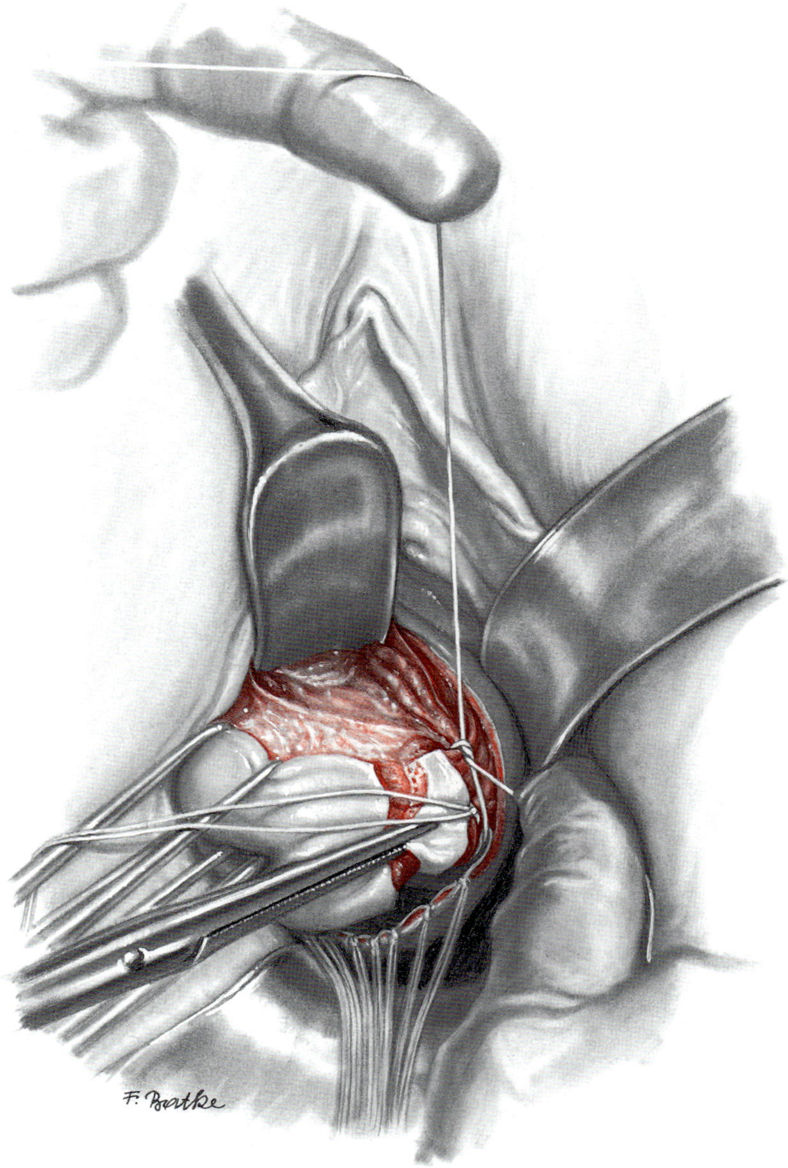

Figure 11.14. Vaginal hysterectomy. Anchoring the second parametrial ligature.

The suture of the first parametrial ligature is drawn over the tenacula to hang freely over the opposite side. Using moderate force, the right assistant grasps the parametrial stump with the right hand and, with a long toothed clamp, pulls it down to the right along with the tenacula.

The second parametrial suture is placed and tied cranially from the first in the groove of the lateral vaginal circumcision. Included in the second suture is the entire lateral and posterior parametrium.

The parametrial tissue bands are severed in the same manner used to create the first parametrial stump, diagonally to the cervical edge. However, the cranial aspects of the lateral parametrium are separated from the cervix only up to the point where the uterine vascular bundle becomes visible at the cervical border. Before its resection, it is once more separately ligated (see Fig. 11.15).

Detail. Left parametrium is doubly ligated and, except for the uterine vascular bundle, severed.

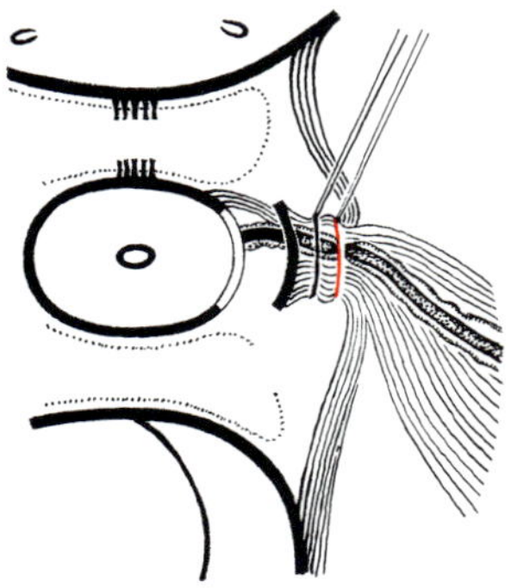

Figure 11.15. Vaginal hysterectomy. Dissecting the uterine vessels separately.

The left parametrium is doubly ligated; the left vaginal wall is *laterally* held back from the pedicle with a lateral retractor.

The unligated uterine vascular bundle is grasped separately with a short, strong, toothed clamp placed transversely to the cervical edge and then divided transversely distally to the clamp.

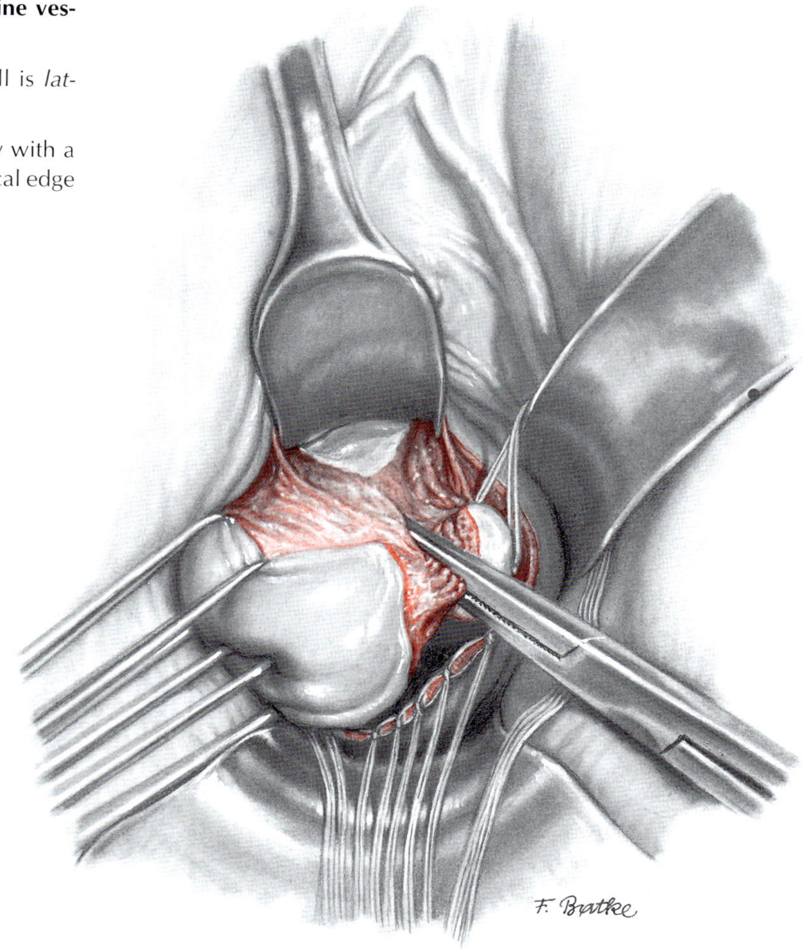

Figure 11.16. Vaginal hysterectomy. Dissecting the uterine vessels separately. Third parametrial ligature.

The uterine vascular bundle has been divided transversely at the cervical border. The clamp holding the end of the stump is turned up by the left assistant's left hand.

The vascular bundle is ligated with silk; however, the suture will not be left as a marker but immediately cut short.

The analogous procedure is performed on the other side to dissect the right parametria.

Detail. Ligation and resection of uterine artery.

The analogous procedure is performed on the other side to dissect the right parametria.

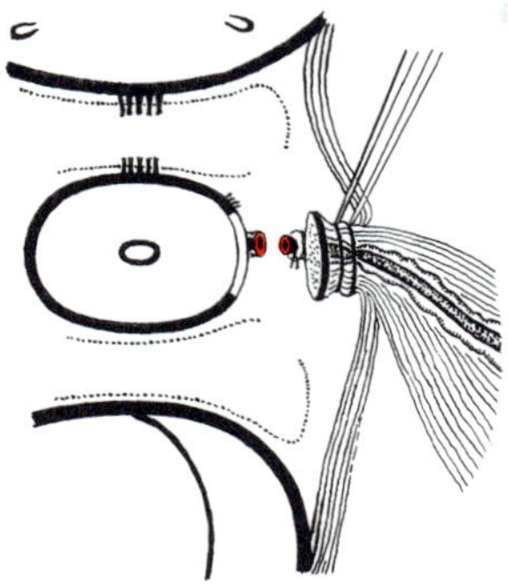

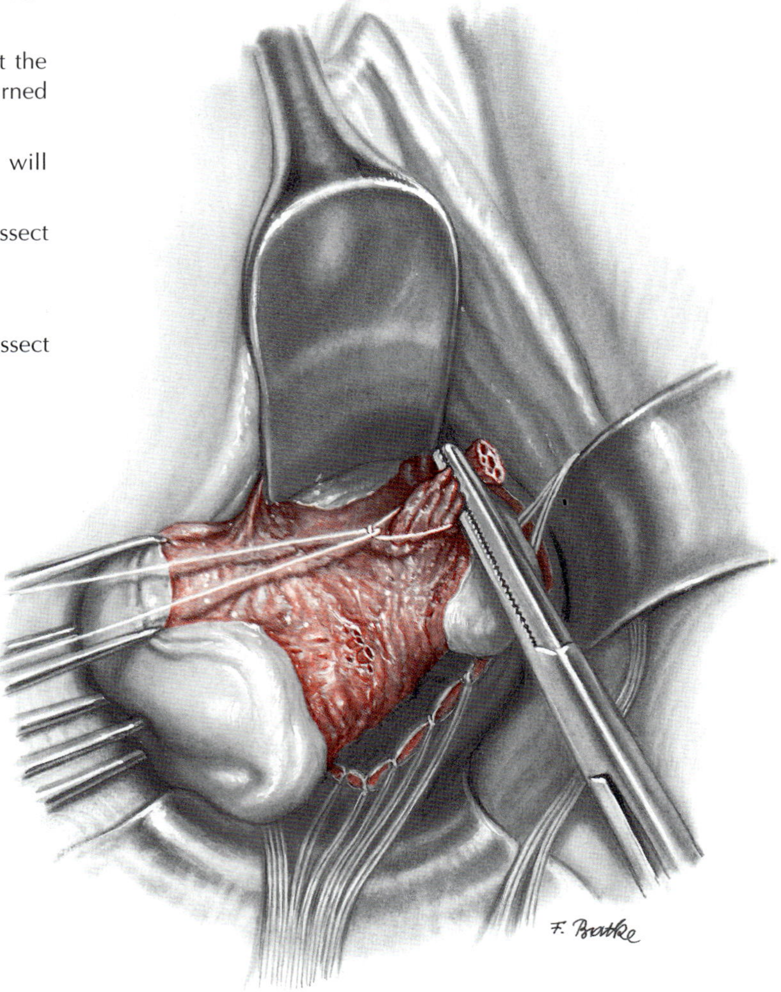

Alternative Techniques

The parametria can also be resected by the clamp method instead of ligating it with the Deschamps needle. For that purpose, strong toothed clamps are placed transversely on the parametrium alongside the cervical border. This approach may be used to advantage when the parametria are very short and rigid (Fig. 11.16).

Ligation of the parametrial tissue with a strong needle is a rewarding method as well. However, both parametrial dissection with clamps as well as suture ligation have the disadvantage that sometimes one cannot clamp or ligate high enough on the cervical border. In addition, sometimes the ligation or clamping may be too close to the edge of the cervix. It is even possible to suture into the cervical stroma or to catch some of the cervix with the clamp; if this happens, the ligature can slip off. Conversely, when one ligates with the Deschamps needle, the dull tip of the instrument is readily inserted high on the border of the cervix. Here, a close interaction between the surgeon's left index finger and the tip of the upward advancing Deschamps needle is desirable. This ensures that the needle can be applied closely to the cervical edge if the surgeon controls its placement carefully by palpation with the left index finger that is inserted in the space of Douglas and holds the parametrium. This is a particularly valuable approach, allowing one to ligate as far from the edge of the cervix as desired. Finally, the Deschamps method permits one to ligate the parametria securely above the uterine vascular pedicle and has the additional advantage that longer parametrial pedicles can be formed as one resects the tissue along the cervical edge. Ligatures applied to these pedicles do not come off easily.

Technical Problems—Figures 11.10–11.16

1. If the entire lateral parametrium and uterosacral ligament are jointly ligated *with one suture* and resected from the edge of the cervix, the pedicle may be so thick that parts of it may later slip out of the ligature. Where the parametria are very thick and foreshortened, we advise ligation of the uterosacral ligament alone and perhaps even suture and division of the lateral parametrium piecemeal before separate ligation of the uterine vessels with an individual suture. Ligating too much at a time risks the possibility of the ligature coming off.

2. Should the parametrial tissue bundle be *ligated too closely to the cervix*, there is great likelihood that the ligature will slip after the parametrium is dissected from the cervix because the pedicle will probably be too short.

3. If the ligated parametrial tissue bundles are *not cut diagonally to the cervical edge* but rather if the scissors blades are held parallel to the edge (Fig. 11.12), the cephalad aspects of the Mackenrodt ligament pedicle will have shorter fibers than the more caudad uterosacral ligament pedicle. This may often cause the ligature to slip away from the pedicles. Other errors that can result in the ligature slipping off the pedicles follow.

- The lateral retractor that *exerts pressure on the parametrial pedicle* may also press on the ligature. The surgeon should therefore take care that this retractor, when inserted by the assistant to spread the vaginal canal, is placed lateral to the parametrial pedicle so that only the vaginal wall is gently pushed aside. Similarly, if the assistant pulls the lateral retractor *upward too vigorously*, the ligature may come off because the uterus is being retracted downward at the same time by the tenaculum held by the other assistant.
- With *incomplete dissection* of the parametria *from the cervical edge*, the ligature can easily slip from the pedicles when the poorly mobilized uterus is rolled forward. This constitutes one of the most common mistakes. During division of the parametrium and the uterine vascular pedicle, one must also always dissect the peritoneum (which covers their posterior surface) carefully from the uterus because otherwise the uterus will adhere to these peritoneal connective tissues and the space in the posterior peritoneum will remain abnormally small, which impedes the progress of the operation.
- While tying the second cephalad parametrial ligature, if no clamp has been applied to the pedicle to pull it, *traction on the first parametrial ligature* may cause it to come off.

4. During division of the doubly ligated parametrium from the cervix, one may injure the *circumcised posterior vaginal wall with the scissors*, endangering the rectum. To avoid the complication, one uses the index finger in the cul-de-sac to ensure that the posterior vaginal edge does not adhere to the posterior cervical wall. If it does, one must push the posterior vagina caudally with the finger. In addition, during the parametrial separation, the tenacula on the cervical portio should be elevated somewhat so that one can visualize the space of Douglas.

5. If *the bladder pillar is included* during the uterine vascular ligation, the ureter coursing there may be at risk by being pulled very close to the operative field. This complication is avoided by the surgeon pushing the stretched medial fibers of the bladder pillars somewhat to either side with the right index finger; this is done after opening the vesicocervical space and subsequent to dissecting the lower bladder pole. This displaces the ureters laterally and upward so that there is no longer any risk that they will be caught in or pulled toward the parametrial ligature.

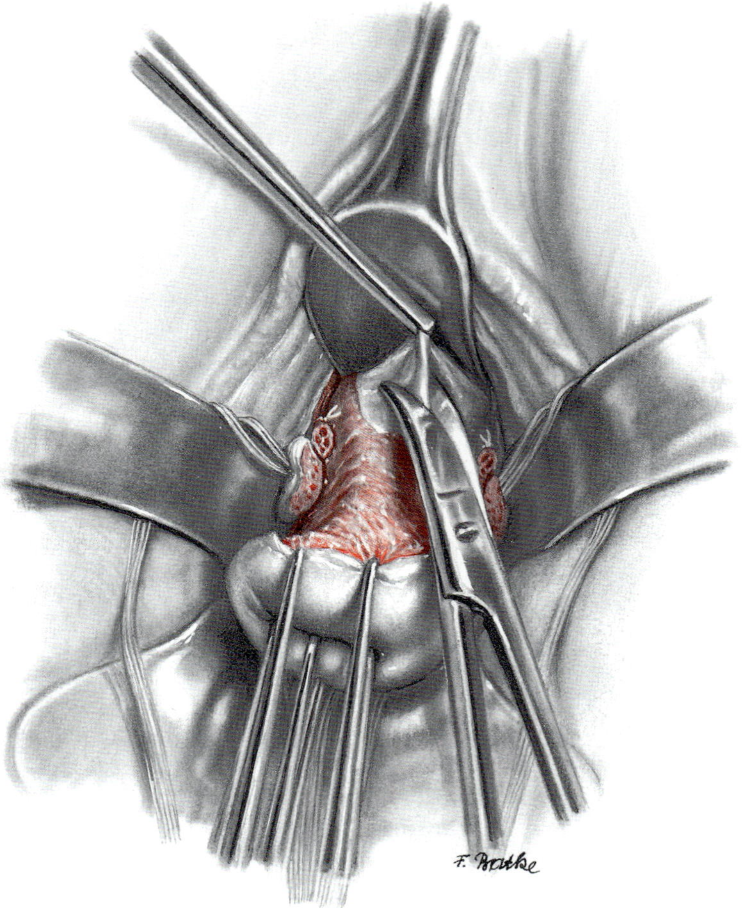

Figure 11.17. Vaginal hysterectomy. Opening the vesicouterine fold (peritoneum of the vesicouterine cavity).

Parametria have been ligated and resected several times on both sides. Long ends of the thread are hanging freely over the two lateral spatulas, which push the vaginal wall (situated laterally to the pedicles) to the side. Sutures of the separately ligated uterine vascular bundles are cut short.

The vesicouterine fold is grasped and lifted with tissue forceps and then incised close to the uterus.

If the peritoneal reflection is located high anteriorly because the vesicouterine excavation is occluded by adhesions from previous surgery or because the bladder peritoneum is fixed to the uterine fundus, the plica (fold) can be brought into view by means of a downward pull on the uterus with a tenaculum placed on the anterior cervical wall.

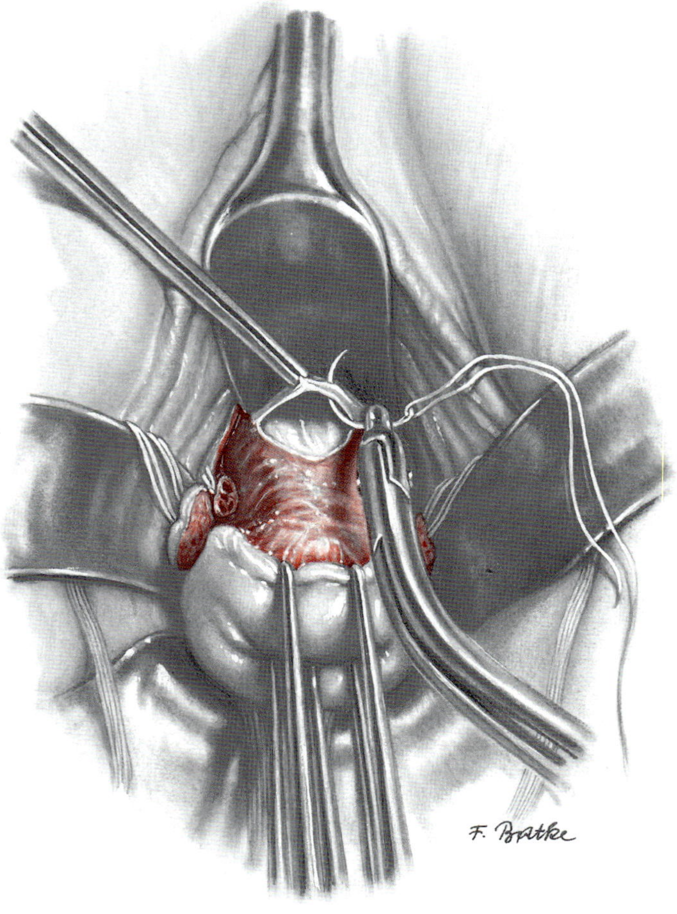

Figure 11.18. Vaginal hysterectomy. Suturing the anterior peritoneal wound edge.

A suture is placed at the vesical cut edge so that the usually retracted peritoneal wound edge can be pulled down later when the peritoneal cavity is being closed.

Because there is usually very little space here, fine silk and a small, delicate needle are used to suture the peritoneum.

An intraperitoneal retractor is inserted next, and a pack is inserted into the abdominal cavity to prevent the bowel from prolapsing.

TECHNICAL PROBLEMS—FIGURES 11.17 and 11.18

1. When the anterior peritoneal reflection is sought too far caudally, one dissects into the anterior cervical wall and is deluded into believing that dense adhesions exist.
2. If the vesicouterine fold was *insufficiently freed* at an earlier stage, some bladder tissue may still remain adherent to it; thus the bladder can be entered when this tissue is lifted with toothed forceps and then dissected with scissors.

The inadequately dissected bladder pole that is fixed to the anterior wall of the cervix may also be torn by excessive pressure on the anterior retractor. Therefore, when there is doubt about whether the tissue held in the forceps is peritoneal reflection or lower bladder pole, one should explore the bladder with a thick sound to locate the lower edge of the bladder pole from the inside.
3. If *silk* used for suture of the anterior peritoneal wound edge is *too heavy*, the peritoneal cut edge will tear at the slightest tug, especially the thin peritoneum of an obese woman.
4. When packing the bowel back, if the *gauze strip is inserted into the peritoneal cavity without retractor support*, the silk suture attached to the anterior peritoneal wound edge may tear out or the peritoneal opening may lacerate laterally.

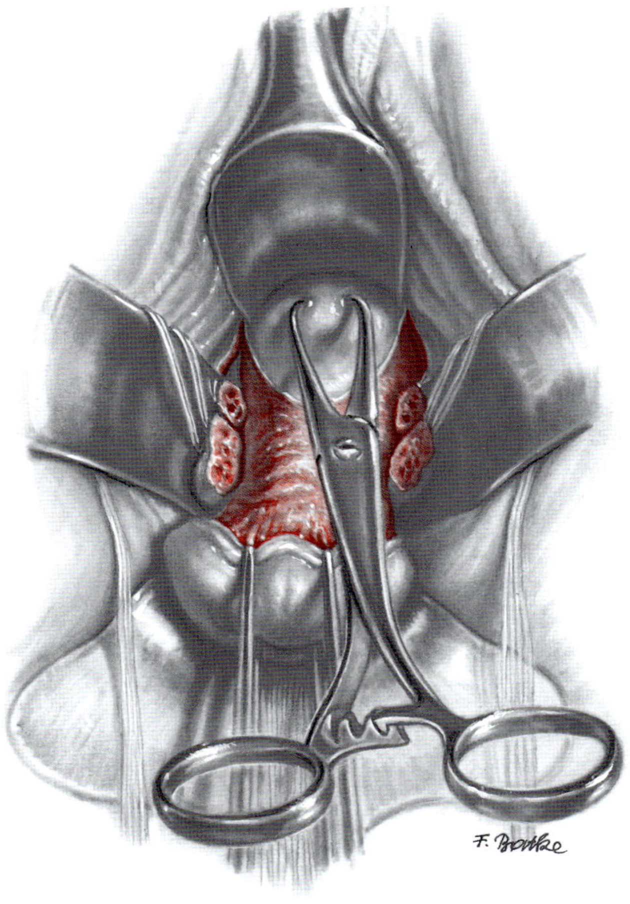

Figure 11.19. Vaginal hysterectomy. Anteverting the uterus.

A retractor inserted intraperitoneally strongly pushes the bladder and the anterior peritoneal wound edge upward. A tenaculum is placed on the anterior uterine wall, and one pulls downward.

For the normally sized uterus, this is successfully done by grasping the anterior uterine wall several times with single-toothed tenacula, progressively climbing upward to the fundus. If the uterus is enlarged, one can facilitate the uterine anteversion by simultaneously pushing the portio back into the abdominal cavity with two tenacula.

If the uterus is considerably enlarged, it is bisected along the entire length of the anterior and posterior wall of the uterine cavity. This will make it easier to antevert its fundus (compare with Fig. 11.34).

TECHNICAL PROBLEMS—FIGURE 11.19

The *parametrial tissue may be incompletely separated* from the cervix: in this case, the uterus is not well mobilized and may only be anteverted with difficulty. In addition, the parametrial suture may come off as a consequence of the resulting rough handling.

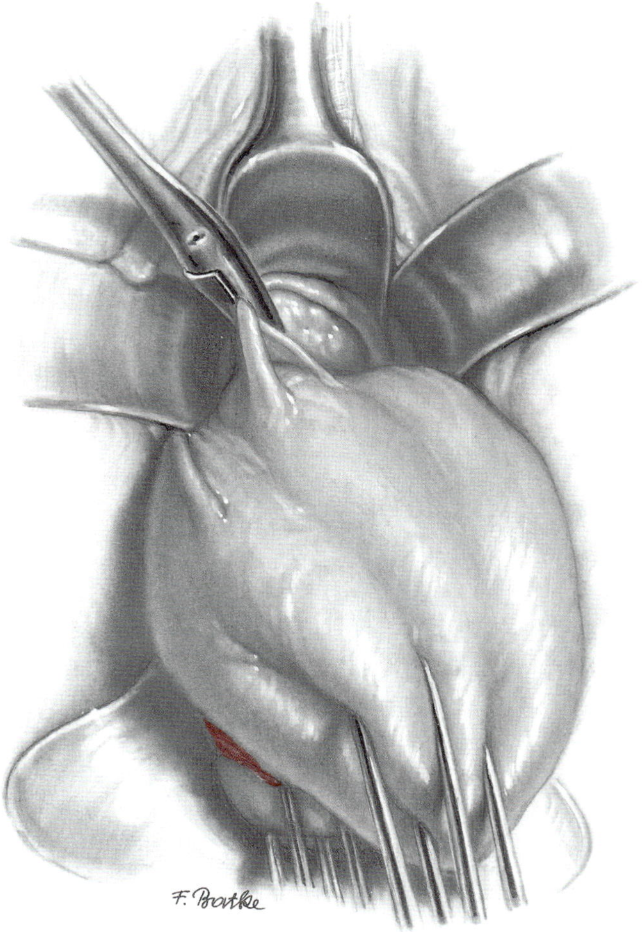

Figure 11.20. Vaginal hysterectomy while leaving the adnexa. Dissecting the right adnexa.

The left assistant pulls the anteverted uterus down to the left with two tenacula attached to its fundus to expose the right adnexal juncture. The right assistant uses a retractor to push the round ligament in lateral direction.

A strong, curved, toothed clamp is placed on the tube and the utero-ovarian ligament close to the uterus and closed, after one is assured that neither bowel nor omentum have been included. The adnexal pedicle can now be severed.

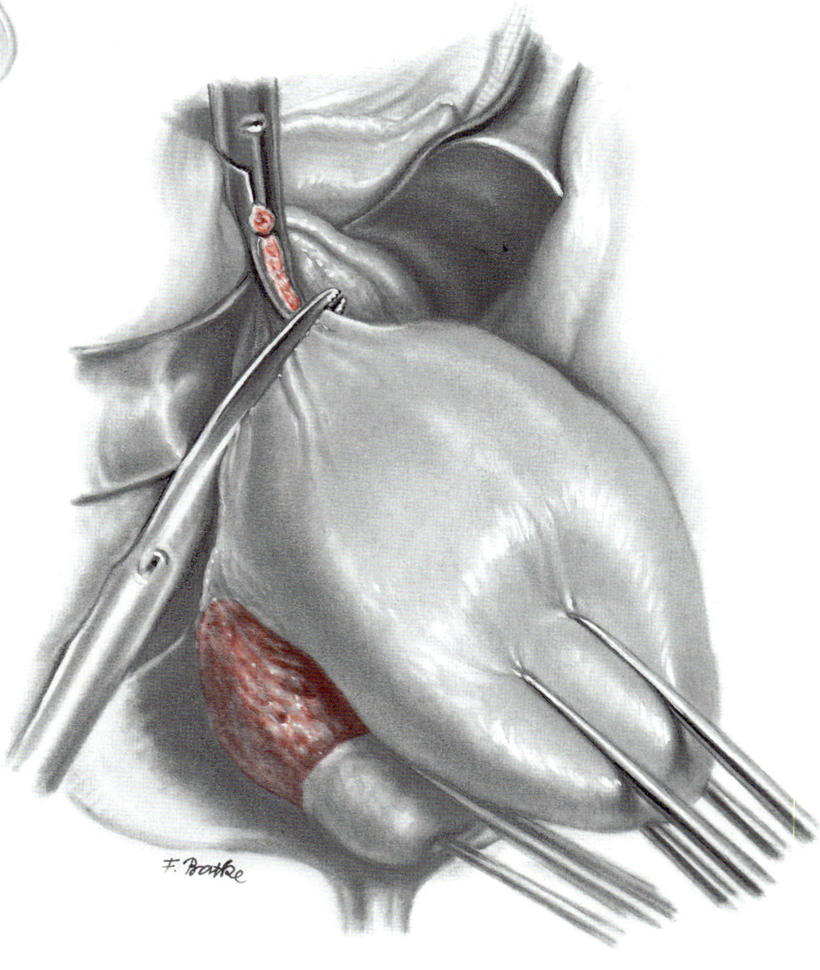

Figure 11.21. Vaginal hysterectomy while leaving the adnexa. Dissecting the round ligament.

Tube and the utero-ovarian ligament have been dissected close to the uterus.

The surgeon grasps the round ligament as well as the remaining undissected part of the ligamentum latum with a second curved clamp applied from below (peritoneal duplication).

After the right adnexa has been dissected, the uterus may be rotated around the still attached left adnexa.

The still attached left adnexa is now in good view. Two clamps are attached in an analogous fashion because the adnexa are to be resected close to the uterine edge.

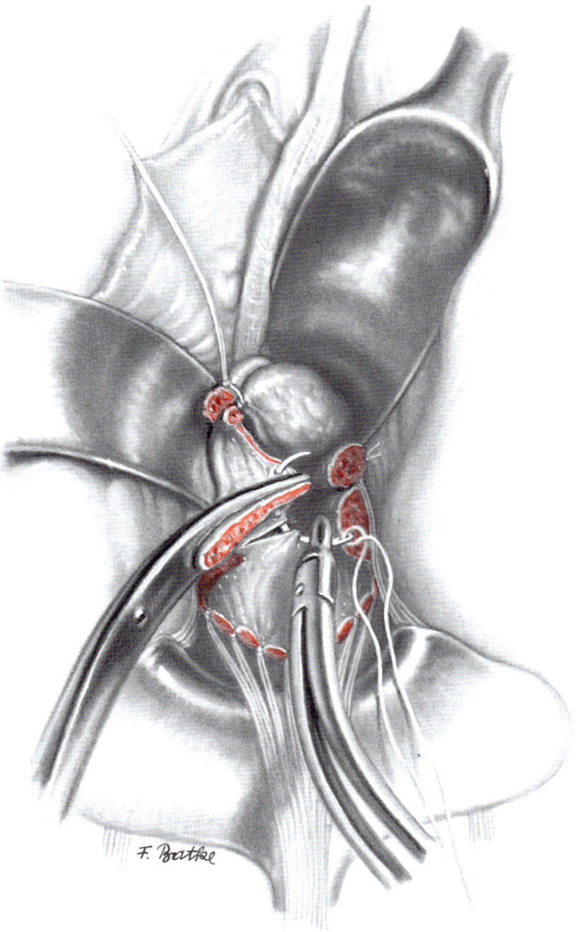

Figure 11.22. Vaginal hysterectomy while leaving the adnexa. Substituting catgut sutures for the clamps.

The left assistant pushes the left adnexa, bladder, and strip used for packing the bowel upward to the left with an intraperitoneal retractor. The right adnexal clamp has already been replaced by purse-string ligation; that concludes the tube and the utero-ovarian ligament dissection.

In the course of replacing the left lower clamp with a catgut suture, one includes, and thereby closes, any coexisting peritoneal laceration present in the cul-de-sac peritoneum.

Suture ends of the adnexa are left long.

Technical Problems—Figures 11.20–11.22

1. When placing the first clamp on the adnexa, if only the tube is clamped because it is situated further anteriorly and better exposed, *the utero-ovarian ligament* (which arises from the posterior uterine wall) *is left unclamped.*
2. If the *clamps* are placed *too close to the uterus*, the adnexal pedicles will be too short and they can slip out of the closed clamp while separating the adnexa from the uterus.
3. Should the tube, utero-ovarian ligament, and round ligament be clamped *only with a single clamp* before division from the uterus, the pedicle will be too thick. Part of the adnexal pedicle can slip out, even when a strong, curved clamp is used.
4. If the *second clamp* applied on the round ligament *incorrectly grasps a portion of the parametrial pedicle*, when the round ligament is severed, the parametrial suture may be cut inadvertently. Bleeding will result from parametrial pedicle vessels.

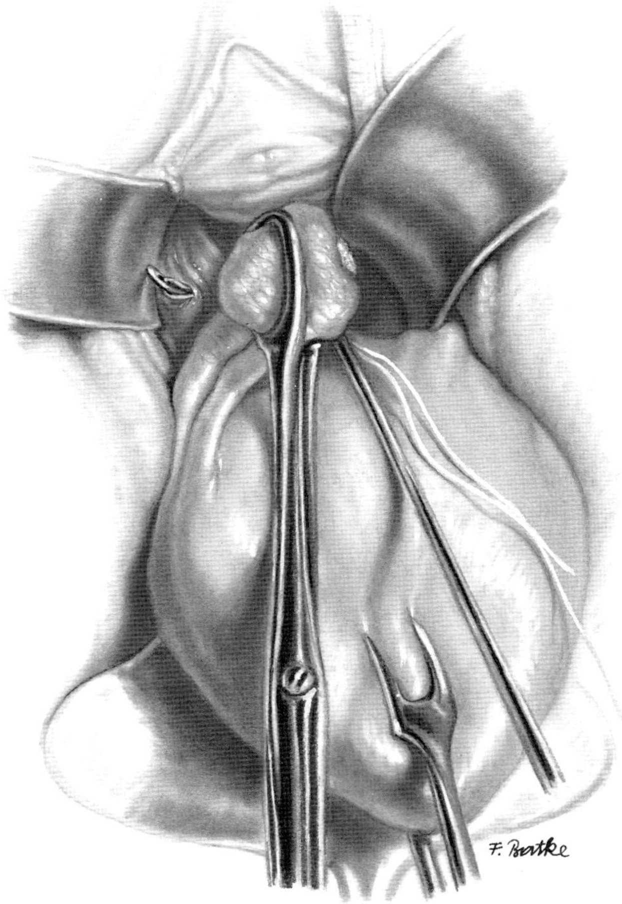

Figure 11.23. Vaginal hysterectomy. Resecting the right adnexa in conjunction with the uterus. Suturing the infundibulopelvic ligament.

One begins the procedure on the side that offers easier access to the adnexa.

The uterine fundus is pulled forward by a Leahy clamp. The right assistant pushes the round ligament to the side using a retractor. The left assistant elevates the bladder up to the left with an anterior retractor inserted into the pelvic cavity.

The surgeon uses tissue forceps to pull the tube out of the abdominal cavity; the tube and ovary are then grasped with an ovarian ring forceps, and the right adnexa is pulled down with moderate force. Simultaneously, the ovarian ring forceps are moved sagitally, lifting the infundibulopelvic ligament a little from the pelvic wall while suturing the ligament and therefore reducing the risk of injuring the ureter that courses behind it.

The right infundibulopelvic ligament is brought into view with its edge facing upward. It is ligated for the first time with a Deschamps needle about 1 cm above the abdominal end of the ovary with the suture applied from the medial to the lateral side.

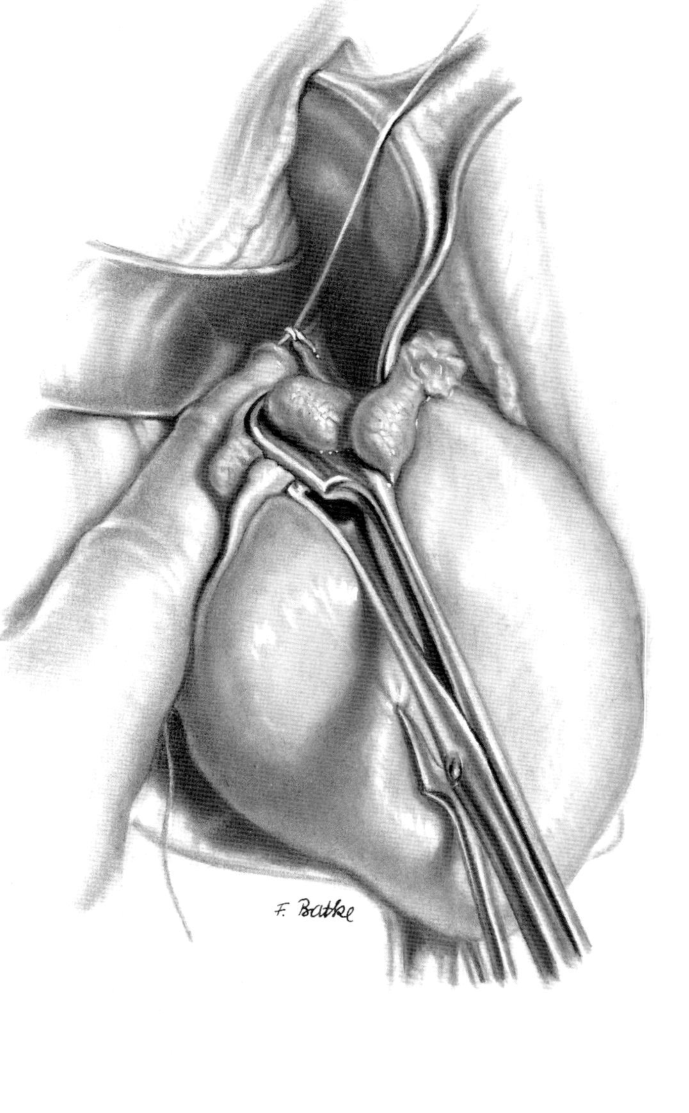

Figure 11.24. Vaginal hysterectomy. Resecting the right adnexa in conjunction with the uterus. Placing the first suture.

The ovarian ring forceps are taken by the right assistant, who holds their fenestrated handles horizontally on the posterior uterine wall. This ensures more room in the operating field and facilitates access to the infundibulopelvic ligament for the surgeon.

The surgeon can easily push the ligature up and cinch it with the index finger. The end of the ligature is left long.

To ensure secure hemostasis of the often large vessels in the infundibulopelvic ligament, another suture should be placed and tied above the first one.

Because the ureter courses downward in the immediate vicinity of the infundibulopelvic ligament, it is even more important here during placement of the second ligature to ensure that the ligament will be lifted from the pelvic wall by placing the ovarian ring forceps once more in the sagittal plane.

This second "safety suture" is cut short so that it cannot be pulled.

Thus hemostasis of the vessels in the infundibulopelvic ligament is afforded: the ligament can be divided from the ligatures on the uterine side. The distal end of the ligature is left long.

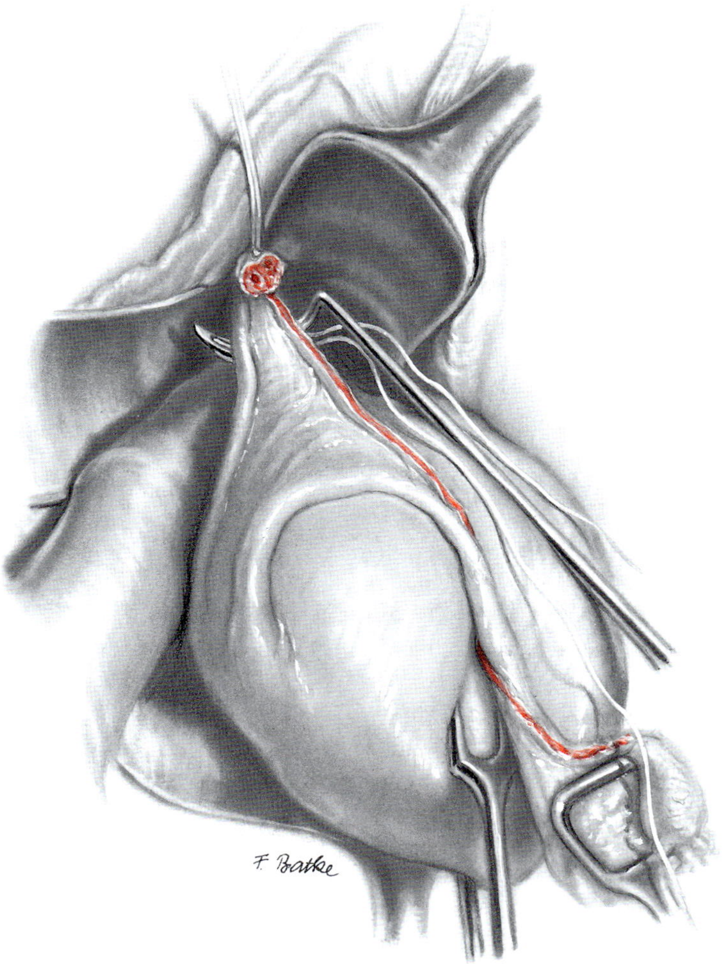

Figure 11.25. Vaginal hysterectomy. Resecting the right adnexa in conjunction with the uterus. Ligating the round ligament.

The doubly ligated infundibulopelvic ligament is now divided.

The surgeon inserts the index finger laterally to the round ligament to push the anterior peritoneal leaf of the broad ligament sacrally. By using a Deschamps needle, the right round ligament and the bordering broad ligament are ligated distal to the infundibulopelvic pedicle (as far removed as possible from the uterus) from medial to lateral.

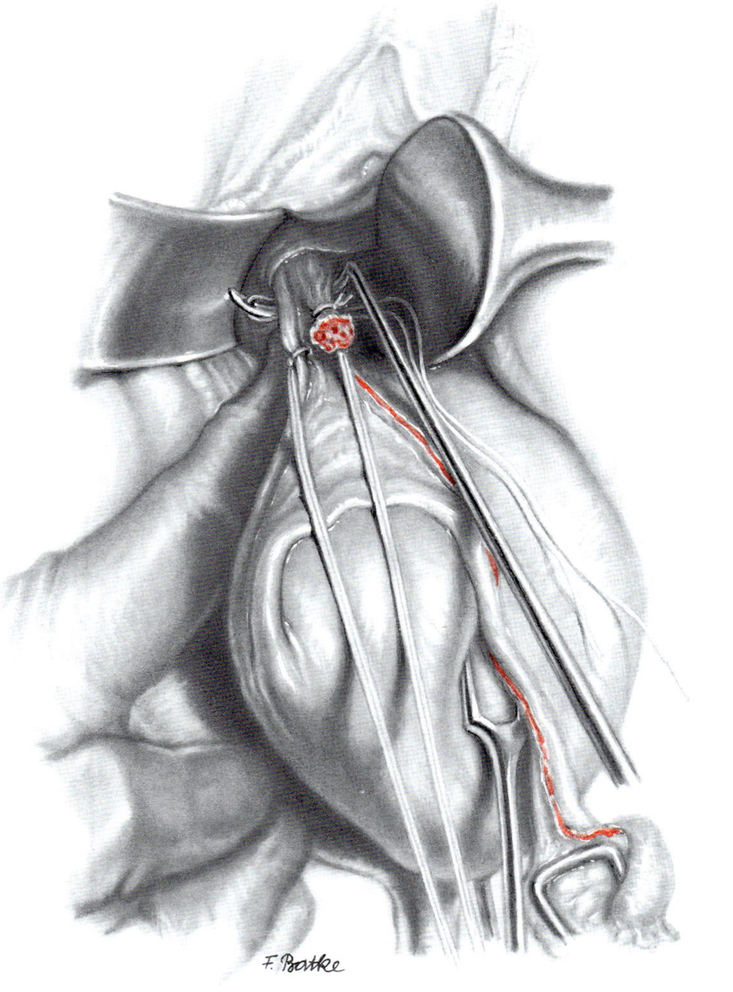

Figure 11.26. Vaginal hysterectomy. Resecting the right adnexa in conjunction with the uterus. Third "safety ligature."

After the round ligament has been ligated in isolation, the infundibulopelvic pedicle and the round ligament are relegated conjointly still further proximally. For that purpose, the distal ligature of the infundibulopelvic pedicle and the ligature of the round ligament are pulled downward, and both ligaments are ligated proximal to the ligature tie from medial to lateral.

This last joint suture with which the round ligament is fixed to the infundibulopelvic ligament is necessary because sometimes small blood vessels that are not secured properly by suturing the ligaments individually course between them. Sutures of this "safety ligature" are cut short. As soon as the round ligament is ligated distally from the ligature tie, the right adnexa are resected together with the uterus.

Technical Problems—Figures 11.23–11.26

1. Should the infundibulopelvic ligament not be ligated close to the vessels it carries but *deeper instead, more tissue is thereby included* in the suture. This can lead to injury or displacement of the ureter that courses nearby. To prevent this, the surgeon must place the handles of the ovarian ring forceps vertically during ligation of the ligament. This will lift the adnexa somewhat away from the pelvic wall. The surgeon should then ligate the ligament close to the vessels.
2. During the ligation of the infundibulopelvic ligament, one must push the round ligament laterally with a retractor so that only the infundibulopelvic ligament is presented for ligation. If the *round ligament is not carefully retracted out of the way*, it will be included in the suture. In that case, considerably more tissue will be placed on the Deschamps needle, and sometimes the ureter may be caught because it lies very close beneath the infundibulopelvic ligament and is covered only by the peritoneum.
3. The infundibulopelvic ligament should not be *sutured too high*; the further away from the ovary the ligature takes place, the more at risk is the ureter that is located in the immediate vicinity of the infundibulopelvic ligament. Therefore, the first ligature is generally placed about 1 cm cranial to the lateral end of the ovary and the second close to the first. Here again it is important to lift the ligament during ligation by appropriate positioning of the ovarian ring clamp (see above) so that it is displaced from the ureter.
4. The first ligature of the infundibulopelvic ligament may be *placed too close to the pelvic pole of the ovary*. If this occurs, the ligature will be too close to the cut edge of the pedicle when the ligament is later divided, and it will come off at the slightest tug.
5. In the event that adnexal adhesions are present, the ovaries and fallopian tubes *must be completely mobilized* before the infundibulopelvic ligament can be ligated because the ureter may be located precariously close to the adnexa. Even after the adhesions are lysed, suturing of the ligament should be especially close to the ovary.
6. If *only one ligature* (whose sutures had been left long to serve as markers) were to be placed on the infundibulopelvic pedicle, and if it comes off as a result of excessively brusque or incorrect traction, massive hemorrhage will occur. Such bleeding is difficult to control vaginally without endangering the ureter because vessels in the ligament will immediately retract upward and become difficult to find. Massive hemorrhage from the vessels that are no longer ligated will dictate immediate laparotomy. To avoid this complication, double ligation of the infundibulopelvic ligament is always performed before it is divided. The distal ligature is left long; however, the proximal suture is always cut short (*caution*: never the reverse). If the distal ligature of the infundibulopelvic ligament comes off because of strong traction, the proximal suture will prevent bleeding; the ligature that came off at the infundibulopelvic pedicle can be replaced without undue haste.
7. If there is *no conjoint ligature* between the infundibulopelvic ligament and round ligament pedicles, bleeding can occur between the two pedicles from small parametrial vessels.
8. *Excessively strong traction* exerted on the adnexa held in the ovarian ring forceps can lacerate the infundibulopelvic ligament during ligation. This may cause the ligament to tear off. It occurs rarely and is most likely to be encountered in older women with fragile tissues.

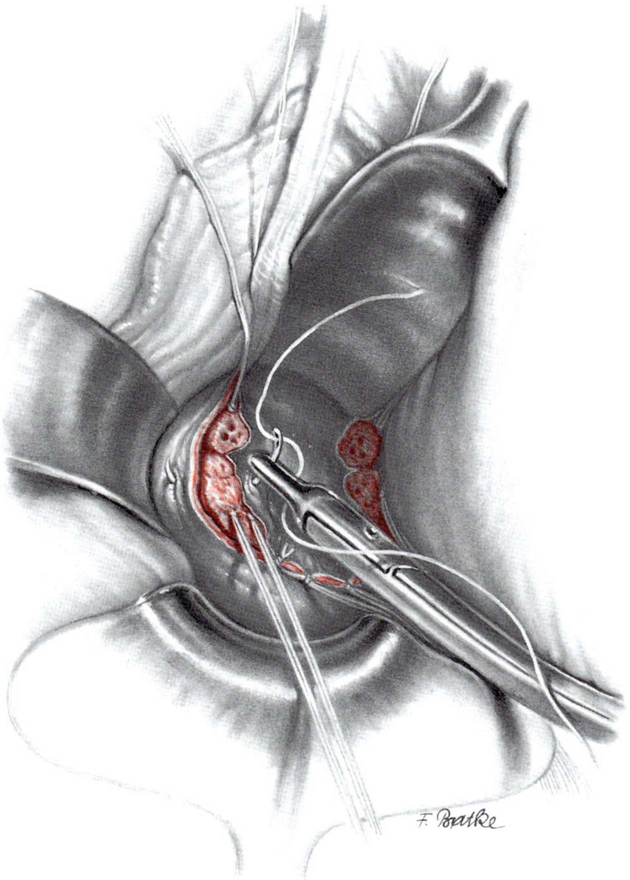

Figure 11.27. Vaginal hysterectomy without adnexa. Fixing the right parametrial pedicle to the lateral vaginal wound edge.

The uterus has been removed; the ligated adnexa were left close to the uterus after dissection.

The left assistant lifts the bladder up to the left with an anterior intraperitoneal retractor and pulls the posterior spaced vaginal sutures down to the left; the right assistant pulls the ligatures of the right adnexal pedicle upward to the right and draws the labia back *laterally* to the vaginal circumcision wound edge with a lateral retractor.

The surgeon pulls the ligatures on the right parametrial pedicle downward and sutures it from medial to lateral.

The parametrial pedicles are fixed to the lateral vaginal edge with a figure-eight suture (Z suture). This contributes to secure hemostasis and a better view of the operational area. It also plays a specific role in anchoring the vaginal cuff. That same suture will include peritoneum medially adherent to the pedicle.

Technical Problems—Figure 11.27

1. When the pedicles are *ligated too broadly*, extensive postoperative tissue necrosis will develop. Delayed healing will prolong convalescence considerably.
2. If *too much of the peritoneum* adherent medially to the parametrial pedicle *is included* in the ligature, only a little of the pedicle is incorporated. This will cause the peritoneum to be pulled forward to the vaginal wall over the pedicle when the suture is tied. Drainage of secretions from the pedicle will be hindered in such a case.
3. Despite meticulous care of the pedicles, some bleeding can still occur, typically from the following three sites.

- At the angle between the adnexal pedicle and the anterior vaginal circumcision edge. Experience shows that most postoperative bleeding occurs here because so far no hemostatic sutures have been placed anteriorly at the vaginal wound edge. In addition, delicate blood vessels of the bladder pillar may have been dissected in this corner. Hemostasis can be secured easily at this time; later, after the anterior repair is conducted, these corners will retract so that they cannot be exposed.
- In the corner between the parametrial pedicle and the adnexal pedicle. A strong catgut suture will staunch bleeding readily.
- In the corner between the parametrial pedicle and the sutures of the posterior circumcision, from the vaginal wound. Fine catgut sutures are used to join the peritoneal cut edge with the vaginal wound edge.

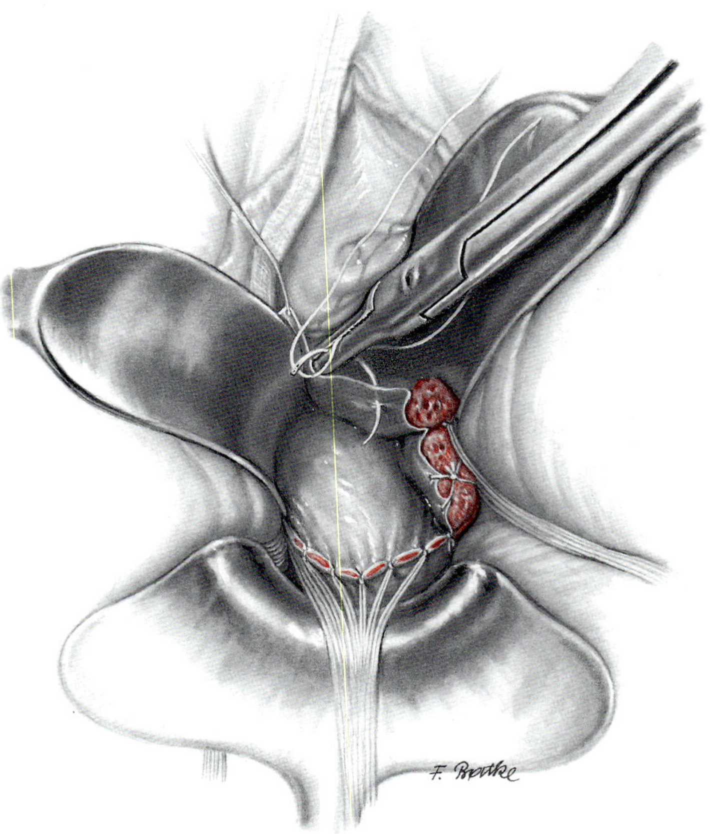

Figure 11.28. Vaginal hysterectomy without adnexa. Closure of the peritoneum and displacing the pedicles extraperitoneally.

Precise closure of the peritoneal cavity with careful extraperitonealization of the pedicles serves as the best prophylaxis against infection and will prevent many postoperative complications (e.g., inflammatory infiltrations, peritonitis, ileus, etc.).

While the left angle suture is being placed, the left assistant pulls down on the ligatures attached to the adnexal and parametrial pedicles, and with a retractor inserted extraperitoneally above the pedicles, the vaginal wound edge and the bladder are pushed to the left. The right assistant, with a retractor inserted intraperitoneally, retracts the bladder upward to the right and pulls the peritoneal wound edge forward by its suture.

Now the left half of the half-purse-string sutures must be placed. The suture is begun at the anterior peritoneal wound edge; the needle is inserted from the outside to the inside first and then continued from above downward.

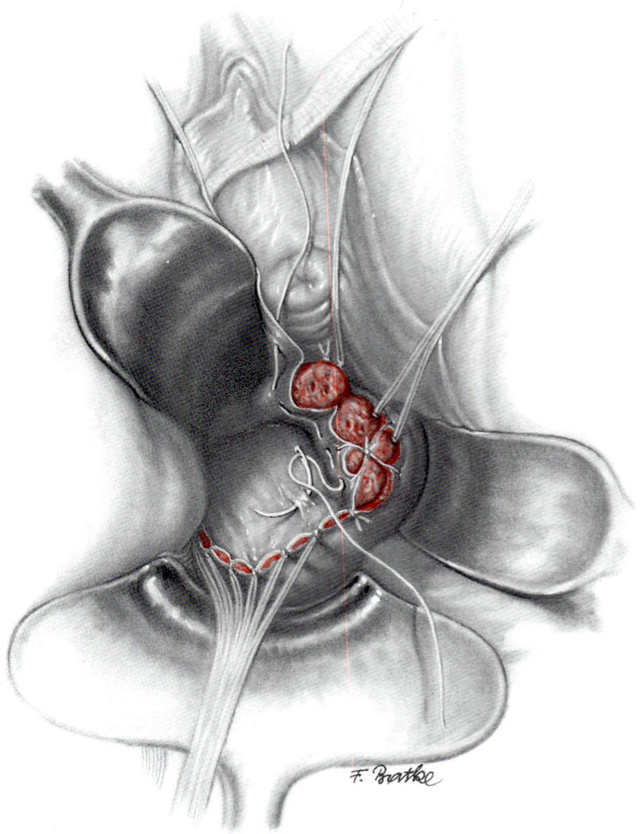

Figure 11.29. Vaginal hysterectomy without adnexa. Placing the left peritoneal angle suture.

After the anterior peritoneal wound edge has been sutured, the needle grasps the peritoneum of the adnexal as well as the parametrial pedicles and sutures along the interior surface of the peritoneum in and out.

During this procedure, the left assistant changes direction of traction on the sutures of the pedicles so that they are directed upward by the right hand, while at the same time pulling the lateral retractor, now in the left hand, downward (change of hands).

The surgeon continues placing the peritoneal suture, applying it laterally from the rectum above the spaced sutures at the posterior vaginal wound edge.

As this half-purse-string suture is being tied, the pedicles displace themselves extraperitoneally.

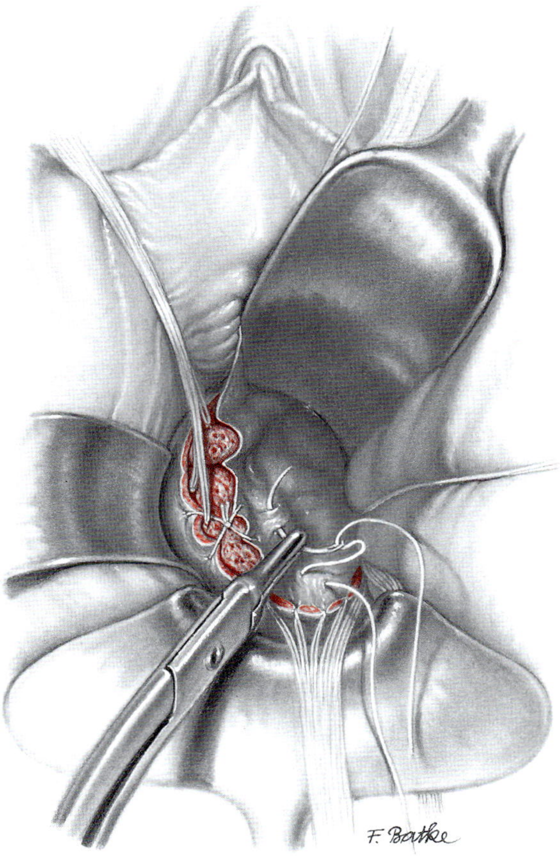

Figure 11.30. Vaginal hysterectomy without adnexa. Placing the right peritoneal angle suture.

With the left hand, the right assistant pulls the ligatures of the adnexal and parametrial pedicles upward and pushes the vaginal wound edge laterally with a lateral retractor. The left assistant pushes the bowel upward with an intraperitoneal retractor.

The analogous half of the purse-string suture is begun at the rectal peritoneum. The peritoneum of the rectum as well as that of the right parametrial pedicle is already grasped by the needle, one continues the suture from below to above.

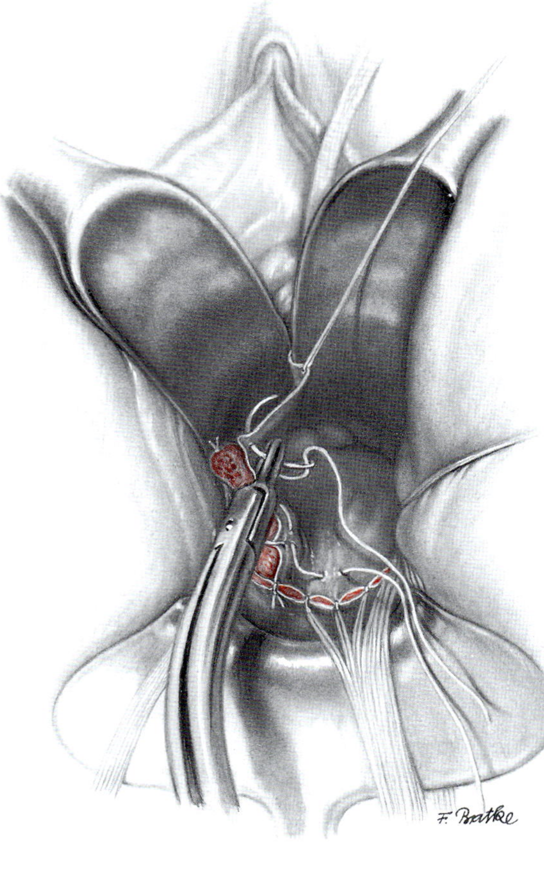

Figure 11.31. Vaginal hysterectomy without adnexa. Continuing the right peritoneal angle suture.

The right assistant has changed hands: the ligatures attached to the right parametrial and adnexal pedicles are pulled down with the right hand, and the bladder is elevated with a lateral extraperitoneal retractor. With the right hand, the left assistant pulls the anterior peritoneal ligatures out and pushes the bowel upward with a retractor.

The posterior peritoneum and that of the parametrial and adnexal pedicles have been sewn. The anterior peritoneal wound edge is now grasped by the needle.

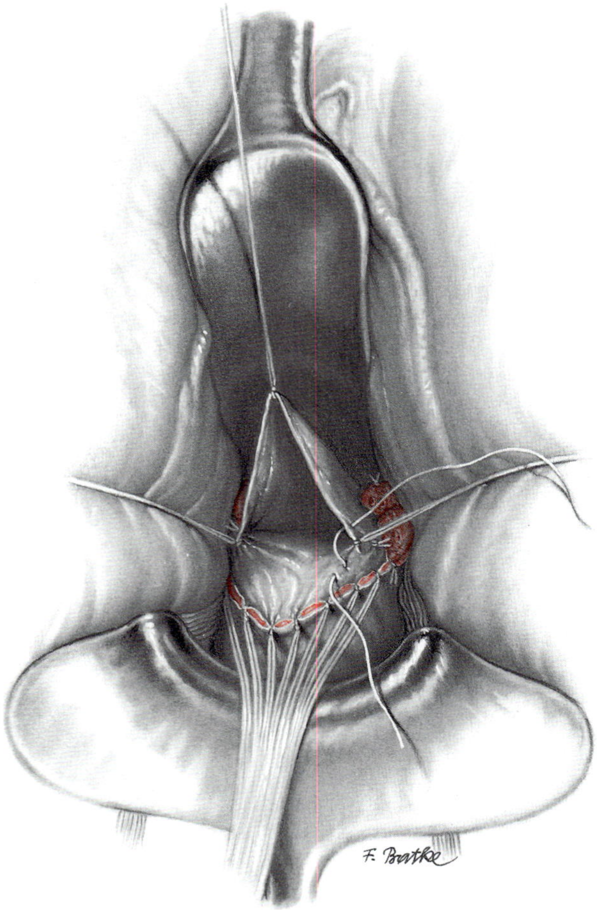

Figure 11.32. Vaginal hysterectomy without adnexa. Closing the peritoneal cavity.

The peritoneal packing strip has been removed. After the angle sutures have been tied on both sides, it is easy to completely close the resting peritoneal opening with interrupted sutures while pulling on the traction sutures that have been left long.

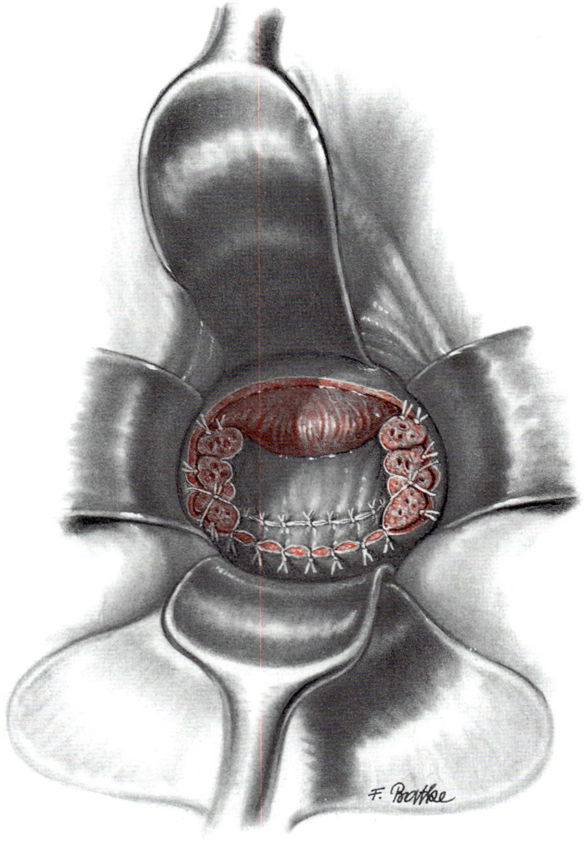

Figure 11.33. Vaginal hysterectomy without adnexa. View at the end of the procedure.

The peritoneum is completely closed. One can see the transverse peritoneal suture, also the parametrial pedicles, fixed to the lateral vaginal wound edges by means of figure-eight sutures and lastly above them the extraperitonealized adnexal pedicles. Hemostasis is secured at the posterior vaginal wound edge by spaced interrupted sutures.

Anterior vaginal hemostatic sutures are not placed in this case, because an anterior colporrhaphy is to be done for the bladder descent; this will involve extensive resection of the anterior vaginal wound edge.

In cases where anterior colporrhaphy is not performed after a vaginal hysterectomy, it would be advisable to place such hemostatic sutures along the anterior vaginal edge or at least at the corners above the adnexal pedicles.

TECHNICAL PROBLEMS—FIGURES 11.28–11.33

1. The *adnexal pedicles* may not be *pulled far enough forward* during placement of the angle suture, or the medially adherent *peritoneum may not be grasped high enough*. If this occurs, a hole is left in the peritoneum after the angle suture has been tied; through it the adnexal pedicles can retract to lie intraperitoneally. Because they would no longer be covered by serosa, the large omentum or a loop of intestine can become adherent, and a bowel obstruction may result.
2. If the needle used for the step-wise angle suture grasps not only the peritoneum but *also deeper tissue*, blood vessels may be punctured, and hematomas may occur.
3. When the peritoneum *is grasped too deeply* in the area of the *adnexal pedicles*, the underlying ureter can be pulled in or even injured.
4. If the *anterior retractor* pushes the bladder extraperitoneally *upward too vigorously* after the angle sutures and the second peritoneal sutures have been placed, the anterior edge of the peritoneum disappears upward so that it can be grasped only with difficulty.
5. If the *catgut sutures* used for closing the peritoneal cavity *are too thick*, they will work their way through the tissues, and the peritoneum will be torn. It is best to use size 0 catgut for the angle sutures and size 00 catgut (or 00 vicryl sutures) for the remaining peritoneal sutures.

Care of the Vaginal Cuff

After the peritoneal cavity has been carefully closed, the vaginal cuff is left wide open to permit drainage of the secretions that are constantly collecting. We tamponade the subperitoneal space for 48 hours, allowing the open vaginal cuff to heal by granulation. We prefer to refrain from joining the adnexal pedicles transversely in the midline because we are not convinced that this practice prevents descent of the vaginal cul-de-sac. We suture the cardinal and uterosacral ligaments laterally into the vaginal circumcision wound, causing the vaginal cuff to be placed on stretch. It would not be advantageous to unite these laterally fixed corners of the vaginal cuff medially.

Usually, no bleeding occurs from the vaginal circumcision wound edges when the circumcision of the portio is done correctly by not incising the lateral part too deeply, thus avoiding entry into the veins coursing in the lateral vaginal fascia. Furthermore, the posterior vaginal wound is made hemostatic by fixing the posterior peritoneal cut edge to the posterior vaginal circumcision edge with spaced interrupted sutures. Should bleeding occur from the anterior vaginal circumcision wound edge, hemostatic sutures are indicated. In most cases such suturing of the anterior vaginal wound edge is not needed to achieve perfect hemostasis, because as a rule (as discussed above) the hysterectomy is followed by an anterior colporrhaphy, which is accompanied by resection of the surplus vaginal mucosa, a step that eliminates the anterior edge of the vaginal circumcision wound. The vaginal cuff must be left wide open for drainage; the vaginal cuff edge closes by itself a few days after removal of the drainage strip or granulates after 2 weeks.

In primary closure of the vaginal cul-de-sac there is no opportunity given for subperitoneal collections of secretions to drain into the vagina. Instead, retention of wound secretions can occur above the closed vaginal cul-de-sac, especially in the presence of infection when it may form a subperitoneal abscess that will extend cranially along the path of least resistance into the loose retroperitoneal connective tissue. This abscess gradually becomes palpable as a sense of resistance in the lateral aspect of the lower abdominal wall above the symphysis. Similarly, a retroperitoneal hematoma can develop caused by postoperative bleeding from the adnexal pedicle or the bladder, which may be undetectable because the vaginal cuff was closed primarily.

For all these reasons it is advisable to leave the vaginal cuff open and to maintain drainage for 48 hours by tamponade. As long as secretions can flow off, there is no danger of ascending infection.

Vaginal Hysterectomy with Myomatous Uterus

Indications

The enlarged uterus may be removed vaginally as long as it can be pulled, at least partially, into the true pelvis and as long as one has access to the uterine vessels. There are two procedures available that work to the patient's advantage (both procedures may be combined):

- Splitting the anterior and posterior wall of the uterus in the midline, which allows its gradual mobilization and makes it easier to pull downward;
- Stepwise resection of myomatous tumor nodules by morcellation.

A primary consideration in the vaginal removal of a myomatous uterus is, however, that the morcellation or bisection must always be performed only under the surgeon's direct vision. Before uterine reduction can happen, the cervix must be separated from its parametrial connections to increase its mobility, and the uterine arteries must be sutured. This may be difficult in cases with deeply seated myomas. Then one may have to make do first with dividing the posterior parametria and ligating the uterine artery.

Bisection Technique

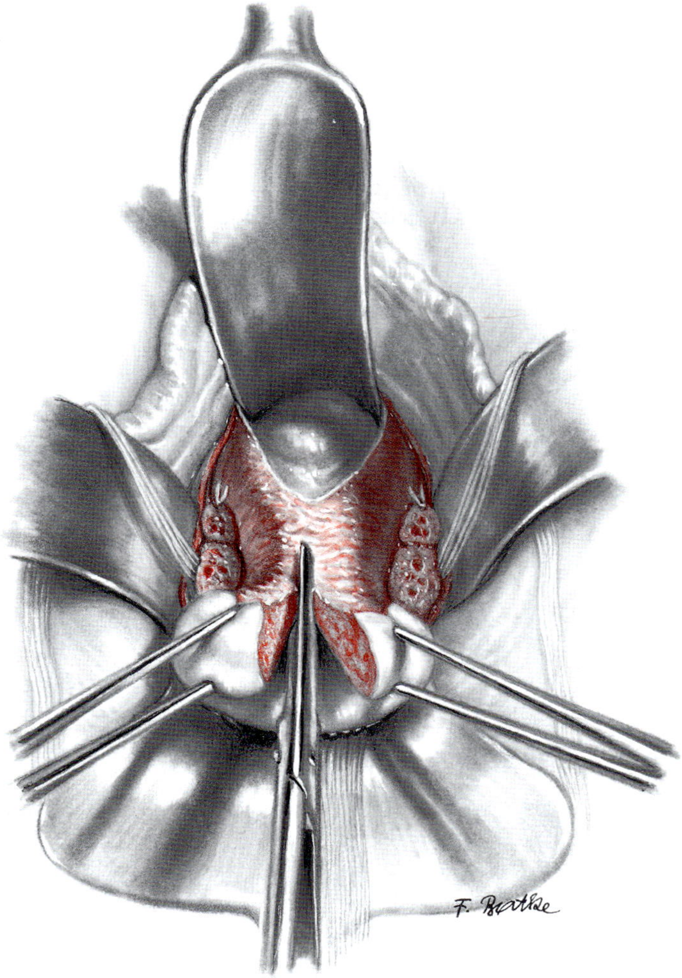

Figure 11.34. Vaginal hysterectomy with myomatous uterus. Bisecting the anterior wall of the cervix.

The parametria have been ligated on both sides and divided, and the peritoneal cavity is open. Two single-toothed tenacula are placed on the portio. An anterior retractor can only partially be inserted into the peritoneal cavity if an anterior wall myoma exists; it serves, however, to protect the bladder during the bisecting procedure.

Bisection is performed with a strong straight scissors.

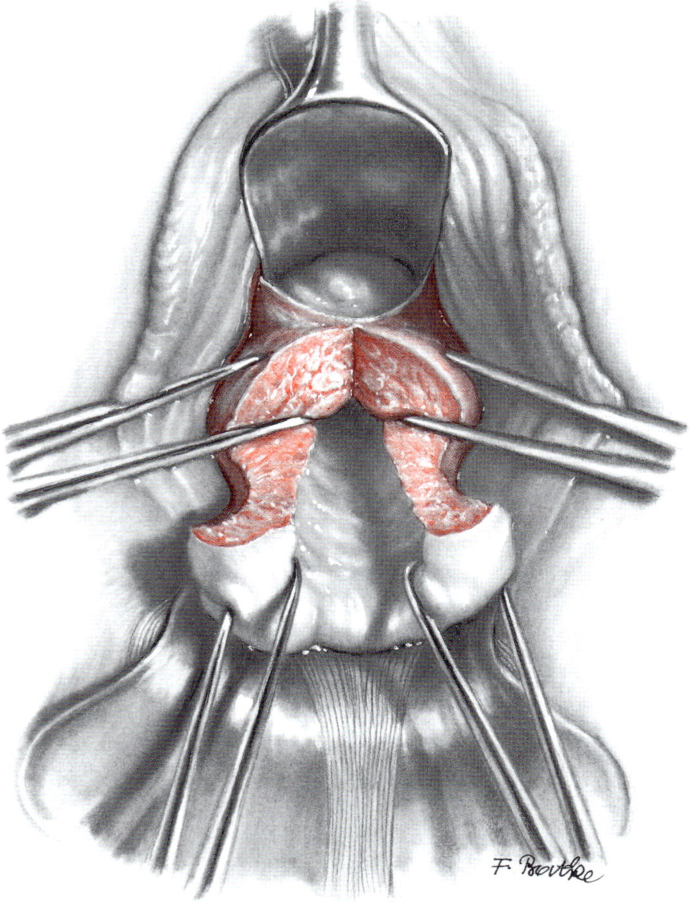

Figure 11.35. Vaginal hysterectomy with myomatous uterus. Bisecting the anterior wall of the corpus.

The anterior cervical wall has already been split, and with a strong pull on the tenacula, the uterus has been pulled further out of the abdominal cavity.

The surgeon grasps the upper wound angle of the cervix with two additional tenacula that are pulled down and outward vigorously by the assistants.

The anterior uterine wall, while fully visible, can be split medially further upward. This procedure is repeated several times by advancing the tenacula progressively upward in stepwise fashion and reattaching each at the highest wound angle.

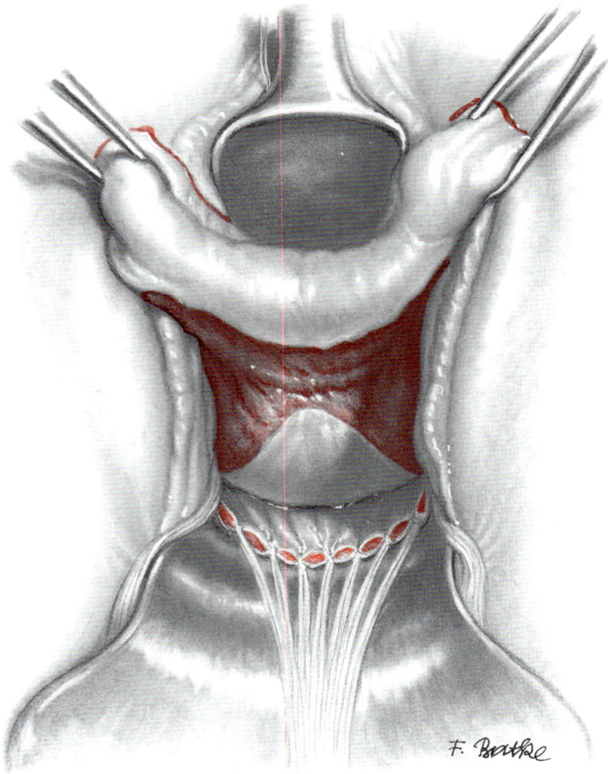

Figure 11.36. Vaginal hysterectomy with myomatous uterus. Bisecting the posterior wall of the cervix.

The anterior wall of the cervix and the corpus have been split as far as they can be seen; the anterior wall cannot be split further at this time because of the size of the myomatous uterus.

The tenacula have been removed from the anterior wound angle, the uterus is pulled straight upward by the tenacula left on the portio.

The anterior intraperitoneal retractor remains in place to protect the bladder. The posterior vaginal wall is exposed with a self-retaining retractor. The posterior peritoneum is opened, the peritoneal wound edges are fixed to the posterior vaginal circumcision wound edge with spaced interrupted sutures.

With continuing good visualization, the surgeon can now split the posterior wall of the cervix and the corpus.

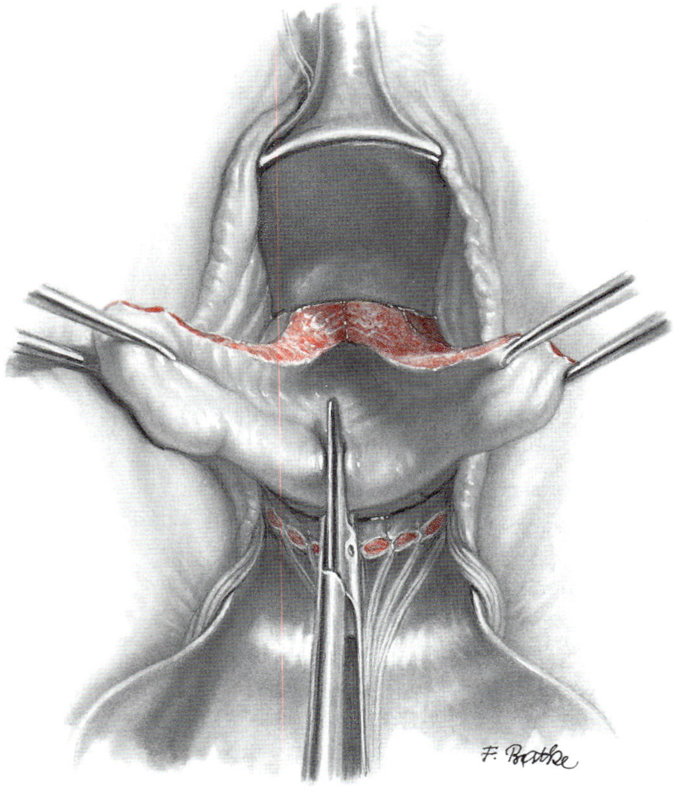

Figure 11.37. Vaginal hysterectomy with myomatous uterus. Bisecting the posterior wall of the cervix.

The operative field is prepared as in Figure 11.36. The pull on the tenacula attached to the portio was changed (the pull is now laterally and somewhat upward) so that the partially split anterior uterine wall is also exposed to view. The surgeon now splits the posterior cervical wall in the midline, which achieves even greater mobilization of the myomatous uterus.

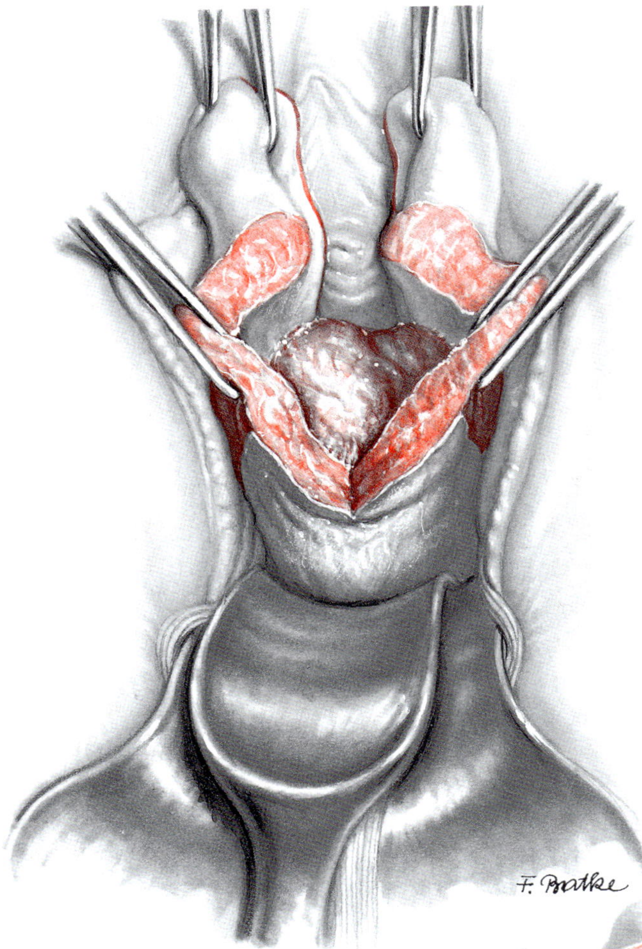

Figure 11.38. Vaginal hysterectomy with myomatous uterus. Bisecting the posterior wall of the corpus.

The posterior wall of the cervix has been split medially. The two new tenacula placed on the wound edges of the cervix together with those on the portio are pulled straight up by the assistants; the posterior uterine wall can now be partially extracted out of the cul-de-sac of Douglas.

The surgeon protects the rectum with a second posterior retractor inserted intraperitoneally. He or she can now split the posterior corpus wall upward in stepwise fashion, using straight scissors. One can already recognize a larger submucous myoma.

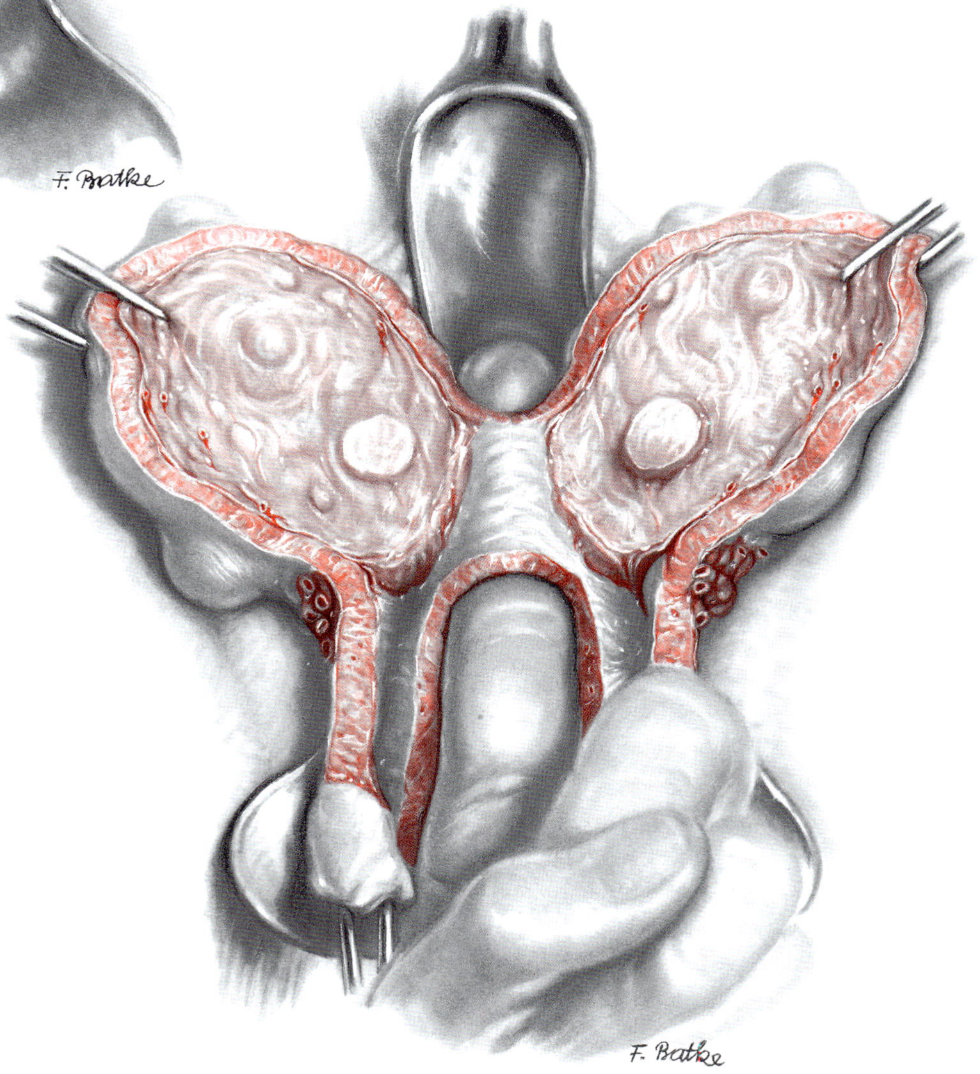

Figure 11.39. Vaginal hysterectomy with myomatous uterus. Complete uterine bisection in two halves.

The deeper the posterior uterine wall has been split, the easier it is to roll the corpus forward out of the space of Douglas. The tenacula have been moved progressively up into the fundus.

At the posterior uterine wall, a narrow intact bridge becomes visible. With the left index finger, the surgeon reaches behind the bridge to protect the bowel during bisection. At the same time, the right assistant pushes the bladder and bowel upward with an anterior intraperitoneal retractor.

It is often unnecessary to split the posterior uterine wall up to the fundus, because the corpus has already been easily mobilized and pulled out of the abdominal cavity.

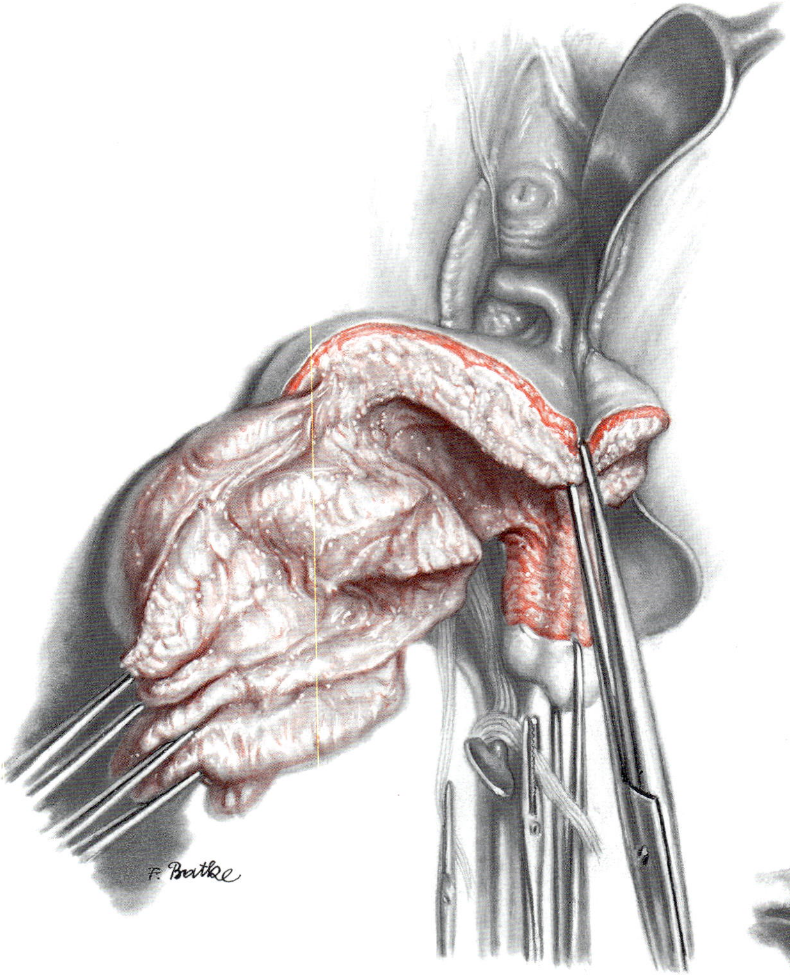

Figure 11.40. Vaginal hysterectomy with myomatous uterus. Exposing the left adnexa.

The right half of the uterus has already been removed; the left half of the corpus is pulled downward to the right; and the left labium minus is pushed back laterally. An additional tenaculum is attached close to the adnexal junction so that the left adnexa may be brought into full view.

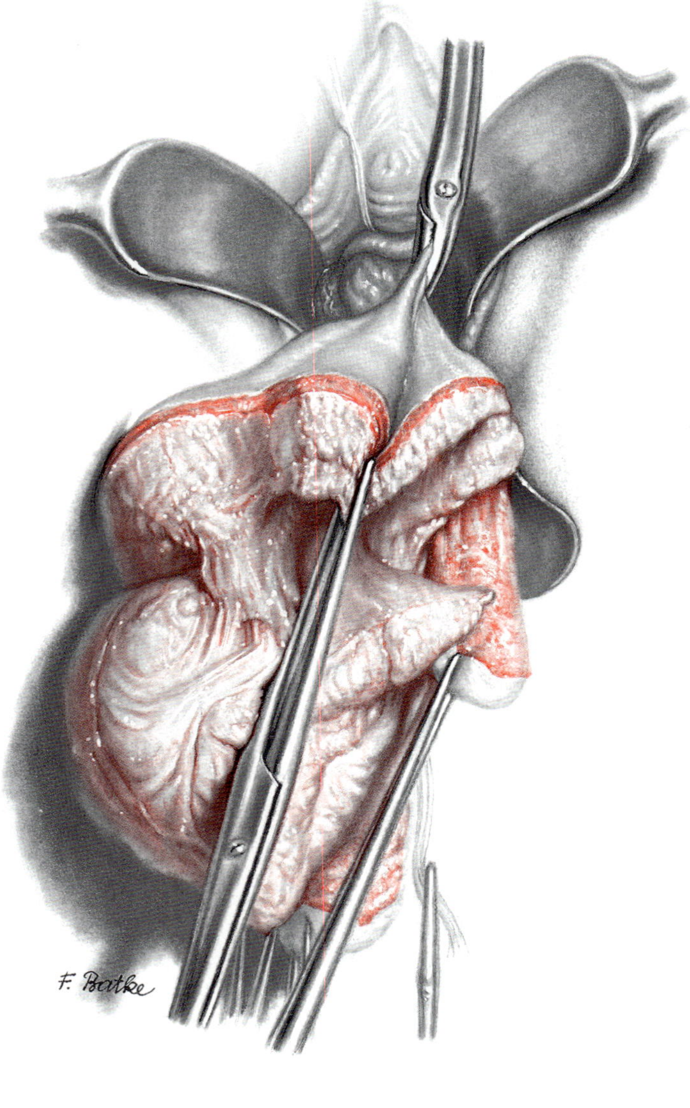

Figure 11.41. Vaginal hysterectomy with myomatous uterus. Dividing the uterus from the left adnexa.

The left half of the uterus has been completely pulled out of the abdominal cavity and placed in front of the vulva. The adnexal junction is in full view.

A heavy curved clamp is applied from above over the tube and the utero-ovarian ligament. This clamp possesses a tooth, which will ensure that tissue held by it cannot slip out of its grasp.

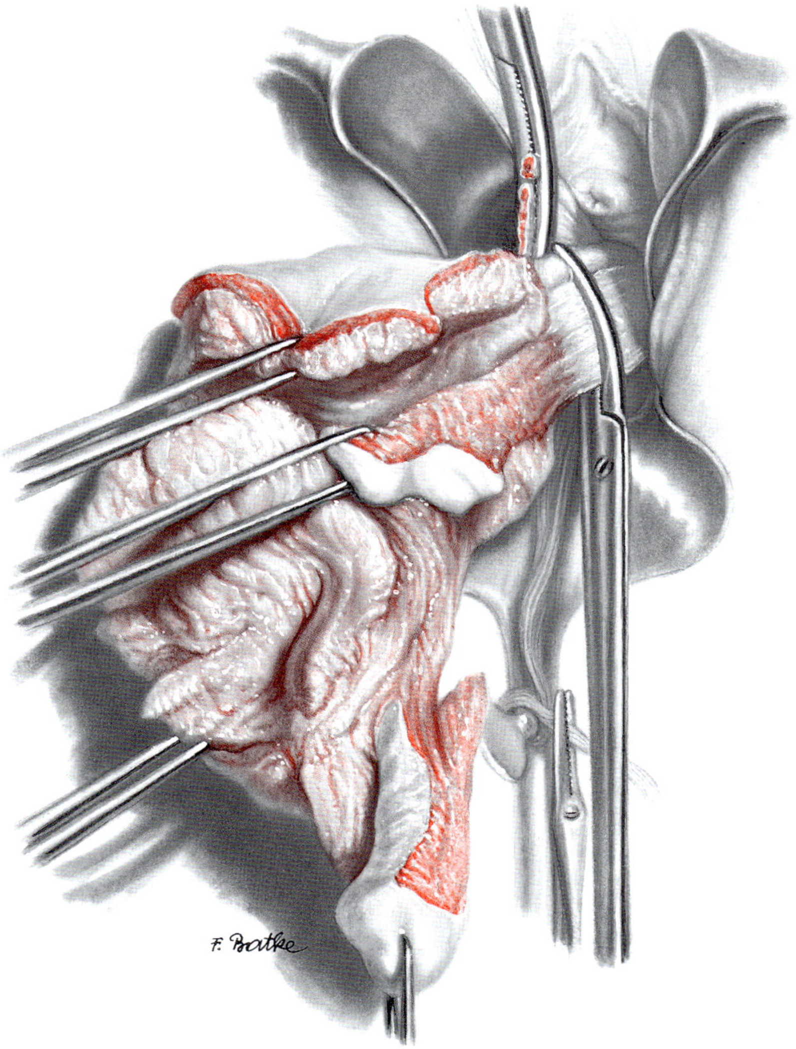

Figure 11.42. Vaginal hysterectomy with myomatous uterus. Extirpating the second half of the uterus.

The left adnexa has been divided close to the uterus. The rolled-out half of the uterus is still attached by the round ligament and the remnants of the broad ligament, which are clamped with a curved clamp.

Morcellation Technique

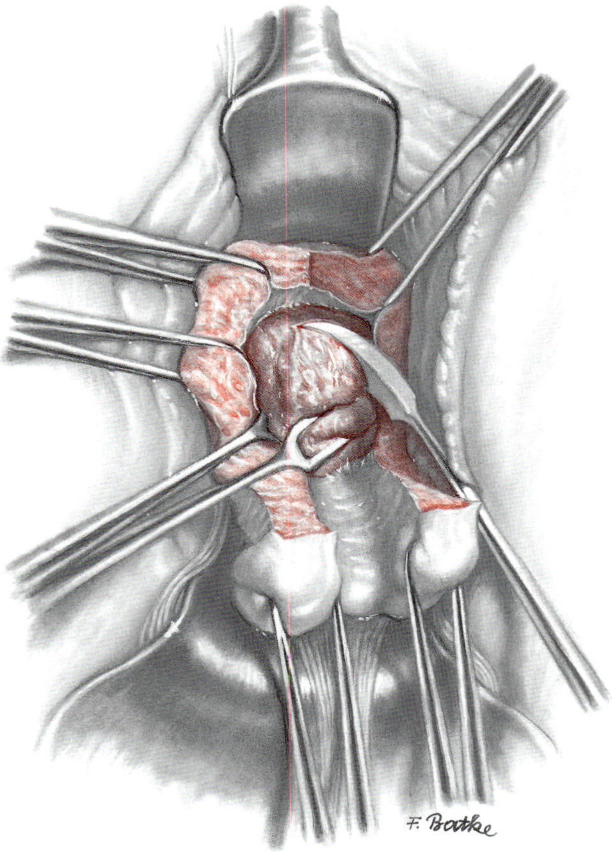

Figure 11.43. Vaginal hysterectomy with myomatous uterus. Morcellation technique.

The uterus is split to the fundus on its anterior wall. Its further bisection up to the fundus is impossible at this time because of the size of a large submucous myoma. The myomatous capsule has already been split. The uterine wound is pulled apart to form a gaping opening by means of several attached tenacula.

The surgeon grasps the visible part of the myoma with a double-toothed claw tenaculum and cuts a piece out of it with a special lancet-shaped double-edged knife. Note the correct positioning of the knife (compare with Fig. 11.44, where knife position is incorrect).

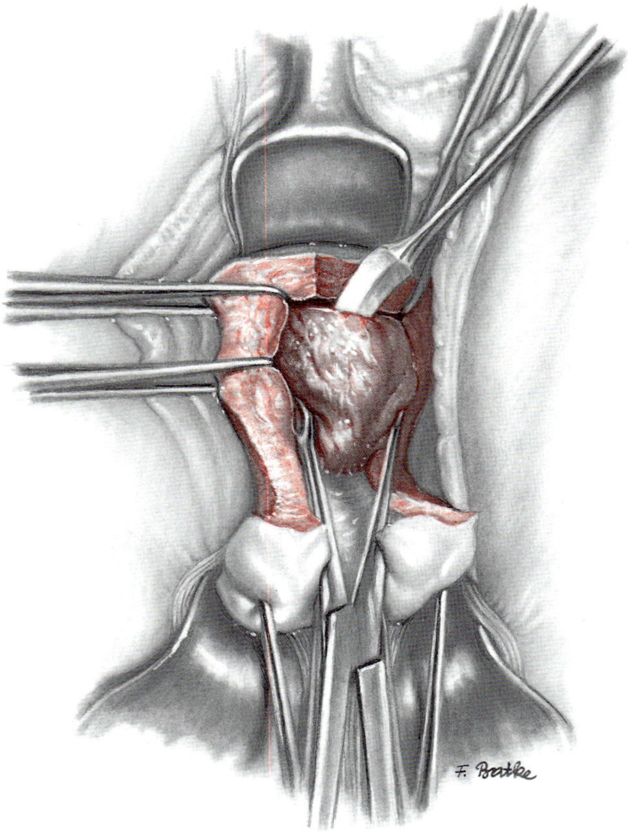

Figure 11.44. Vaginal hysterectomy with myomatous uterus. Incorrect positioning of the knife during morcellation.

If the tip of the morcellation knife cannot be seen as it is pushed through the myoma, it can perforate the posterior wall of the uterus and injure the bowel.

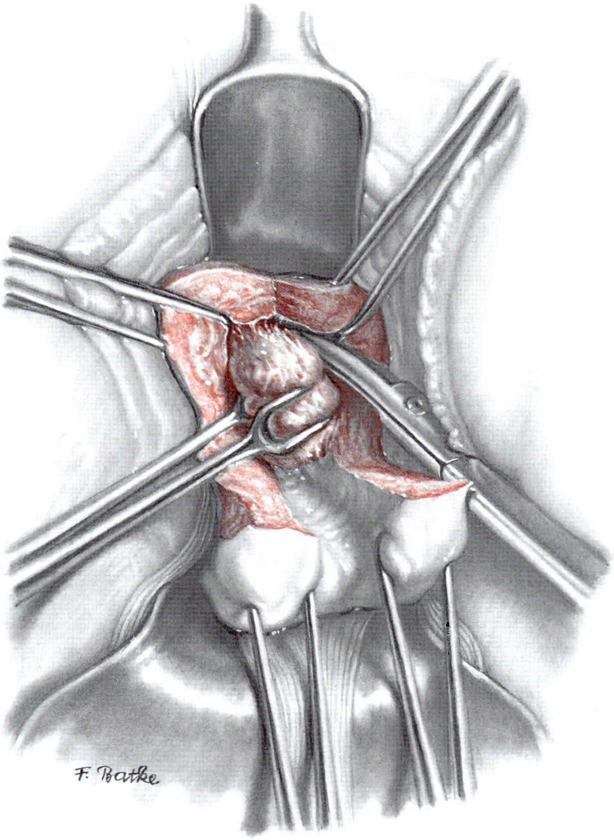

Figure 11.45. Vaginal hysterectomy with myomatous uterus. Morcellation technique.

A portion of the submucous myoma nodule has already been removed by morcellation; the rest of the nodule is grasped once more with a claw tenaculum.

The surgeon pulls the myoma nodule downward and to the right and mobilizes intracapsularly the upper aspect of the nodule.

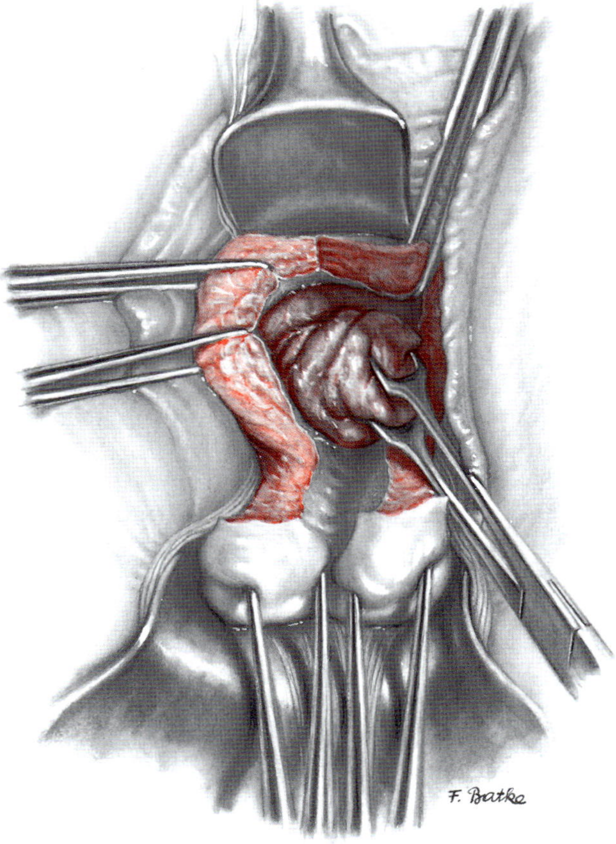

Figure 11.46. Vaginal hysterectomy with myomatous uterus. Morcellation technique.

The myoma nodule, which had been partially mobilized by scissors, can be avulsed with the attached claw tenaculum.

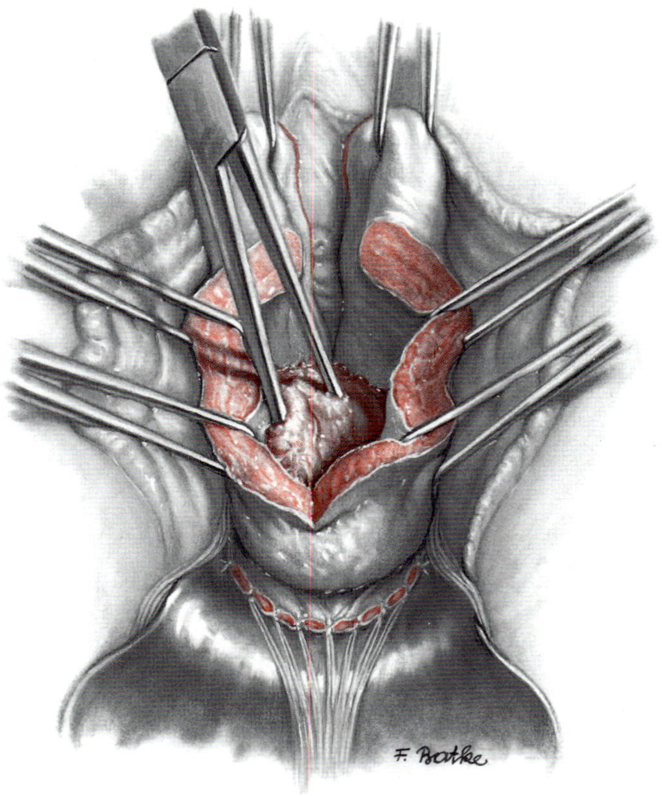

Figure 11.47. Vaginal hysterectomy with myomatous uterus. Morcellation and bisection.

The uterus is split medially at its anterior and posterior wall. An additional, somewhat larger myoma nodule is exposed and removed through morcellation.

In this way the large myomatous uterus is reduced in a step-wise manner until it can at last be rolled forward out of the abdominal cavity.

Technical Problems—Figures 11.43–11.47

1. Should the uterine wall covering the *myoma not be split wide enough* up to the lower pole of the myomatous nodule, access for morcellation will be inadequate. However, it is unnecessary to split the uterus up to the fundus immediately; it is only necessary to dissect that section which is accessible.
2. It is difficult to roll out the uterus if the *tenacula* attached to the wound edges and those on the portio *are pulled simultaneously*. One should therefore pull only on the uppermost tenacula.
3. The cervix that is *insufficiently separated from its connection with the parametrium* will limit uterine mobility. The presence of larger myomata may make it impossible to dissect the parametria from the cervix edge at first; it is imperative to correct this deficiency as soon as the uterus has been mobilized by partial reduction in its size. If this is not done, severe hemorrhage can occur from the unligated uterine artery.
4. It is dangerous to *enucleate* a large myoma in toto because one can cut through the uterine wall while sharply dissecting the upper aspect with the double-edged morcellation knife, thereby risking injury to adjacent organs. Moreover, it may be impossible to remove a large myoma because of the immobility of the uterus. It is preferable to excise several conical segments in a stepwise manner always under direct vision.
5. If the *dissecting knife approaches too closely to the uterine wall* and is not directed *in parallel to the serosal surfaces*, it may perforate through the wall and damage neighboring structures.
6. It is important *not to be impatient* when reducing the size of a large myomatous uterus. One should morcellate small pieces until the uterine mass is small enough to be rolled out of the abdominal cavity.
7. *When performing a hysterectomy, the vaginal route should not be pursued* unduly long. As soon as it is determined that the vaginal procedure cannot safely be continued (because of adnexal changes, broad adhesions between the bowel or the omentum, uterine immobility, or underestimated uterine size), one should not hesitate to discontinue this approach (because the indication was wrong) and proceed abdominally.

Vaginal Hysterectomy in Total Prolapse

In patients with total vaginal prolapse, the anterior and posterior vaginal walls are completely inverted. Within the vaginal sac is the uterus, usually with an elongated, thinned cervix. The bladder reaches far down caudad under the anterior vaginal wall; its lower pole has sometimes sunk almost all the way to the portio.

With total prolapse, one should try to avoid injury to the bladder by localizing the lower bladder pole with a probe inserted into the bladder. The procedure is continued with a median colpotomy to expose the bladder. Only then is the hysterectomy performed, and finally the prolapsed bladder is plicated.

Technique

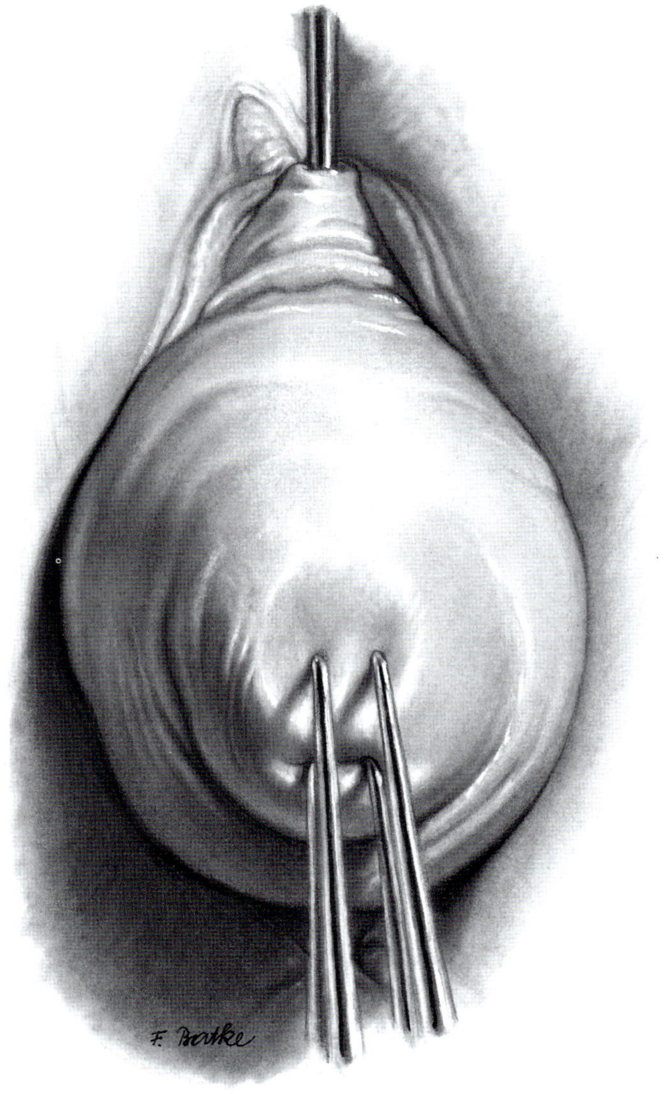

Figure 11.48. Vaginal hysterectomy in total prolapse. Locating the lower bladder pole.

Two tenacula have been placed on the anterior cervical lip and are being pulled by the left assistant, who draws the prolapsed uterus downward. The interior vaginal wall is completely inverted.

By means of a probe in the bladder, the surgeon determines how far the bladder reaches beneath the anterior vaginal wall. The tip of the probe deflects the anterior vaginal wall forward somewhat to recognize the lowermost border of the bladder: the lower pole of the bladder reaches almost to the tenacula.

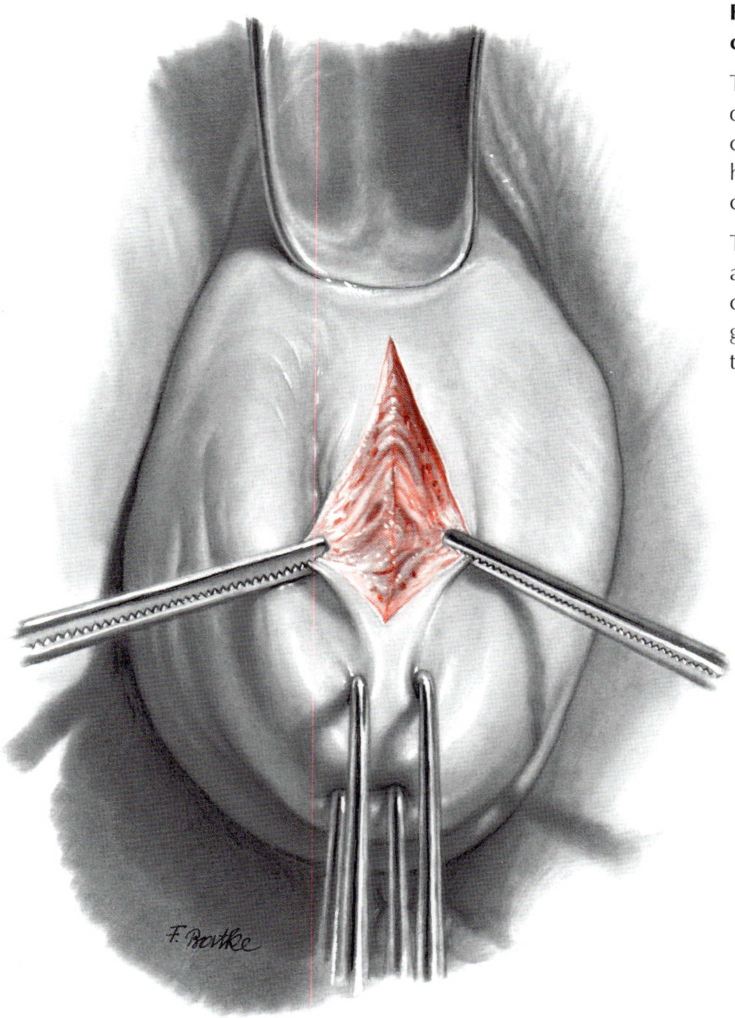

Figure 11.49. Vaginal hysterectomy in total prolapse. Median colpotomy.

The prolapsed uterus and inverted anterior vaginal wall are pulled downward with the two tenacula attached to the anterior lip of the cervix; traction is made on the tenacula by the left assistant's left hand. The right assistant stretches the anterior vaginal wall with counterpressure applied through an anterior retractor.

The median colpotomy is begun by severing the vaginal mucosa and fascia; this opens the vesicovaginal space. The colpotomy incision extends caudally almost to the portio. The wound edges are grasped with toothed clamps that are pulled down and outward by the assistants.

Figure 11.50. Vaginal hysterectomy in total prolapse. Dissecting the bladder free on the right side.

The median colpotomy is extended from the portio to just under the urethral meatus. The tenacula on the portio are pulled sacrally by the surgeon. The wound edges of the fascial flaps of the vaginal wall are grasped with toothed tenacula.

The left assistant pulls up only on the clamp at the uppermost wound angle using the right hand. In addition, the clamps attached to the left vaginal wound edge are held parallel with each other in his or her left hand. The right assistant fans out the clamps placed on the right wound edge with both hands.

At the right side, the mucosa and fascia have already been dissected free of the bladder. The mobilized bladder balloons forward.

Detail. Layers of the vaginal wall (see also Fig. A.18).

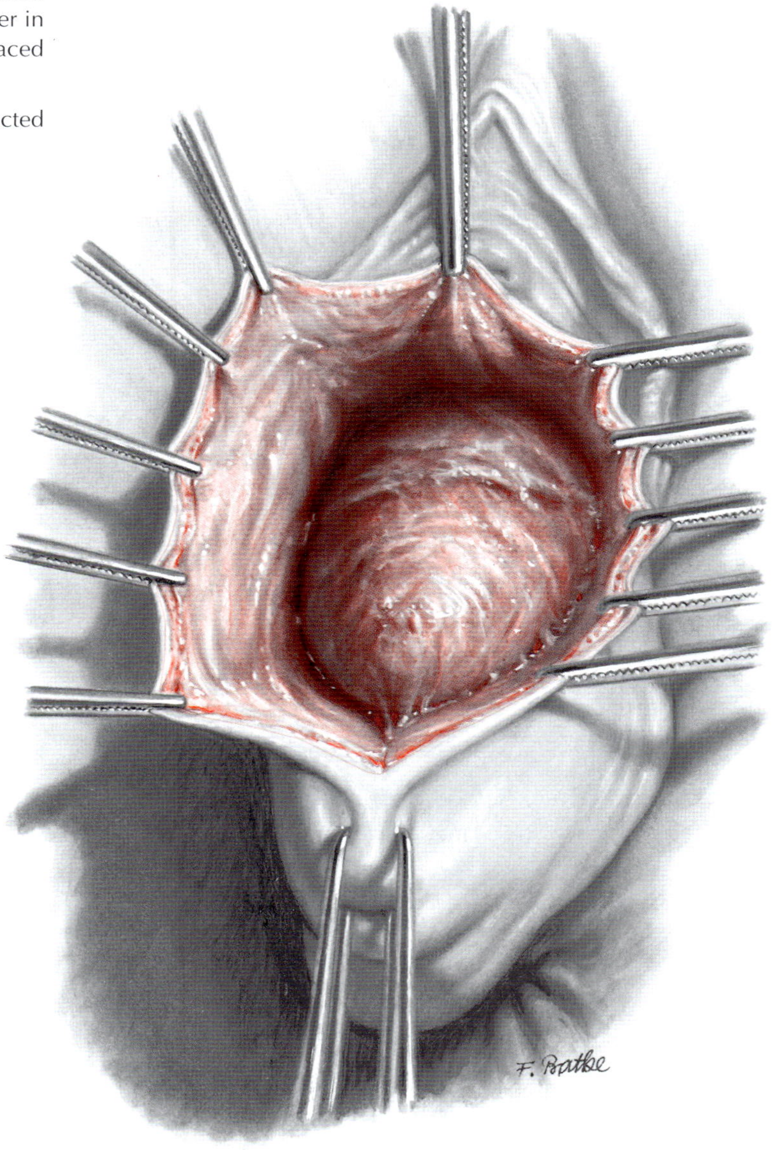

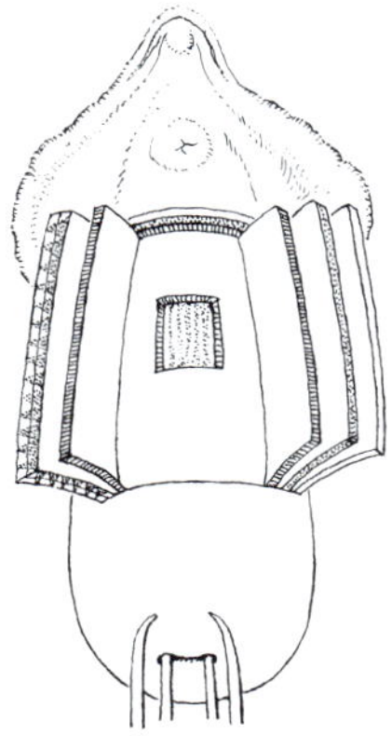

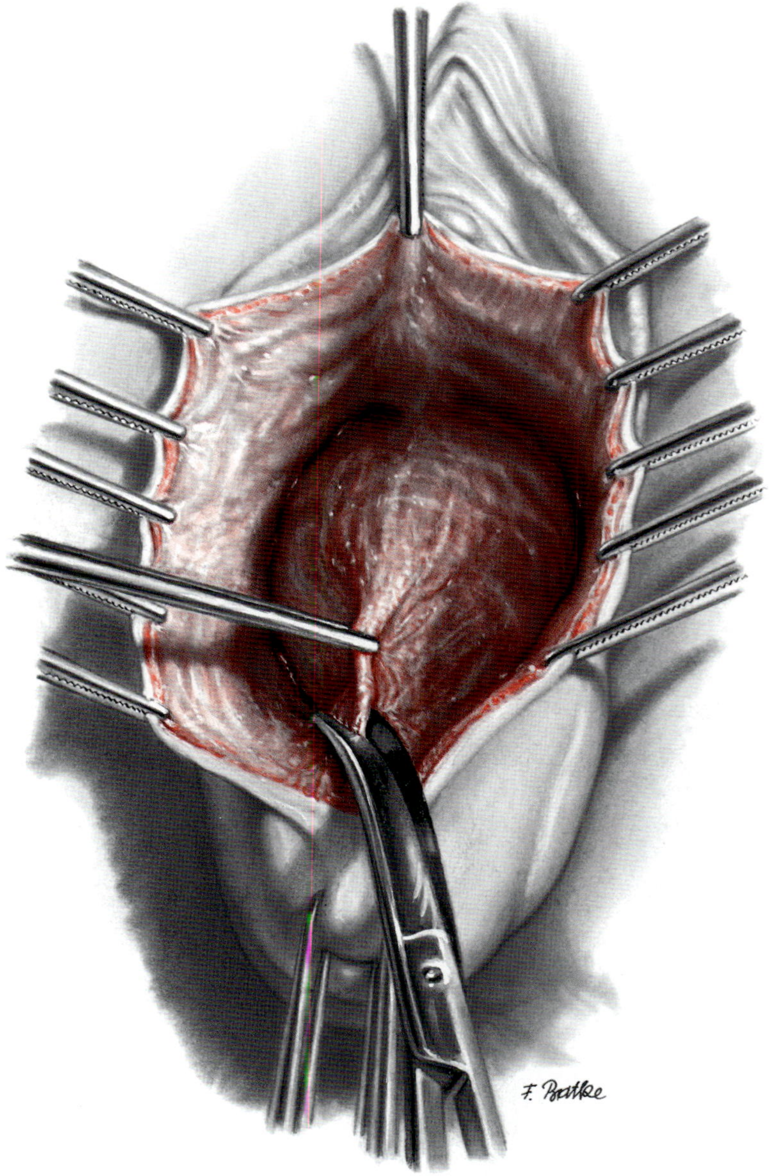

Figure 11.51. Vaginal hysterectomy in total prolapse. Dividing the supravaginal septum.

The left assistant's left hand pulls the tenacula down, while the right assistant's left hand pulls the clamp grasping the uppermost wound angle up. Both assistants hold the wound edge clamps in parallel under slight lateral traction.

The bladder is completely freed bilaterally; the bladder neck and urethra are exposed.

The surgeon lifts the lower pole of the bladder (which reaches far caudally) with toothed tissue forceps and severs the supravaginal septum; tips of the scissors point toward the cervix.

Figure 11.52. Vaginal hysterectomy in total prolapse. Mobilizing the lower bladder pole.

The bladder is entirely freed laterally on both sides. The vesicocervical space is opened. The surgeon inserts the right index finger here to elevate the lower pole of the bladder above the peritoneal reflection.

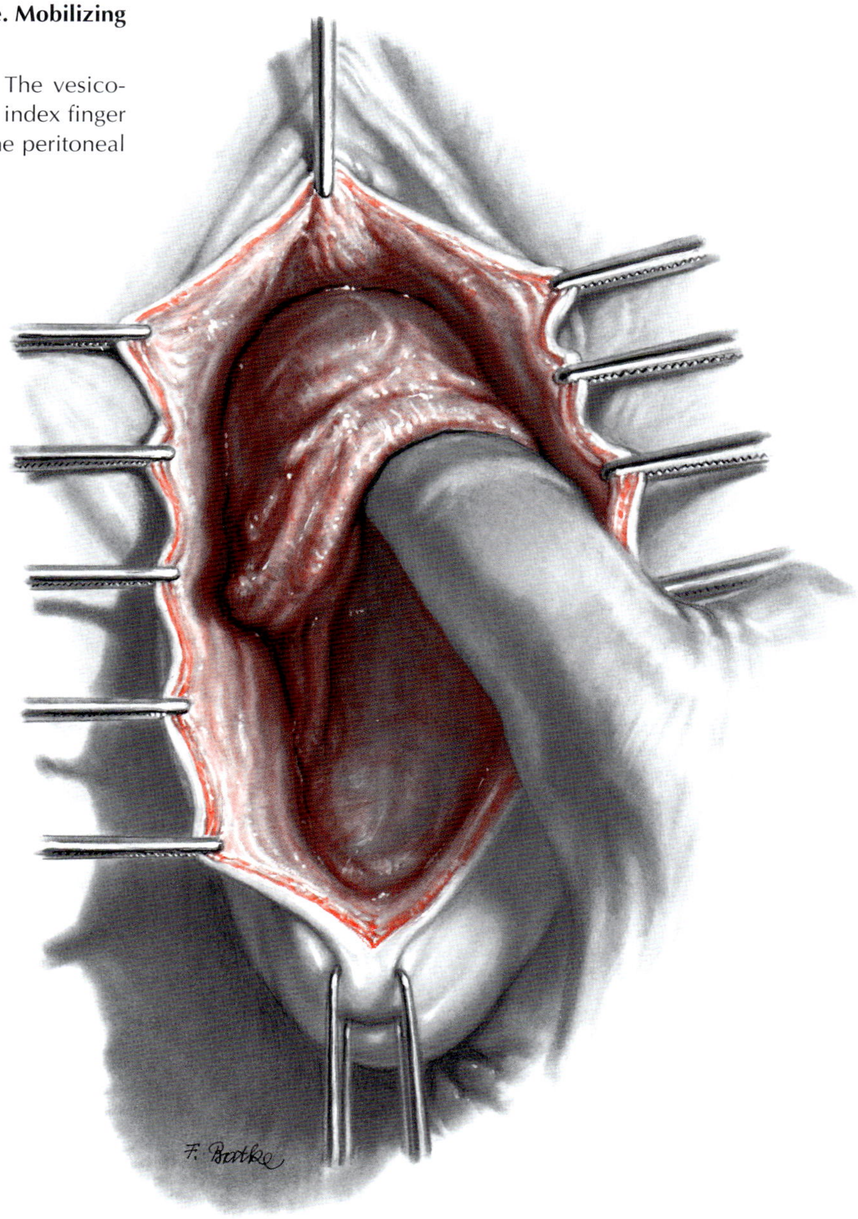

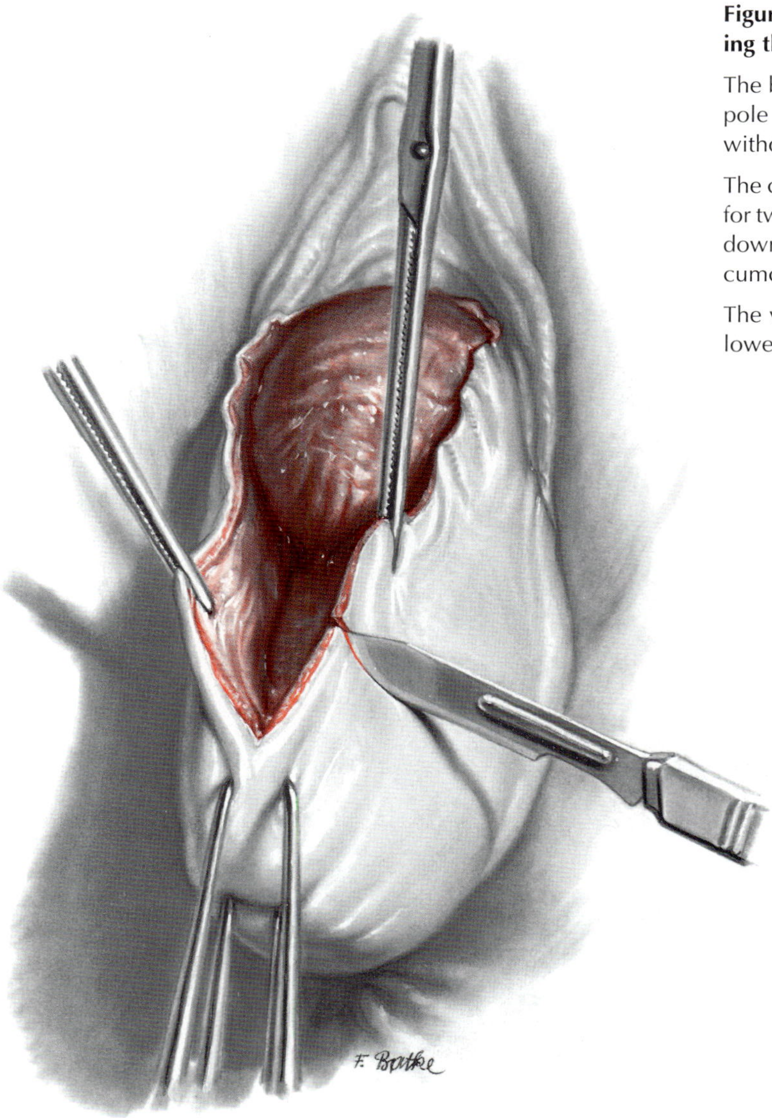

Figure 11.53. Vaginal hysterectomy in total prolapse. Circumcising the vagina.

The bladder has been completely mobilized and the lower bladder pole moved upward. The vaginal circumcision can now be done without risk of bladder injury.

The clamps on the vaginal wound edges have been removed except for two; those are pulled upward by the assistants. The surgeon pulls down on the tenacula attached to the anterior cervical lip and circumcises the inverted prolapsed vaginal canal with a scalpel.

The vaginal circumcision is performed about 2 cm cranially to the lowest angle of the colpotomy incision.

Figure 11.54. Vaginal hysterectomy in total prolapse. Ligating the left parametrium.

The right assistant pulls the portio downward with the tenacula and lifts the mobilized bladder to the right with a retractor inserted in the vesicocervical space; this stretches the left bladder pillar in which the ureter courses.

On the right side the parametrium has already been doubly ligated and divided from the cervix. The left prolapsed vaginal wall is completely dissected from the bladder and is turned outward by a toothed clamp fixed to its edge.

The cul-de-sac peritoneum is already opened and fixed to the posterior vaginal wound edge by spaced sutures (three are visible on the left side).

On the anterior uterine surface one can see the peritoneal reflection; the cervix is noticeably elongated and thin.

The surgeon places the left index finger into the opened cul-de-sac of Douglas to grasp the uterosacral and Mackinrodt ligaments. The lateral and posterior parametrial tissue bundles are ligated far caudad from the visible peritoneal reflection, but near the cervix, with a Deschamps needle.

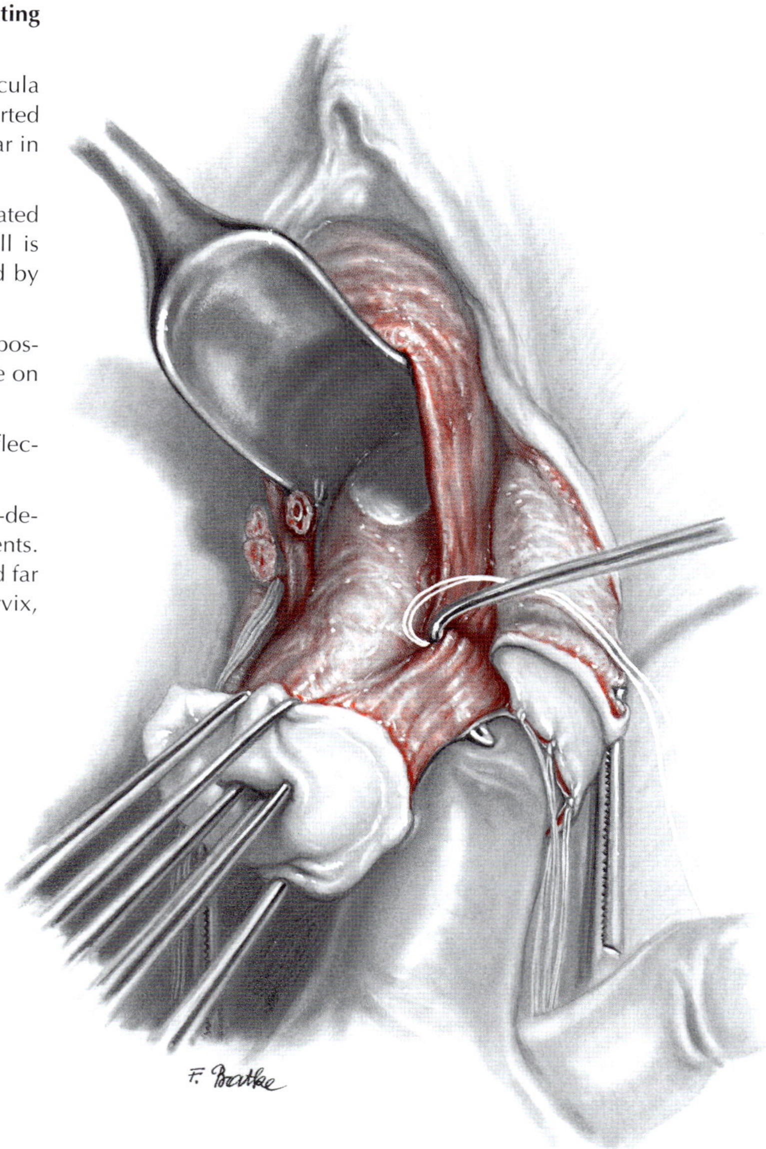

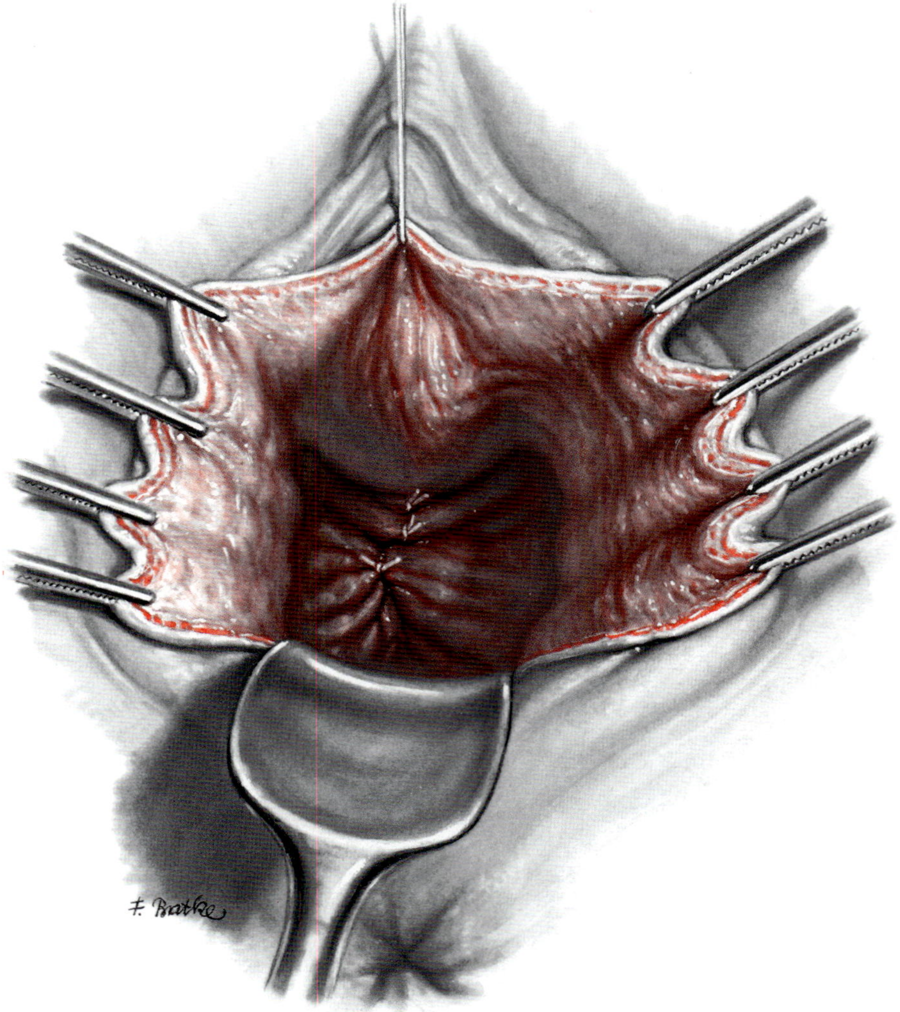

Figure 11.55. Vaginal hysterectomy in total prolapse. Plicating the bladder.

The uterus and the adnexa have been removed, and the peritoneal cavity is closed. The fascial flaps of the vaginal wall are again grasped with toothed clamps, which are retracted to the sides to expose the operative field. A posterior retractor provides better visualization by depressing the posterior vaginal wall sacrally.

Two purse-string sutures have been placed at the neck of the bladder. The remaining part of the descended bladder has been gathered with another half-purse-string suture. There is a distinct angulation between the urethra and the plicated bladder neck.

Technical Problems—Figures 11.48–11.55

1. *Circumcision* of the prolapsed vagina should not be done *without first freely mobilizing the lower bladder pole* via a median colpotomy. This may lead to injury of the bladder because it almost reaches to the external cervical lip.
2. Should the *parametrial ligatures be placed too high* on the tautly stretched parametria during their ligation, the ureter may be included because it reaches down in this region.
3. *Plication sutures of the bladder that reach too far laterally* can badly dislocate or even incorporate the juxtavesical portions of the ureter.

12/ Anterior Colporrhaphy

Indications

The anterior colporrhaphy is used for reconstructing the supporting structures of the bladder floor and the urethra; it is a component of surgical treatment for vaginal prolapse. It is seldom carried out alone; rather it is usually combined with a colpoperineoplasty (reconstruction of the pelvic floor). The anterior repair unites the supporting tissue where it has separated laterally under the bladder and urethra, elevates the descending lower bladder pole, and tightens the vagina. If simultaneous urinary incontinence occurs, the urethrovesical junction must be plicated and supported precisely and extensively in the area of the internal urethral orifice by means of periurethral tissue (pubovesical fascia).

For choice of surgical method and its extent the following must be considered:

- Degree of vaginal prolapse;
- Size of the uterus;
- Occurrence or lack of bladder impairment;
- Retaining the reproductive capability;
- Age of the patient.

With regard to women in childbearing age, we must note, however, that subsequent pregnancies and childbirths are to be seen as potentially damaging for any vaginal repair.

We will follow the approach to anterior colporrhaphy that in the past has been regarded as the classical method; numerous modifications of this technique are found in the literature.

Technique

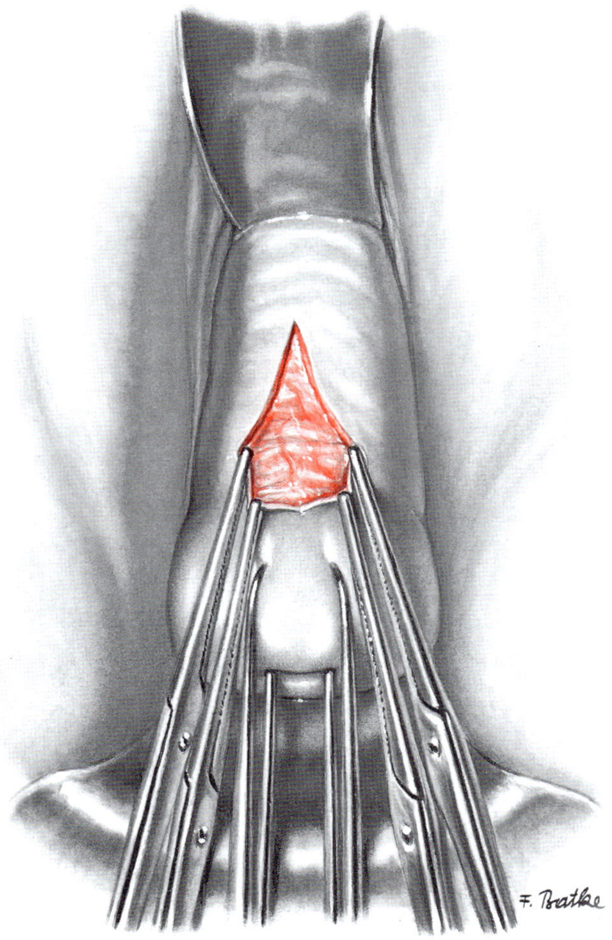

Figure 12.1. Anterior colporrhaphy. Median colpotomy.

A posterior retractor pushes the posterior vaginal wall toward the sacrum. The cervix is grasped with two tenacula and pulled forward in front of the vulva.

In our opinion, a median longitudinal colpotomy incision leads to fewer problems in the later dissection of the vaginal mucosa from its fascia or from the bladder than the alternative technique involving excision of the vaginal wall by means of an elliptical incision.

The incision begins just above the cervix and is continued upward for a few centimeters. One severs only the vaginal mucosa, leaving the underlying fascia intact.

The vaginal wound edges are grasped with delicate toothed clamps, two on each side. The right assistant pushes the inverted vaginal wall upward with a retractor, stretching it further with this motion.

The median colpotomy is extended upward.

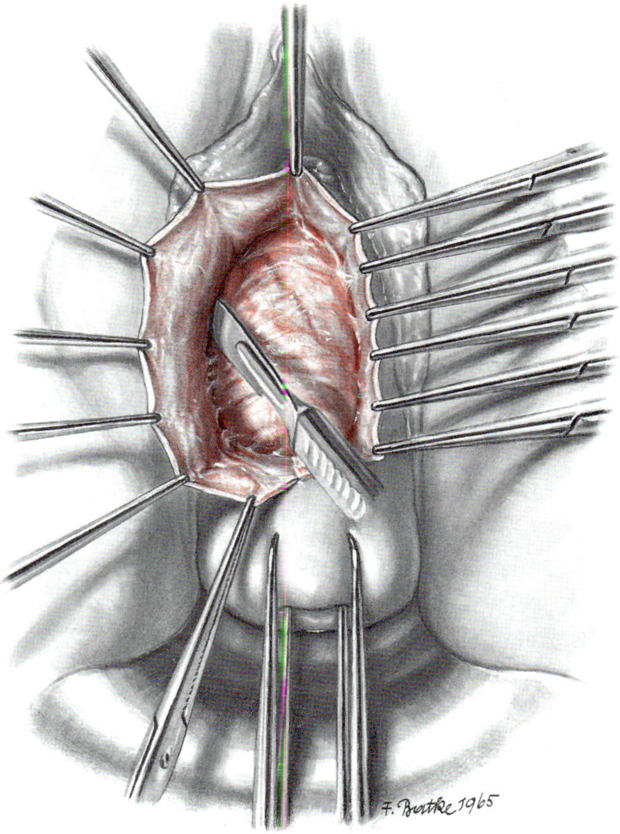

Figure 12.2. Anterior colporrhaphy. Dissecting the vaginal wall on the right side.

The median colpotomy incision has been extended from the cervix to just beneath the external urethral meatus.

The left-sided clamps are held in parallel and pulled slightly to the left by the assistant, who places a single clamp at the upper wound edge and pulls it upward with the right hand. The assistant on the right fans out the clamps with both hands.

Using a scalpel, the surgeon dissects laterally between the vaginal fascia and the mucosa and separates the vaginal wall from its fascia (the vaginal fascia remains attached to the vesical fascia on the bladder).

There is essentially no bleeding with this procedure because none of the small blood vessels coursing in the vaginal fascia are opened in the process. However, this approach, in which the mucosa is separated from the fascia and the bladder with its vaginal fascia are later plicated, is applicable only when a small cystocele is present. For greater degrees of cystocele, the median colpotomy incision must be carried through the vaginal mucosa and deepened through its fascia. This permits the surgeon to mobilize the bladder more extensively (compare with Fig. 12.7).

Figure 12.3. Anterior colporrhaphy. Dissecting the vaginal wall on the left side.

The right vaginal flap has been dissected. The right assistant takes over the midline clamp in the left hand and pulls it upward; in addition, he or she holds the clamps on the dissected vaginal wound edge to the side in parallel. Using both hands, the assistant fans out the clamps on the left vaginal wound edge.

The surgeon grasps the bladder with tissue forceps and pulls medially. Sharp dissection mobilizes the bladder laterally in analogous fashion to the procedure on the right side.

The better the vaginal wall is fanned out by traction on the attached clamps, the easier it is to dissect with curved incisions in the correct layer. After initial sharp dissection of the vaginal wall from its fascia, continuing lateral blunt dissection with sponge forceps is possible because the lateral aspects of the bladder are no longer fixed to the vaginal fascia.

Blunt dissection at the bladder neck or at the urethra is not possible because the vesical and vaginal fascias are closely adherent to one another. In this area one should dissect sharply with small incisions, and the vaginal fascia is left on the vesical fascia.

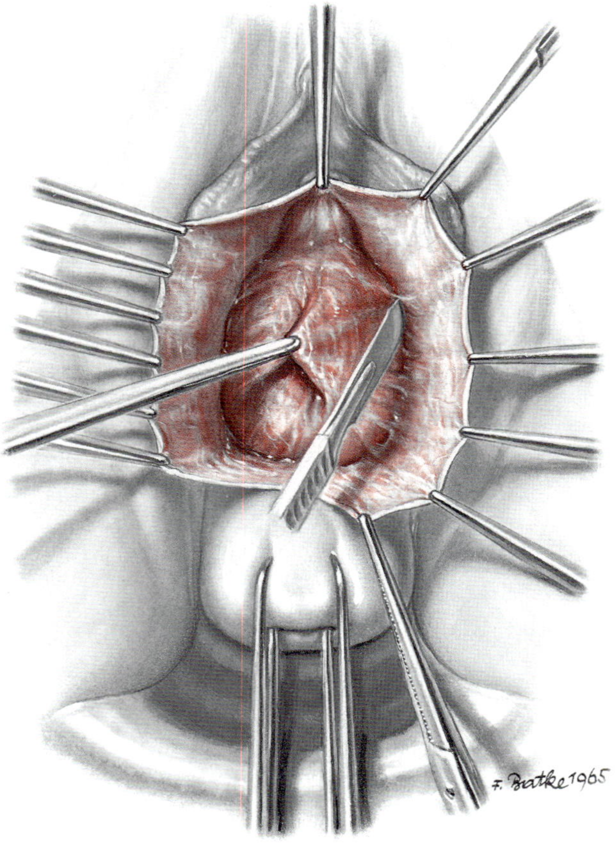

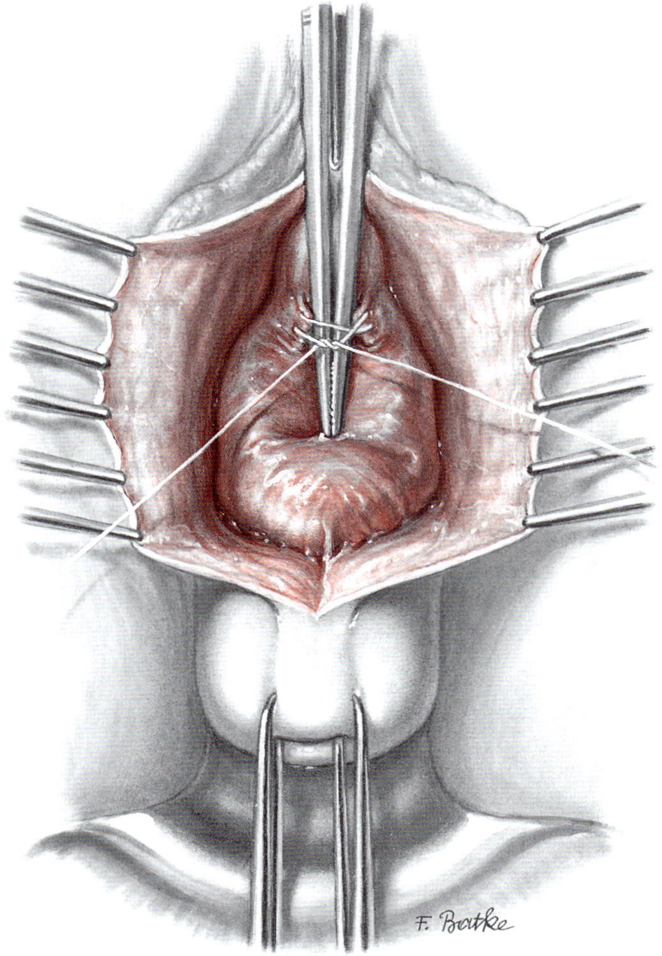

Figure 12.4. Anterior colporrhaphy. Suburethral plicating suture.

The vaginal wall has been dissected from the bladder bilaterally.

Clamps on the vaginal wound edges are held horizontally by the assistants on either side. The left assistant has taken hold of the uppermost midline clamp with the right hand and is pulling it upward.

A generous amount of paraurethral tissue is plicated at the urethrovesical juncture. While this suture is being tied, the tissue of the bladder neck is pushed back by tissue forceps and thus invaginated.

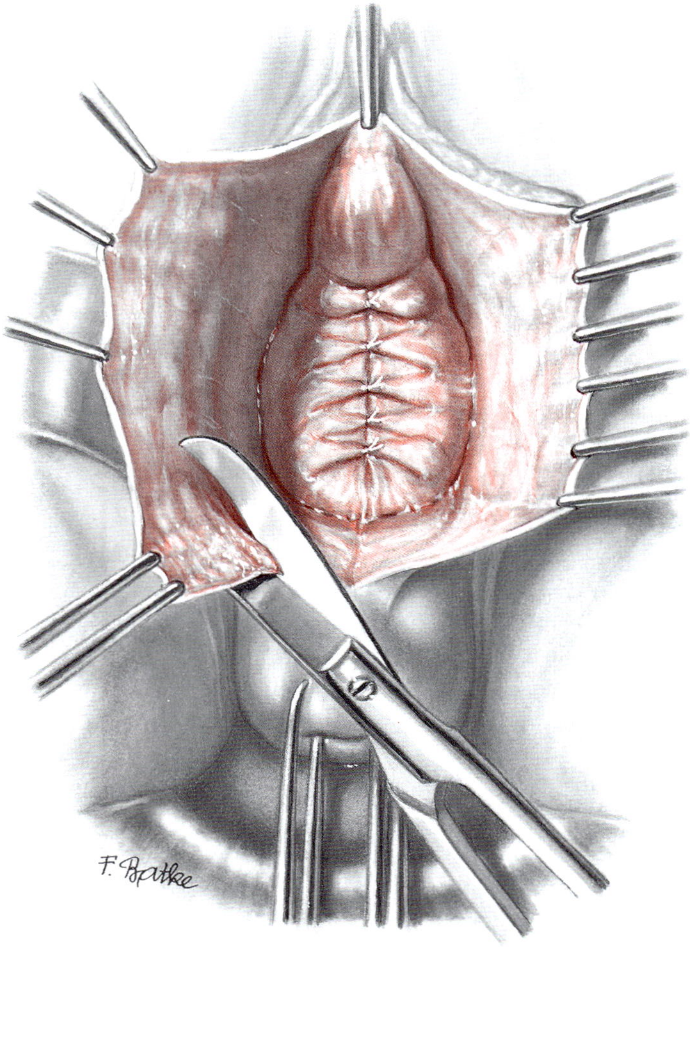

Figure 12.5. Anterior colporrhaphy. Resecting the superfluous vaginal mucosa.

At the level of the internal urethral orifice a tissue cushion has been formed by the suburethral plication suture; this produced angulation at the urethrovesical junction that somewhat narrows the urethral lumen, which will favorably affect any existing incontinence. The vaginal fascia is plicated by a sagittal tier of horizontal mattress sutures (the lowest bladder plication suture is fixed to the anterior wall of the cervix to form a supplementary "supravaginal septum").

An elliptical resection of the excess vaginal mucosa is performed with scissors. For this, the surgeon pulls down on two of the lowest clamps, and the assistant fans out the upper clamps and holds back the labia with a lateral retractor.

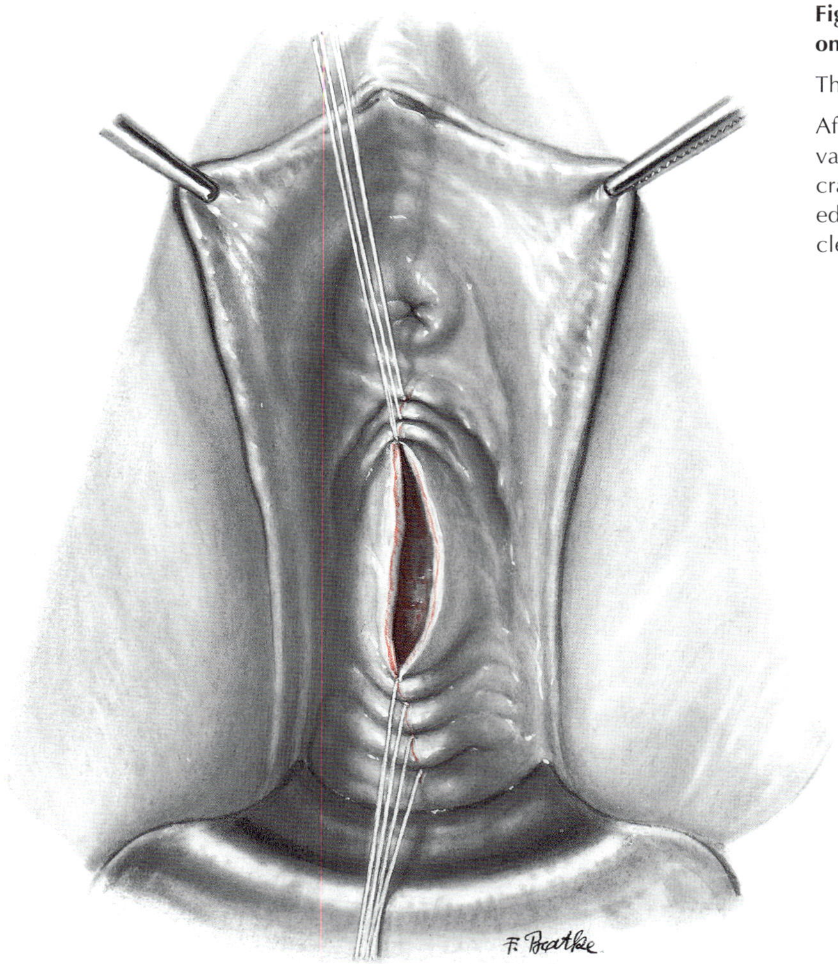

Figure 12.6. Anterior colporrhaphy. Closing the colpotomy wound.

The excess vaginal wall has been resected.

After the clamps have been removed from the cervix, the vaginal wound edges are sutured from the caudal end to the cranial. A pull on the lower sutures will present the wound edges retracted at the uppermost colpotomy region more clearly.

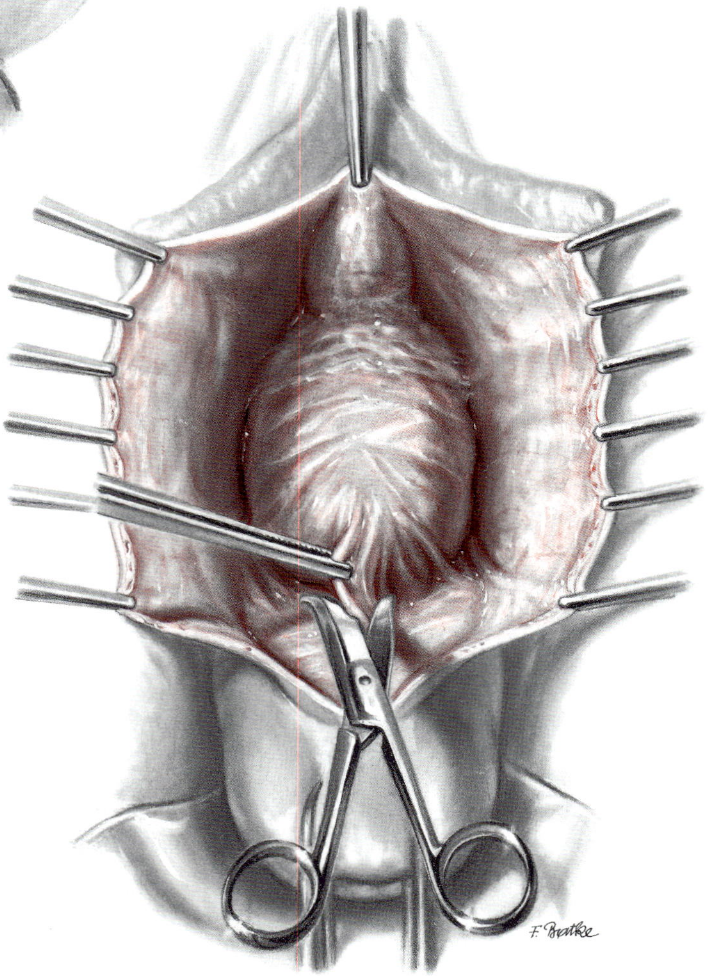

Figure 12.7. Anterior colporrhaphy with extensive cystocele. Dividing the supravaginal septum.

During the median colpotomy the vaginal wall and also its vessel-bearing fascia have been incised. The lower bladder has been well mobilized laterally by sharply dissecting in lateral direction between the vaginal and bladder fascia.

To avoid injuring the bladder or the urethra, the vaginal fascia was left adherent to the bladder fascia in the vicinity of the bladder neck because in this area both blend into a connective tissue layer that extends to the region of the upper third of the urethra (urethrovaginal septum).

To mobilize the lower bladder pole the bladder is lifted, and the stretched connective tissue bands of the supravaginal septum are severed close to the cervix; tips of the curved scissors point toward the cervix.

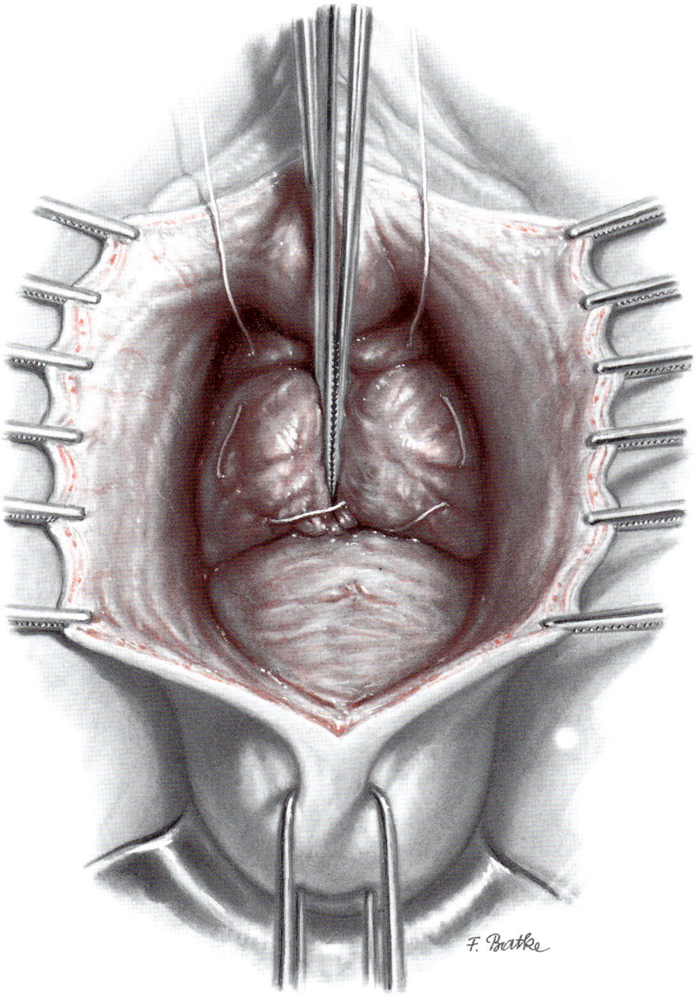

Figure 12.8. Anterior colporrhaphy with extensive cystocele. Plicating the bladder.

After the supravaginal septum had been dissected and the vesicovaginal space opened, the lower bladder pole was advanced to the peritoneal reflection. Remnants of the dissected supravaginal septum can be seen still attached to the anterior wall of the cervix.

The first suburethral plication suture has been performed near the bladder neck.

For further plication of the bladder, a half purse-string suture is placed, beginning on the left side at the site of the first suburethral suture and reaching caudally to the lower bladder pole; it is then continued on the right side upward to the first suburethral plication suture.

While this suture is tied, the assistant invaginates the bladder with tissue forceps.

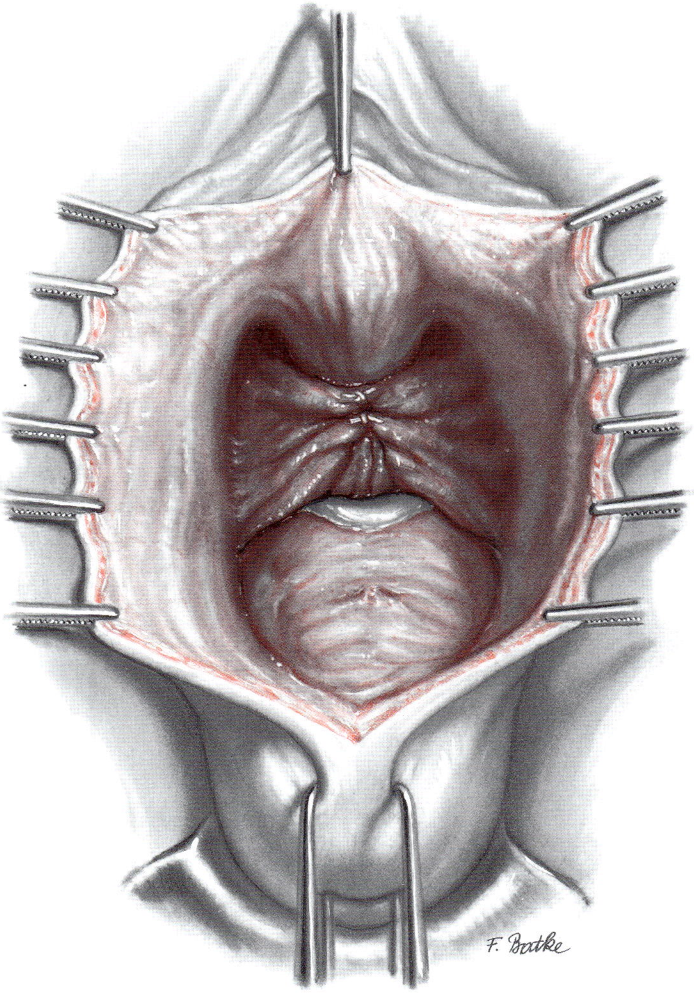

Figure 12.9. Anterior colporrhaphy with extensive cystocele. View after plicating the mobilized bladder.

The suburethral plication suture and the purse-string suture have been placed and tied. This not only plicated the bladder but also elevated it as well. The lower pole of the peritoneal reflection is in view.

Resection of the superfluous vaginal mucosa and closing of the colpotomy wound follow.

Technical Problems

1. During dissection of the vaginal flaps, the toothed clamps attached to the wound edge might be fanned out properly by the assistants, but they may have *retracted the flaps too far laterally* so that they are bent over. In this case the surgeon may enter the wrong tissue layers and ''buttonhole'' the vaginal wall, despite a gentle, stroking movement on the tissue with the scalpel. It can generally be avoided by ensuring that the assistant does not pull the flap too strongly in a lateral direction; instead it should be retracted up by pulling more in the sagittal direction. Simultaneously, the surgeon should retract the bladder medially with tissue forceps.

2. *One should avoid insufficiently mobilizing the vaginal wall at the upper end* of the median vertical incision. Especially with cases of urethrocele it is important that extensive lateral dissection be performed on the vaginal wall in the area of the bladder neck and urethra so that enough periurethral and perivesical tissue is exposed for later plication. Because of the dense interconnection here between the bladder and vaginal fascias, dissection must be performed sharply with a scalpel, and the vaginal mucosa must be separated from its fascia with small stepwise cuts. For this the left assistant has to lift the upper angle clamp with moderate force precisely in the midline. The surgeon must direct the blade of the scalpel so that it is slanted laterally, thus avoiding injury to the urethra. He or she always dissects close to the vaginal wall and leaves the vaginal fascia in this area attached to the fascia overlying the urethra and the bladder neck. After correctly dissecting in this region, one can recognize the urethrovesical transition that forms a distinctive angulation at the internal urethral orifice where the urethra exits from the bladder.

3. If *dissection is conducted too far laterally in the upper third of the vaginal wall*, the lateral aspects of the space of Retzius are entered. Some of the many veins draining the bladder may be injured here. Even a vaginal tamponade performed later cannot stop the resulting hemorrhage; instead, ligations must be used for that purpose. The needle for such ligatures should always be pointed laterally away from the urethra toward the pubic arch; it must be applied in the reverse direction, or the urethra may be punctured.

4. If *the supravaginal septum is divided incompletely* in the case of a noticeably prolapsed bladder, the lower pole of the bladder cannot be adequately mobilized, and the bladder cannot be advanced up to its original location. To avoid this complication it is occasionally necessary to incise the laterally stretched, tense bladder pillars near the cervix.

5. The excess vaginal mucosa can be *too extensively resected*, especially in its lateral aspects. In this case, the vaginal wound edges will be under too much tension when they are united, and that will lead to postoperative dehiscence. Even if the colpotomy wound *could just barely be closed without apparent tension* on the catgut mattress sutures it is still possible that too much of the vaginal wall has been resected. This situation will only be recognized at the end of the procedure: after reconstruction of the perineum, the vaginal canal is even more tightened with the colpoperineoplasty, causing coital problems.

It is better to excise too little than too much. It is not essential that the excess vaginal wall be resected generously to correct urinary incontinence; more important are the correct placement of the suburethral and vesical plication sutures, reconstruction of the relaxed pelvic floor by uniting the freed edges of the levators, and rebuilding the perineum.

6. The vaginal canal may be made too narrow by the anterior colporrhaphy and colpoperineoplasty procedures (it should be able to comfortably accommodate at least two fingers). If one finds at the conclusion of the perineal reconstruction that sexual intercourse will probably not be possible as a result of the excessive vaginal narrowing, it is advisable to make small lengthwise releasing incisions at 5 and 7 o'clock, respectively, in the lateral vaginal walls and then suture them transversely. This technique is not ideal, but it does enlarge the vaginal lumen without having to cut the sutures that have just been placed to reconstruct the perineum, which, after all, is especially important for alleviating incontinence.

7. With regard to *delayed scarring with stenosis* we recommend colpoperineoplasty (see point 18 under ''Technical Problems'' in Chapter 13).

13/ Colpoperineoplasty

Indications

The posterior colporrhaphy and perineorrhaphy procedures serve to reconstruct the pelvic floor. As a general rule, they are combined with an anterior colporrhaphy in patients with vaginal descensus. In cases with more severe grades of descensus and prolapse, combined with a moderate degree of urinary incontinence (''stress incontinence''), the patient's age and wish to retain menstruation and parity must determine above all the choice of surgical method.

For young women hoping to have children, the method of choice is an anterior colporrhaphy combined with a colpoperineoplasty. However, the disadvantage with this method is that renewed dilation of the birth canal during birth might render ineffective the result achieved from the prior surgical procedure to correct stress incontinence.

For older women, for whom conception is no longer desired nor even possible (see ''Indications'' under ''Basic Operation'' in Chapter 11), best results are achieved with a simple vaginal hysterectomy (while retaining the adnexa), followed by a colporrhaphy and a colpoperineoplasty. This procedure is particularly advised for patients also suffering from stress incontinence.

A colpoperineoplasty alone is rarely indicated. For patients with a large myomatous uterus that must be removed abdominally, this procedure may be performed after a hysterectomy for prophylaxis of a vaginal cuff prolapse.

Technique

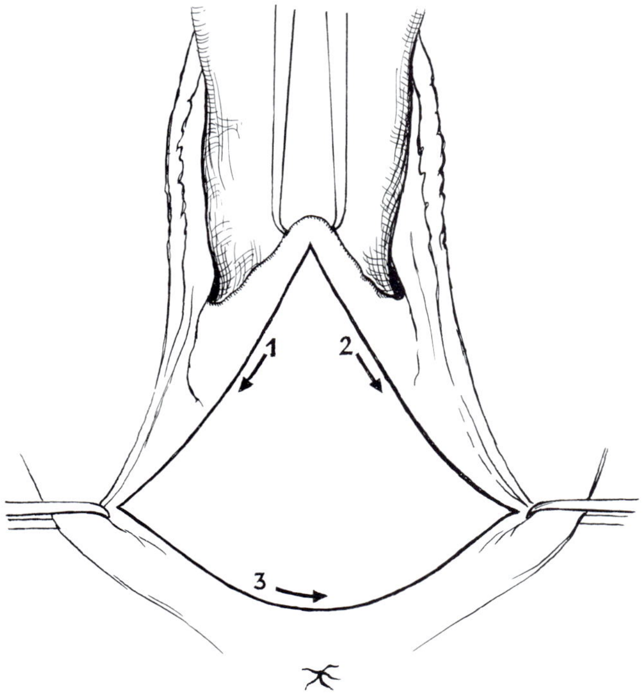

Figure 13.1. Colpoperineoplasty. Hegar plasty procedure.

The vagina is tamponaded with a gauze pack. Extent of the Hegar plasty is shown with three lines (*numbered arrows*).

Two tenacula are placed laterally on the posterior commissure. The distance between the lateral tenacula must be wide enough to allow two fingers to pass comfortably between them. An additional tenaculum is placed in the midline of the posterior vaginal wall. If a severe rectocele is present, the tenaculum must be placed higher up on the posterior vaginal wall.

In the presence of a large rectocele, recognizable by the saccular ballooning of the posterior vaginal wall, we recommend instead that a delicate silk traction suture (size 000) be placed to avoid injury to the rectum.

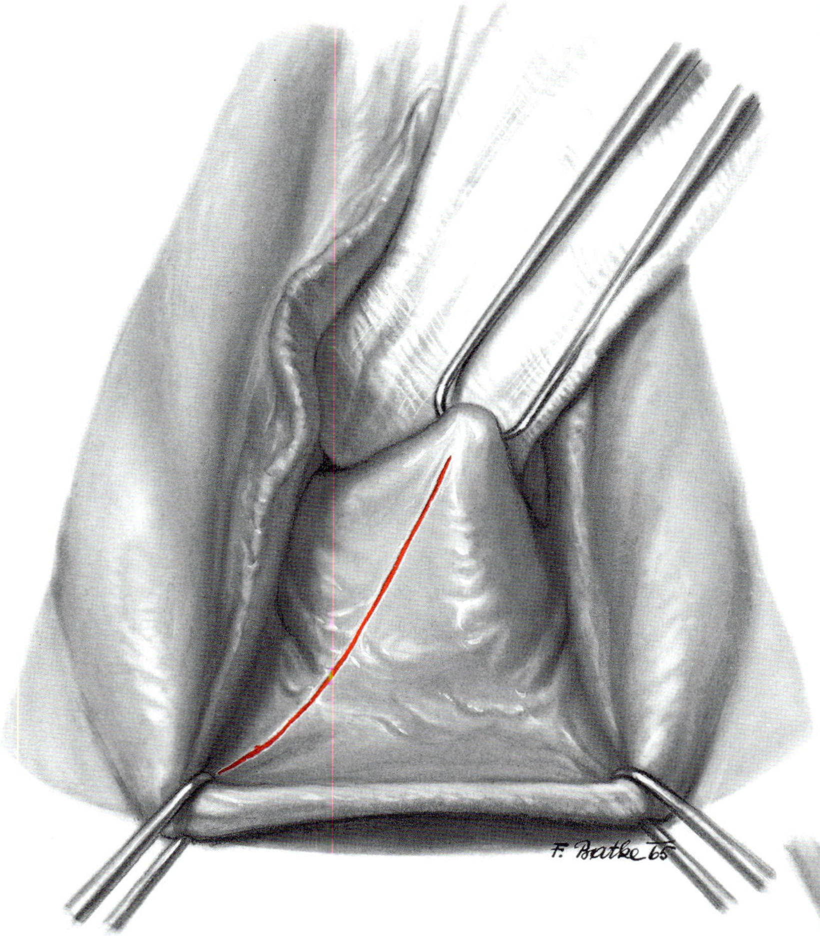

Figure 13.2. Colpoperineoplasty. Hegar plasty procedure.

To proceed with the right vaginal incision, the lateral tenacula are pulled downward, and the right hand of the left assistant pulls the median tenaculum upward to the left.

The incision is carried only through the vaginal mucosa; the underlying vaginal fascia is left intact at this point.

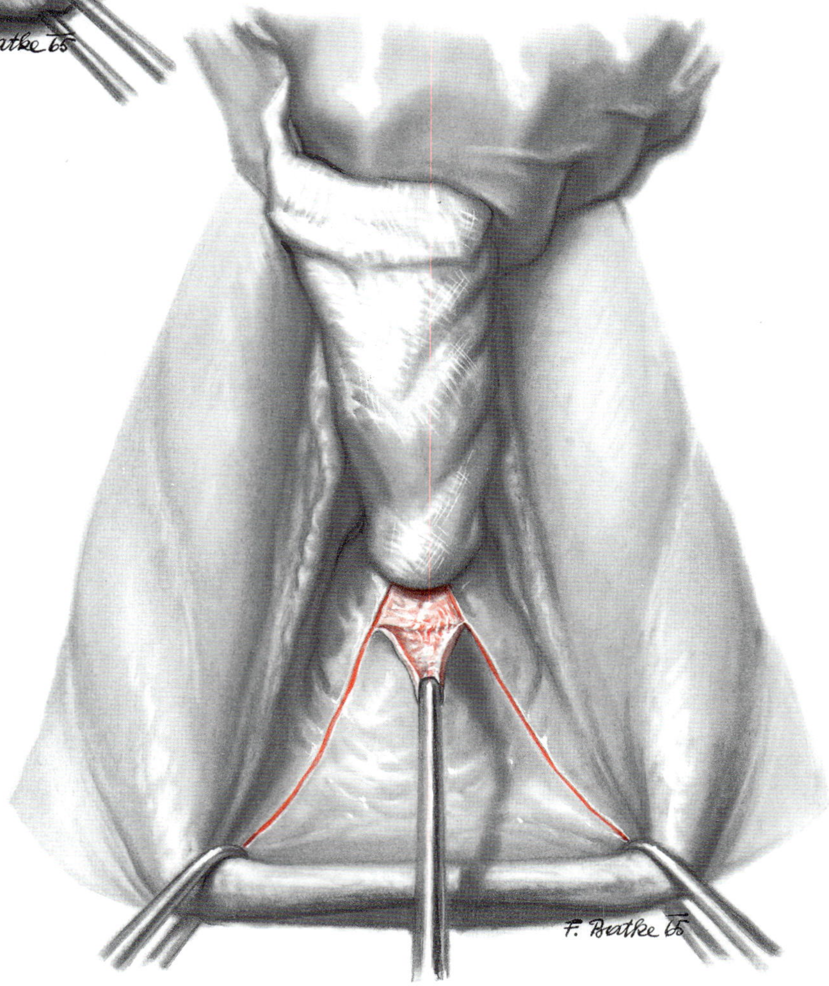

Figure 13.3. Colpoperineoplasty. Dissecting the mucosa within the Hegar triangle.

At this point, the vaginal mucosa alone is excised with a scalpel. To protect the rectum, the vaginal fascia is left intact on its anterior wall.

The right assistant makes it easier to execute this step. The anterior rectal wall is gently pushed back with his or her gauze-wrapped left index finger. This places fibers of the rectovaginal connective tissue on stretch so that they can be readily severed sharply without injury to the vaginal fascia on the anterior rectal wall or to the rectum itself.

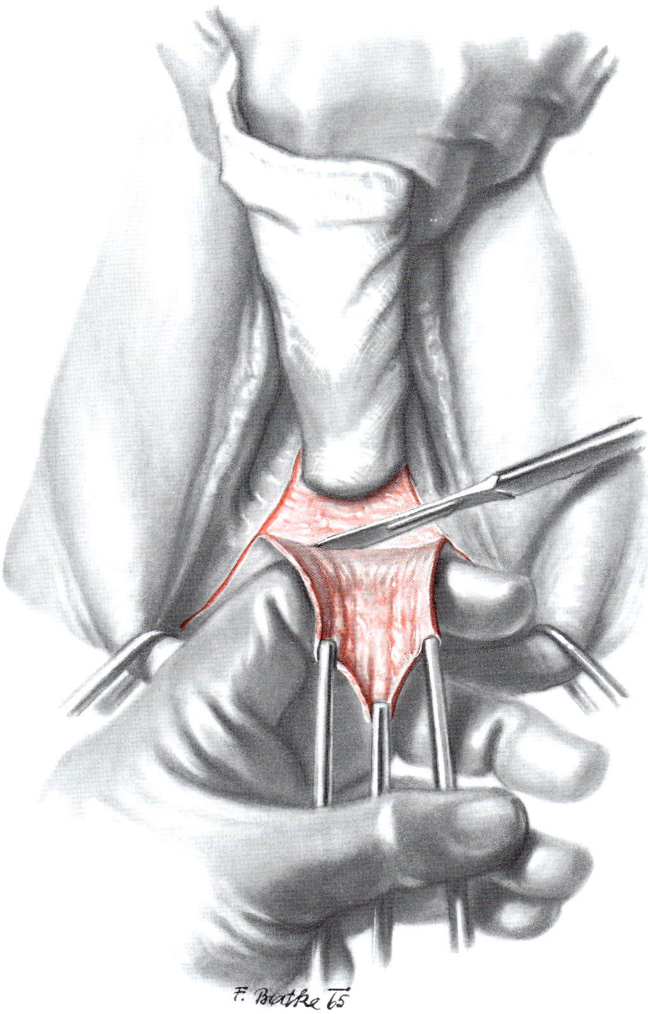

Figure 13.4. Colpoperineoplasty. Dissecting the posterior vaginal wall within the Hegar triangle.

The partially dissected mucosal flap is grasped with three toothed clamps and is inverted.

The surgeon positions the left index finger (acting as a buffer) under the dissected flap and pulls the mucosa downward by the clamps, thereby stretching the tissue. The dissection can now be continued with light transverse incisions. As before, the right assistant pushes the rectum back with the index finger. In this way, the vaginal wall is freed to the posterior commissure without ever endangering the rectum.

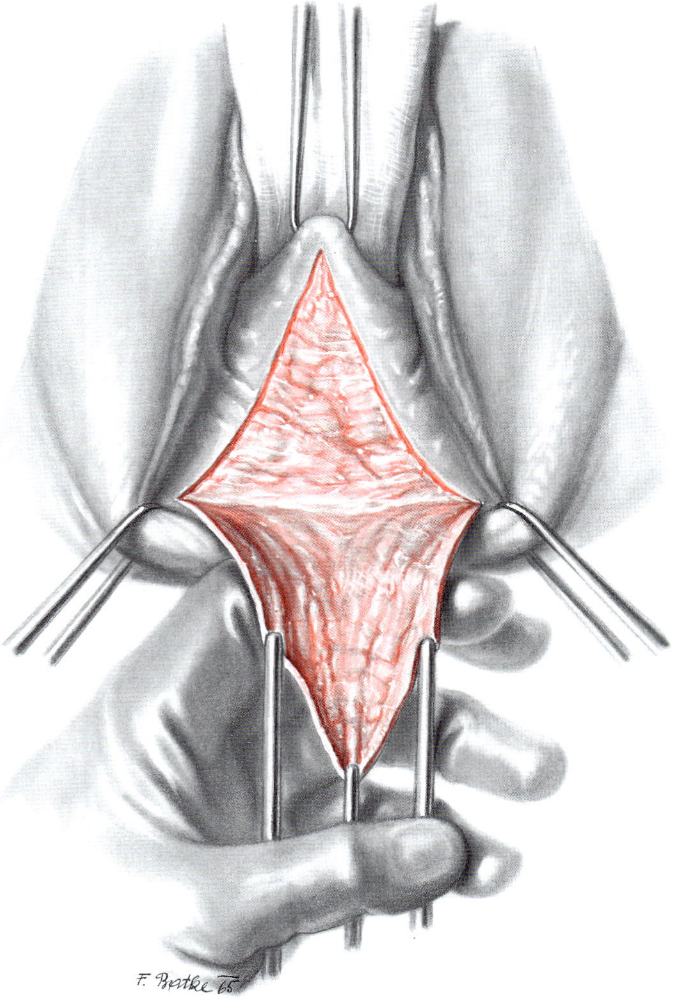

Figure 13.5. Colpoperineoplasty. Conditions after dissection of the vaginal flap to the posterior commissure.

Injury to the anterior rectal wall practically never happens with this dissection method.

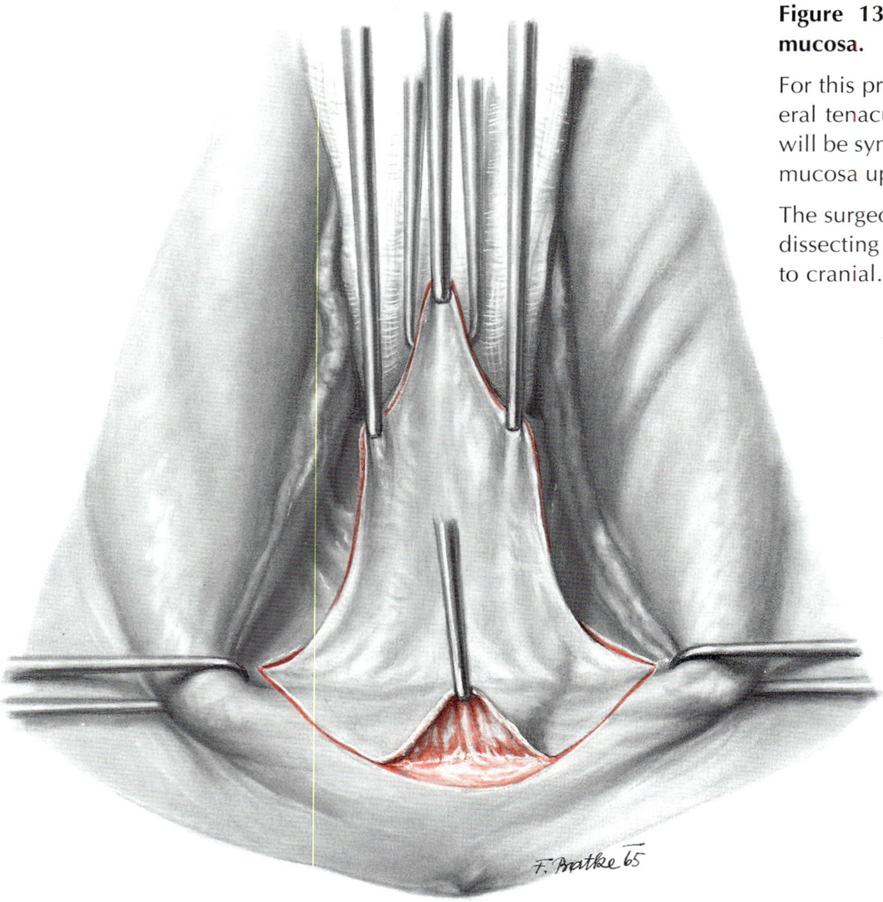

Figure 13.6. Colpoperineoplasty. Dissecting the perineal mucosa.

For this procedure, exact horizontal pull is exerted on the lateral tenacula to ensure that the curved perineal skin incision will be symmetrical. The right assistant pulls the flap of vaginal mucosa upward with three toothed clamps.

The surgeon begins on the lowest point of the triangle, sharply dissecting the perineal skin with a scalpel moving from caudal to cranial.

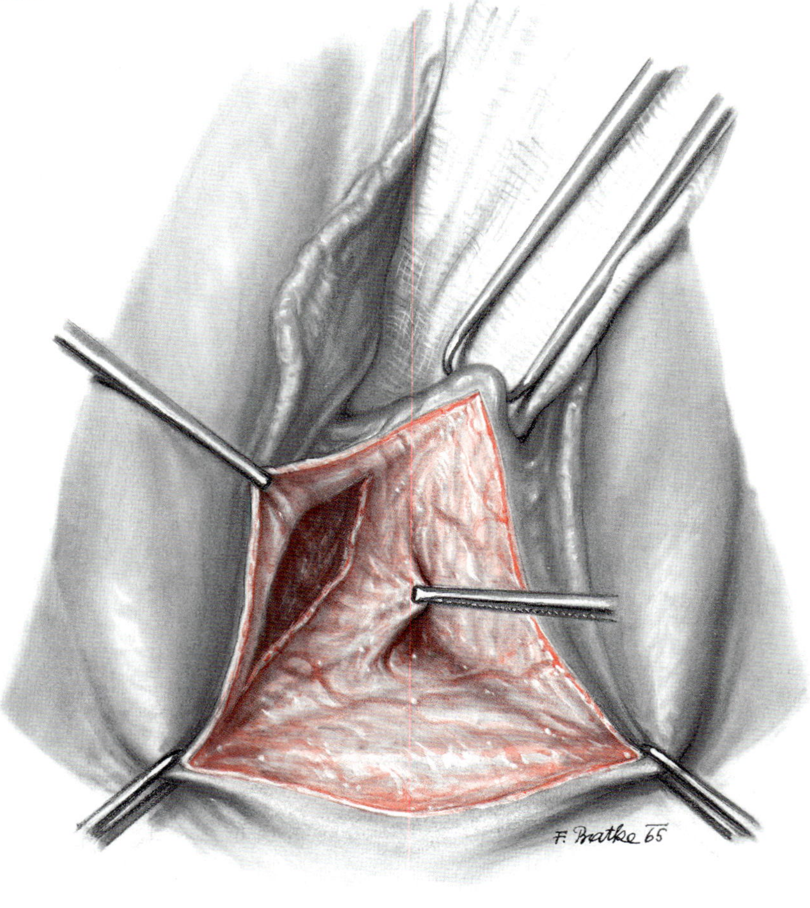

Figure 13.7. Colpoperineoplasty. Opening the rectovaginal space on the right side.

The skin is completely removed in the triangular incision area.

The right perineal tenaculum is pulled to the right and down and the median tenaculum to the left and upward; the toothed clamp placed on the right vaginal wound edge is pulled gently up and out.

The surgeon pulls the vaginal fascia toward the midline and severs it in parallel with the right vaginal wound edge until the rectovaginal space is opened.

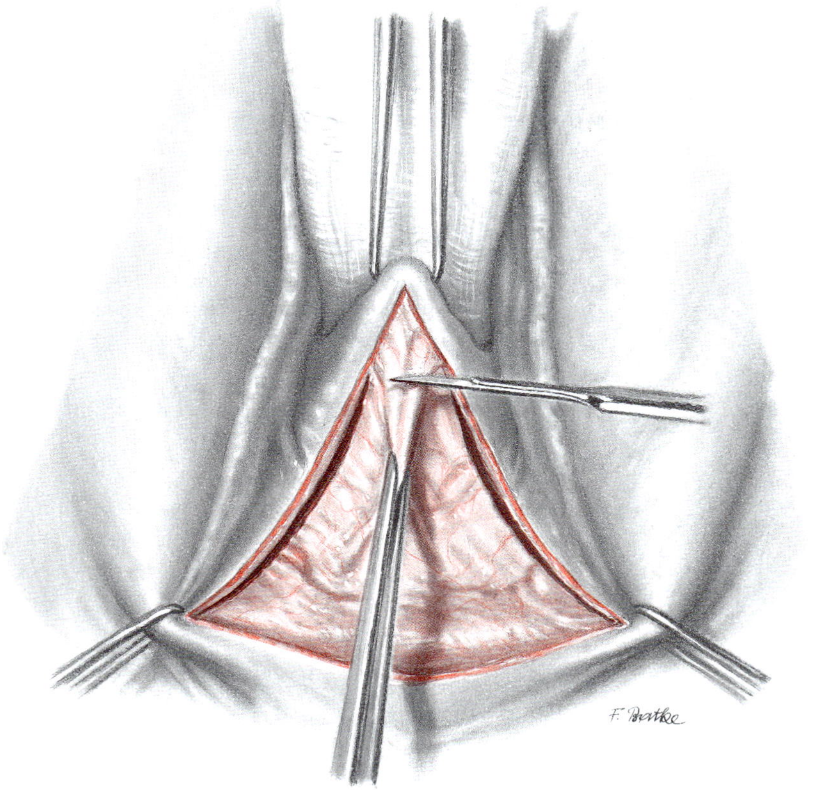

Figure 13.8. Colpoperineoplasty. Opening the rectovaginal space.

The vaginal fascia has been incised bilaterally parallel to the vaginal wound edge (laterally placed mucosal clamps are omitted here for clarity).

To open the rectovaginal space completely, the vaginal fascia must still be cut at the uppermost apical wound angle. It is usually easy to separate the anterior rectal wall bluntly from the cephalad portions of the posterior vaginal wall.

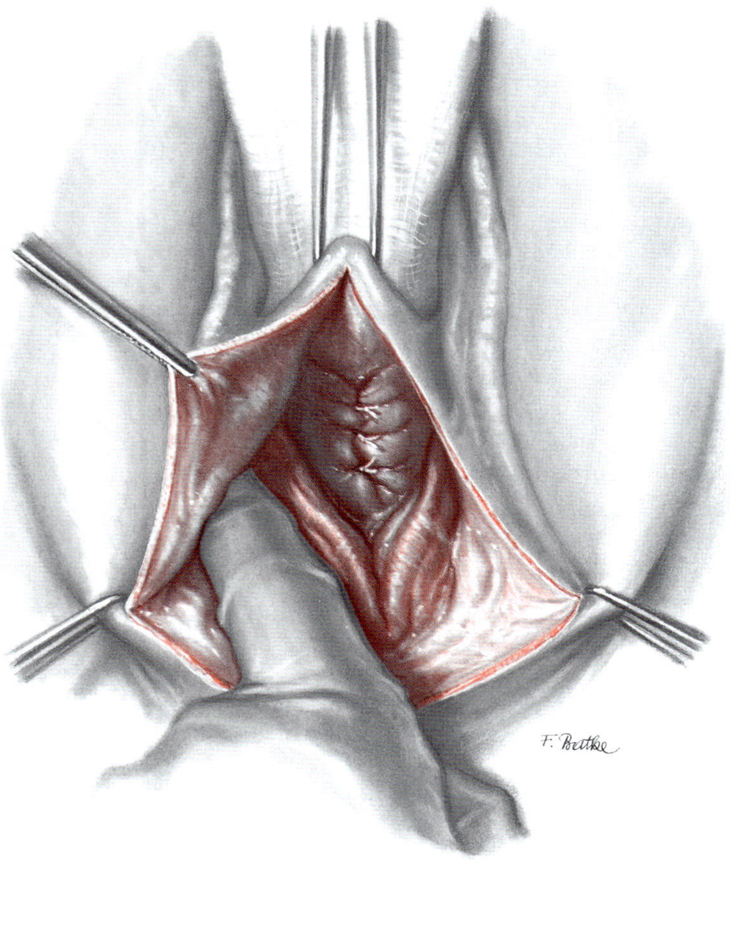

Figure 13.9. Colpoperineoplasty. Preparing the levator borders.

The forward ballooning anterior rectal wall is plicated with a sagittal row of catgut mattress sutures.

Levator fibers (puborectal muscle) are adherent laterally to the rectum; they can be dissected bilaterally by blunt pressure with an index finger applied laterally alongside the distal segment of the rectum, advancing into the cavity between the levator and the bulbocavernosus tissue. The finger should not be carried too deeply, or the levator lamina may be penetrated and the ischiorectal fossa will be opened; this will be recognized when the ischiorectal fat becomes visible.

The novice can identify the stretching of the levator borders on either side of the rectum by pulling on the anal sphincter because the levator fibers terminate in the external anal sphincter.

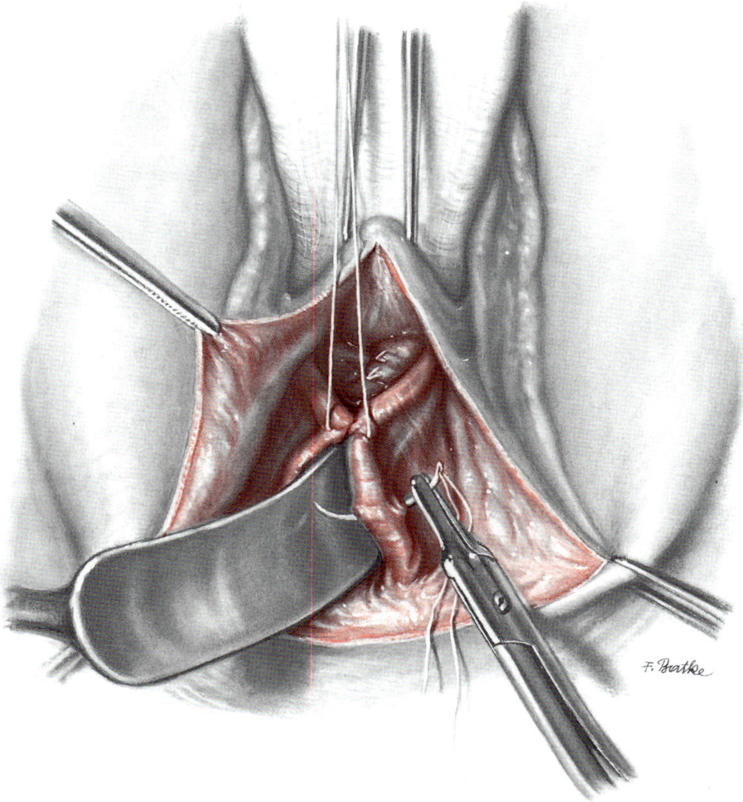

Figure 13.10. Colpoperineoplasty. Median approximation of the levator borders.

The puborectal fibers of the levator ani muscle adhere to the sidewalls of the rectum; they may appear, depending on their condition, either as a coarse muscular bundle or as a delicate strand. The levator borders are united with two or three interrupted catgut sutures placed in stepwise fashion from cephalad to caudad.

The uppermost levator suture is already in place but not yet tied. Instead the sutures are clamped and used to lift the suture upward. This allows distal aspects of the levator pillars to become more clearly visualized and makes it easier to place a second suture.

If a severe rectocele exists, the anterior rectal wall must be pushed back with a retractor for protection.

Figure 13.11. Colpoperineoplasty. Joining the bulbocavernosus tissue and perineal reconstruction.

The anterior rectal wall has been plicated with several interrupted catgut sutures. In the next layer, the levator borders were medially united with three catgut mattress sutures.

To construct a long perineum, the bulbocavernosus tissues on both sides are united in the midline with several sutures to form a flat layer. (This is the first suture.)

After the uppermost bulbocavernosus suture has been tied, one should check to ensure that the vagina still accommodates two fingers comfortably; if the reconstruction of the subfascial perineal tissue is too extensive, a step-like stricture of the posterior vaginal wall can result. The vaginal wound edges are then sutured from cephalad to caudad, up to the posterior commissure at first.

During reconstruction of the subfascial perineal tissue, one must be careful to unite the deep tissue layers of the wound with buried sutures to ensure that no dead space remains. That is often accomplished with a multilayered closure of the perineal tissue.

The perineal skin is sutured with interrupted silk sutures or with an absorbable material in a caudocranial direction; this allows exact juxtaposition of the perineal wound edges, which is more important than apposition of the vaginal mucosa. Once this is complete, the last of the vaginal mucosa can be closed with two or three catgut sutures.

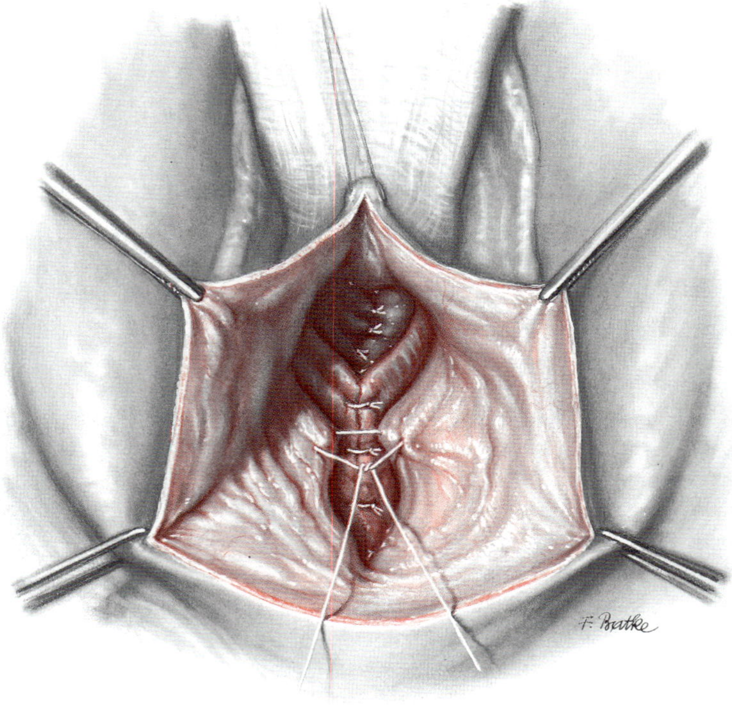

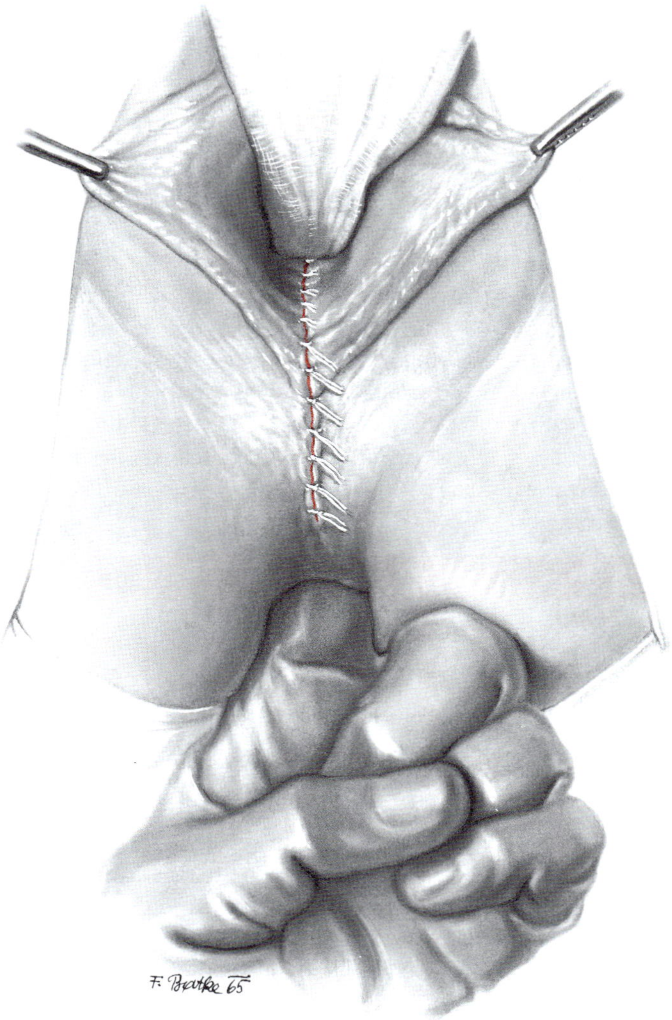

Figure 13.12. Colpoperineoplasty. View of the operative field at the end of the procedure.

The perineal skin edges were approximated with silk sutures; the vaginal wound was closed with catgut sutures. The vagina is tamponaded with a gauze strip.

A digital examination to the rectum should demonstrate that the reconstructed perineum can be felt as a thick, fleshy tissue layer. In addition, one must ensure with palpitation that the rectal wall has not, by any chance, been punctured while the levator sutures were applied. Should this be the case, it must be immediately corrected.

Technical Problems

1. If *the lateral tenacula are placed too far laterally* on the posterior commissure, the incision will be too wide, and later the introitus will be too narrow when the vaginal incision is closed.
2. When *the midline tenaculum is not placed high enough* on the posterior vaginal wall in association with extensive rectocele, the vaginal incision will not reach sufficiently far upward, and the rectocele will soon recur.
3. Should *the levator pillars in the triangular posterior vaginal wall incision be placed too far laterally* in the upper region, vaginal stenosis can occur when they are united.
4. During dissection of the perineal skin, the connective tissue fibers of the rectovaginal space may not be stretched because *counterpressure is not being applied* by the right assistant's index finger. If this should occur, the surgeon may approach too closely to the anterior wall of the rectum while dissecting the vagina from its fascia.
5. In the course of making the curved perineal skin incision, if the lateral *tenacula are not pulled precisely in a horizontal direction*, the incision on the perineum will be distorted, and consequently the perineal repair will be crooked.
6. The *rectovaginal space may be insufficiently opened* by the incision of the vaginal fascia that is placed parallel to the vaginal incision edges. If that is the case, the puborectal fibers of the levators are displaced laterally and are not visible.
7. If the *vaginal fascia* in the apical wound angle *is not divided*, and the rectovaginal septum is not completely opened, the rectum cannot be well mobilized from the posterior vaginal wall, nor can it in some cases be plicated properly with interrupted or purse-string sutures.
8. After incision of the vaginal fascia, the *surgeon's index finger* may penetrate too far laterally during dissection of the levator borders and *perforate the levator lamina*, opening the ischiorectal fossa.
9. *Dissection of the levator borders may be carried too far cephalad*. This will cause bleeding that can be stopped only with difficulty. If hemostasis is inadequate, the perineal skin overlying the reconstructed area will become ecchymotic by 24 hours postoperatively. Intervention is unnecessary with a slight hematoma; if conservative measures are observed, gradual absorption will occur, and the posterior repair will hold. However, when very active bleeding occurs, the hematoma will cause dehiscence of the wound a few days after the operation.
10. When *the midline approximation of the dissected levator borders is carried too far cephalad*, excessive narrowing of the vagina may result with the formation of a ringlike stenosis. This causes pain particularly during intercourse.
11. The *levator borders may not be well dissected and united* because only the vaginal fascia and the bulbocavernosus tissue were brought together with buried sutures. As

a consequence, there is no levator support, and descent of the posterior vaginal wall will recur in time. This is the most common cause of recurrence.

12. In severe rectocele, the triangular incision in the posterior vaginal wall has to extend above the sac-like protrusion and must be made larger than usual; moreover, the rectum should be dissected from the lateral vaginal wound edges so that the ballooning rectal wall can be plicated with several sutures. Then the lateral vaginal wound edges will be elevated away from the rectum and become freely mobile in the operative field. Despite the forgoing extensive triangular excision of mucosa, there generally appears to be much superfluous vaginal wall left. However, it is essential that one refrain from undertaking another *resection on the lateral sides of the triangular incision* because the appearance of excessive vaginal mucosa is an illusion, and circular vaginal stenosis may result.

13. If the *deep tissues* at the upper vaginal wall are *too widely plicated*, a very serious stenosis of the vagina will be produced. This can be avoided by uniting only the vaginal wound edges in this region with interrupted sutures; the perineal tissue should be plicated only farther down.

14. *Dead spaces* should not be left in the course of the layered closure of the perineum. Bleeding can occur into these spaces because the perineal tissue was not completely closed, and thus there was inadequate hemostasis.

15. The interrupted silk sutures placed to bring the delicate perineal skin edges together *must not be tied too tightly*, or they will cut through after a few days.

16. If the patient's *legs are overly abducted*, tension my develop while tying the perineal skin sutures. This is easily avoided by changing the patient's position (leg abduction and stretching of the hip joint) so that the legs are brought closer together.

17. Tamponading the narrowed vaginal canal at the conclusion of the anterior colporrhaphy and colpoperineoplasty must be done gently; *forceful packing* will cause dehiscence of the wound.

18. Occasionally, one discovers during the postoperative examination that the *vaginal introitus* or canal has become *too narrow*. One should await complete healing of all wounds, a period of at least 3 months after the first operation, before proceeding to correct the problem. One divides the troubling introital or vaginal band of scar tissue with two small lateral longitudinal incisions and then joins the gaping wound edges transversely with delicate sagittally placed interrupted catgut sutures. However, for a less severe vaginal stenosis, one can widen the vaginal canal immediately after finishing the colpoperineoplasty with small lateral longitudinal incisions. If this does not produce a well-functioning result, the stenosis and/or the excised scar tissue must be replaced with interposition of healthy tissue at a later time (flap plasty).

Surgical Treatment of Enterocele

In patients who have an enterocele, the posterior vaginal incision must reach all the way to the posterior vaginal fornix. Dissection of the vaginal wall begins at the uppermost wound angle. The hernia sac of the ballooning space of Douglas is not opened but is plicated with a light purse-string suture because even when the peritoneum is opened with great care, there is the risk of injuring the bowel that is often affixed to the cul-de-sac by adhesion strands. In our opinion, resection of the hernia sac is unnecessary. We advise that the peritoneal connective tissue, which has receded laterally in the presence of a large enterocele, be plicated. After this, the levator muscle is freed and sutured medially (possibly also bringing fibers of the rectal pillars together in front of the rectum with interrupted catgut sutures), and an extensive posterior repair performed.

14/ Amputation of the Cervix

Indications

Since the introduction of diagnostic and therapeutic conization of the cervix, partial amputation of the cervix is less common because satisfactory results can be achieved with conization alone. High amputation of the cervix, however, is still performed occasionally for the patient with a hypertropically enlarged, plump, and elongated cervix as well as the patient with extensive dysplasia. These conditions generally cannot be effectively treated nor histologically cleared up with conization. ''Carcinoma-in-situ'' also represents an indication. In Chapter 15 we detail how the cervical wound surface is covered. However, because the manner in which the needle is guided and directed during isolated cervix amputation is somewhat different with Sturmdorf sutures, we are presenting a summary of this method immediately after our discussion of amputation, dissection of bladder and rectum, and construction of a vaginal cuff. In most cases we use a medium-strong, nonabsorbable suture that must be removed postoperatively after 2 weeks.

Technique

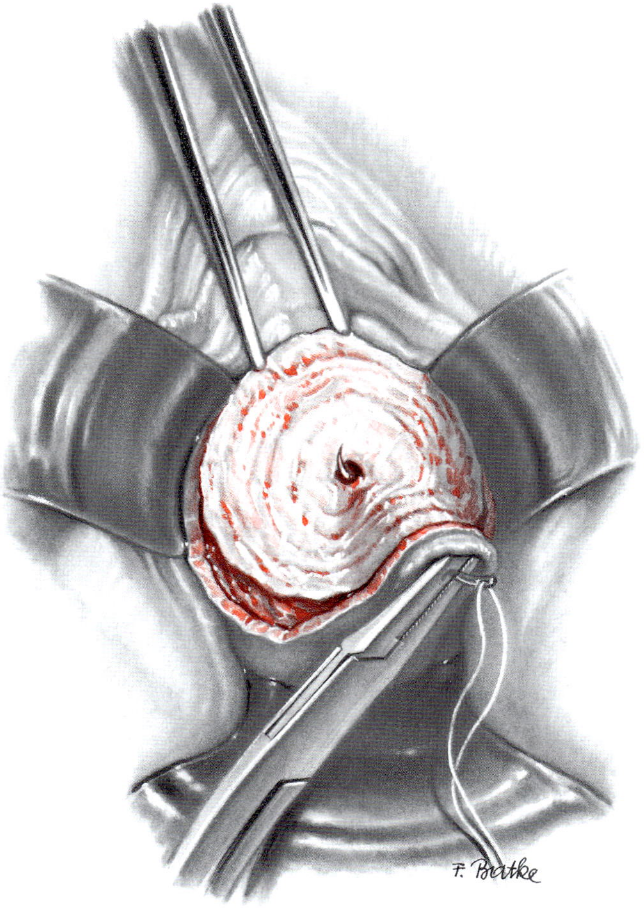

Figure 14.1. Cervical amputation. Posterior Sturmdorf suture.

The needle enters into the left paramedial vaginal cuff about 2 cm from the wound edge, goes through the posterior vaginal and cervix wall, and exits into the cervical canal.

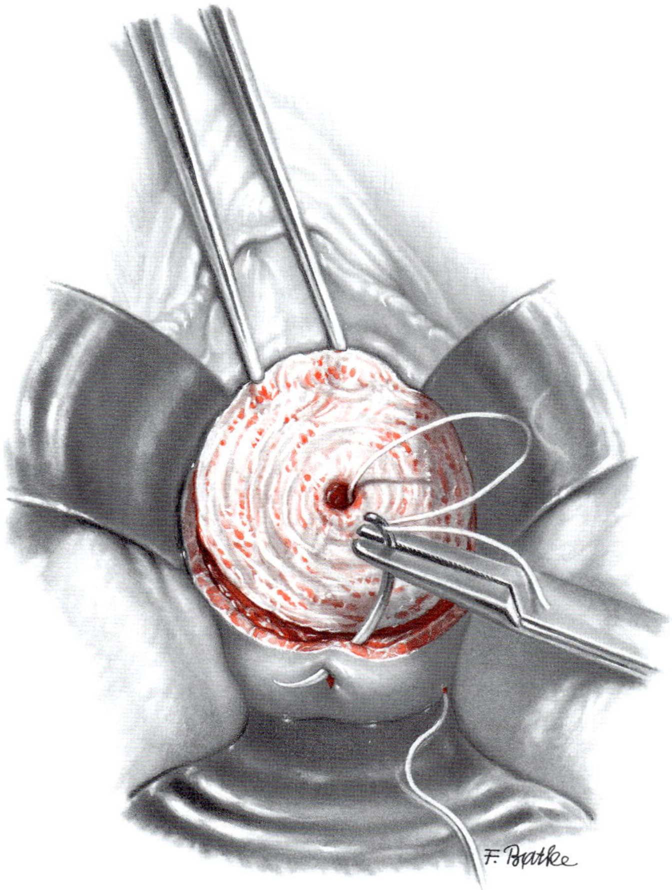

Figure 14.2. Cervical amputation. Posterior Sturmdorf suture.

The posterior vaginal wound edge is sutured in the midline with the needle directed from the inside out.

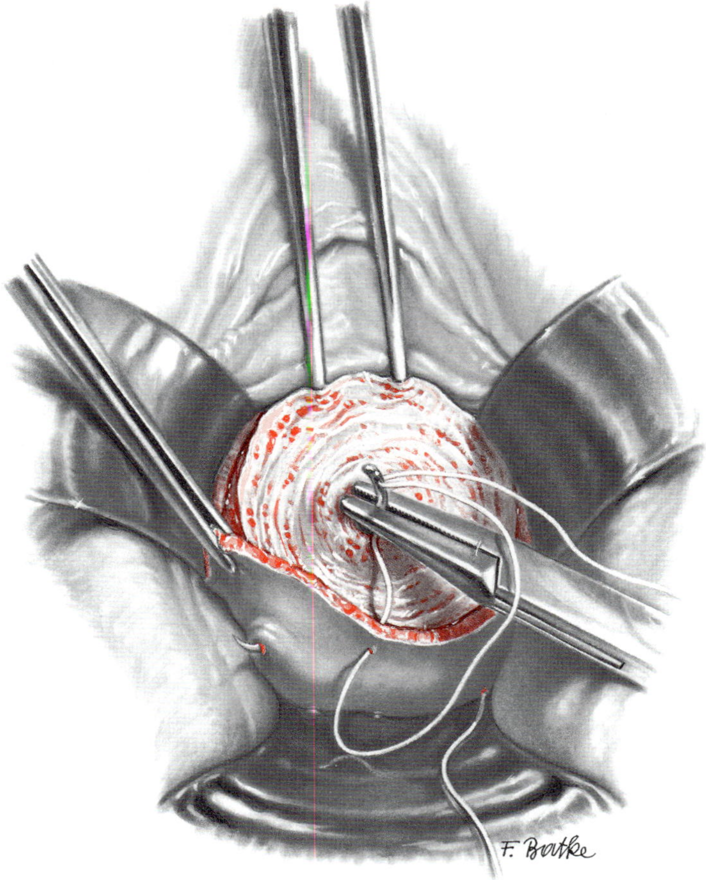

Figure 14.3. Cervical amputation. Posterior Sturmdorf suture.

The needle is inserted back into the cervical canal and correspondingly guided in a right posterolateral direction through the cervical stroma until the tip of the needle emerges from the right paramedial vaginal cuff.

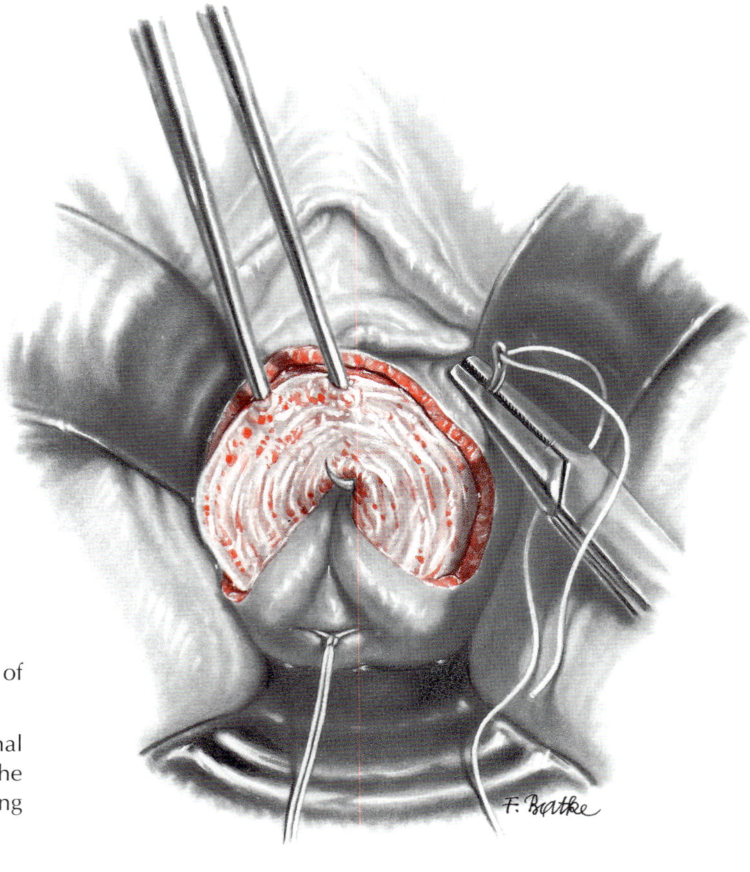

Figure 14.4. Cervical amputation. Anterior Sturmdorf suture.

The posterior Sturmdorf suture is tied, thereby pulling a tongue of vaginal cuff into the cervical canal.

The anterior Sturmdorf suture begins at the left paramedical vaginal cuff about 2 cm from the wound edge; it is passed through the vaginal cuff and cervical tissue, with the tip of the needle emerging in the cervical canal.

Figure 14.5. Cervical amputation. Anterior Sturmdorf suture.

The needle is pulled out of the cervical canal and stitched through the anterior vaginal wound edge in the midline from the inside out.

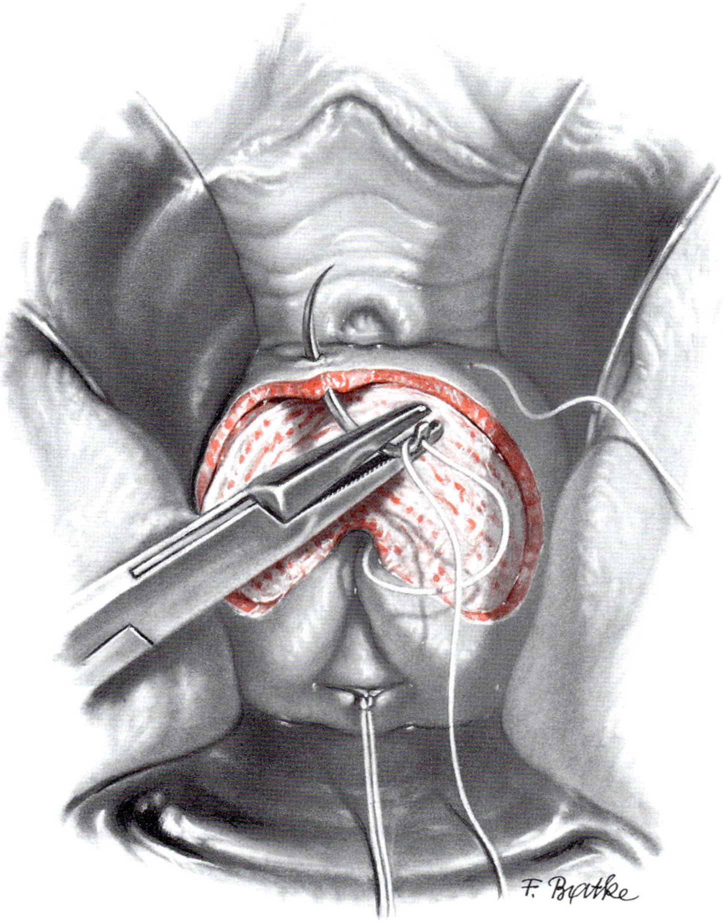

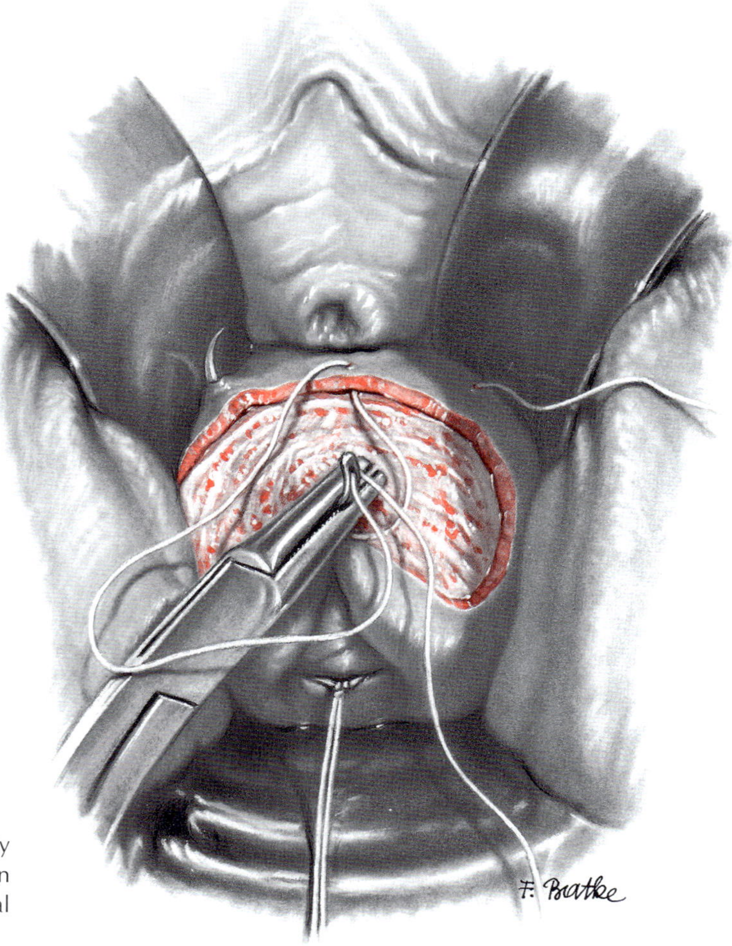

Figure 14.6. Cervical amputation. Anterior Sturmdorf suture.

The needle is reinserted in the cervical canal and correspondingly guided through the cervical tissue in a right anterolateral direction until the tip of the needle emerges from the right paramedial vaginal cuff.

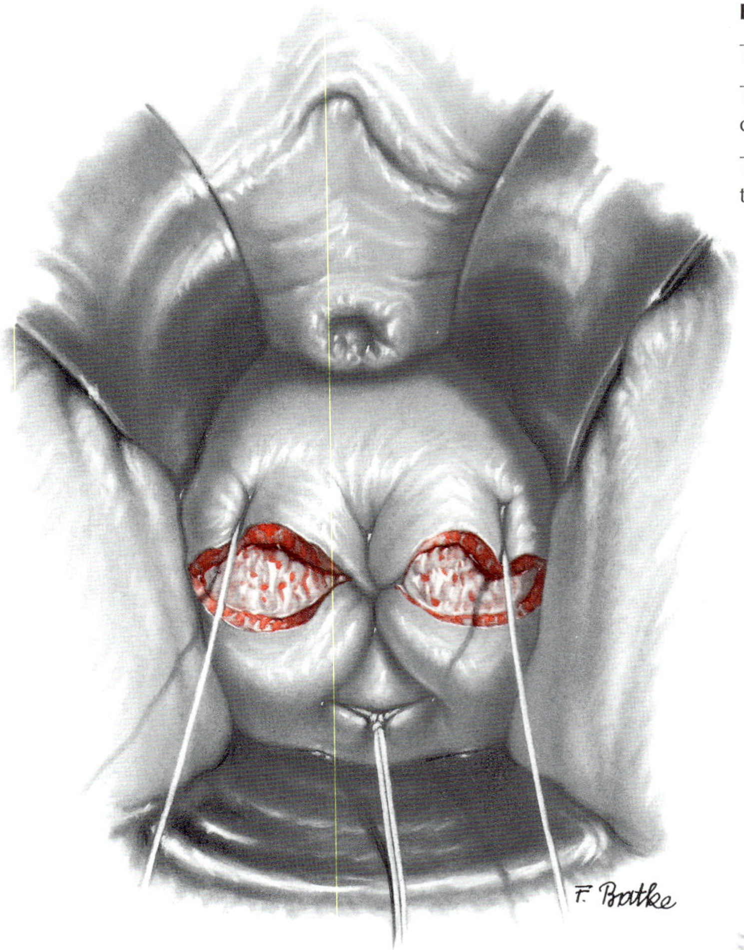

Figure 14.7. Cervical amputation. Sturmdorf suture.

The posterior Sturmdorf suture has been tied.

Traction on the anterior suture draws a tongue of anterior vaginal cuff into the cervical canal.

The lateral portions of the vaginal wound edge must also be joined together by interrupted catgut sutures.

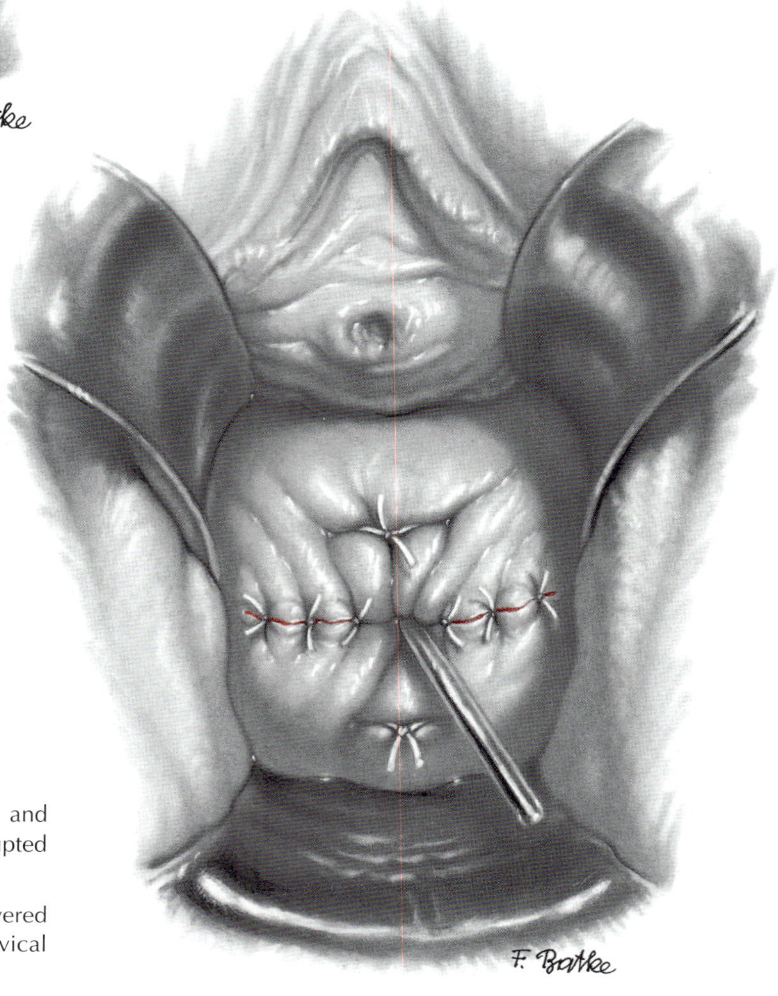

Figure 14.8. Cervical amputation. Sturmdorf suture.

The anterior and posterior Sturmdorf sutures have been tied, and the lateral vaginal wound edges have been united with interrupted sutures.

The wound surface of the amputated cervix is completely covered with vaginal mucosa. A Hegar dilator is inserted into the cervical canal to demonstrate that the rest of the canal is patent.

Technical Problems

1. Insufficient dilation of the cervical canal will make it difficult to apply Sturmdorf sutures. With sufficient dilation at the beginning of the procedure there will be no danger of postoperative cervical stenosis.
2. If high amputation is required to remove all diseased tissue, the *lower bladder pole must be mobilized* and the rectum moved caudally before the procedure is begun. We also recommend ligating the blood vessels at the lateral edge of the cervix. This is performed by suturing the cervical tissue bilaterally.
3. The ends of the Sturmdorf sutures *should not be tied too tightly*. This will cause the sutures to cut into the tissue. They are removed 2 weeks after the operation. By that time the vaginal mucosa covering the cervical wound is usually well healed.

15/ Manchester Operation (Donald-Fothergill)

Indications

This procedure was originally devised by Donald (who combined anterior colporrhaphy and colpoperineoplasty with amputation of the cervix) and by Fothergill (who added fixation of the freed cardinal ligaments to the anterior wall of the cervix). It is useful for treating vaginal prolapse with urinary incontinence when cervical hypertrophic elongation and uterine retroversion exist simultaneously. The operation is usually performed on women of childbearing age who desire uterine retention. In Anglo-American countries it is also a standard procedure for uterovaginal prolapse in menopausal women for whom hysterectomy is not indicated. However, in most hospitals the Manchester procedure is rarely used, even though this method retains the potential for conception. This may be due to the fact that the risk of abortion and premature delivery is considerably higher, and that scar formation might cause dyspareunia.

Technique

The Manchester operation consists of a combination of different surgical procedures that, if not conducted in the correct sequence, are technically difficult to execute. The sequence to be observed in performing individual operational segments follow:

(*a*) Dilation of the cervical canal up to Hegar no. 7 and sounding the uterus to determine elongation of the cervix;
(*b*) For pre- and postmenopausal women endometrial curettage should be performed separately to preclude the existence of an asymptomatic endometrial carcinoma;
(*c*) Anterior colporrhaphy with mobilization and plication of the bladder, also resection of the excess anterior vaginal mucosa;
(*d*) Circumcision of the cervix and reconstruction of the vaginal cuff;
(*e*) Separation of the parametria from the cervix;
(*f*) Amputation of the cervix;
(*g*) Placement of the posterior Sturmdorf suture;
(*h*) Fixation of the parametrial stumps to the anterior cervical wall (Fothergill suture);
(*i*) Placement of the anterior Sturmdorf suture;
(*j*) Closure of the anterior colpotomy;
(*k*) Possibly a colpoperineoplasty.

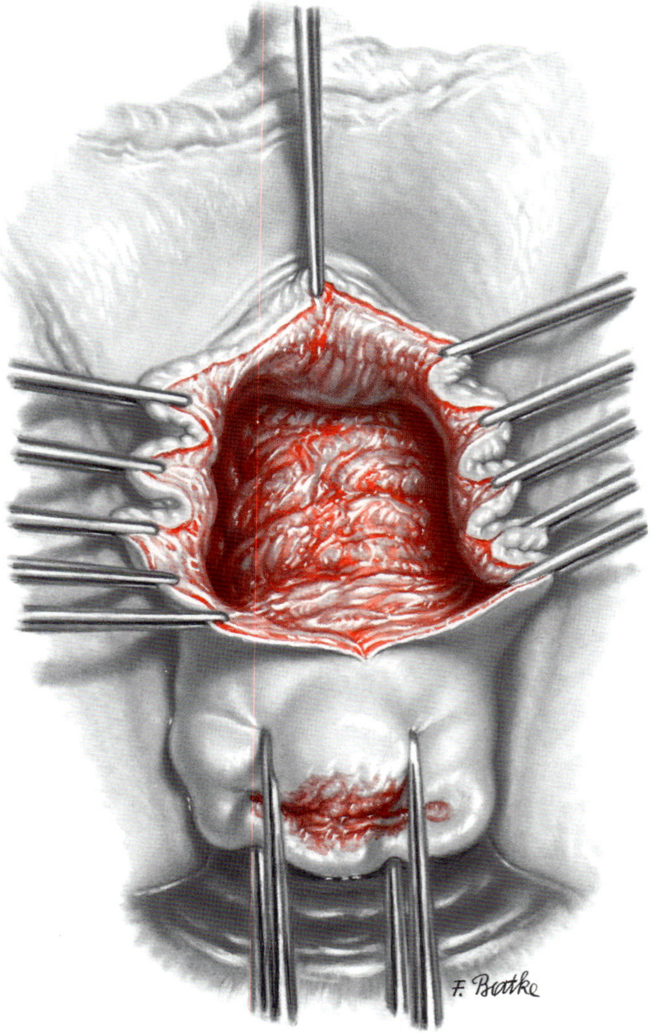

Figure 15.1. Manchester operation. Anterior colporrhaphy.

For a midline colpotomy, the incision cuts through the entire thickness of the vaginal wall, including both the fascia and the vaginal wall. Vaginal walls are dissected free in the usual manner in a lateral direction until the bladder neck is exposed.

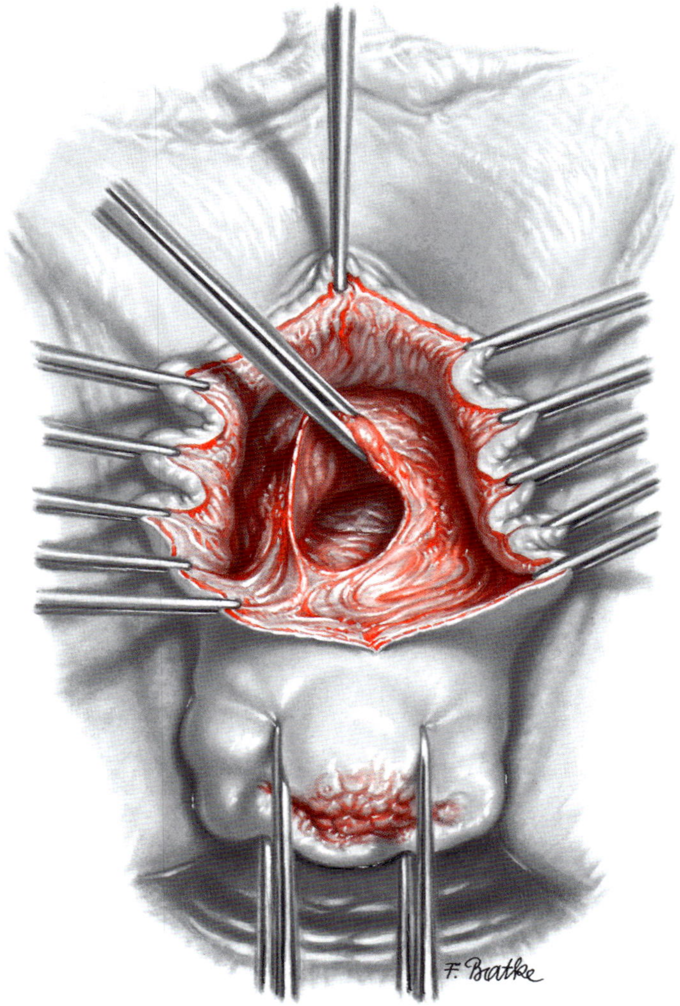

Figure 15.2. Manchester operation. Mobilizing the lower bladder pillars.

The supravaginal septum is severed; the vesicocervical space is widely opened; and the lower pole of the bladder is displaced bluntly. The anterior peritoneal reflection, which remains unopened, is now visible deep within the vesicocervical space.

The lower bladder pole is lifted upward; this stretches the bladder pillars laterally so that they can be dissected from the edge of the cervix with several small incisions.

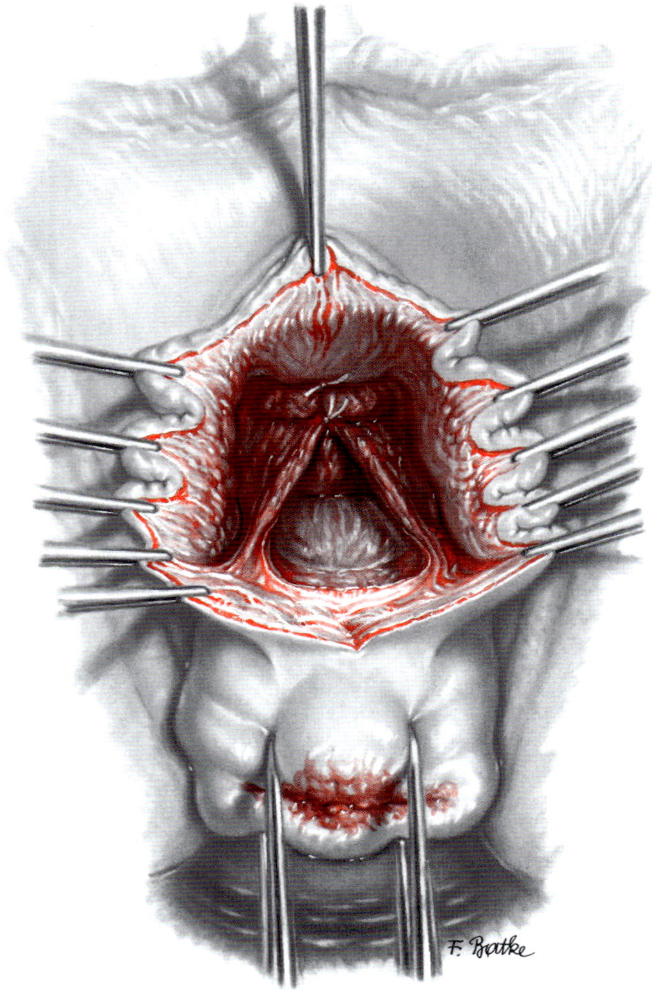

Figure 15.3. Manchester operation. Plicating the bladder neck and the bladder.

The bladder neck is plicated by a suture that angulates the urethrovesical junction.

The rest of the cystocele wall is plicated with a half purse-string suture and is advanced upward.

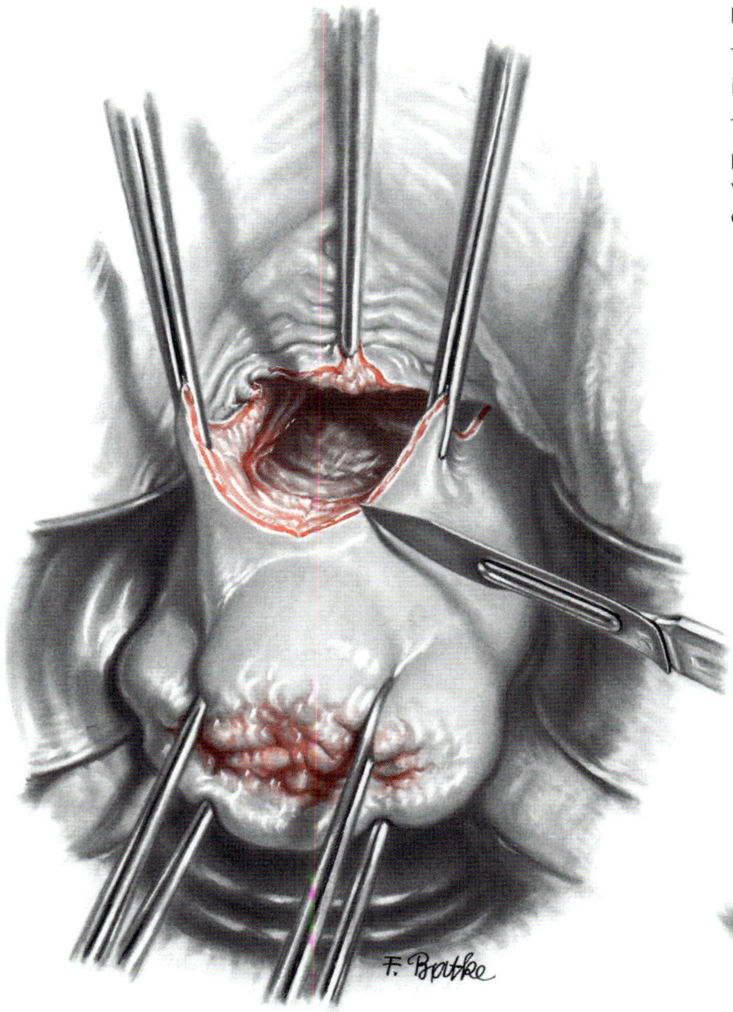

Figure 15.4. Manchester operation. Circumcising the cervix.

The bladder has been plicated and the redundant vaginal wall sparingly resected.

The incision line of the circumcision should be located laterally and posteriorly at the level of the peritoneal fold between the mobilized vaginal wall and the smooth vaginal mucosa that is fixed to the cervix.

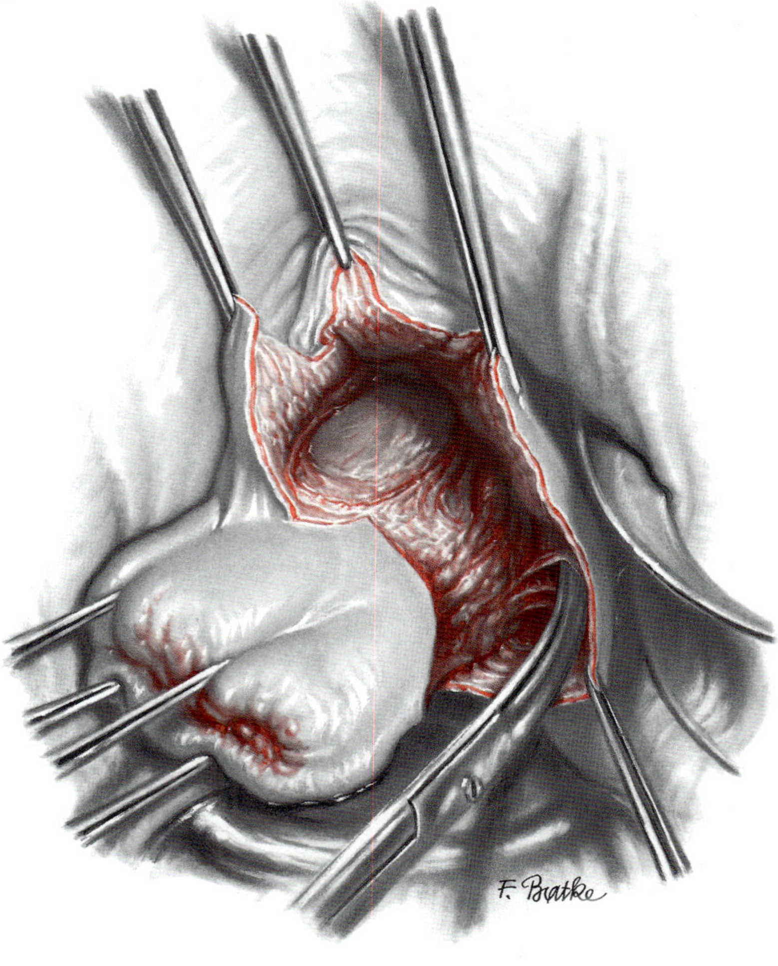

Figure 15.5. Manchester operation. Mobilizing the vaginal cuff.

The circumcisional wound edge is dissected off posteriorly and laterally for 2–3 cm with scissors. This step is aided by a pull on the cervix toward the opposite side.

Freeing the vaginal cuff laterally is of particular importance for exposing the elongated cardinal ligament (lateral parametrium) on the border of the cervix. The rectum is also dissected off the posterior wall of the cervix caudally.

The stretched parametrial tissue is now visible at the left border of the cervix.

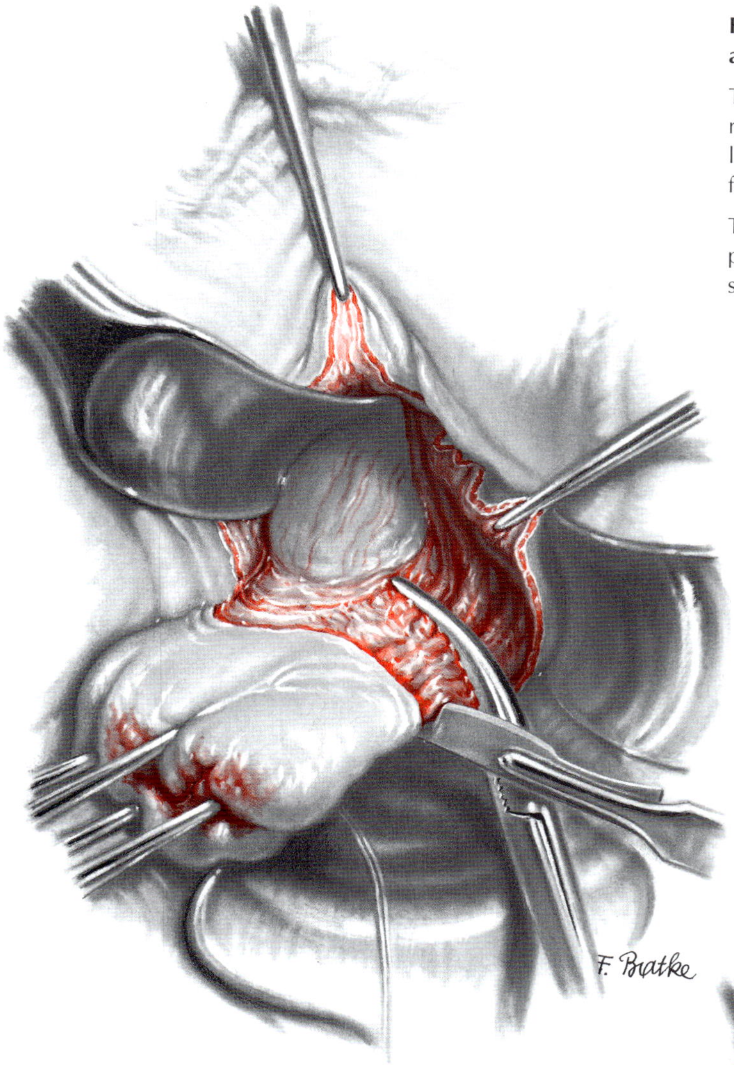

Figure 15.6. Manchester operation. Dividing the left cardinal ligament and the uterosacral ligament.

The left vaginal cuff has been dissected from the cervix and is being retracted laterally with a lateral retractor. The plicated bladder is lifted somewhat with an anterior retractor. The anterior peritoneal fold is clearly visible.

The parametrial tissue is grasped with a strong toothed clamp applied right at the edge of the cervical border and divided with a scalpel in a distal direction.

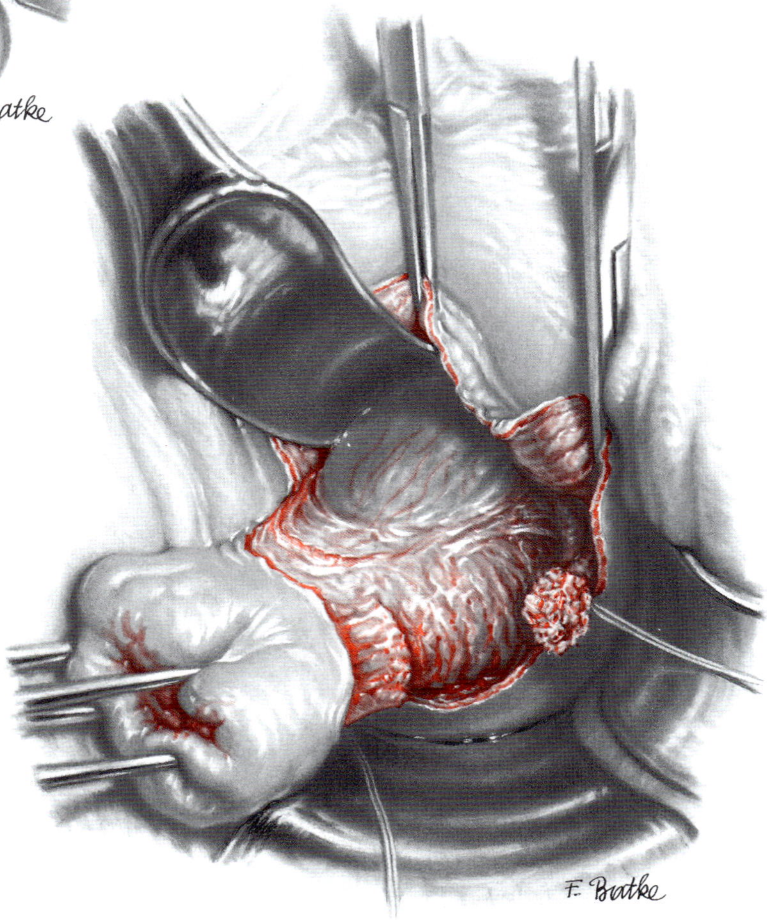

Figure 15.7. Manchester operation. Mobilizing the divided cardinal ligament.

The doubly ligated parametrial tissue band is separated further from the cervix. This will make it easier later to attach to the anterior cervical wall at the level of the internal cervical os (Fothergill suture).

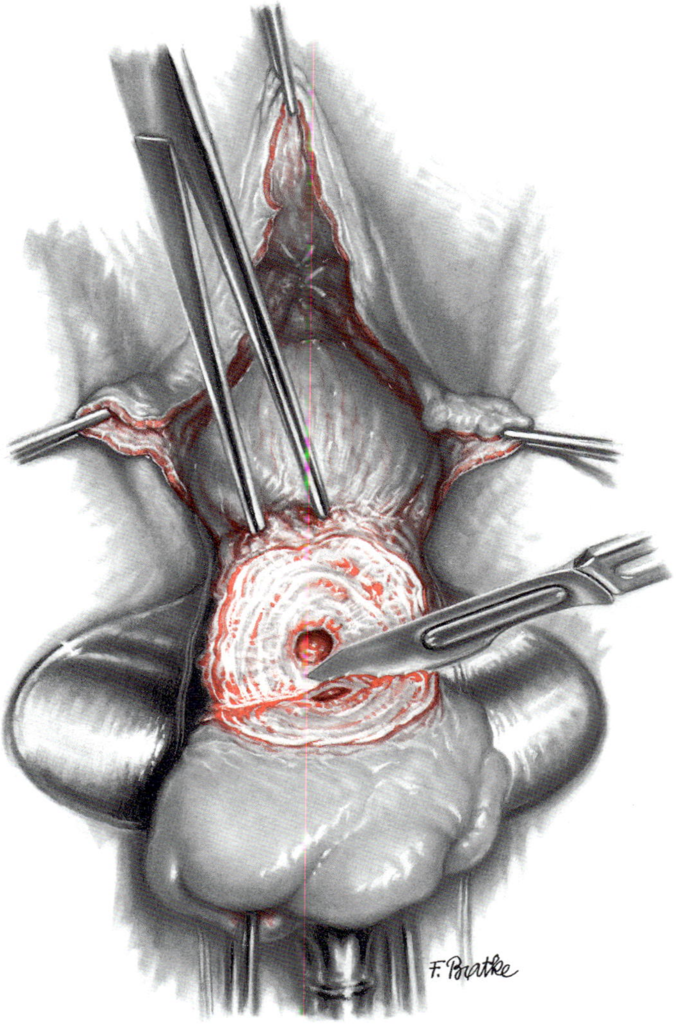

Figure 15.8. Manchester operation. Amputating the cervix.

The anterior wall of the cervix is grasped with a tenaculum, and the cervix is pulled down with two tenacula.

The level at which the cervix is transected depends on the degree of hypertrophy. The point of reference is the internal cervical os.

In general, the cervix is amputated about 1 cm distal to the internal os with a slightly conical incision. In young women, the level chosen is about 2 cm distal to the internal os to ensure functional uterine competency in the event of a future pregnancy.

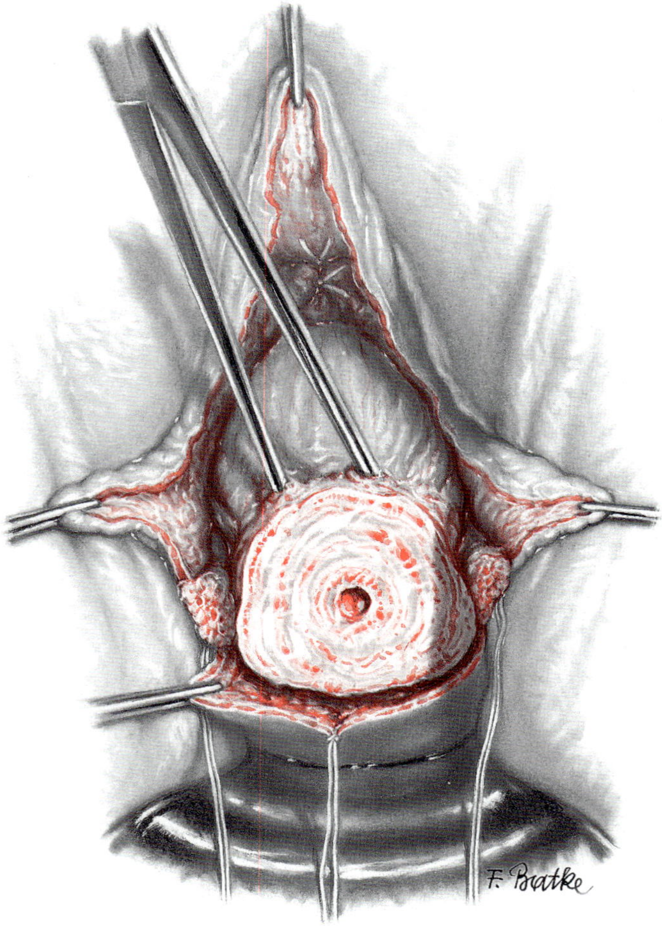

Figure 15.9. Manchester operation. Posterior Sturmdorf suture. First step.

The elongated cervix has been amputated; the bladder has been plicated; and the stumps of the cardinal ligaments have been separated from the cervix.

The stump of the cervix is covered with vaginal mucosa. For technical reasons, the Sturmdorf sutures are first placed posteriorly because the stump at this moment is still freely mobile. This will no longer be the case after the anterior half of the cervical wound has been covered.

The posterior vaginal cuff is ligated in midline with a medium strong, nonabsorbable traction suture (for the posterior Sturmdorf suture).

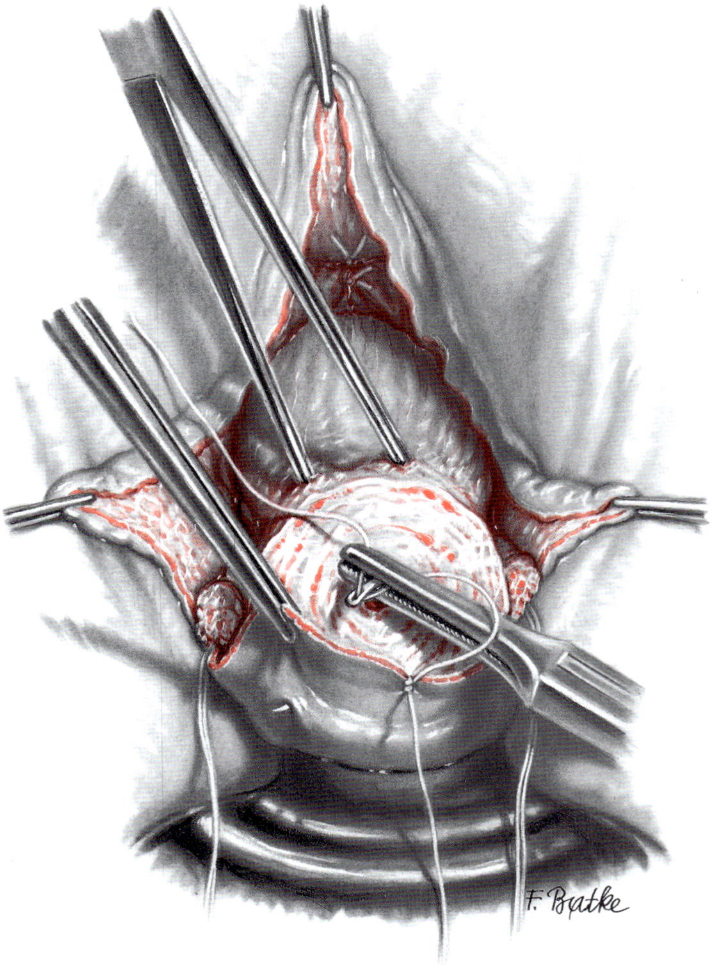

Figure 15.10. Manchester operation. Posterior Sturmdorf suture. Second step.

One end of the posterior Sturmdorf suture is threaded into a sharp needle.

The needle is placed from the cervical canal and guided through the right posterior wall of the cervix so that its tip emerges to the right about 2 cm from the free edge of the posterior paramedial vaginal cuff.

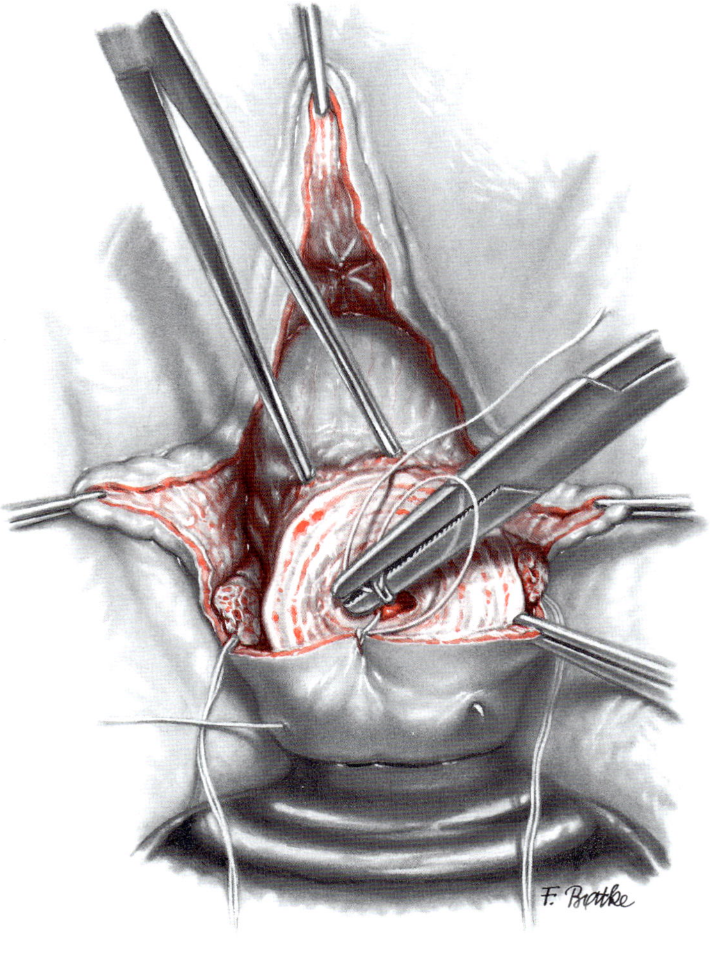

Figure 15.11. Manchester operation. Posterior Sturmdorf suture. Third step.

The other end of the posterior Sturmdorf suture is threaded into a needle. That needle is placed from the cervical canal and guided through the left posterior wall of the cervix so that its tip (in analogous fashion to the right side) emerges 2 cm to the left of the midline.

Figure 15.12. Manchester operation. Fothergill suture.

After the posterior Sturmdorf suture has been tied, the free edge of the tip of the posterior vaginal cuff is pulled into the cervical canal so that the posterior half of the cervical wound is covered with vaginal mucosa.

With a strong suture, at the level of the internal os, the stumps of the cardinal ligaments are united and affixed to the anterior wall of the cervix. This produces traction, and the cervical stump retracts noticeably in the cephalad and posterior direction after the suture has been tied.

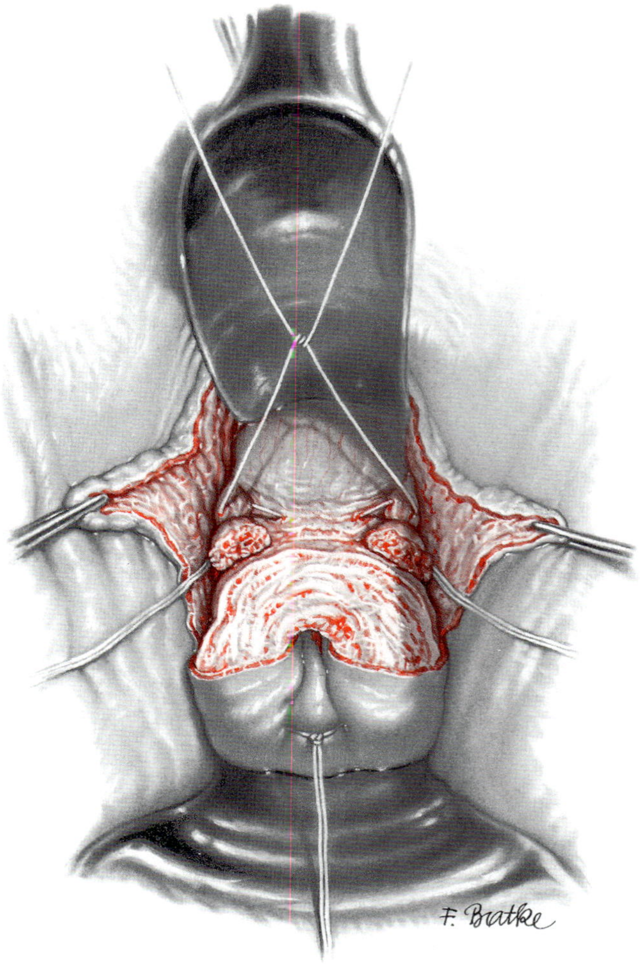

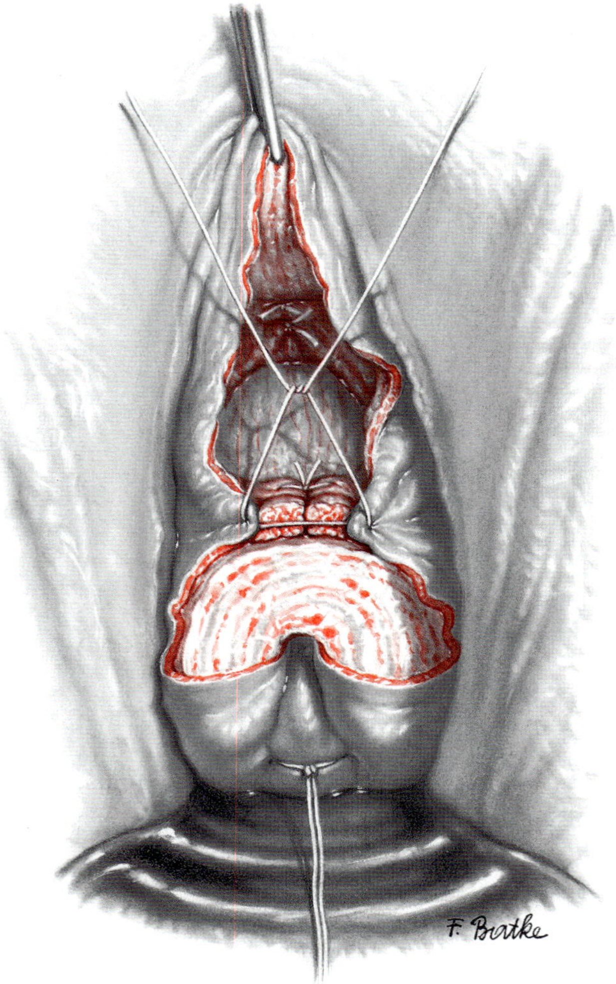

Figure 15.13. Manchester operation. Anterior Sturmdorf suture. First step.

The cardinal ligaments are fixed to the anterior wall of the cervix; the bladder is plicated; and the redundant anterior vaginal mucosa is resected.

The anterior Sturmdorf suture unites the lower wound angles of the anterior colpotomy.

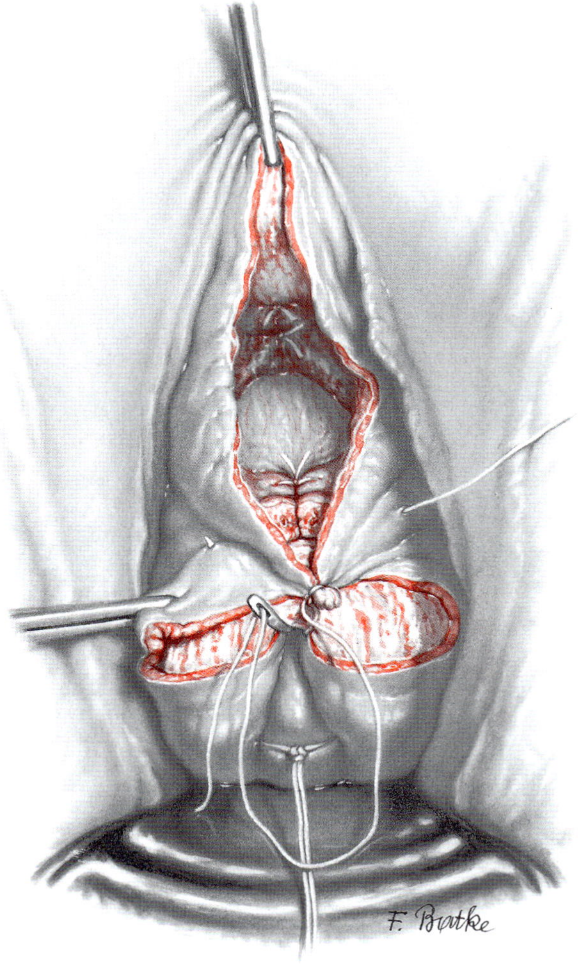

Figure 15.14. Manchester operation. Anterior Sturmdorf suture. Second step.

The ends of the anterior Sturmdorf suture are placed on needles.

The sharp needles are directed from the cervical canal through the posterior wall of the cervix in a fashion analogous to the posterior Sturmdorf suture.

On the left side, one suture end has already been pulled through the left paramedian anterior vaginal cuff. To the right appears the point of the needle, which is inserted via the cervical canal through the right anterior cervical wall, exiting from the vaginal cuff 2 cm from the vaginal wound edge.

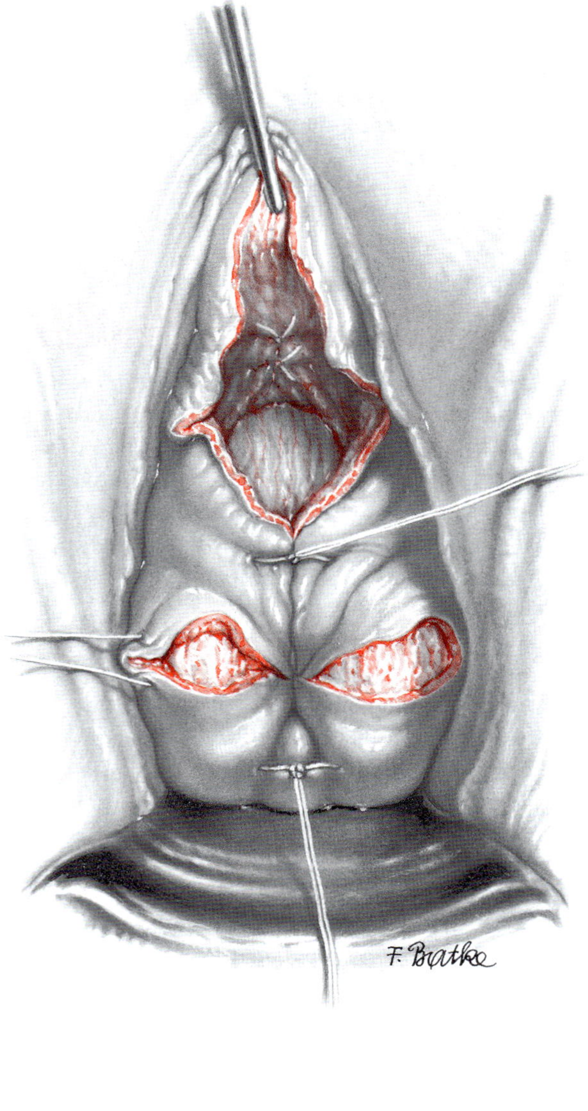

Figure 15.15. Manchester operation. Closing the vaginal wound edges.

The posterior and anterior Sturmdorf sutures have been tied so as to pull tongue-like projections of the anterior and posterior vaginal walls into the cervical canal.

To cover the wound surface of the cervix completely, the lateral vaginal wound edges at the circumcision site are joined together with additional interrupted catgut sutures (chromic catgut no. 1). One such suture has already been placed in the right wound angle.

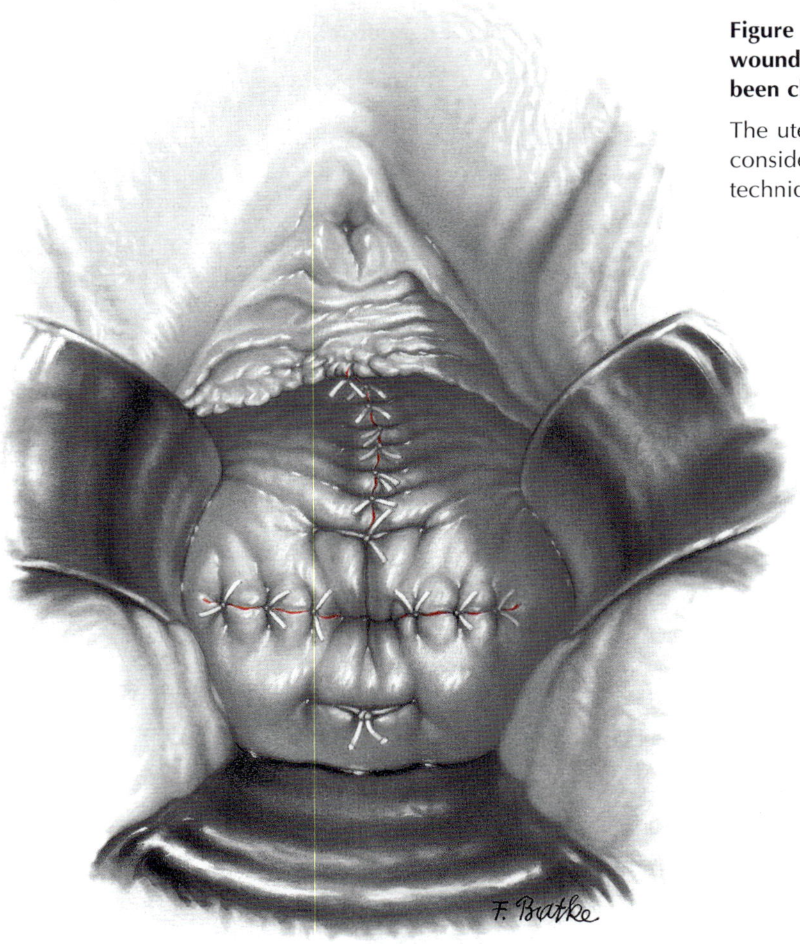

Figure 15.16. Manchester operation. View after the cervical wound surface has been covered and the anterior colpotomy has been closed.

The uterus has retracted into the vagina. At this point, one might consider continuing with an additional colpoperineoplasty (for technique see Chapter 13).

Technical Problems

1. *The operation has not been conducted in the correct sequence*. For example, if the Fothergill suture had been placed immediately after the amputation of the cervix, the cervical stump would be repositioned and elevated prematurely and thereby become inaccessible for the Sturmdorf suturing.
2. If the *circumcision of the cervix is performed too far from the external os of the cervix*, the vagina will be foreshortened.
3. Should the circumcised *vaginal wall not be dissected well laterally*, so that the parametria are not properly exposed, the pedicles of the parametria will be too short when they are separated from the edge of the cervix.
4. The *cardinal and uterosacral ligaments may not have been mobilized* after they were transected from the edge of the cervix. This too will yield pedicles that are too short; after the cervix is amputated, they can be reattached in the midline only under tension to the remaining anterior cervical wall.
5. The *parametria might not have been doubly ligated.*
6. *Cervical amputation may be performed at too high a level*. This may open the cul-de-sac of Douglas peritoneum (particularly if there is a coexisting enterocele). In addition, the internal os may be damaged, leaving the cervix incompetent to retain a subsequent pregnancy.
7. The *freed stumps of the parametria should not be fixed too high* on the anterior wall (i.e., at or above the internal os), or the uterus will be elevated but not anteverted. Instead, the corpus uteri is displaced toward the sacrum. The indication for a Manchester operation was wrong if the cardinal ligaments of the retroflected uterus have not straightened, despite the proper level of their fixation.
8. The *Sturmdorf sutures must not be placed with tapered needles*. They might break when pushed through the tough cervical tissue. Strong, cutting needles should be used for this segment of the procedure.
9. If *too much vaginal wall is resected near the anterior colpotomy*, insufficient mucosa may be left to cover the anterior cervical wound surface, and a circular vaginal stenosis might develop.

16/ Colpocleisis

Indications

If vaginal function is no longer vital for a patient, colpocleisis is indicated to avoid long-term use of a pessary in elderly women in poor general condition. The original methods have been modified many times. In our experience, four occlusion procedures proved to be of particular value:

Labhardt partial colpocleisis;
Neugebauer-Le Fort partial colpocleisis;
Doederlein cross-bar colporrhaphy;
Conill colpocleisis.

None are considered to be stressful procedures; they may at times be performed under local anesthesia.

Labhardt Partial Colpocleisis

Indications

We combine the partial Labhardt colpocleisis with a perineorrhaphy, which allows us to designate this surgical method as a partial "colpoperineocleisis." The vaginal introitus is almost completely occluded up to the urethral meatus by the formation of a tissue wedge. This tissue wedge is considerably strengthened by the additional posterior repair, which reduces the possibility of recurrence. The urinary control mechanism is unaffected.

Technique

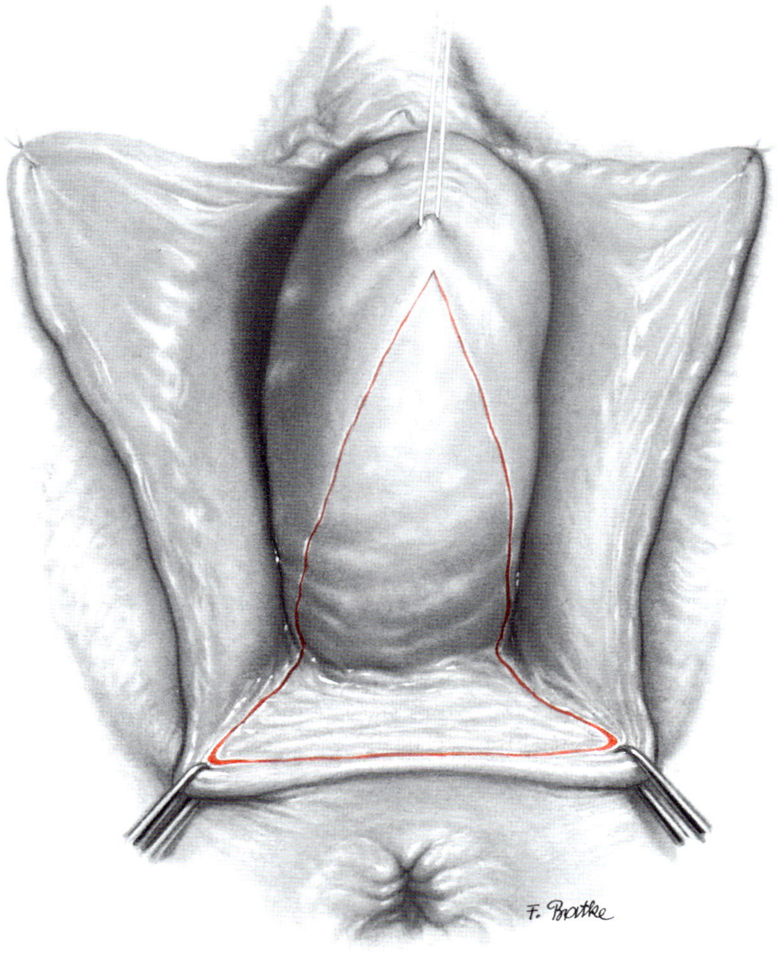

Figure 16.1. Labhardt partial colpocleisis. Hegar incision. The labia minora are sutured to the skin of the labia majora for better exposure.

Two tenacula are placed at the posterior commissure and used to cause the vaginal introitus to gape wide open. A silk traction suture is applied near the prolapsed posterior fornix. The prolapsed uterus is lifted upward by pulling on this traction suture.

The surgeon incises a triangular segment of the posterior vaginal mucosa, extending upward to the posterior fornix.

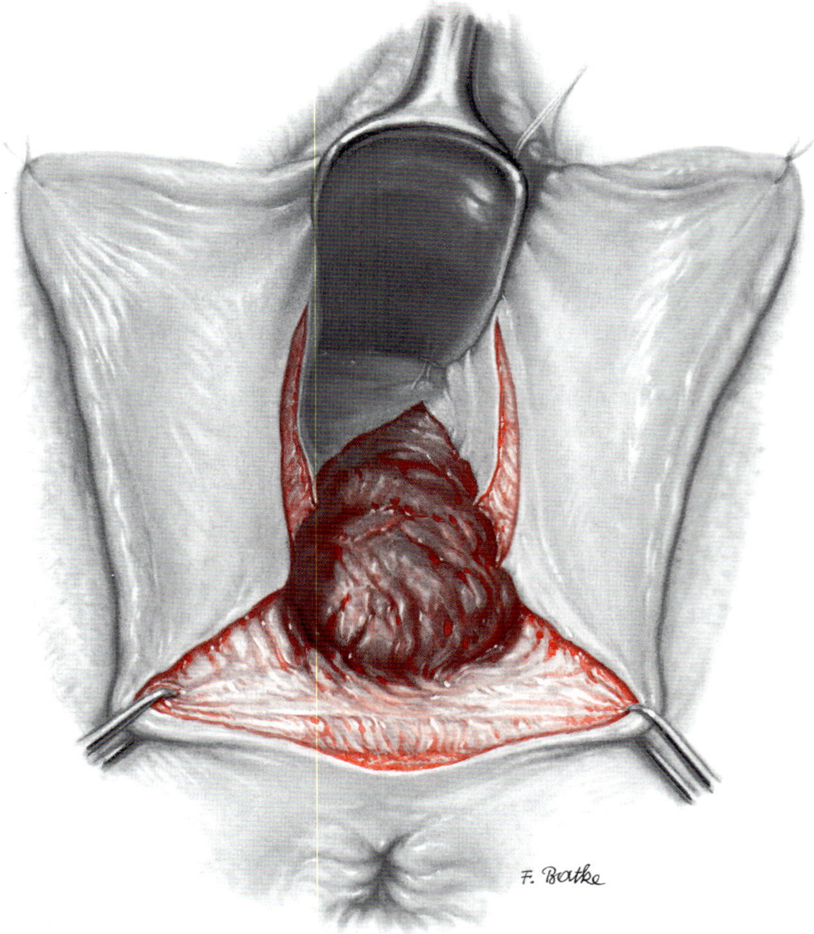

Figure 16.2. Labhardt partial colpocleisis. Additional triangular incision.

The vaginal and perineal mucosa have already been removed from the incised triangular area; the anterior wall of the rectum is exposed. The prolapsed uterus and the anterior vaginal wall are elevated with a retractor.

Another acutely angled triangle is incised at the inner aspect of the labia minora bilaterally up to the level of the urethral meatus. The labial mucosa is dissected free within these triangular areas. The bases of these small triangles lie about halfway between the posterior commissure and the apex of the posterior vaginal incision; the labial incisions run perpendicular to the vaginal incision edges.

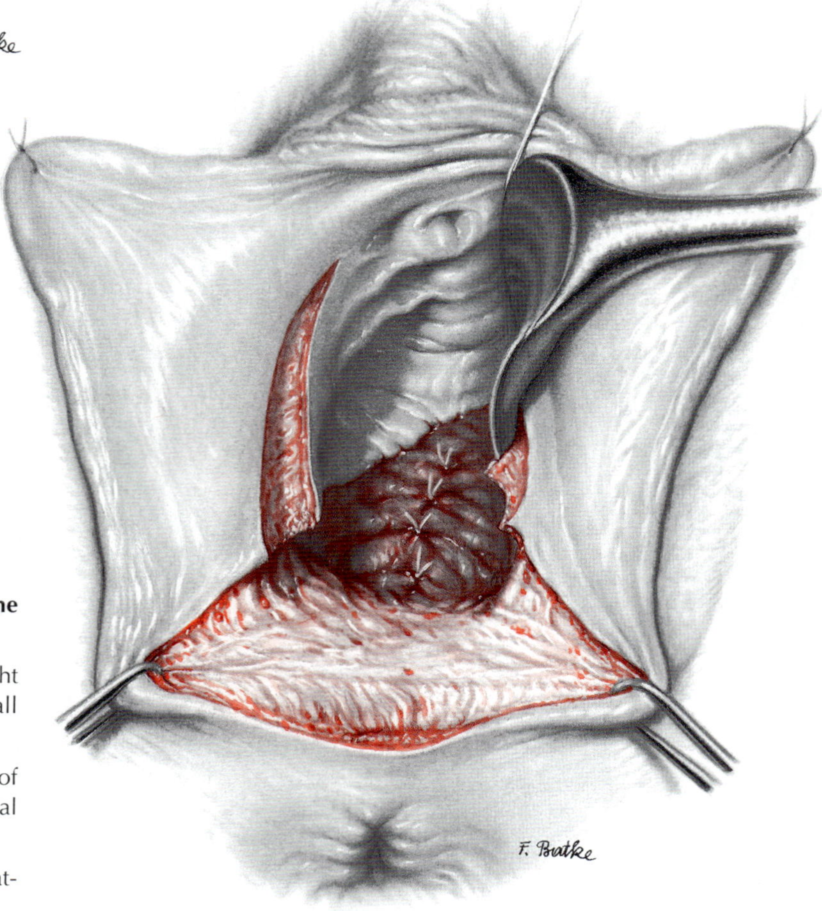

Figure 16.3. Labhardt partial colpocleisis. Plicating the pararectal tissue.

All triangular incisions have been performed, and the right side is exposed; a retractor pushes the anterior vaginal wall upward to the left.

One can see that the small triangle on the interior side of the right labium minus reaches up to the level of the external urethral orifice.

The pararectal tissue is plicated with several interrupted catgut sutures.

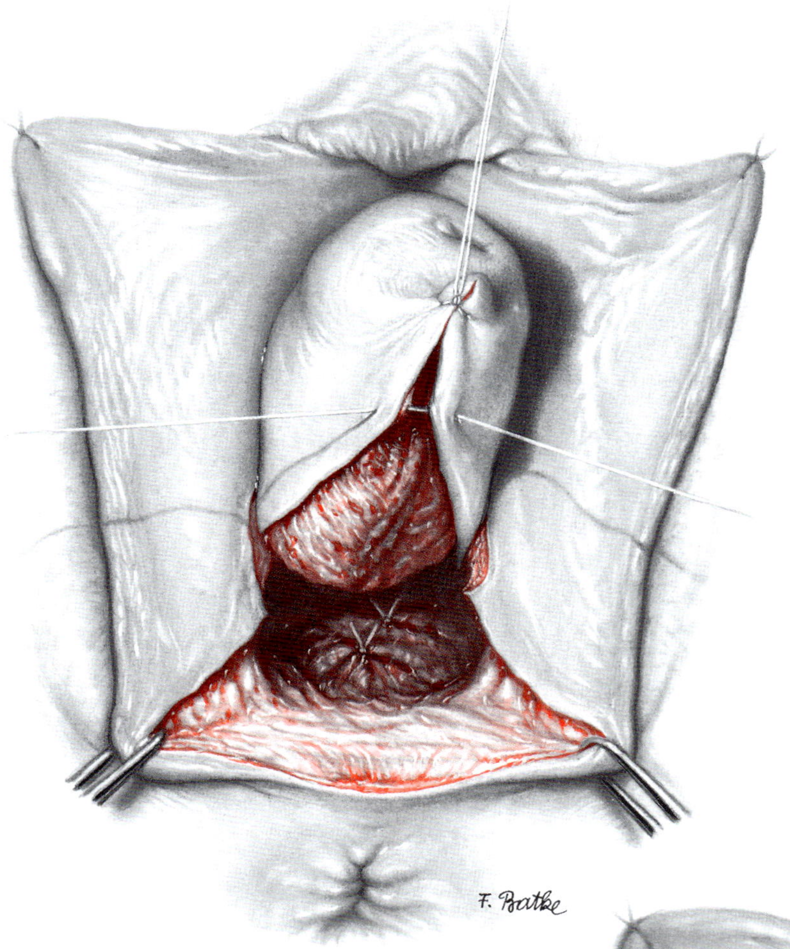

Figure 16.4. Labhardt partial colpocleisis. Suturing the inner vaginal incision edges.

At the apical angle of the vaginal incision, the wound edges have already been joined by a suture, the ends of which have been left long. They are being pulled upward by the left assistant to elevate the prolapsed uterus.

This exposes the posterior vaginal wound edges, which can be united with additional interrupted catgut sutures.

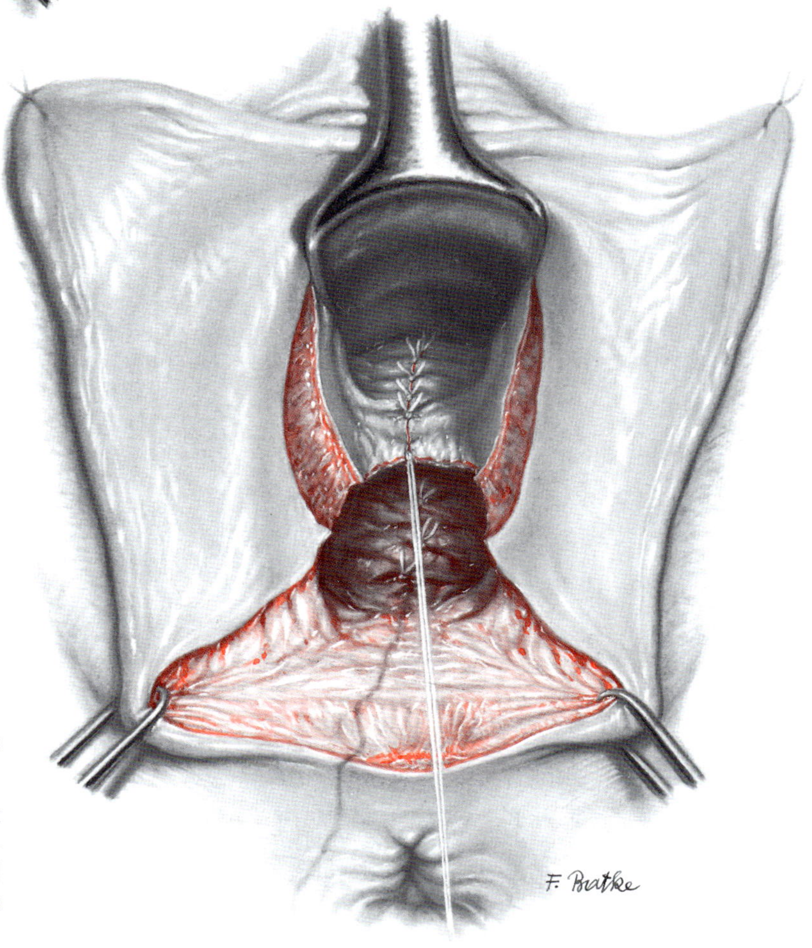

Figure 16.5. Labhardt partial colpocleisis. Suturing the inner vaginal wound edges.

The upper part of the vaginal wall triangle is closed almost to the labial incisions with several interrupted catgut sutures. The lowest of these sutures is left long and pulled caudally. An anterior retractor holds the prolapsed uterus back.

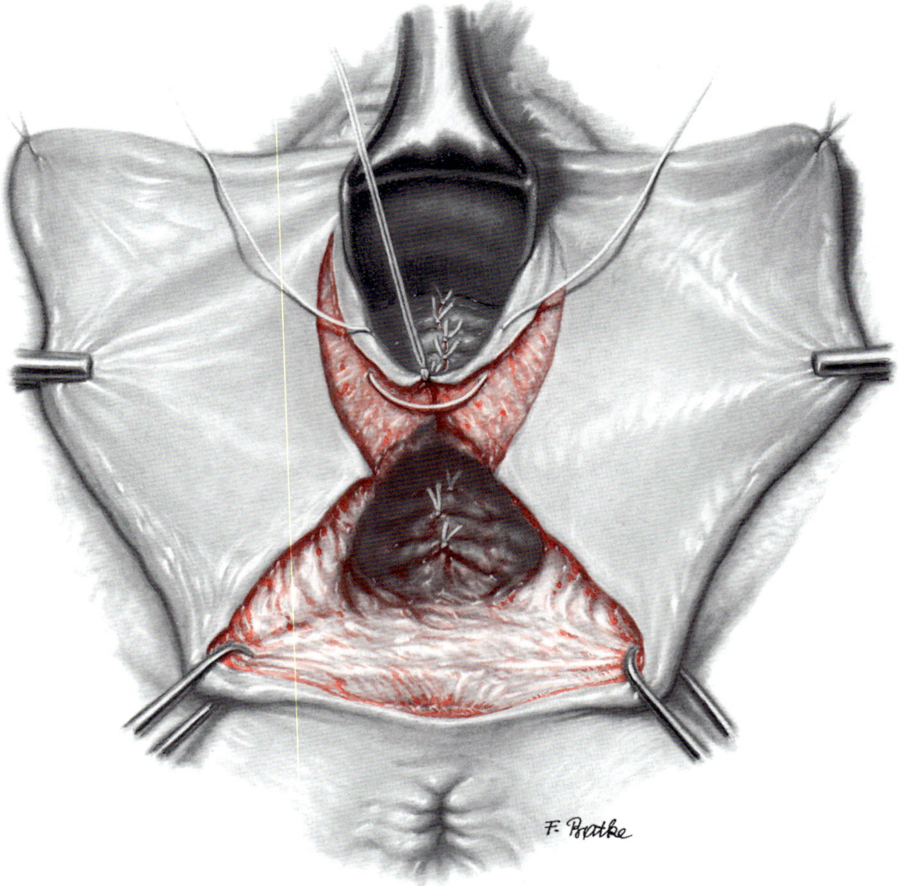

Figure 16.6. Labhardt partial colpocleisis. Ligating the inner labial wound edges.

The triangular posterior vaginal wound is completely closed with interrupted sutures up to the lateral labial incisions; the last of these sutures is pulled upward. An anterior retractor lifts the uterus upward; the hypertrophic labia minora are held apart by two tissue forceps.

The surgeon begins to join the inner edges of the labial incisions by placing another suture.

Make sure that the suture on the left leads from the vaginal side to the wound surface; the reverse is true on the right. In this way, the knot will face the vaginal canal after the suture has been tied.

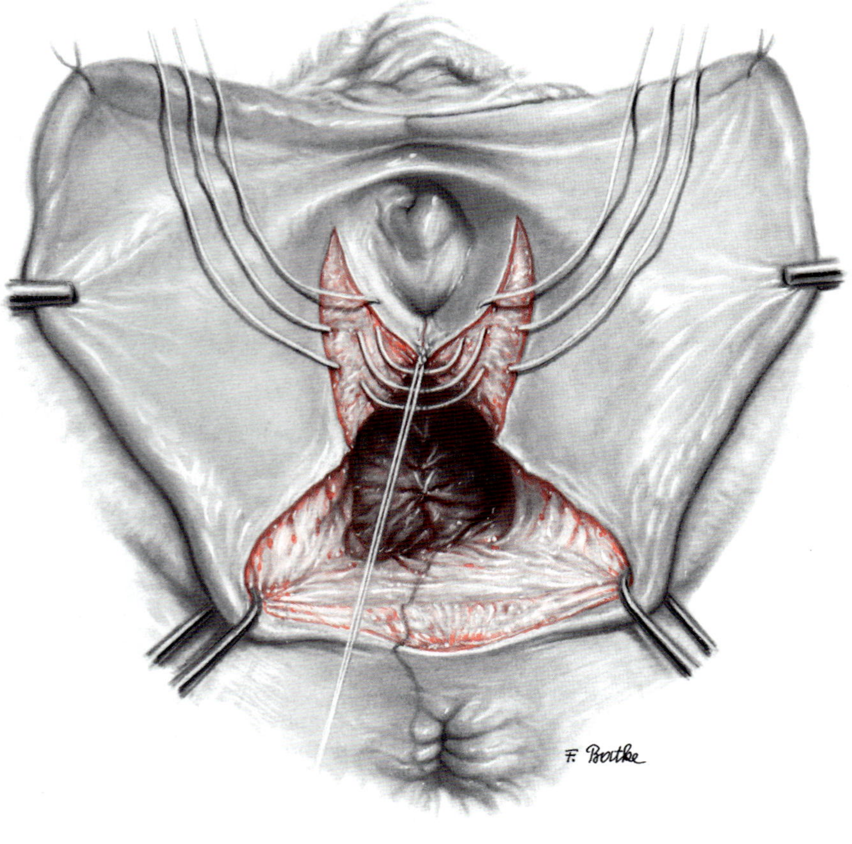

Figure 16.7. Labhardt partial colpocleisis. Uniting the wound surfaces.

The inner edges of the labial wounds are partially joined (one suture is tied and pulled downward, and a second one is placed). Two subcutaneous sutures are applied to approximate the wound surfaces of the labia minora.

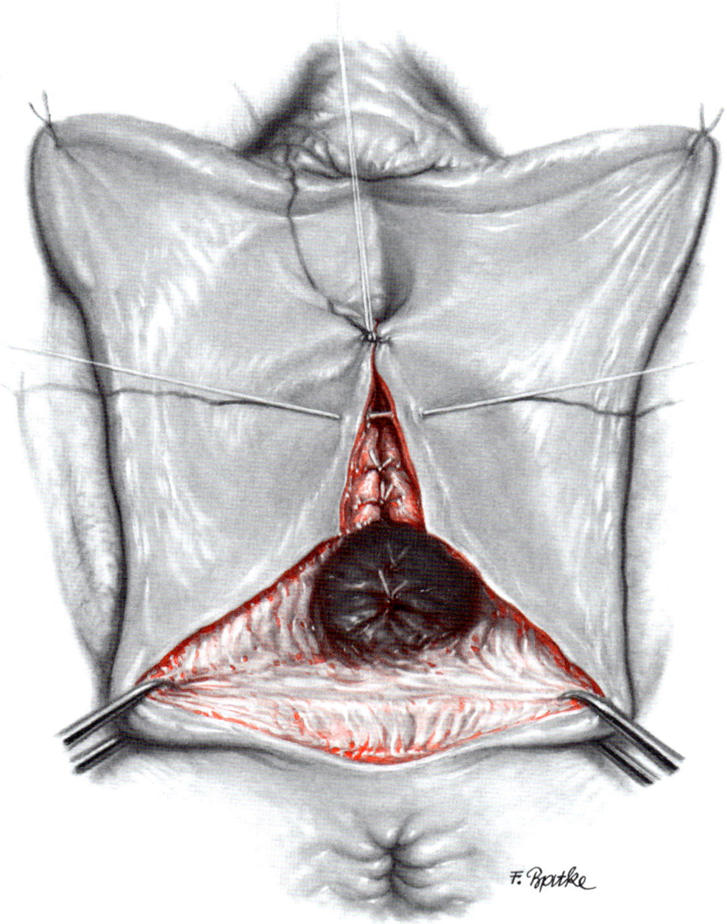

Figure 16.8. Labhardt partial colpocleisis. Ligating the outer incisional edges.

All inner wound edges are sutured, and the triangular labial incision edges are approximated with two catgut sutures.

The uppermost suture on the outer labial wound edges is pulled upward at the level of the external urethral orifice. The wound edges of the labia minora can now be joined together with additional sutures.

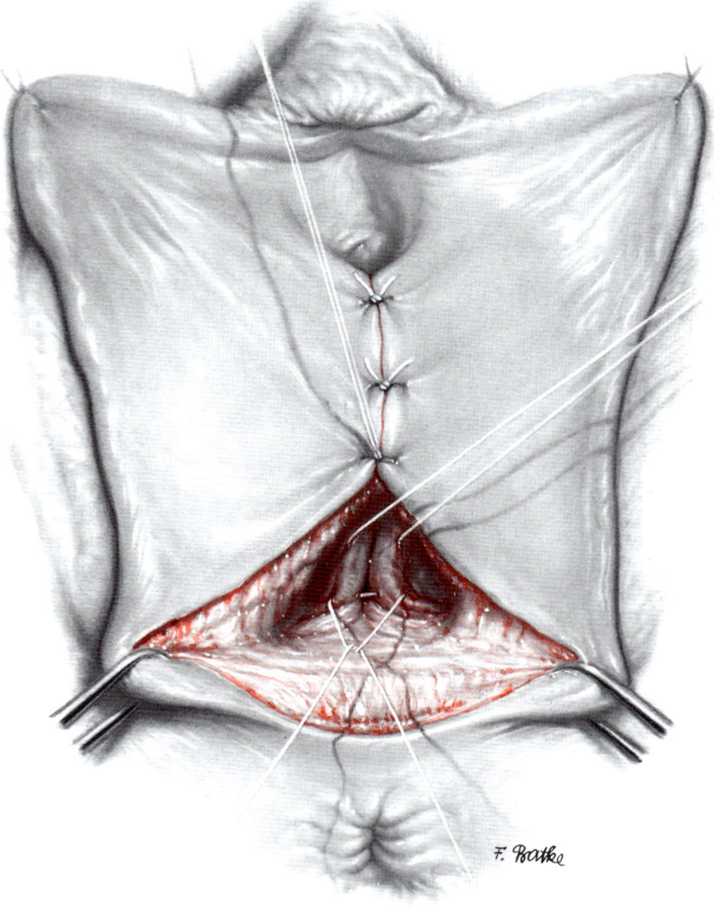

Figure 16.9. Labhardt partial colpocleisis. Supplementary colpoperineoplasty.

The labial wound edges are united with interrupted catgut sutures. The most caudal of these is lifted upward.

To construct a long perineum, the borders of the levator have been dissected free and are joined together in the midline with two sutures.

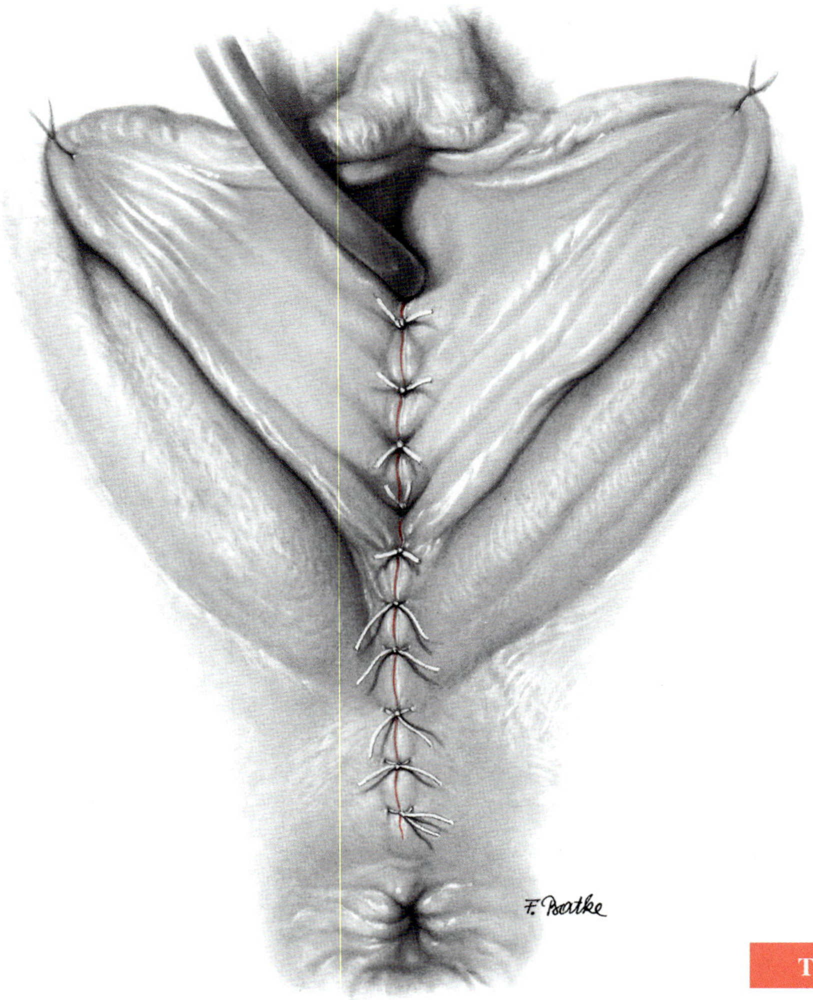

Figure 16.10. Labhardt partial colpocleisis. Completing the procedure.

After the long perineum has been constructed, the labial suture line will lie on a level with the perineal wound. The vaginal opening is almost completely closed. An indwelling catheter is inserted into the bladder.

Technical Problems—Figures 16.1–16.10

1. If the entire vaginal and perineal *incision to form the five-point star is made immediately*, before any part of the vaginal wall is excised within the first triangular incision, one creates great technical difficulties because exposure and the development of proper tension become tedious and inexact. It is preferable to excise the posterior vaginal triangle first, then cut the perineal skin with a bow-shaped incision and remove it, and finally make the acutely angled triangular incisions bilaterally along the inner aspects of the labia minora and dissect the narrow triangles of mucosa in this area.
2. Should the bilateral acutely angled labial incisions be *extended cranially above the urethral orifice*, apposition of the corresponding wound edges will close the vaginal introitus too far cephalad, covering the urethral opening. This will cause the urine to be directed partially into the remaining vaginal canal during micturition.
3. The *bilateral acutely angled triangular incisions should not be made too narrow*, or recurrence of the prolapse can be expected to result because the tissue barrier that closes the vaginal canal will be too thin to provide adequate support.

Neugebauer-Le Fort Partial Colpocleisis

Technique

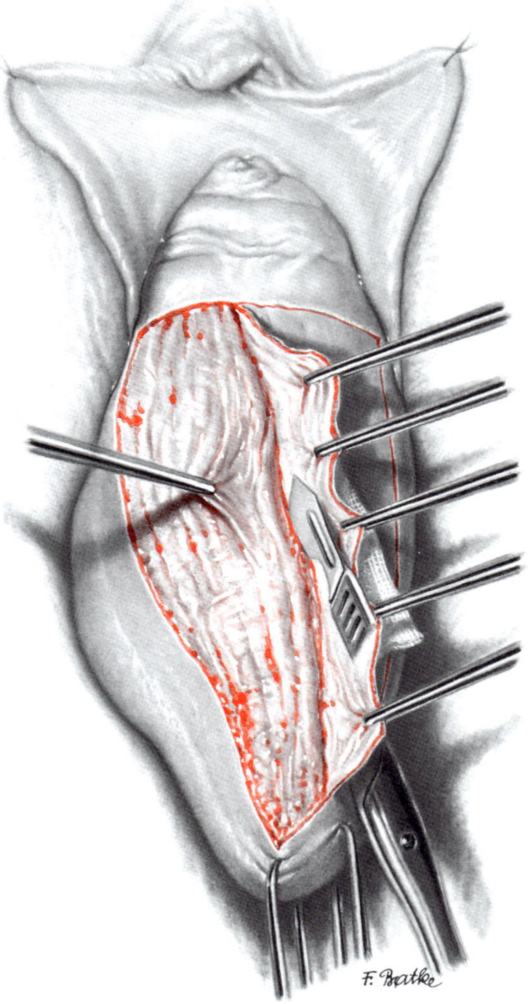

Figure 16.11. Neugebauer-Le Fort partial colpocleisis. Anterior rectangular incision. Dissecting the vaginal mucosa.

The prolapsed uterus lies in front of the vulva; it is being pulled down by two tenacula applied to the cervix, which exposes the anterior vaginal wall.

The rectangular incision of the anterior vaginal wall extends from the cervix up to about two fingerbreadths beneath the urethral orifice.

The mucosal flap has been partially dissected off and is pulled to the left by the assistant using toothed clamps. The surgeon lifts the wound surface tissue to the left with forceps, causing the mucosal flap to become stretched. The superficial dissection of the mucosa can now be continued in the correct plane.

Because there is a considerable cystocele present, the left assistant, using a sponge, pushes the bladder back behind the partially folded vaginal flap.

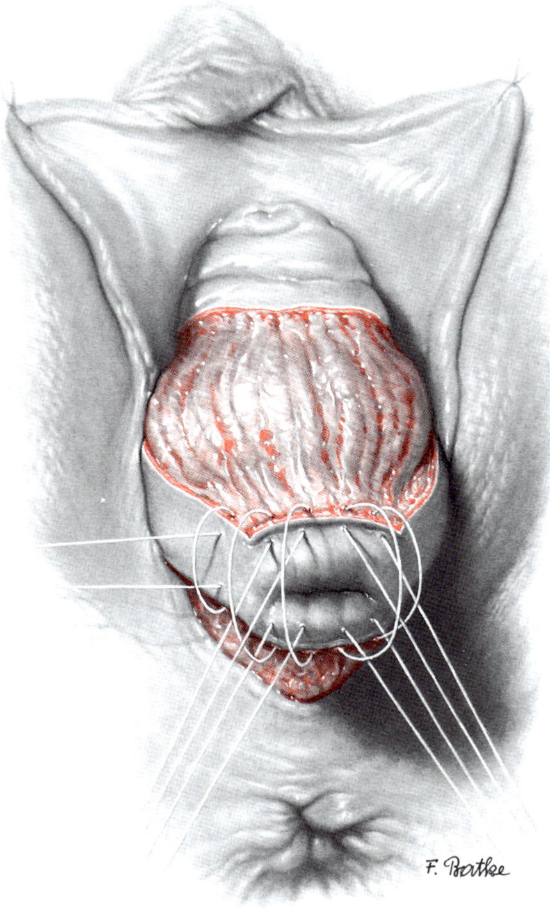

Figure 16.12. Neugebauer-Le Fort partial colpocleisis. Closing the wound edges near the cervix.

The mucosa has been removed from both the anterior and posterior rectangular incisions. A large cystocele and rectocele are present.

Four sutures are placed to join the anterior transverse wound edge with the corresponding posterior mucosal edge. An additional suture is applied to the right side for apposing the lateral wound edges.

Note the suturing technique: to ensure that the knot faces the cervix, the needle is inserted at the anterior wound edge from the mucosa to the wound surface and posteriorly from the wound surface to the mucosa.

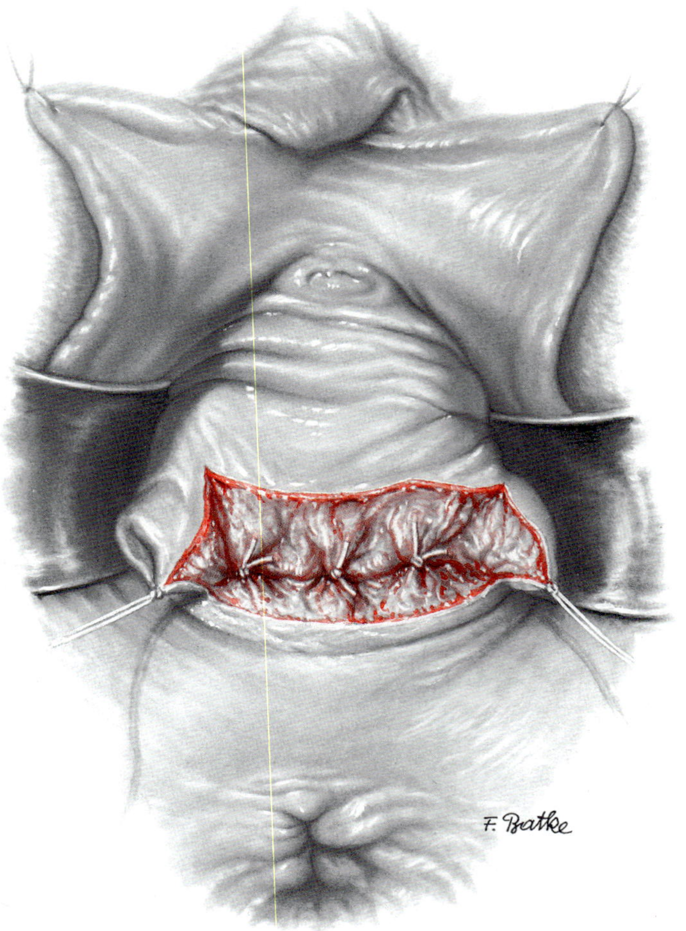

Figure 16.13. Neugebauer-Le Fort partial colpocleisis. Closing the wound surfaces.

The rectangular wound surfaces are sutured widely with multiple tiers of sutures. The repositioned uterus is supported by constructing a broad tissue septum.

The lateral wound edges have been extensively sutured; the last sutures are left long for traction and pulled laterally. On the right side, one can recognize a umbilicated lateral indentation that represents the opening of the lateral vaginal canal.

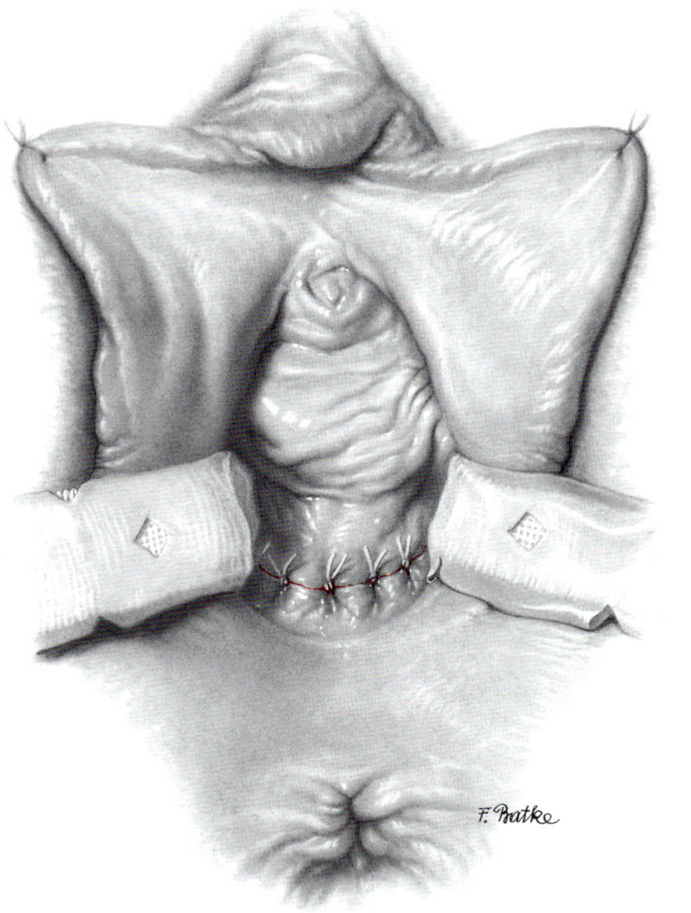

Figure 16.14. Neugebauer-Le Fort partial colpocleisis. Final view.

Wound edges and surfaces are united so that the vagina is closed except for the lateral mucosal canals. The vaginal canals are drained with Penrose drains that remain in place for 48 hours.

The transverse vaginal wound is located about two to three fingerbreadths from the urethral orifice to prevent scarring of the urethra. However, a new cystocele or urethrocele may develop later above the transverse vaginal scar.

Technical Problems—Figures 16.11–16.14

1. The *anterior rectangular incision may reach too close to the urethral orifice*. If it does, at the end of the operation excessive tension will be needed to join the anterior and posterior transverse vaginal wound edges. The subsequent pull on the scar may result in urinary incontinence.
2. Should the *incisions be extended too far laterally*, the remaining lateral vaginal tissue bridges will be too narrow. They may become necrotic after the wound edges have been ligated.
3. The Neugebauer-Le Fort procedure *cannot relieve urinary incontinence* associated with total prolapse. In fact, urine loss may be much increased by the postoperative scarring that will adversely affect the bladder control mechanism; alternatively, stress incontinence may first develop postoperatively. The original Neugebauer-Le Fort technique has therefore been frequently modified. One of these modifications is the Doederlein cross-bar colporrhaphy.

Doederlein Cross-Bar Colporrhaphy

Indications

The most significant difference from the Doederlein procedure is that, after having first united the two rectangular wound surfaces in the prolapsed anterior and posterior vaginal wall, the anterior rectangular incision is carried upward in an acute angle toward the exterior urethral orifice. This will leave the bladder neck and the urethra completely free, and the operation can therefore be combined with an exact plication of the bladder neck. An additional perineorrhaphy is also possible in this case.

Technique

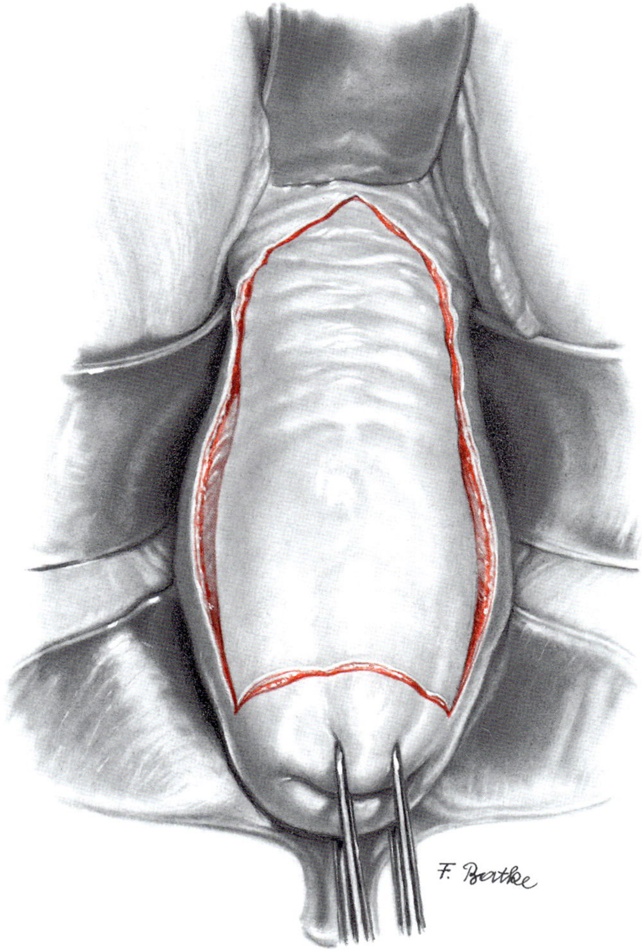

Figure 16.15. Doederlein cross-bar colporrhaphy. Anterior vaginal incision.

The uterus is pulled down by two tenacula attached to the cervix.

The anterior vaginal wall is inverted. A rectangular incision, which is angulated at the top, is made.

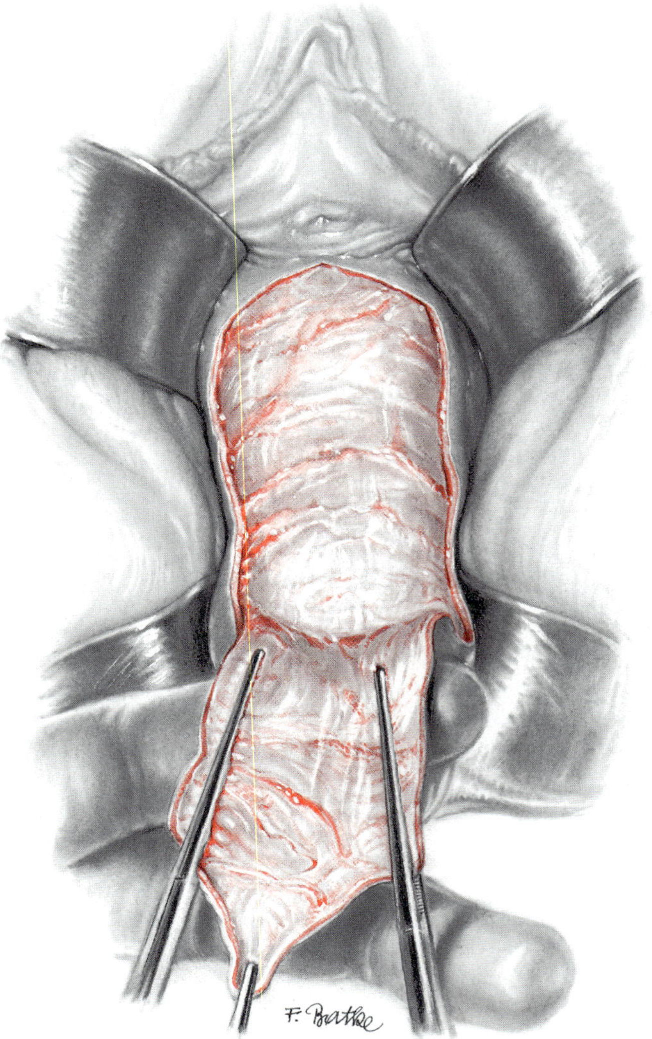

Figure 16.16. Doederlein cross-bar colporrhaphy. Dissecting the anterior vaginal mucosa. The anterior wall incision extends cranially to just below the urethral meatus.

To be able to separate the mucosal flap as superficially as possible (without touching the vaginal fascia), the surgeon stretches the dissected flap, held in clamps, over the left index finger. This makes it easier to dissect in the correct plane.

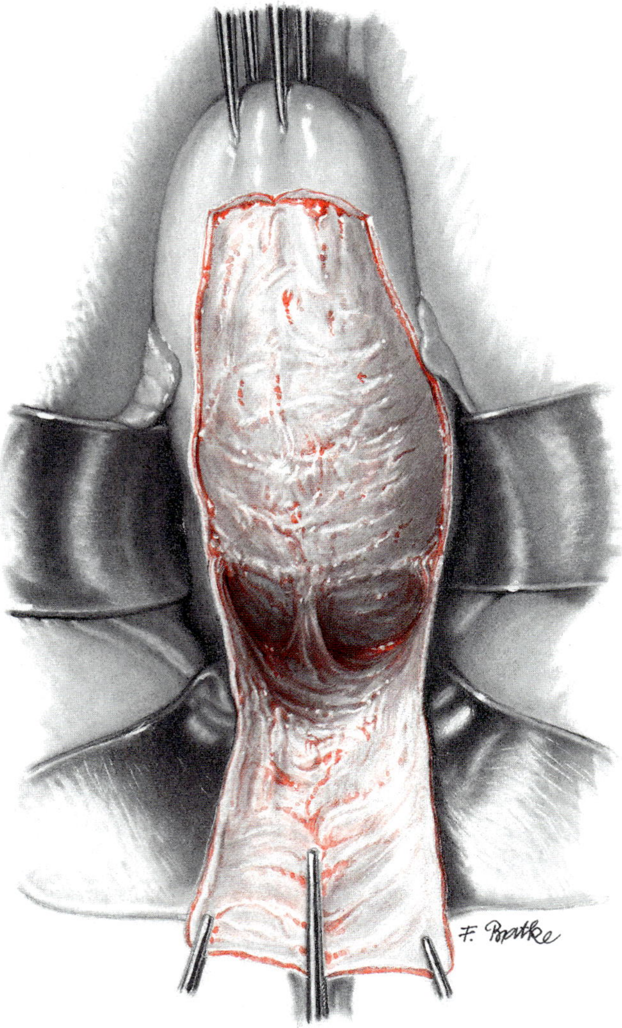

Figure 16.17. Doederlein cross-bar colporrhaphy. Dissecting the posterior vaginal mucosa.

The uterus is pulled straight upward. The flap of the vaginal mucosa in the region of the posterior rectangular wall incision has been separated superficially and is being pulled down with three clamps.

Dissection of the mucosa in its more caudal aspects necessitates moving progressively further away from the rectum as one approaches the posterior commissure.

The rectangular wound should end about 4 cm above the posterior commissure.

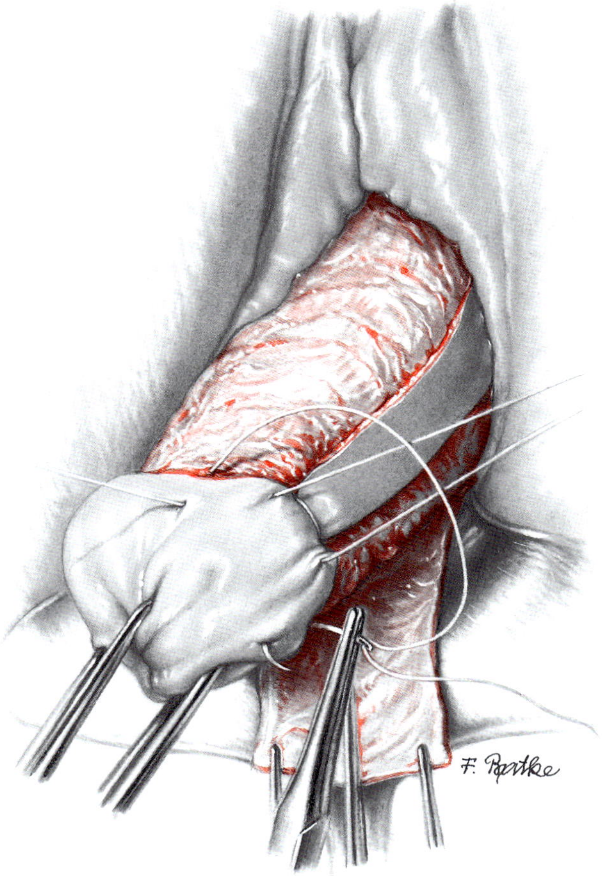

Figure 16.18. Doederlein cross-bar colporrhaphy. Burying the cervix.

The uterus is pulled down to the right by the attached tenacula. Rectangular portions of mucosa have been resected anteriorly and posteriorly. The posterior mucosal flap is being retracted by three clamps. Laterally between the anterior and posterior wound surfaces, there is a bridge of vaginal mucosa about 2 cm wide.

To unite the transverse vaginal wound edges near the cervix, the left corner suture has already been placed, and a second suture is being placed. Note the suture technique: anteriorly, the needle is directed from the vaginal mucosa toward the anterior wound surface, whereas posteriorly it is directed from the wound surface to the mucosa, thereby ensuring that the knot will lie in the vagina when the suture is tied.

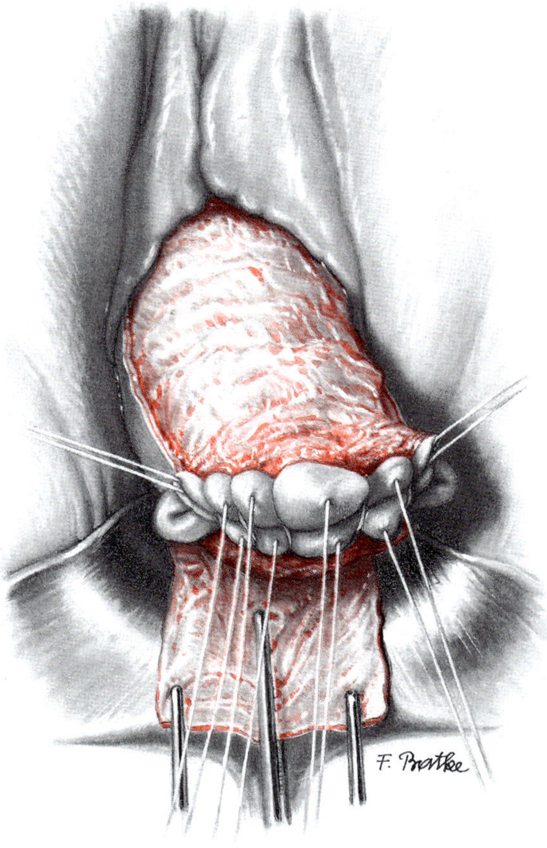

Figure 16.19. Doederlein cross-bar colporrhaphy. Closing the anterior and posterior wound edges.

This will ensure that the cervix is buried. Lateral to the corner sutures, the openings to the future lateral vaginal canals can be seen.

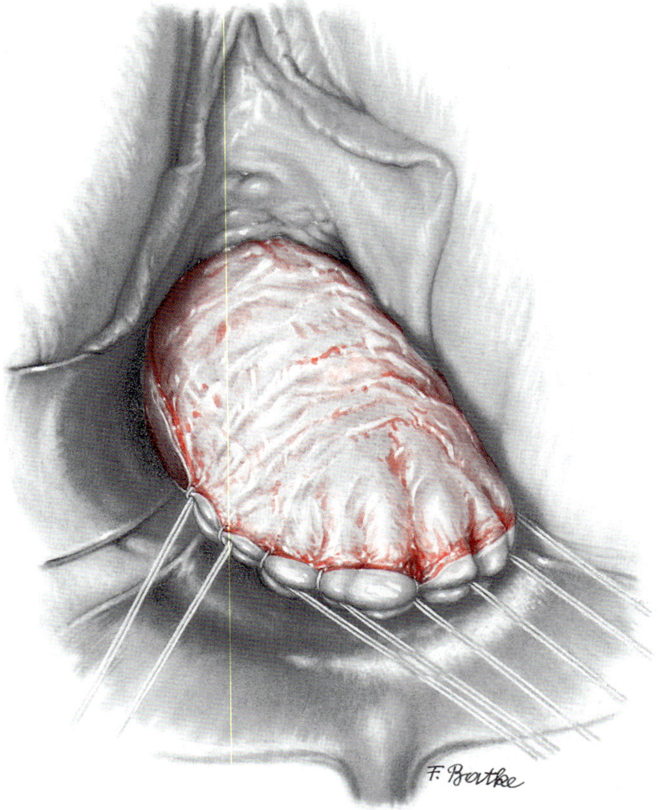

Figure 16.20. Doederlein cross-bar colporrhaphy. Closing the lateral vaginal wound edges.

The transverse vaginal wound edges near the cervix have been joined by interrupted sutures. Suture ends are left long. They are being pulled downward and to the left; their knots lie within the vagina, facing the cervix that is now completely buried.

Two sutures have been placed at the lateral vaginal wound edges on the right side. The suture technique here is the same as that shown in Figure 16.18.

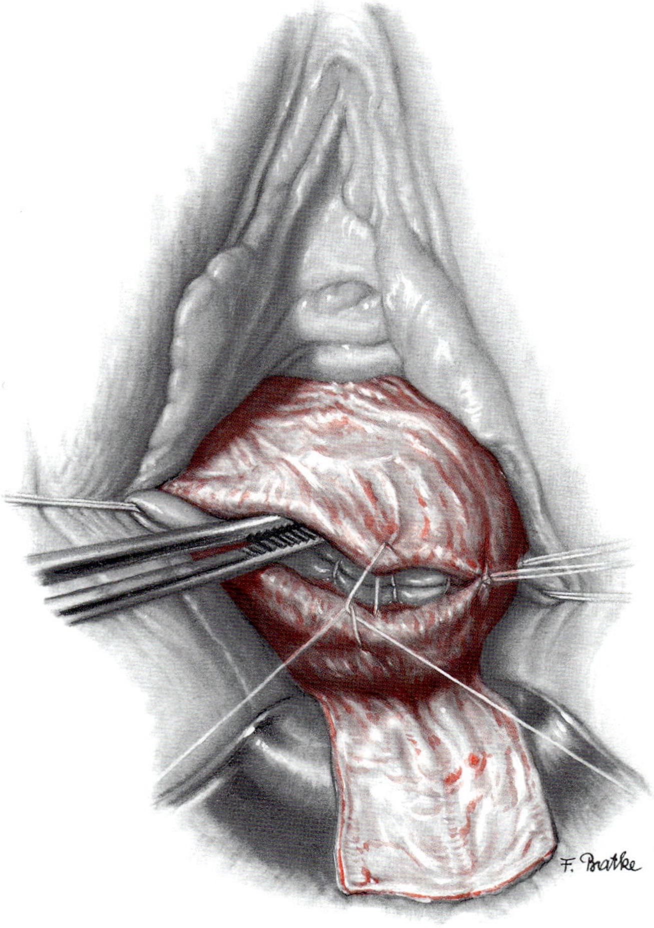

Figure 16.21. Doederlein cross-bar colporrhaphy. Closing the wound surfaces.

The vaginal wound edges have been joined, and the uppermost sutures are left long for now to serve for lateral traction.

The anterior and posterior wound surfaces are united with wide sutures. As these are being tied, the assistant pushes the exposed transverse vaginal wound edges upward with tissue forceps.

Figure 16.22. Doederlein cross-bar colporrhaphy. Supplementary bladder neck plication.

The anterior and posterior rectangular wound surfaces have already been joined with widely placed sutures. The outermost sutures on the lateral mucosal bridges are left long, and the ends are being pulled downward. The rectal wall is held back with a gauze strip.

In the acutely angled part of the anterior vaginal wall dissection, the vaginal mucosa is grasped with a series of toothed clamps and fanned out as shown. The bladder neck is plicated with three sutures (for technique see Chapter 12).

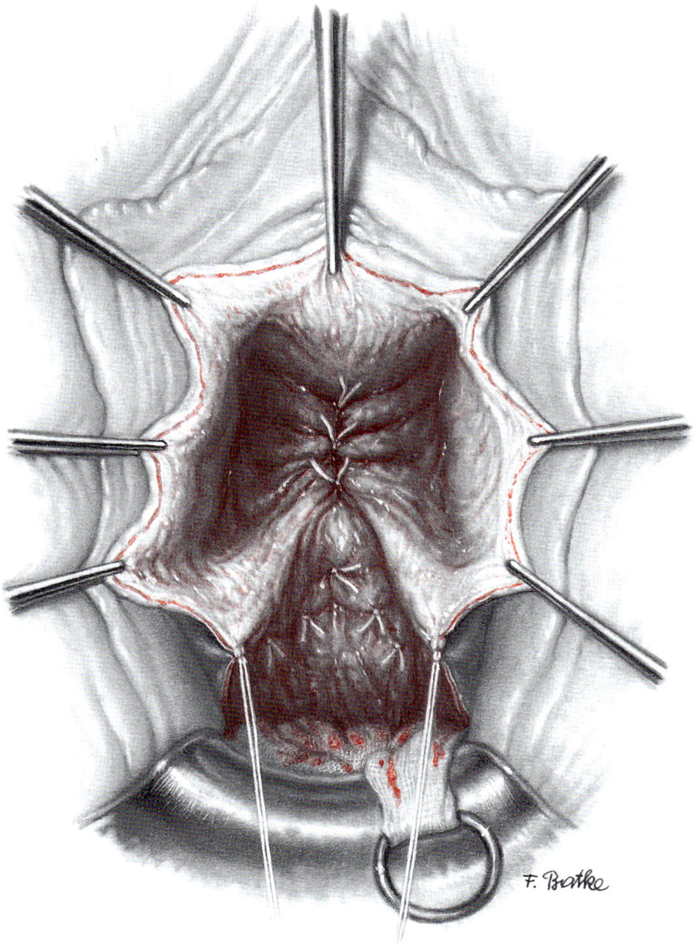

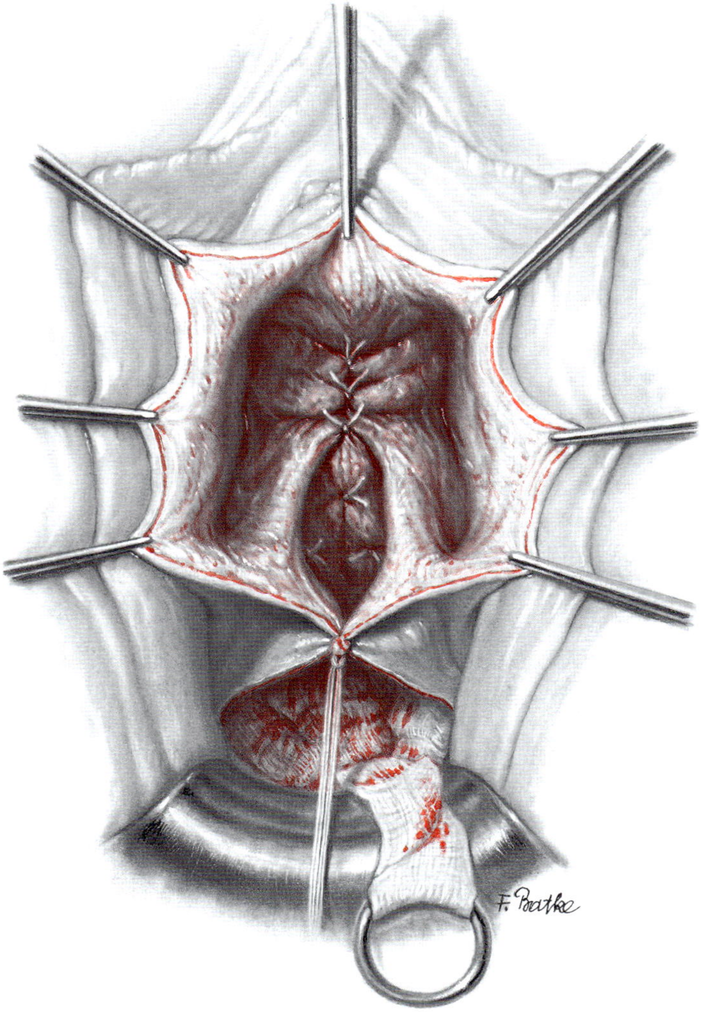

Figure 16.23. Doederlein cross-bar colporrhaphy. Tying the corner sutures.

Plication of the bladder neck is complete. The prolapsed uterus has been completely repositioned by the approximation of the anterior and posterior vaginal wound surfaces.

The corner sutures demarcating the lateral vaginal mucosa bridges are tied together. Lateral to the now medially located tied corner sutures, the entrances to the lateral vaginal canals can be seen.

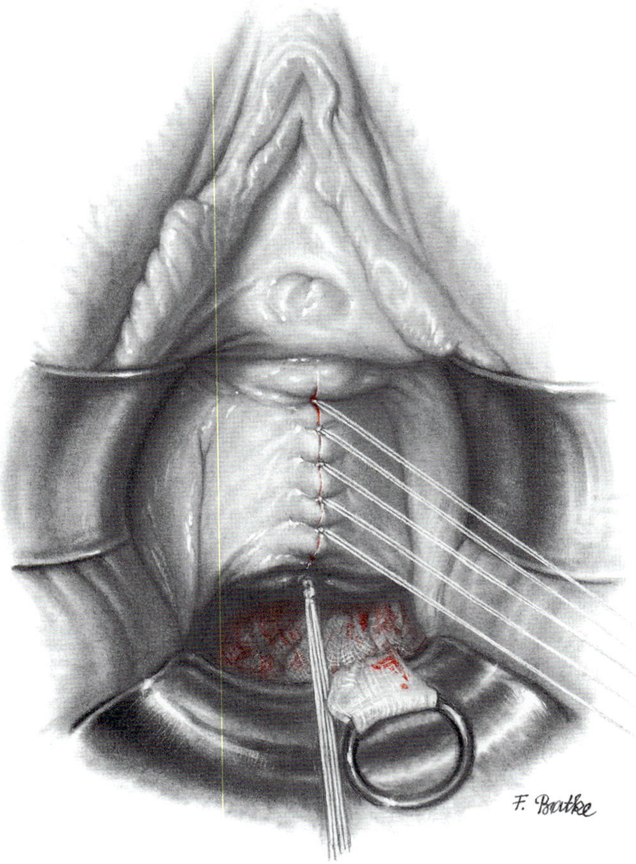

Figure 16.24. Doederlein cross-bar colporrhaphy. Closing the anterior colporrhaphy.

The anterior colporrhaphy wound is closed by a longitudinal row of interrupted catgut sutures. The rectal wall is held back with a gauze strip. The corner sutures of the lateral mucosal bridges have been tied in the midline; the openings of the lateral vaginal canals are visible as umbilicated indentations just lateral to the midline knots.

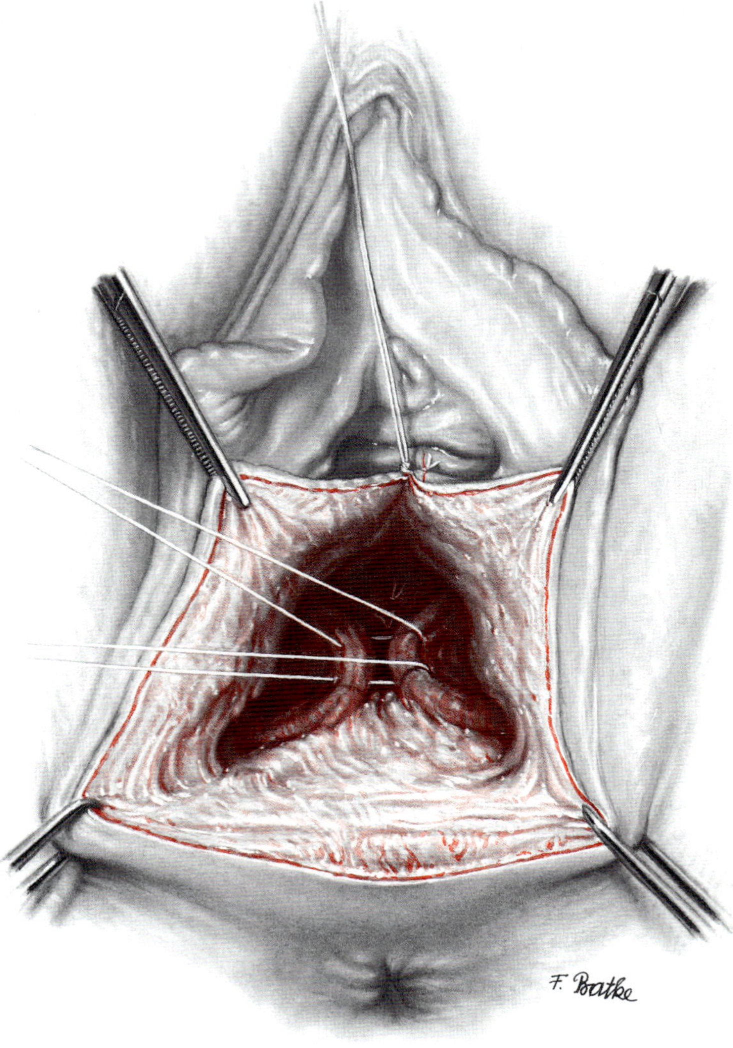

Figure 16.25. Doederlein cross-bar colporrhaphy. Levator plication.

The anterior rectal wall is plicated with two sutures visible in the depths of the field.

The levator borders are dissected free and are united above the rectum with two sutures (for technique see Chapter 13).

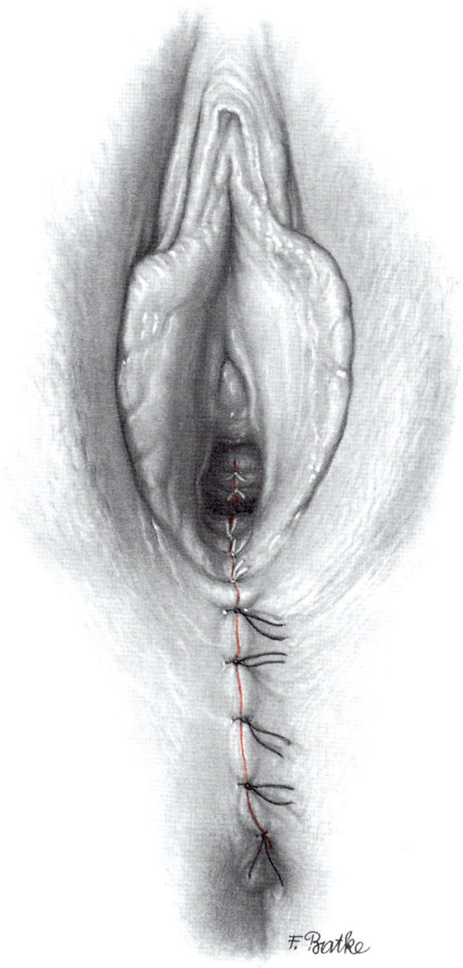

Figure 16.26. Doederlein cross-bar colporrhaphy. Closing the perineal incision.

The cross-bar colporrhaphy is completed, including the supplementary procedures of bladder neck plication and levator plasty. The vaginal wound was sutured with catgut and the perineum with silk. A short vaginal cul-de-sac has been created.

Technical Problems—Figures 16.15–16.26

1. The *rectangular excisions of vaginal mucosa should not reach too far laterally* because otherwise the outermost sutures placed to form the lateral canals can only be tied together in the midline under tension.
2. The *cross-bar tissue obstruction should not extend too close to the cervix*. The lower transverse incision of the rectangle must not be made on the fixed mucosa of the cervix but is placed instead in the nearby mobile mucosa of the fornices. Otherwise, one might encounter difficulty in uniting the anterior and posterior transverse wound edges and burying the cervix.
3. The *flap of vaginal mucosa may not be dissected superficially enough*. As a result, the underlying fascia, which is needed to serve as a supporting structure, will be removed, and the blood vessels coursing in this layer will be opened.
4. If *painstaking hemostasis is not obtained* in the area of the rectangular wound surfaces, a hematoma may form and disrupt the joined wound surfaces within a few days after the operation.
5. The *vaginal wound edges near the posterior fornix may hemorrhage into the depth of the operative field if not approximated precisely*. Such complications tend to arise in patients improperly selected for the Doederlein procedure, e.g., those who do not have total prolapse of the vagina. If partial prolapse of the posterior wall has occurred, the posterior fornix lies high up and is accessible only with difficulty when the posterior rectangular incision is performed. As a result of the poor exposure, union of the wound edges is inexact, and hemostasis is inadequate.

Conill Colpocleisis

Indications

This operation consists of a simple, logical combination of the cross-bar plasty and an introital closure. It may be undertaken even in the oldest patients with total prolapse without significant risk because it can be performed under local anesthesia.

Technique

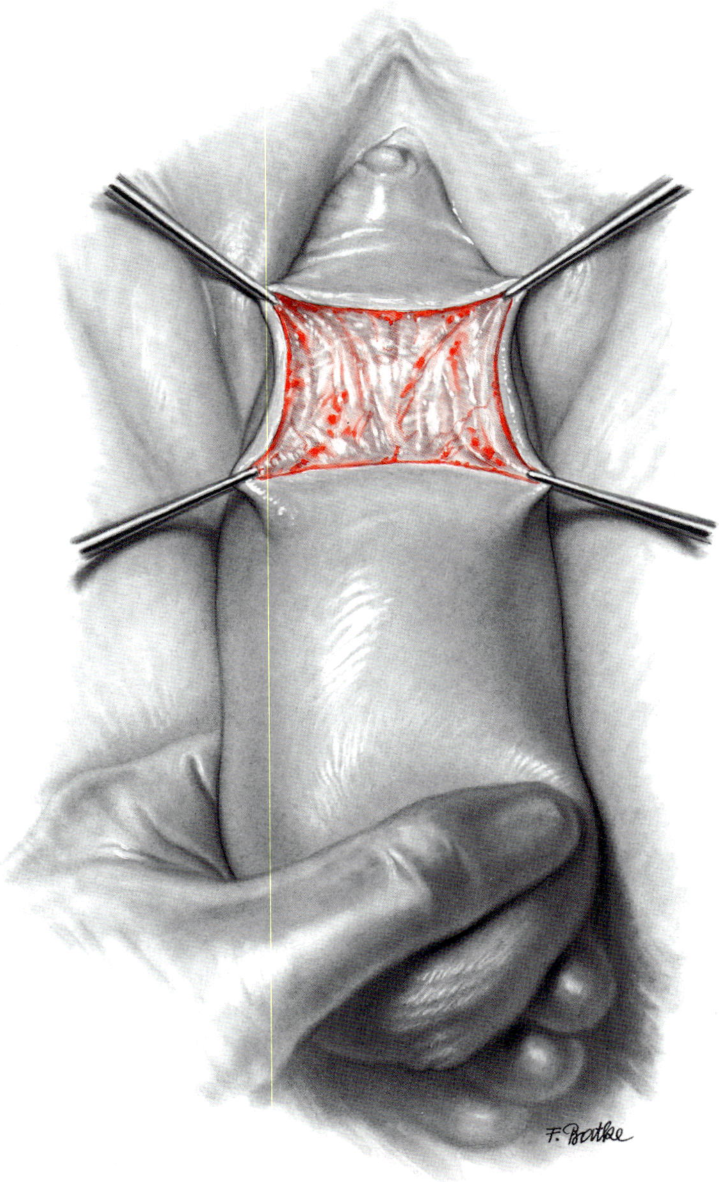

Figure 16.27. Conill colpocleisis. Rectangular anterior vaginal incision.

The prolapsed uterus is pulled downward.

A rectangular incision is made in the upper third of the inverted anterior vaginal wall. The wound edges are retracted apart with clamps. The upper margin of the wound surface extends to 2 cm from the urethral meatus.

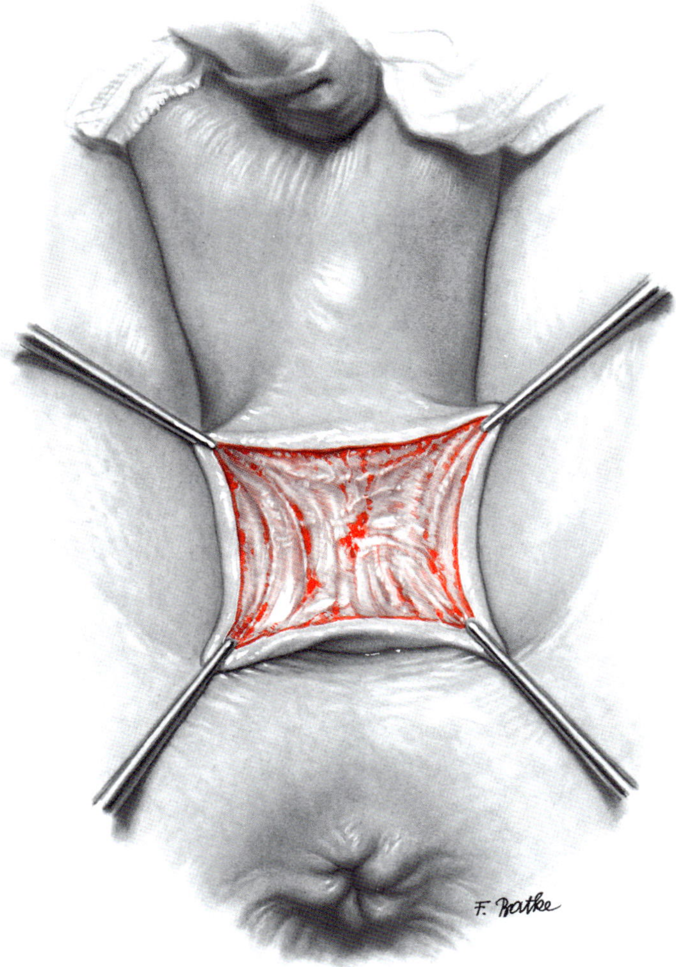

Figure 16.28. Conill colpocleisis. Posterior rectangular vaginal incision.

The totally prolapsed uterus is pulled upward. A rectangular incision is executed in the lower third of the inverted posterior vaginal wall, corresponding in size to the anterior wall incision. The lower margin of this incision should be about 2 cm from the posterior commissure.

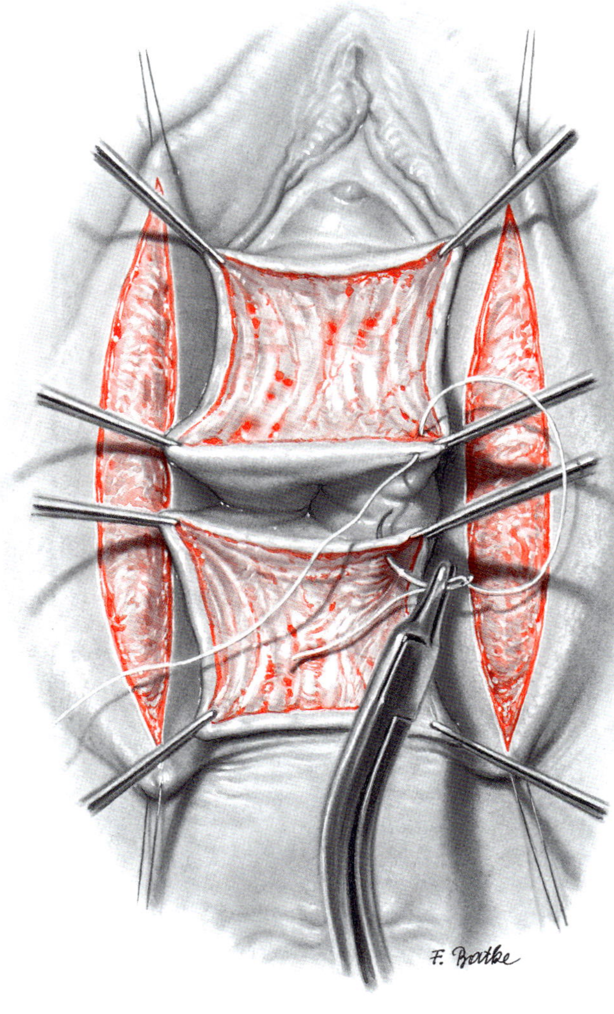

Figure 16.29. Conill colpocleisis. Uniting the lower wound edge of the anterior with the upper wound edge of the posterior wound surfaces. Incising the labia majora bilaterally.

The prolapsed uterus has been repositioned. The anterior and posterior wound edges, held with clamps, are juxtaposed and sutured together to form one large rectangular wound surface. Note that the needle was inserted anteriorly from the vaginal mucosa to the wound surface and posteriorly in the reverse direction so that the knots will lie in the vaginal lumen.

The skin on the inside of the labia majora is stretched bilaterally with two silk traction sutures, and an elongated skin flap is excised from the skin of the labia majora, extending beyond the vaginal wound surfaces by 1 cm both caudally and cranially. These skin flaps reach almost up to the urethral orifice cephalad.

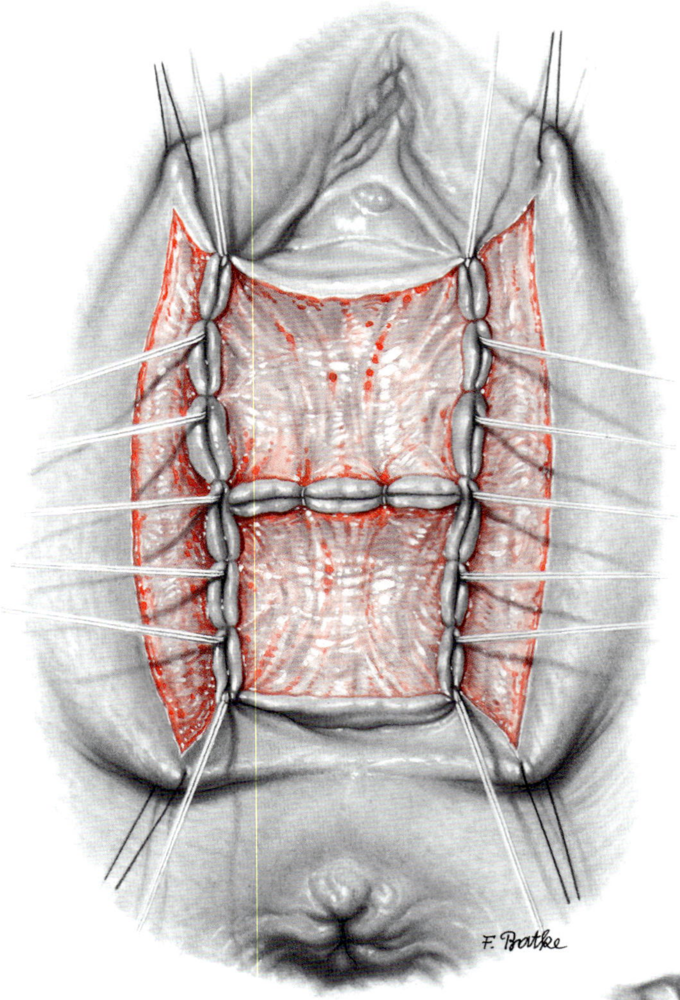

Figure 16.30. Conill colpocleisis. Partial closure of the lateral vaginal and median labial wound edges.

The upper and lower angle sutures serve for traction. Because of the analogous nature of the suture technique used, the knots of the remaining sutures lie in the vaginal lumen and are therefore not visible.

The labial wound surfaces exceed the vaginal wound surfaces somewhat in both cephalad and caudad directions.

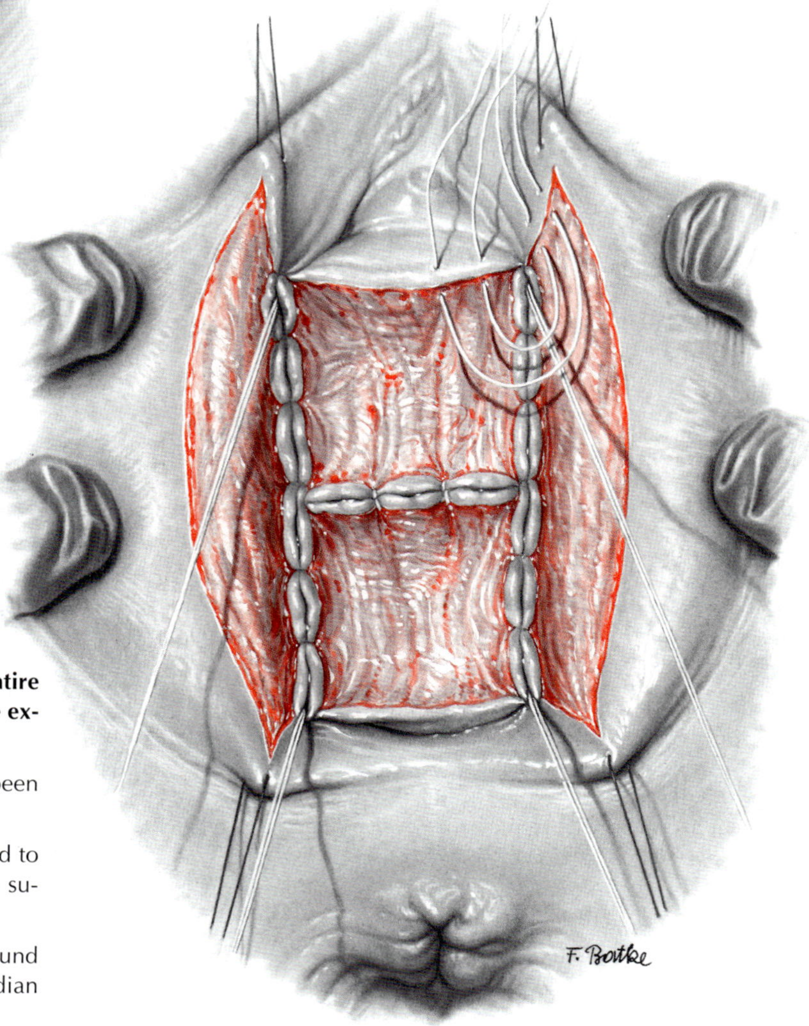

Figure 16.31. Conill colpocleisis. Approximating the entire upper and lower transverse vaginal wound edges with the excess of the median labial wound edges.

Most of the lateral vaginal and labial wound edges have been joined.

The anterior transverse vaginal wound edge is now sutured to the cranial excess of the left labial wound edge. Two such sutures are in place on the left side.

The remaining transverse upper and lower vaginal wound edges are then apposed to the excess remainders of the median labial edges.

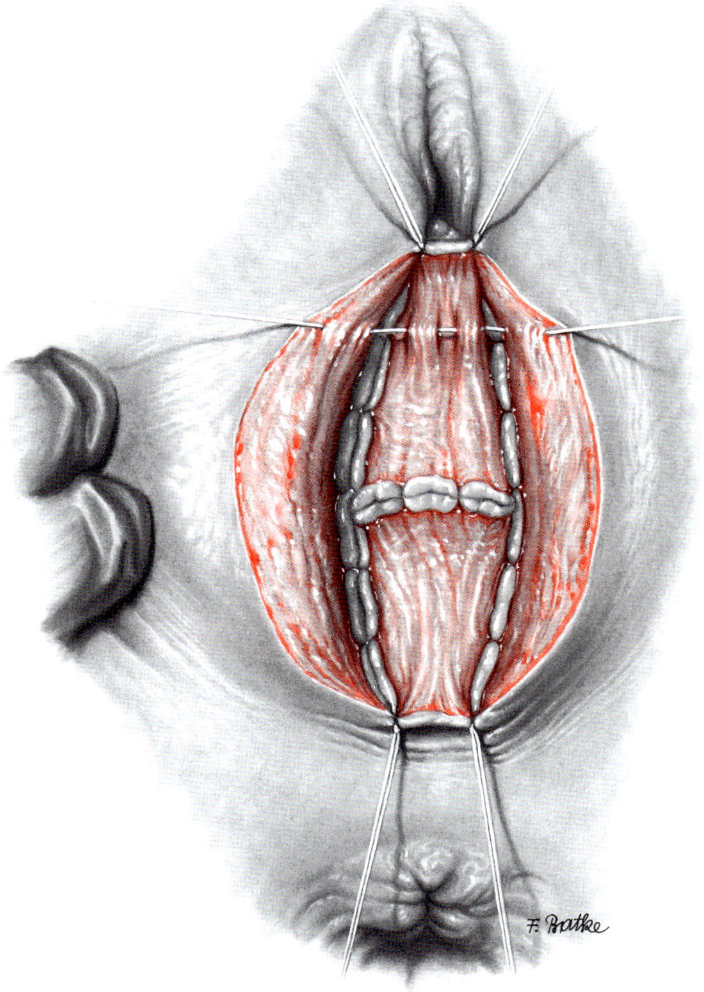

Figure 16.32. Conill colpocleisis. Closing the wound surfaces. First suture.

The labial and vaginal wound edges are joined with interrupted catgut sutures; to retain a clear view, these should be left untied until all are in place.

Approximation of the large wound surfaces will form a broad, weight-bearing septum for occluding the vaginal introitus.

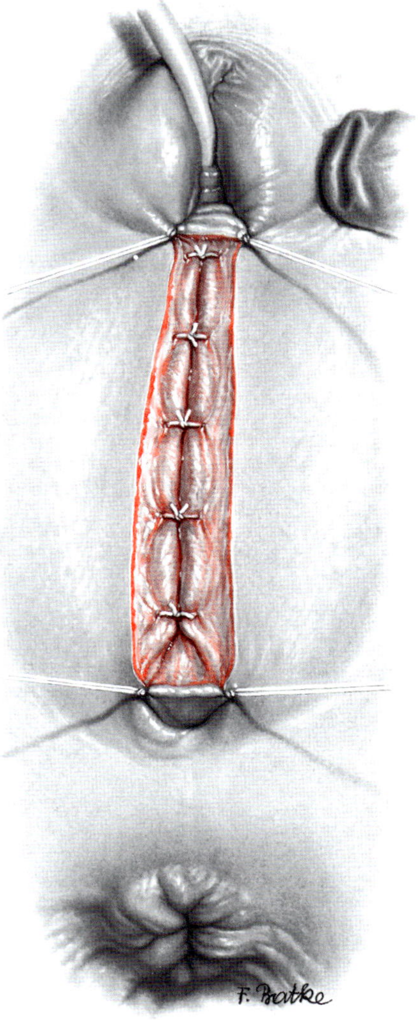

Figure 16.33. Conill colpocleisis. Closing the wound in layers.

Through approximation of the wound surfaces a broad, weight-bearing septum has been formed; this will close the vaginal introitus. An indwelling catheter is inserted into the bladder.

Note that the upper end of the newly formed tissue wedge terminates about 1 cm caudad to the urethral meatus, and the lower end reaches to about 1 cm from the posterior commissure.

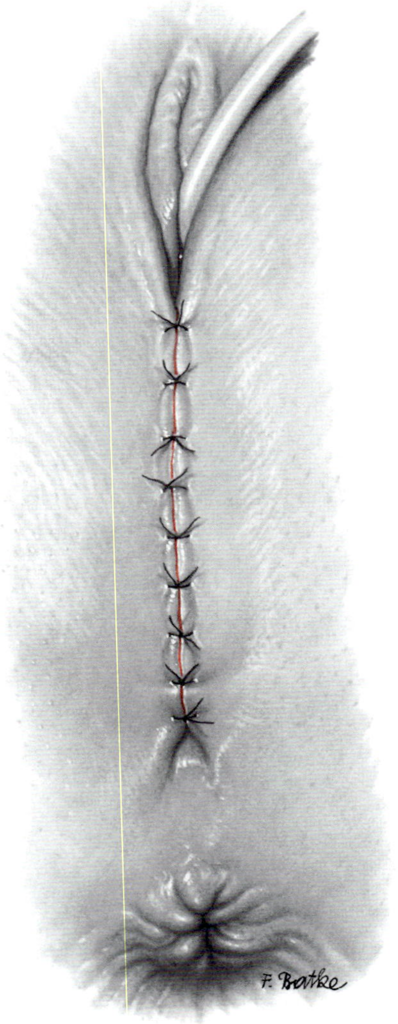

Figure 16.34. Conill colpocleisis. Completing the procedure.

The colpocleisis is completed by uniting the lateral labial skin edges with silk button sutures.

Technical Problems—Figures 16.27–16.34

1. The *vaginal and labial wound surfaces may be insufficient in breadth*. As a result, the tissue wedge formed to close the vaginal introitus will be too narrow and not strong enough, possibly leading to wound dehiscence.
2. If the *mucosal flap is performed too far cranially* at the edge of the labia majora, the urethral meatus will be covered when the wound surfaces are united. This will hinder spontaneous emptying of the bladder.

17/ Surgical Treatment of a Perineal Laceration

Indications

The posterior vaginal wall is always involved whenever an obstetrical laceration of the perineum occurs. Three degrees of severity are distinguished according to the extent of the laceration:

- First degree: vaginal laceration and laceration of the posterior commissure;
- Second degree: laceration extends through the mucosa to include the perineal musculature (without damage to the external anal sphincter);
- Third degree: laceration of the perineal musculature as well as external anal sphincter (can include the anterior rectal wall).

All perineal lacerations must be sutured. Even small tears of the frenulum should be repaired with catgut sutures so they heal more rapidly. Those that are not repaired may become infected by lochial contamination. Ulceration may develop and take weeks to heal. A second degree laceration that remains unsutured will likely give rise to vaginal prolapse. Those patients sustaining complete (or third degree) lacerations of the perineum with injury to the anterior rectum will be incontinent of stool and flatus. Fresh lacerations of the perineum demand immediate attention.

Repair of an Old Third Degree Perineal Laceration

Indications

Results of the repair of an old third degree perineal laceration are not as good as those of the repair of a fresh one of equal severity.

If the freshly repaired third degree laceration does not heal primarily, we highly recommend waiting at least 6 months before secondary repair is attempted to allow healing of local inflammatory changes. Even the unrepaired third degree tear should not be repaired before 6 months postpartum. Before undertaking the procedure, the bowel must be thoroughly emptied. On each of two preoperative days, the patient takes a laxative together with a liquid diet, and a purging enema is given.

Technique

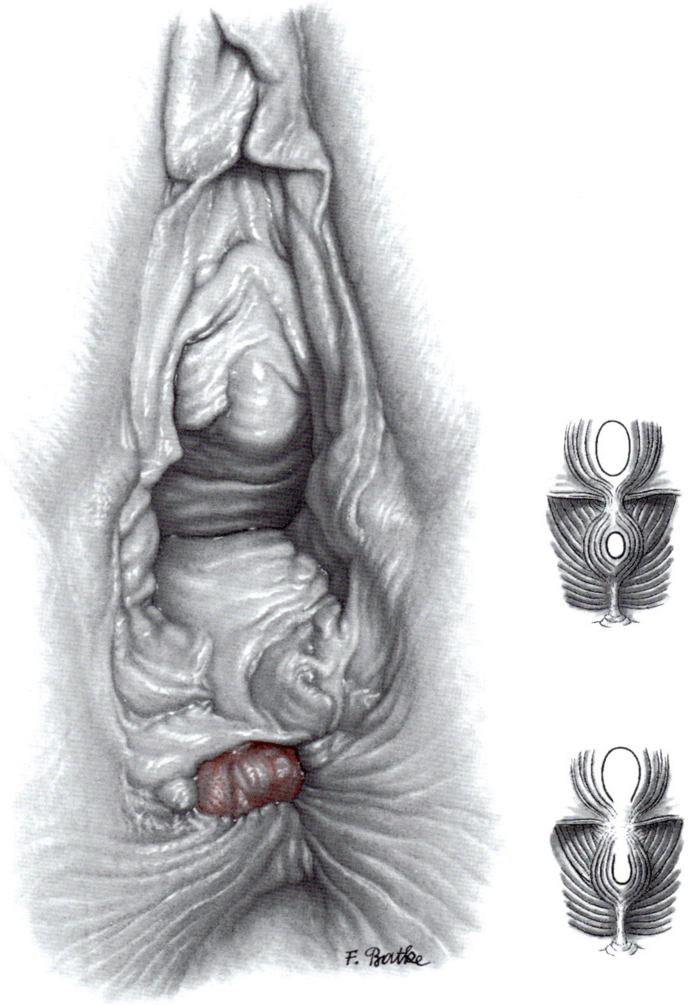

Figure 17.1. Repair of old third degree perineal laceration. Original condition.

The perineum is completely absent, and the posterior vaginal mucosa juxtaposes the rectal mucosa; extensive scar tissue is apparent between the two. Because of the torn external sphincter ani muscle, radiating folds of perineal skin are only present posteriorly.

Details. Pelvic and urogenital diaphragms are shown with undamaged perineum (*upper*) and third degree perineal laceration (*lower*).

Figure 17.2. Repair of old third degree perineal laceration. Initial incision.

The posterior vaginal wall is grasped with a tenaculum in the midline approximately 3–4 cm cranially from the region of scar tissue. The connective tissue at the posterior commissure is pulled laterally by tenacula placed on either side of the scarred area.

A vaginoperineal incision is made to include only the scarred area of the perineum—but no more—extending up the posterior vaginal wall to form a triangular area for excision.

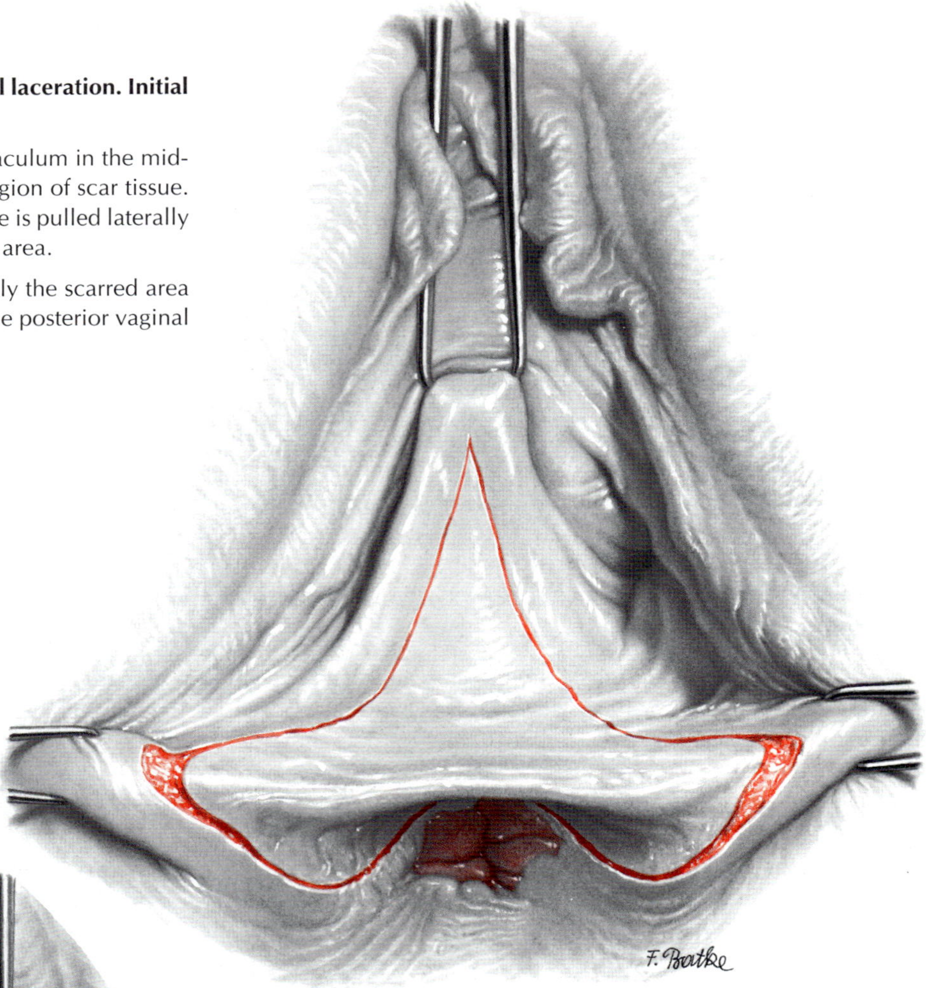

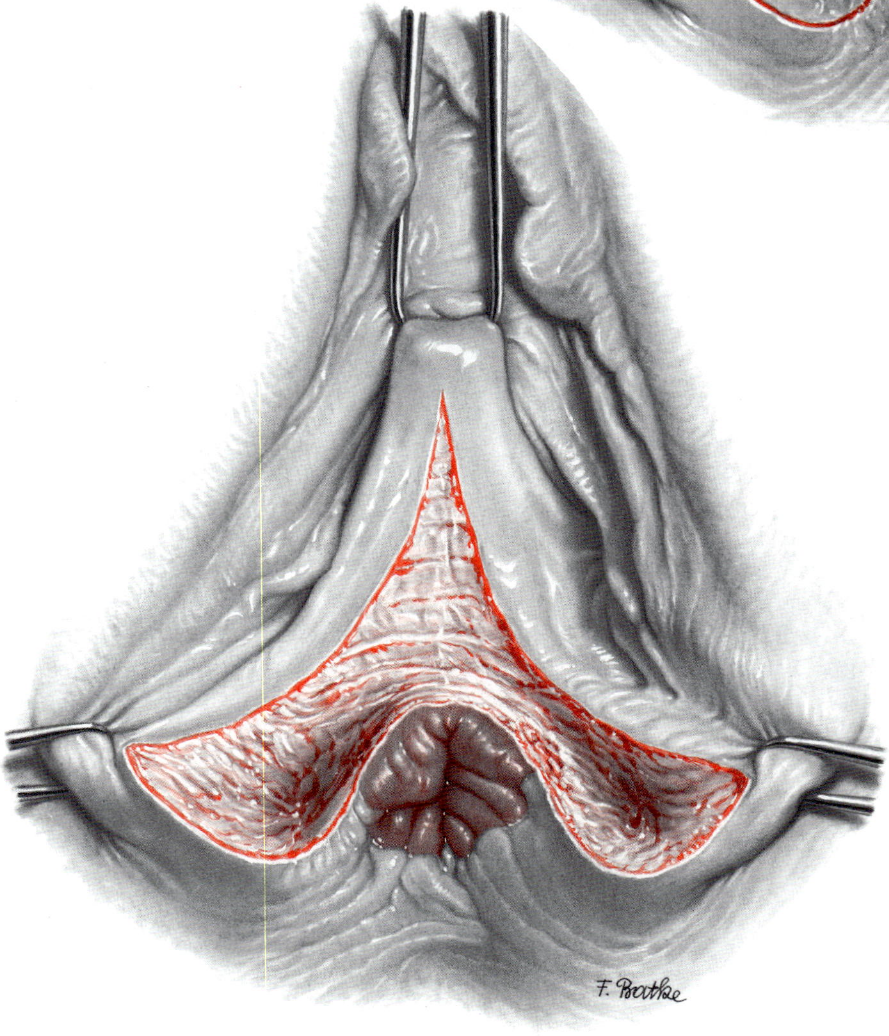

Figure 17.3. Repair of old third degree perineal laceration. Excising the scar.

The incision begins in the posterior vaginal wall just beneath the apical tenaculum. It courses laterally along the proximal edge of the scarred area and caudally to the laterally placed tenaculum. From there it runs in a convex curve posteromedially, bowing around the prolapsed rectal mucosa and including both sphincter dimples.

As soon as the entire scar tissue has been excised within the mucosal incision, the scissors are advanced within the rectovaginal septum before isolating the vaginal incision surface from the rectum. During this step, one should dissect as close as possible to the vaginal wall to avoid damage to the anterior rectal wall.

The rectum and the vagina must also be separated from each other laterally so that the retracted muscle portions of the perineum and the external anal sphincter can be dissected free and pulled together later.

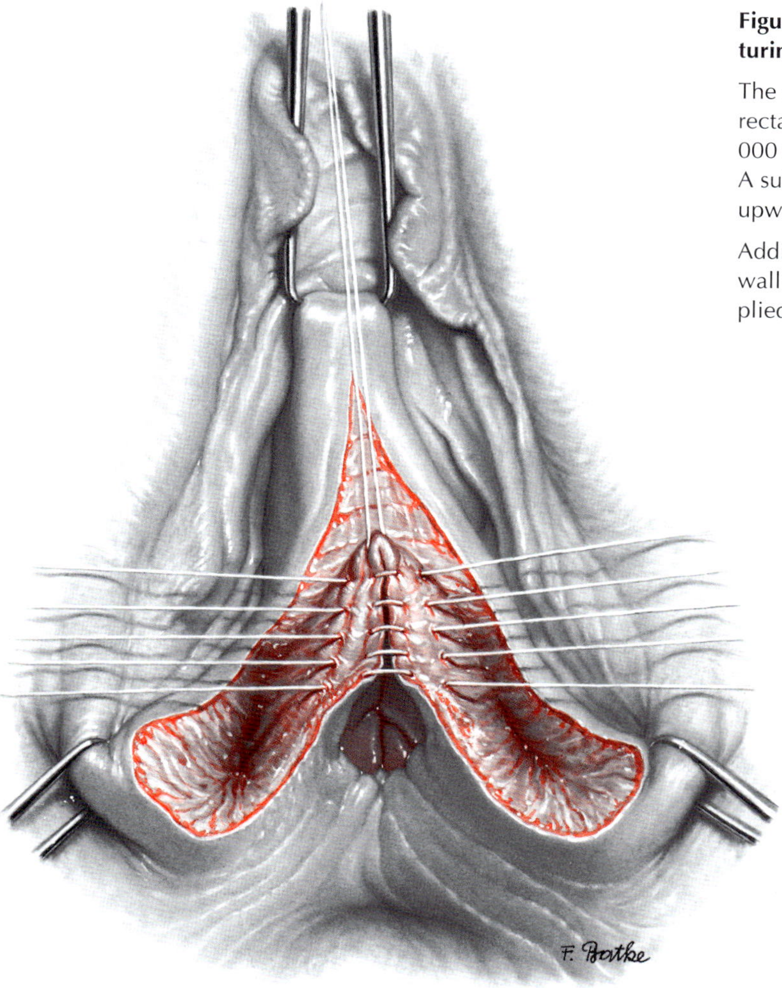

Figure 17.4. Repair of old third degree perineal laceration. Suturing the rectal wall.

The rectal aspects of the laceration are repaired by uniting the perirectal tissues with several sutures (using atraumatic needles and size 000 chromic catgut), making sure not to include the rectal mucosa. A suture is placed first at the uppermost wound angle and retracted upward. This exposes the entire length of the rectal tear.

Additional sutures are placed to bring the lacerated anterior rectal wall edges together. A second identical row of sutures is then applied to secure the first row of rectal sutures.

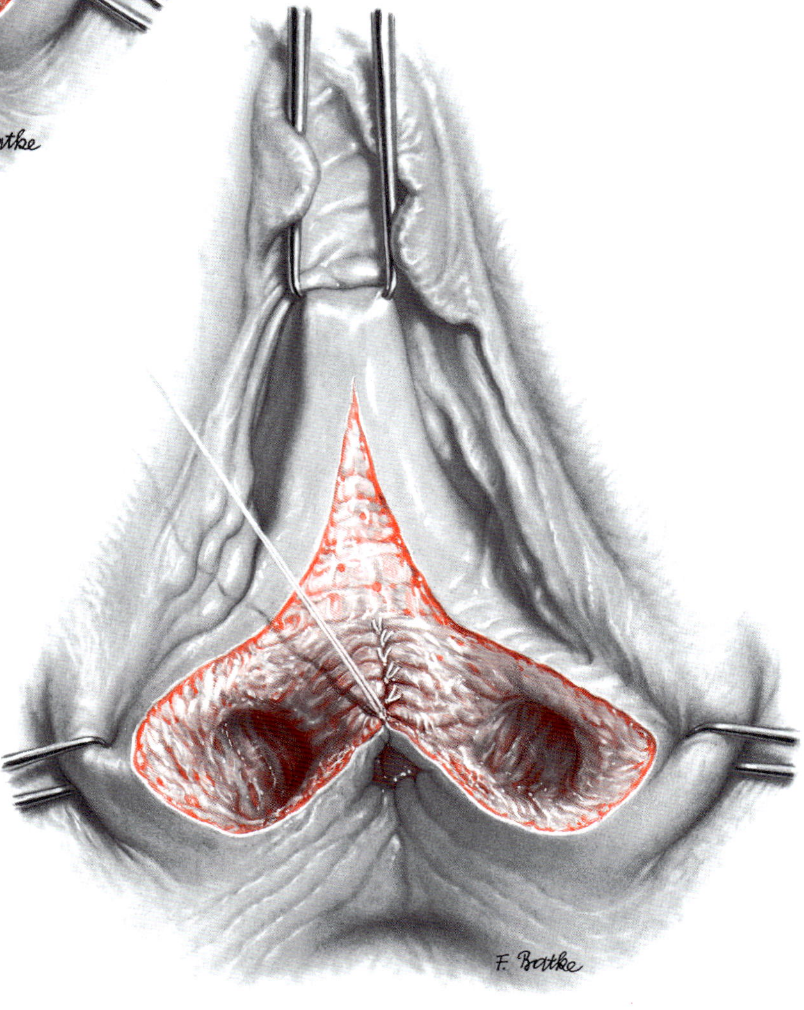

Figure 17.5 Repair of old third degree perineal laceration. Performing the sphincter repair.

The tear in the anterior rectal wall has been closed, and the rectal mucosa has been reapposed. The lowermost suture has been left long for traction.

On both sides of the newly constructed anus one can see within the dimpled area the retracted fibers of the lacerated external anal sphincter muscle.

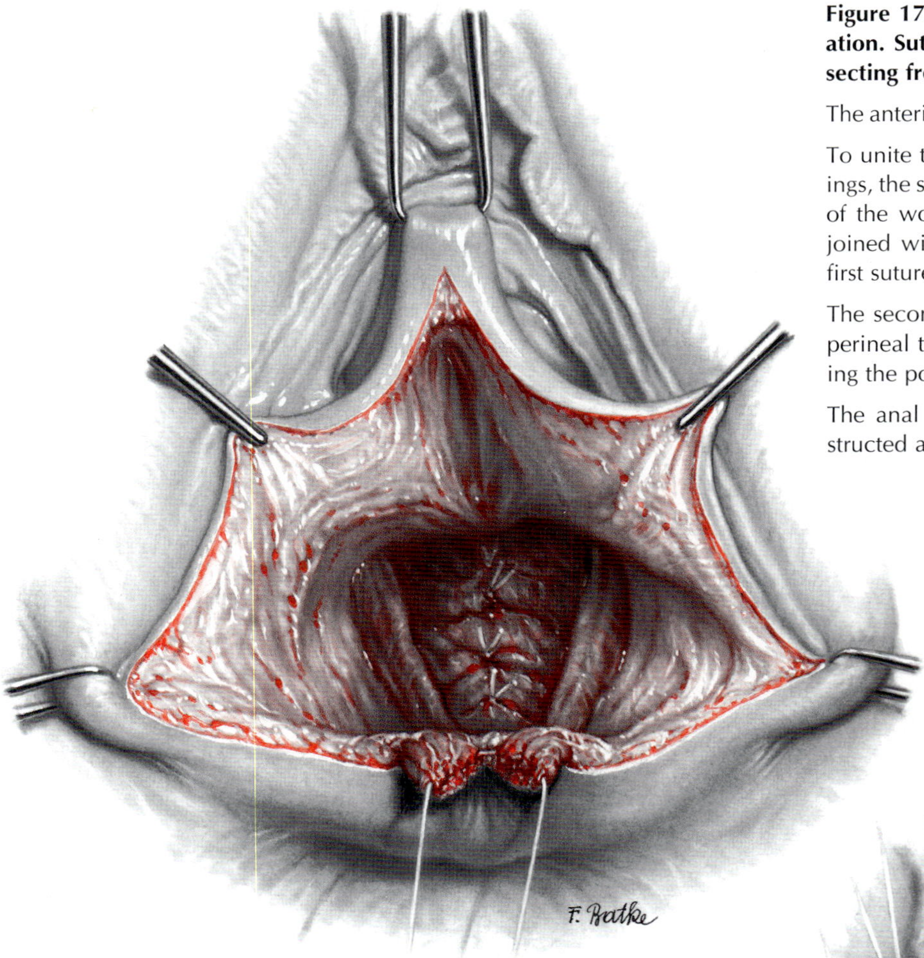

Figure 17.6. Repair of old third degree perineal laceration. Suturing the external anal sphincter muscle. Dissecting free the levator borders.

The anterior rectal wall has been closed by several sutures.

To unite the retracted sphincter ends and their surroundings, the sphincter ends are pulled out of the deep recesses of the wound with delicate mouse-toothed clamps and joined with two U-shaped chromic catgut sutures. (The first suture has been placed.)

The second suture is placed above the first suture in the perineal tissues adherent to the rectum, thus reconstructing the posterior part of the perineal wedge.

The anal closing mechanism is now completely reconstructed and can be tested by digital examination.

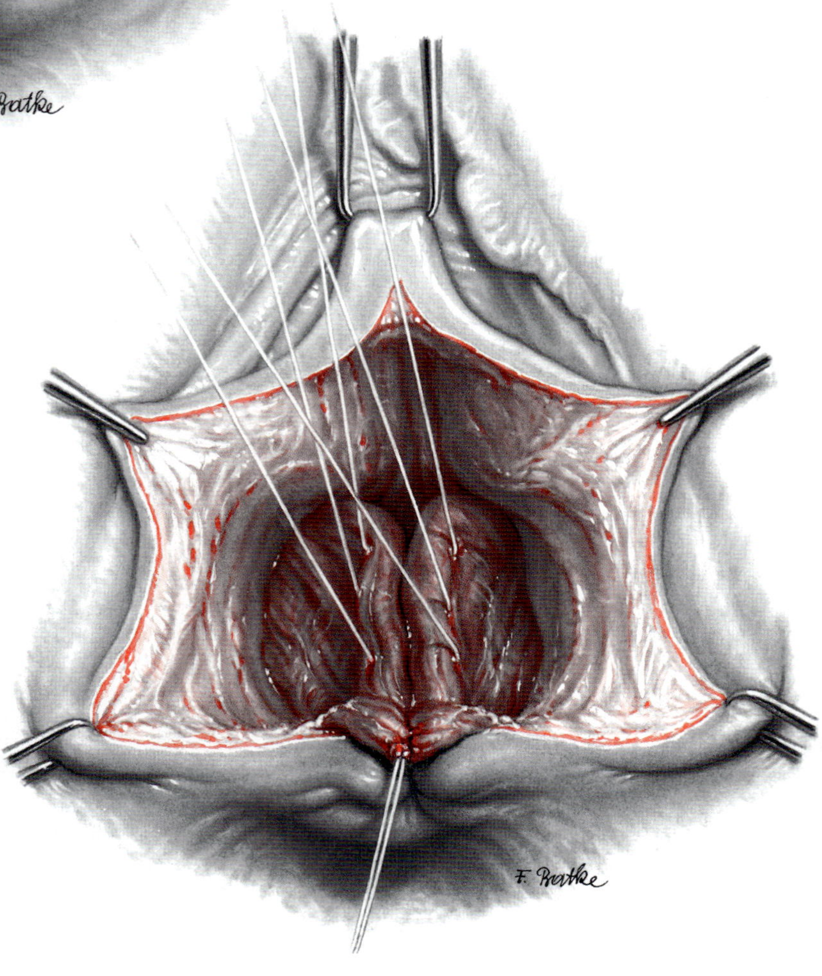

Figure 17.7. Repair of old third degree perineal laceration. Apposing the levator borders.

The ends of the anal sphincter have been united in the midline. The freed levator borders have been plicated with three sutures that cover the rectal sutures.

The next step is closure of the vaginal mucosa and perineal skin.

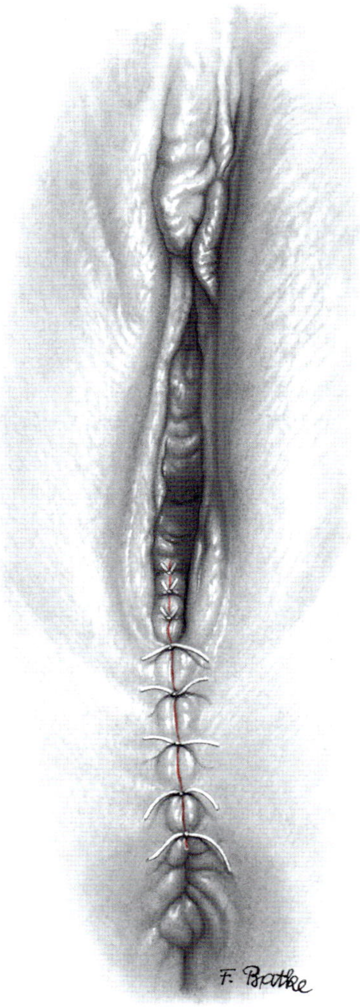

Figure 17.8. Repair of old third degree perineal laceration. Final view.

After a long perineal reconstruction has been accomplished, the vaginal wound edges are brought together with catgut sutures, and the perineal skin is closed with silk sutures.

Technical Problems—Figures 17.1–17.8

1. If the *scarred area is not completely resected*, it will be difficult to find the torn ends of the external anal sphincter; one must also remember that scar tissue heals poorly.
2. The *rectum and the vagina may be insufficiently separated from each other*. Should this occur, not enough tissue can be brought in from the sides. The rectal sutures will then be under tension, and wound dehiscence may occur. Furthermore, the perineum cannot be well reconstructed in this case.
3. If the *sphincter suture pulls* the external anal sphincter muscle ends together *too tightly*, the rectal canal may be made excessively narrow postoperatively. This may lead to excessive stretching of the rectum through backed-up contents of the bowel. Anal patency should be tested by inserting the index finger into the rectum.

Special postoperative care. After the repair of first and second degree lacerations, the patient will get up within the first 12 hours after surgery. The digestive process will be set in motion by usual means. For patients with third degree repair, we recommend that the bowel function be delayed for 5–6 days after the procedure to allow time for the rectal wound to heal. This is achieved by the administration of opiates (15 drops of tincture of opium three times a day for three days), a low residue fluid diet, and strict bed rest. On the fifth postoperative day, the stool is softened by use of laxatives, and on the sixth day bowel movement is brought about but without using an enema.

Suture of a Fresh Third Degree Perineal Laceration

Technique

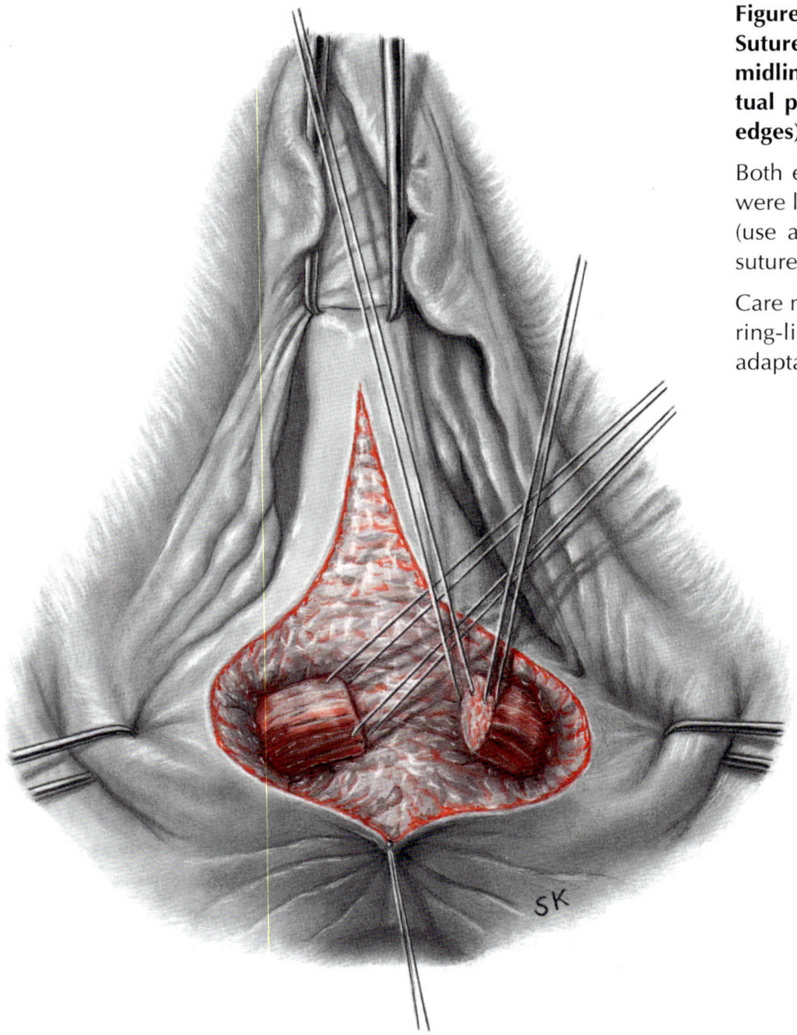

Figure 17.9. Repair of a fresh third degree perineal laceration. Suture of the external anal sphincter muscle, depicted here after midline episiotomy with severing of the sphincter muscle (an actual perineal tear would have involved laceration of the wound edges).

Both ends of the sphincter muscles have been dissected free and were ligated with thin sutures through the outer layers, respectively (use atraumatic needles with size 000 absorbable monofilament suture).

Care must be taken to include the cranial and dorsal aspects of the ring-like musculature to ensure an all-encompassing secure adaptation.

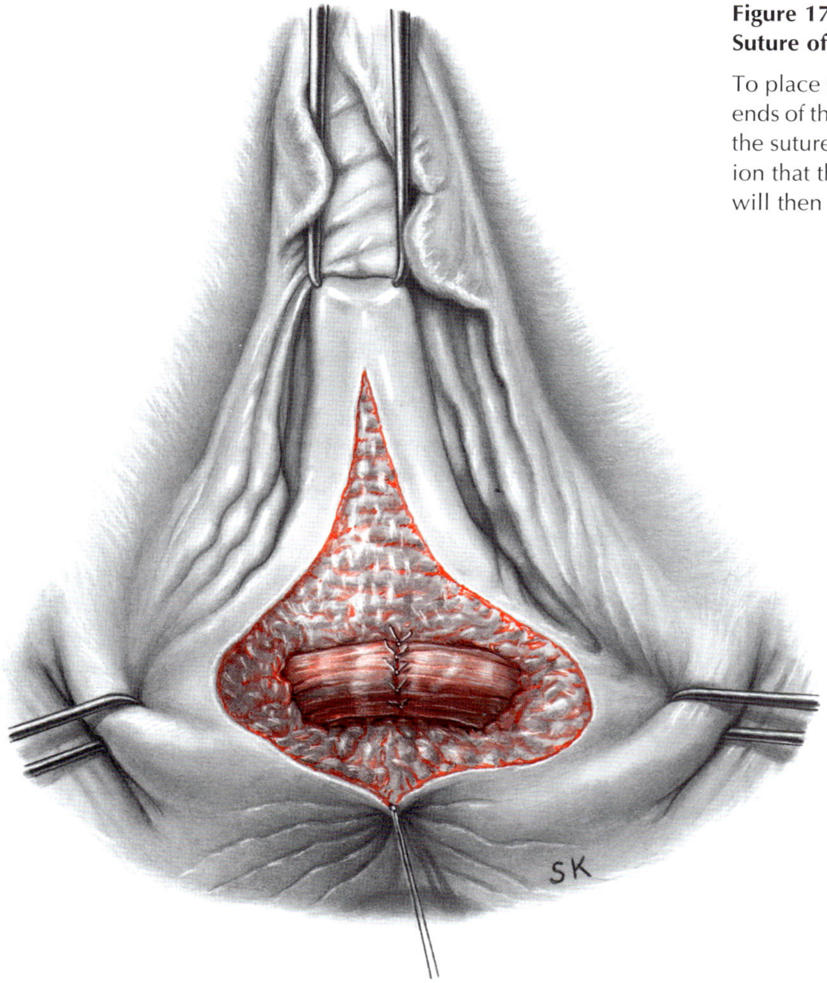

Figure 17.10. Repair of a fresh third degree perineal laceration. Suture of the external anal sphincter muscle.

To place the interrupted sutures, the needle is pushed through both ends of the muscle in U-shaped motion. Where the needle emerges, the suture is tied—not too tightly—over the one side in such a fashion that the wound surfaces obtain good contact. The anal mucosa will then once again be surrounded by radiating folds of the skin.

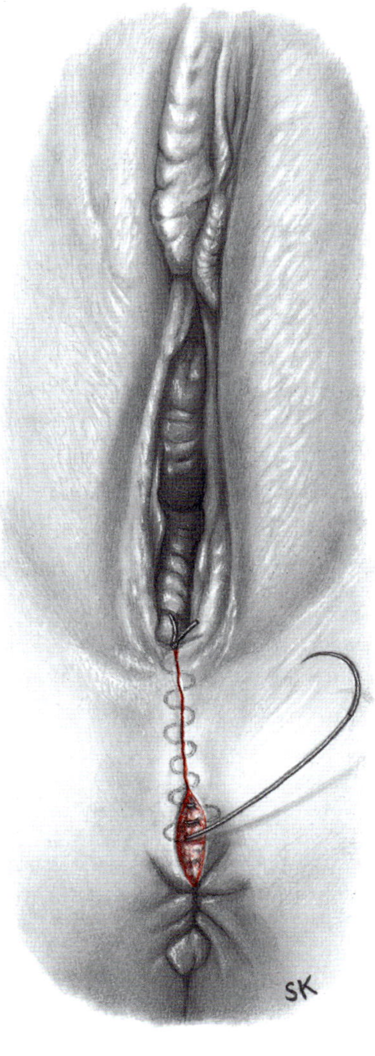

Figure 17.11. Subcuticular suture after median episiotomy or with a fresh third degree perineal laceration.

Beginning at the upper wound angle, the needle is guided in a back and forth motion through the skin of the two wound edges. This is performed after the subcutaneous fatty connective tissue has been apposed with interrupted sutures (cf. Figs. 7.4 and 7.5). Atraumatic needles and absorbable suture size 000 should be used (with very sensitive patients size 00 catgut could be used).

The knots, which might feel irritating on the skin, may be removed on the eighth day after surgery.

18/ Surgical Treatment of Vesicovaginal Fistula

Indications

The *Füth* repair of a fistula is indicated

- For closing small and medium-sized fistulas that are not located too high;
- For the closure of fistulas when the uterus is still in place.

The *Martius* bulbocavernosus flap repair is indicated for surgical care of large complicated vesicovaginal fistulas to provide a supplementary bolster.

The *Symonds-Knapstein* is indicated for myocutaneous bulbocavernosus repair.

The *Latzko* fistula repair is indicated for highly placed small fistulas located in the vaginal cuff, mostly found above the transverse scar in the anterior vaginal wall.

Doederlein rolled-flap fistula repair is indicated

- For closing large fistulas;
- For care of recurrent fistulas.

Patient preparation. When deciding the right time to close a postoperative vesicovaginal fistula caused by injury to the bladder wall, or by necrosis from local ischemia, one might argue that it can never be postponed too long. However, consider that constant involuntary urinary flow gradually becomes an unbearable condition for the patient. No attempt should be made to close fistulas that develop as a result of a surgical procedure before 3–4 months after the operation, since healing is inhibited because of persistent inflammation of the fistula tract.

Fistulas developing after radiation therapy should not be operated on for 1 year. Before beginning treatment of a fistula, a thorough gynecological examination and urinalysis, including cystoscopy and intravenous pyelography, must be conducted. A cystoscopy may be performed when the vagina is tamponaded with gauze. This will elucidate the position of the fistula in relation to the ureteral ostia and the character of the tissues surrounding the fistula. Cystoscopy will also uncover the true extent of the mucosal defect, which is usually larger than the scarred fistulous opening seen from the vaginal side.

In the presence of large defects, general anesthesia might be recommended when performing this procedure. An excretory pyelogram might enable timely detection of a possibly coexisting fistula of the ureter—developed after radical surgery for carcinoma of the cervix.

Any existing urinary tract infection must be treated before surgery. In addition, the bacteriological examination of the urine must include study of the antibiotic sensitivity of organisms discovered. This will facilitate targeted antibiotic therapy after surgery, but one cannot always achieve bacteria-free urine before surgery. Local vaginal inflammations and encrustation of the fistulous tract are treated with daily vaginal irrigations of a lactic acid solution (1 teaspoon lactic acid concentrate to 1 liter fluids) and boric acid water irrigations of the bladder. To build up the vaginal epithelium, we recommend preoperative daily injection of 1 mg i.m. estradiol benzoate for 1–2 weeks. If the skin of the external genitalia is inflamed as a consequence of constant irritation by urine, warm sitz baths are useful several times daily with Kamillosan (chamomile extract) added to the solution. Acute inflammation can be successfully treated with an antibiotic ointment (e.g., gentamicin ointment). After this, the skin should be covered with zinc paste.

The optimal time for the operation arrives when the fistulous tract has been completely cleaned, the urinary encrustations have been alleviated, and the inflammatory processes in the vagina and external genitalia have healed. It can take more than 4 months to achieve these conditions.

Postoperative treatment. The vaginal tract is loosely tamponaded with a gauze pack for 24 hours. To ease pressure on the bladder suture, transurethral bladder drainage is conducted for 2 weeks. We recommend a Pezzer catheter that keeps the bladder completely empty at all times, because its head lies at the bladder's lowest point right above the internal urethral orifice. Irrigate the bladder twice daily with 50 ml lukewarm 3% boric acid solution. Subsequently, 10 ml antibiotic solution are instilled for 30 minutes while the catheter is clamped off. At all other times, the catheter is left open constantly and the urine collected into a sterile plastic container. This container is a disposable unit and is to be changed every 24 hours.

The degree of severity of the fistula operation determines when the patient will be allowed to get up; for all patients we prescribe at least 5 days of strict bed rest.

Beginning on the 10th day after surgery, the catheter is clamped off daily, initially for 20 minutes and progressively prolonging the duration until the 2-hour mark is reached. The catheter is completely removed on the 14th postoperative day. At that point, the patient is advised to empty her bladder hourly on the first day; later it is to be emptied every 2–3 hours. The residual must be checked often for complete emptying.

The healing process can be aided by injecting small dosages of estrogens (5 mg i.m. weekly).

If the wound is dry after the catheter has been removed, the patient can be discharged a few days later. A cystoscopic examination is performed 6 weeks after surgery.

Füth Plastic Repair of Rolled Fistula

Technique

The operation is performed more easily with the patient in lithotomy position. Adequate lighting, long delicate instruments, and atraumatic needles are just as important for closing a fistula as is thorough and careful mobilization of the fistulous bed. Rough tissue handling will lead to failure and subsequent enlargement of the existing fistula.

If the vagina is narrow because of atrophy, it is advisable to enlarge access to the fistula by means of an episiotomy or a vaginoperineal levator incision (Schuchardt incision, see Chapter 22). In the case of a badly scarred fistula fixed to the symphysis or the pubic bone, the bladder should be mobilized well away from the side with a Schuchardt incision, and the paravesical space opened (for technical details see Chapter 22). A suprapubic incision is usually not needed.

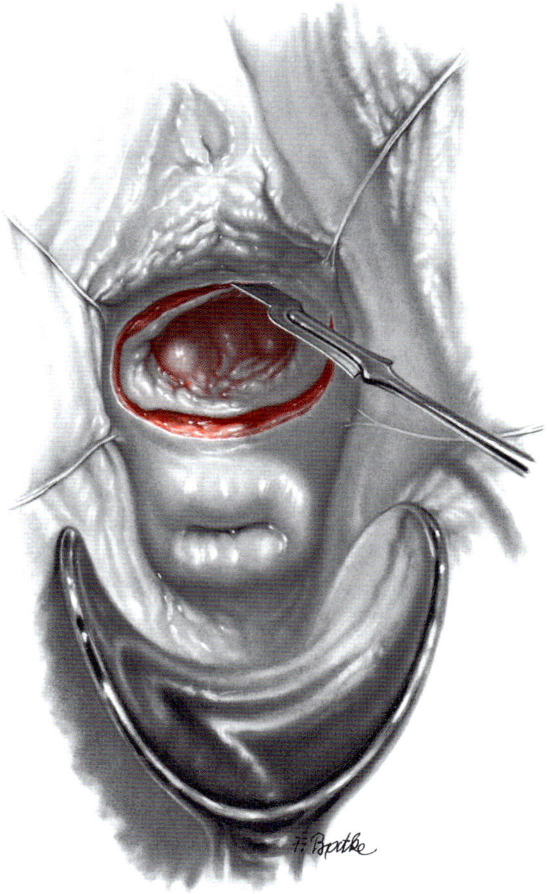

Figure 18.1. Füth fistula repair. Circumcising the fistula.

At a distance of 2 cm from the edge of the fistula, four silk traction sutures are symmetrically placed in the vaginal wall. These sutures are used to draw the fistula forward; this will make circumcision easier.

The circumferential incision is begun posteriorly approximately 1 cm from the edge of the fistula and continued anteriorly.

The circumcised vaginal wall must be mobilized well enough on all sides to allow formation of a fistula collar.

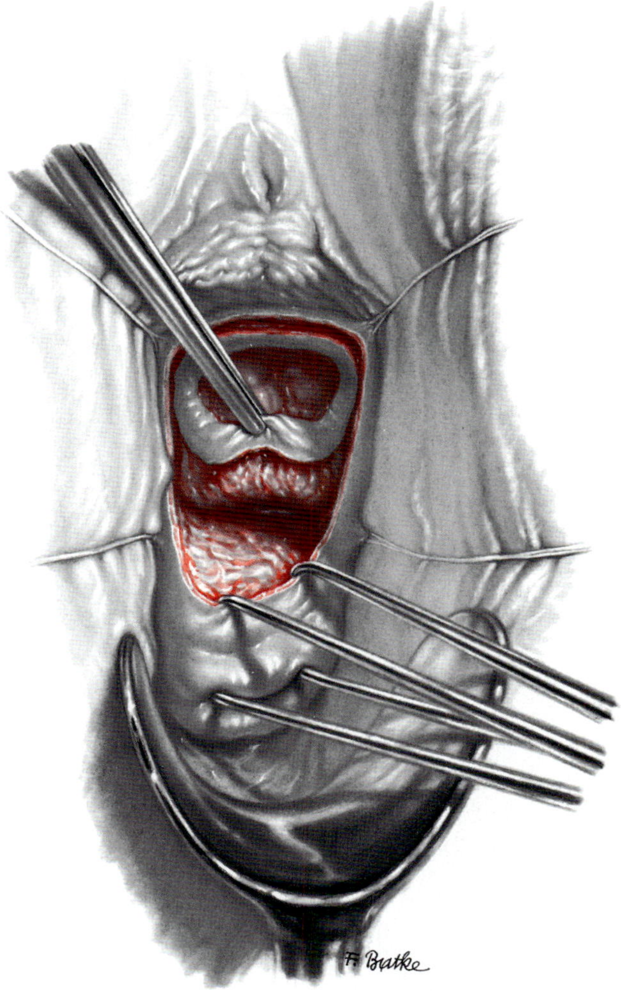

Figure 18.2. Füth fistula repair. Mobilizing the bladder.

The fistula collar is mobilized well on all sides, and the circumcised vaginal wall dissected away widely. The uterus is pulled downward by two retractors placed on the anterior lip of the cervix.

The lower pole of the bladder is dissected from the anterior cervical wall up to above the peritoneal reflection. Deep in the wound, the anterior peritoneum is just visible.

This creates a larger bladder wound surface in the area of the posterior circumcision, so the fistula can then be closed completely by a tier of multilayered bladder sutures.

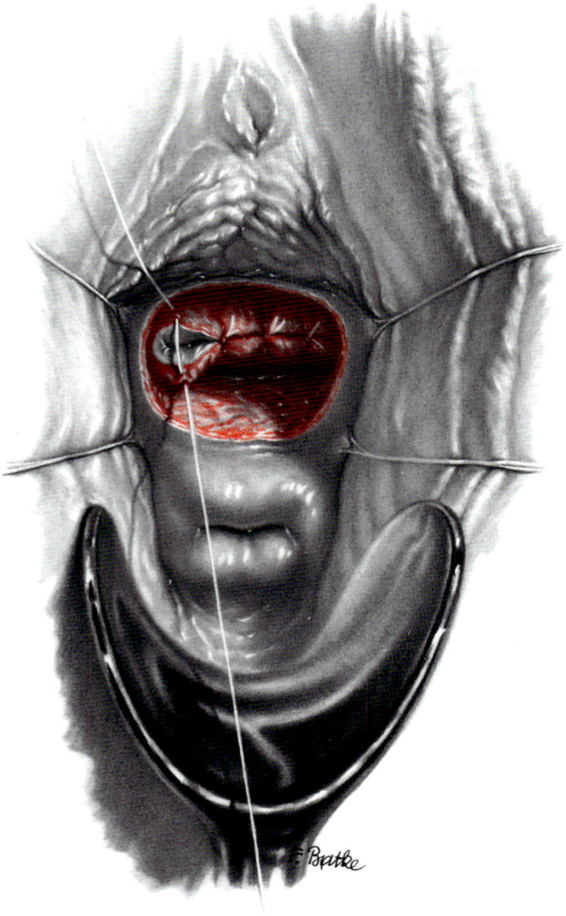

Figure 18.3. Füth fistula repair. Closing the fistula. First row of sutures.

The fistula collar inversion is accomplished as follows: the first transverse row of the bladder sutures is placed with sagittal interrupted sutures (size 00 chromic catgut, atraumatic needle) over the fistula without inserting the needle into or through the fistulous bed.

The bladder should already be watertight after the first row has been placed; this can be tested by filling the bladder slowly with 100 ml saline solution.

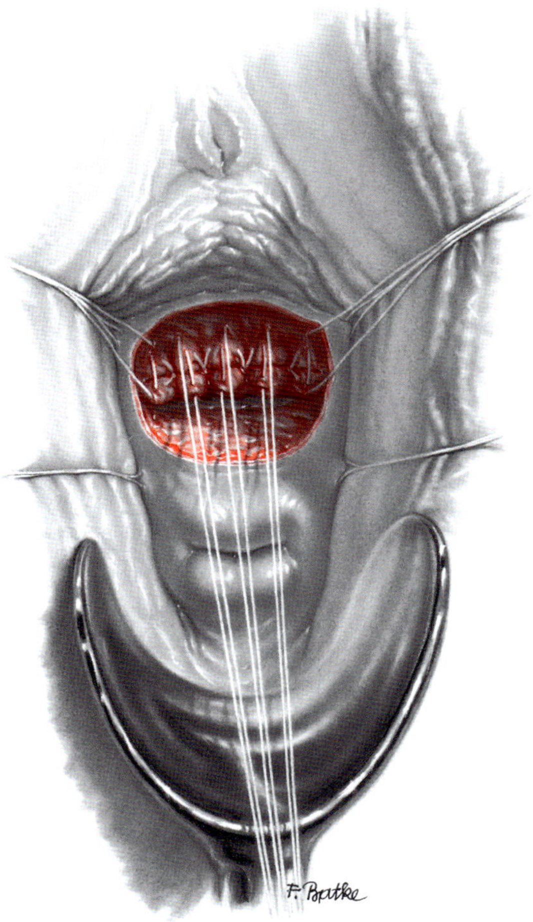

Figure 18.4. Füth fistula repair. Closing the fistula. Second row of sutures.

As the second layer of bladder tissue is approximated transversely, the second tier of lateral sutures extends far beyond the limits of the first row so that the corners of the first row are covered safely. All sutures are first placed and then tied.

Then the vaginal wall is closed lengthwise with strong chromic catgut sutures.

Technical Problems—Figures 18.1–18.4

1. If the *circumcision* at the edge of the fistula is performed while the *vaginal wall is insufficiently stretched*, the circumcision will be irregular and the circumcised vaginal wall will appear fringed. Subsequently, the fistulous bed will also be resected irregularly.
2. If *the vaginal wall is inadequately mobilized from the bladder*, the wound surface that is created will not be wide enough and not enough of the bladder can be sewn together. As a consequence, a two-tiered closure can be accomplished only with difficulty.
3. Dissection of the bladder may cause excessive bleeding, because the *bladder fascia* and the blood vessels coursing in it may be *injured*. The bladder fascia should remain attached to the bladder as much as possible; the sutures will hold better in this fascia than in bladder musculature.
4. During the mobilization of *the fistulous bed*, it is important *not to dissect too deeply* toward the bladder. If this happens, one may again perforate into the bladder. If too little bladder tissue is available for the two-tiered covering of the fistula after dissection of the fistula, one should dissect the bladder from the external vaginal wound edge to mobilize it more fully. This is particularly needed at the lateral, but at times also the anterior, aspects of the fistula.
5. If the *lateral bladder sutures are not placed far enough laterally*, the inverted edges of the fistula will not be covered completely.
6. The *bladder sutures* lying in the two-layered closure *should not be placed too closely* together, or ischemia will occur and necrosis can develop. A new fistula may form under such conditions. This error is often made as a consequence of fear that one will not make the repair sufficiently watertight.
7. If the *vaginal wound edges were to be joined transversely* analogous to closure of the bladder tissue, the vaginal wall would be severely shortened. Conversely, if one closes the vaginal wound edges with a longitudinal suture tier, the vaginal canal will only be shortened slightly. Unfortunately, it is not always possible to achieve a lengthwise closure.

Martius Bulbocavernosus Flap Repair

Technique

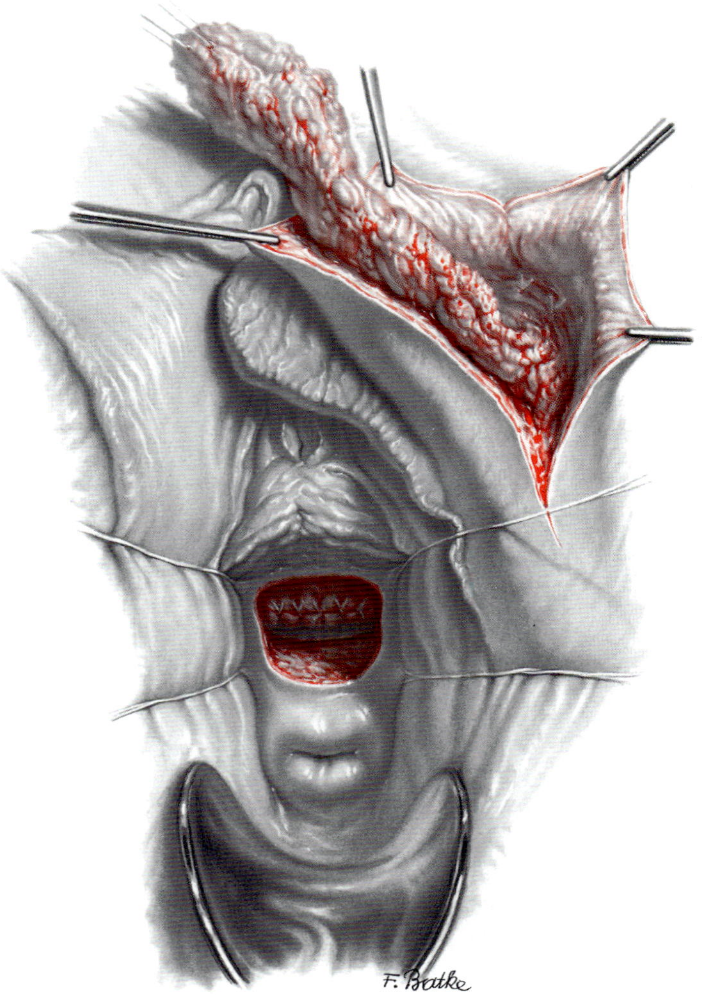

Figure 18.5. Martius bulbocavernosus flap repair.

The bladder fistula has been closed with a two-layered suture. The lower pole of the bladder is mobilized to above the peritoneal reflection.

A bulbocavernosus tissue flap is used for bolstering and to cover the bladder sutures.

An 8-cm longitudinal incision is made in the skin of the left labium major (the incision reaches anteriorly approximately to the level of the clitoris). The incision edges are pulled apart with small clamps.

The fatty muscular flap is dissected in its upper two-thirds aspects all the way to the fascia. Care must be taken to ligate several venous vessels in the process. Two catgut sutures are placed at the flap's uppermost aspect. Toward the back, the flap is left attached at its base as a pedicle.

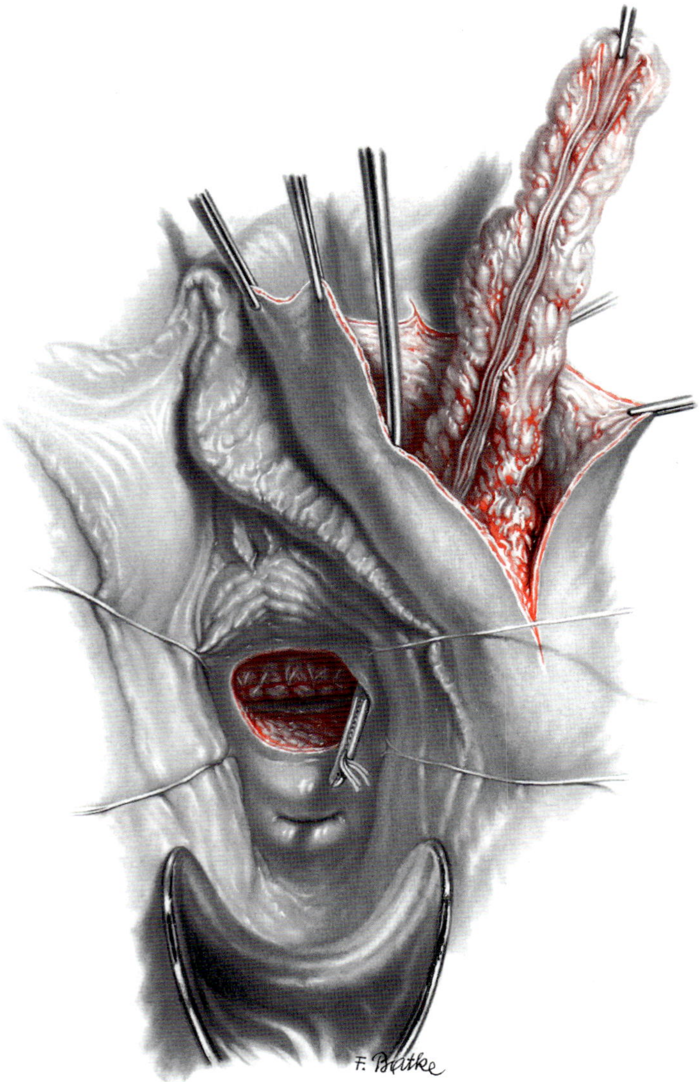

Figure 18.6. Martius bulbocavernosus flap repair.

The bulbocavernosus tissue flap has been extensively mobilized in its upper two-thirds portion.

A tunnel was created under the skin bridge from the labial to the vaginal wound areas with delicate dressing forceps. Ligatures attached to the end of the pedicle were left long; these are drawn through the tunnel into the vaginal wound with the dressing forceps. It is technically easier to advance the forceps bluntly from the vulvar wound area to the vaginal rather than in the reverse direction.

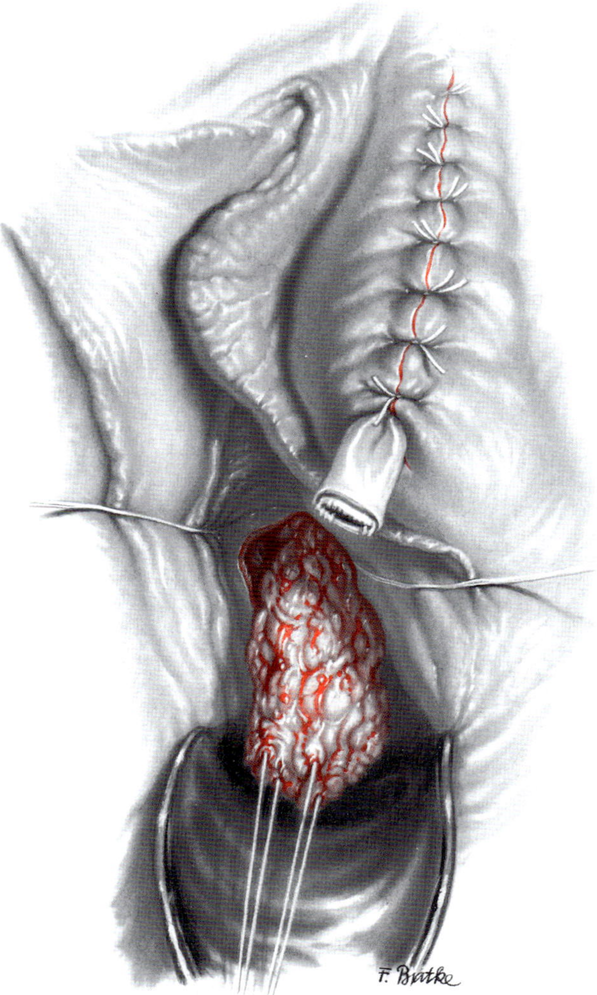

Figure 18.7. Martius bulbocavernosus flap repair.

The bulbocavernosus flap is drawn through the tunnel into the vagina with catgut sutures.

The labial wound can now be drained with a Penrose drain and the skin edges of the wound closed with silk sutures.

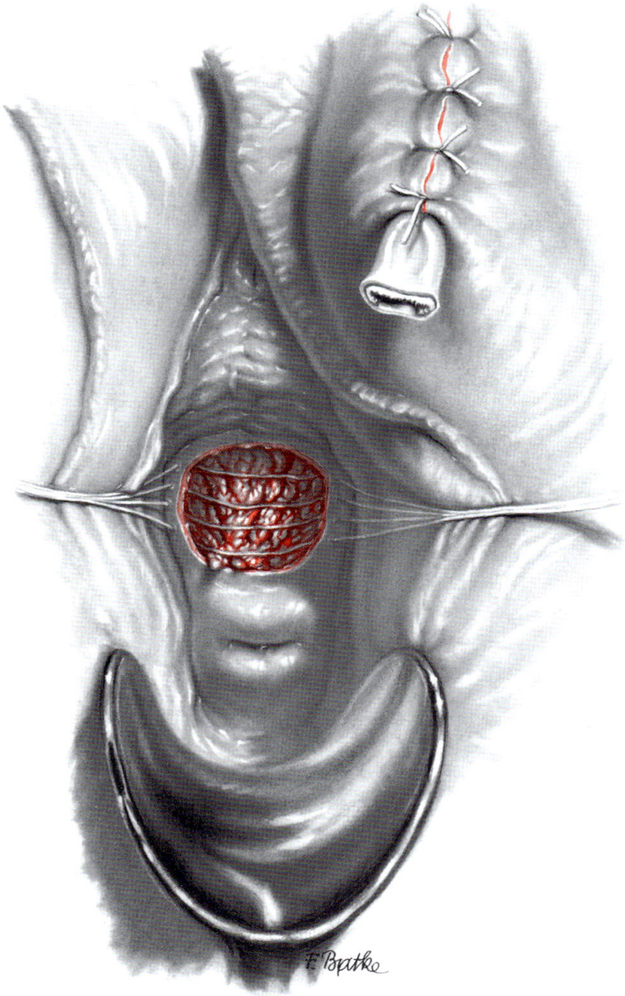

Figure 18.8. Martius bulbocavernosus flap repair.

The bulbocavernosus flap is spread out as filler and supporting tissue under the fistula repair site and fixed to the bladder fascia with interrupted catgut sutures.

Technical Problems—Figures 18.5–18.8

The *tunneling of the mucosal bridge must be carried widely. Inadequate tunneling* can easily result because the vaginal wall is firmly adherent in this area to the urogenital diaphragm. This will result in a tunnel that is too narrow and will severely compress the flap as it is pulled through. Under such circumstances the flap can become necrotic.

Symonds-Knapstein Myocutaneous Bulbocavernosus Repair

Indications

The effect of the reliable bulbocavernosus flap repair may be significantly improved and the indication expanded if a skin graft from the vulvar region is inserted along with the fatty-muscular pedicle into the subvesical vaginal defect. The fatty-muscular pedicle serves in this case as the vascular source for the transplanted skin flap. In effect we are dealing with a ''myocutaneous skin graft repair.''

In the original Füth method, a relatively large defect of the anterior vaginal wall remains after the fistula has been closed. Primary wound edge apposition by means of interrupted button sutures may cause stenosis of the upper third of the vagina (cf. Fig. 18.8). This may be avoided by replacing the defective area with the skin graft. Furthermore, the primary healing process of the fistula closure will be expedited, and the chance for relapse will be greatly reduced by bolstering the bladder wall with two additional well-perfused tissue layers consisting of muscle, subcutaneous fat, and skin.

Additional indications for this very reliable method are postoperative stenosis or shortening of the vagina after an incorrect anterior colporrhaphy, after oncologic surgical procedures such as the Wertheim-Meigs procedure, after radiation, or after an unsatisfactory neovaginal construction for the Rokitansky-Küstner syndrome or rectovaginal fistulas. If needed, bilateral skin flaps may be mobilized.

Technique

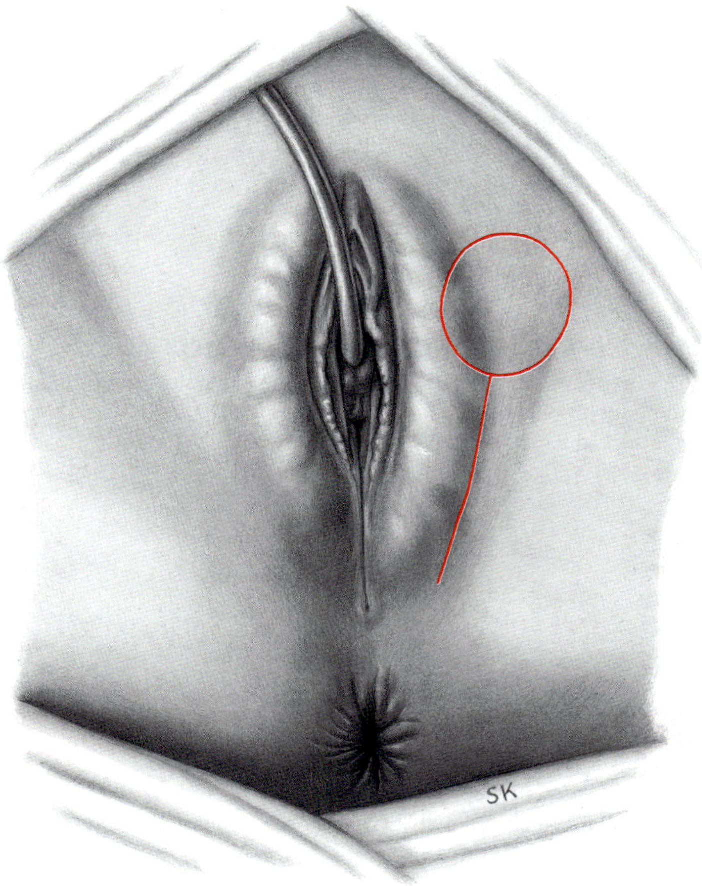

Figure 18.9. Symonds-Knapstein myocutaneous bulbocavernosus repair. Plastic incision figure in the ventral perivulvar region and longitudinal incision along the lateral third of the labium majus.

A circular skin graft is excised from the ventral perivulva, corresponding in size to the extent of the vaginal defect. Its size will be approximately 4 × 2 cm in most cases.

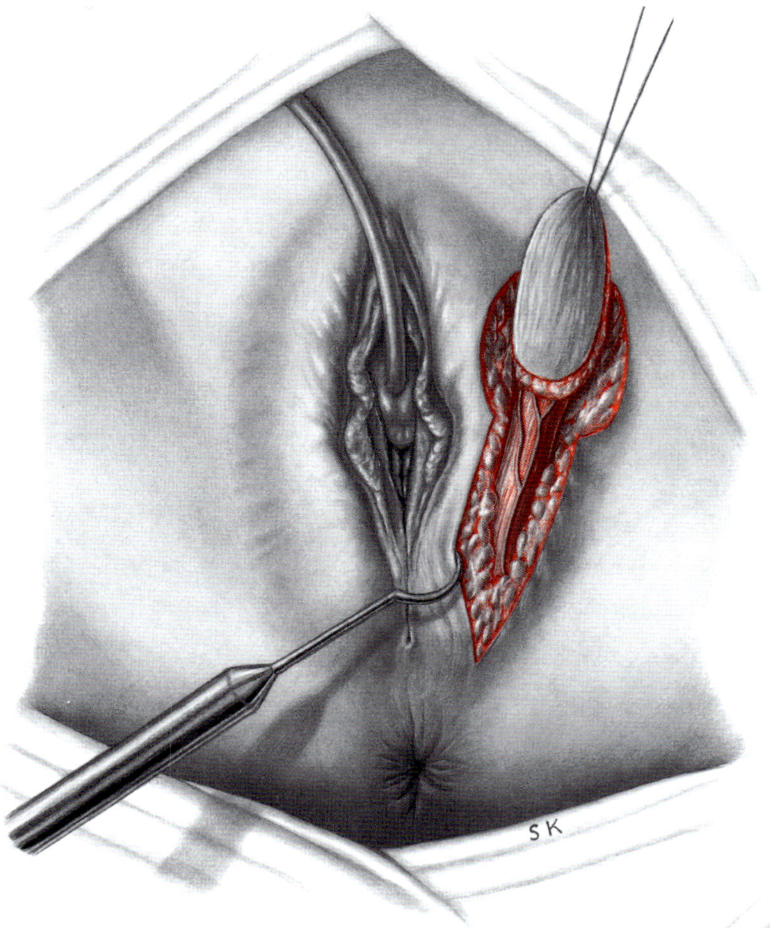

Figure 18.10. Symonds-Knapstein myocutaneous bulbocavernosus repair. Cutting around the skin island and preparing the bulbocavernosus muscle with surrounding adipose tissue and blood vessels.

A longitudinal incision is made in the lateral third of the labium majus. The bulbocavernosus muscle is identified and dissected free posteriorly up to the level of the perineum.

Skin flap vascularization remains intact if the dissection plane of the fatty-muscular pedicle is selected immediately beneath the labium majus skin. Laterally entering blood vessels can be severed, but the main branches coming from the internal pudendal vessels at the base of the pedicle must remain intact (cf. Fig. A.6). A fine, monofilament traction suture is placed on the tip of the skin graft.

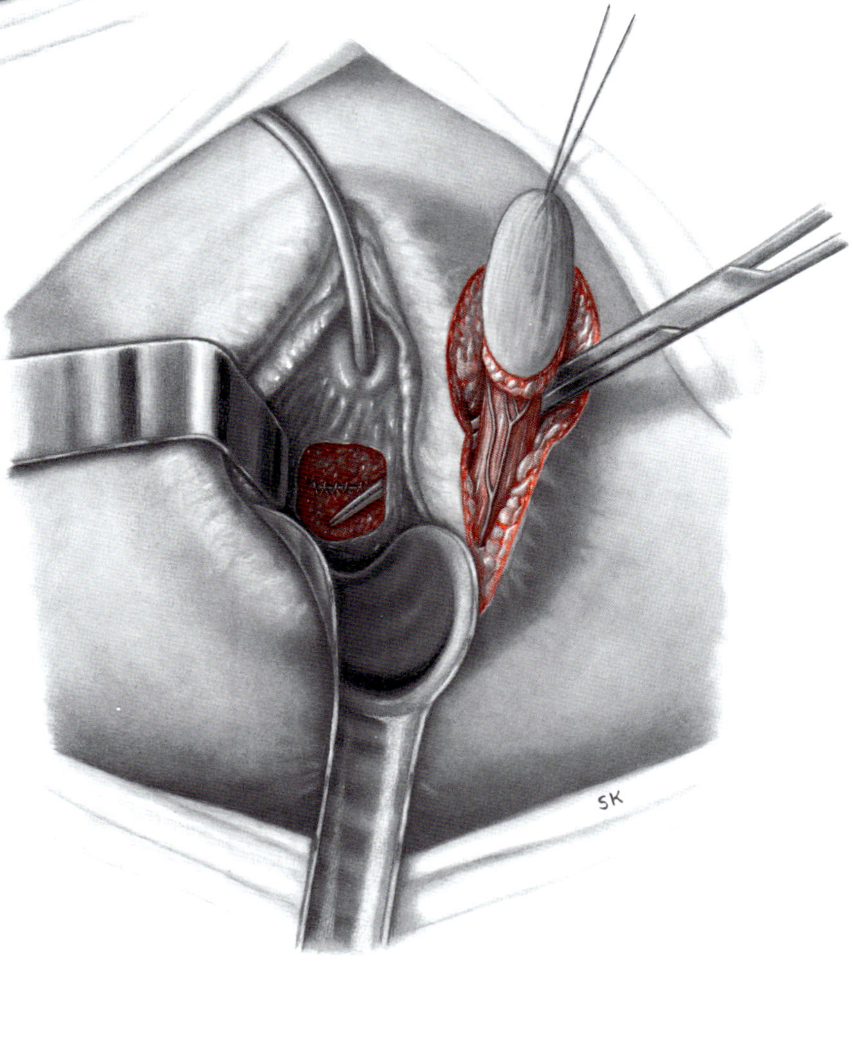

Figure 18.11. Symonds-Knapstein myocutaneous bulbocavernosus repair.

A subcutaneous tunnel is created using a combination of sharp (with scissors) and blunt (with Schmitt's clamp) dissection. The tunnel starts at the donor wound and leads to the vaginal defect; it must be wide enough to allow the skin flap to be pulled through comfortably. Any bleeding resulting from this must be checked carefully.

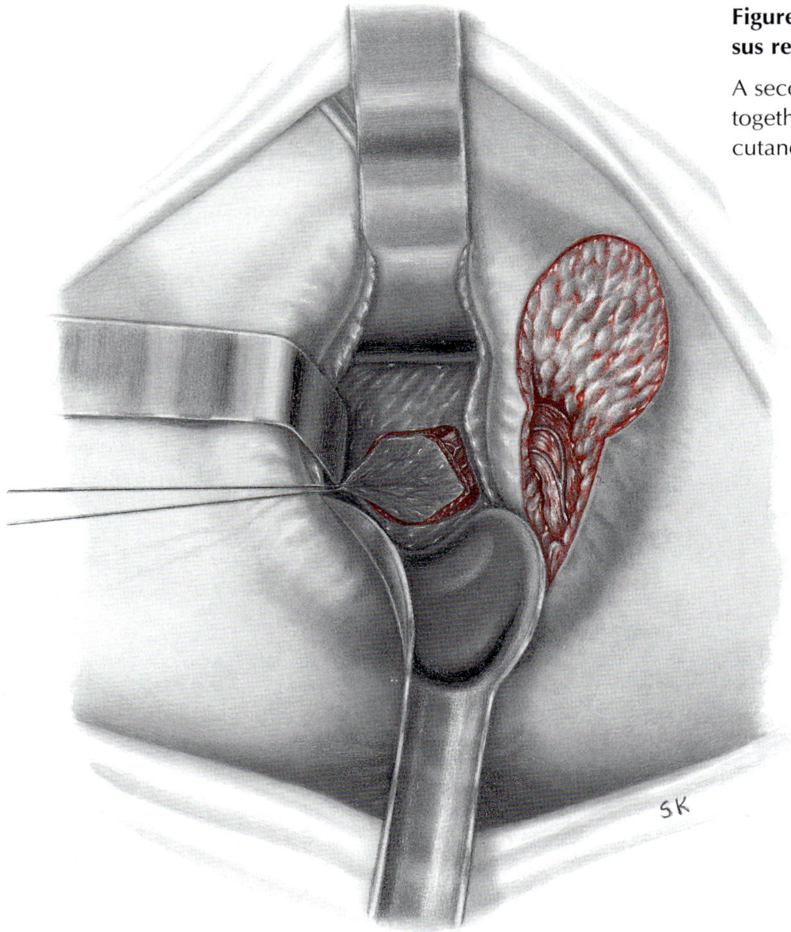

Figure 18.12. Symonds-Knapstein myocutaneous bulbocavernosus repair.

A second clamp grasps the traction suture at the tip of the flap and, together with the fatty muscular pedicle, pulls it through the subcutaneous tunnel into the vagina.

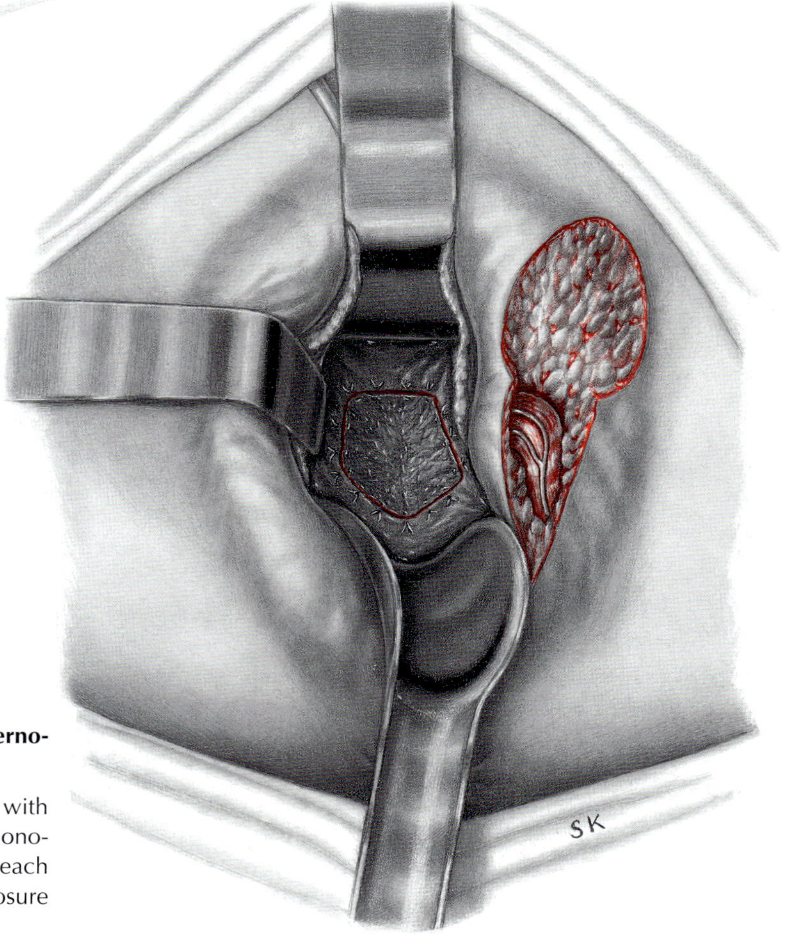

Figure 18.13. Symonds-Knapstein myocutaneous bulbocavernosus repair.

The skin flap is fixed onto the margins of the vaginal wound with interrupted mattress sutures (use size 000 to 0000 absorbing monofilament suture). These two supplementary tissue layers, each served by a separate vascular system, will secure the fistula closure of the bladder.

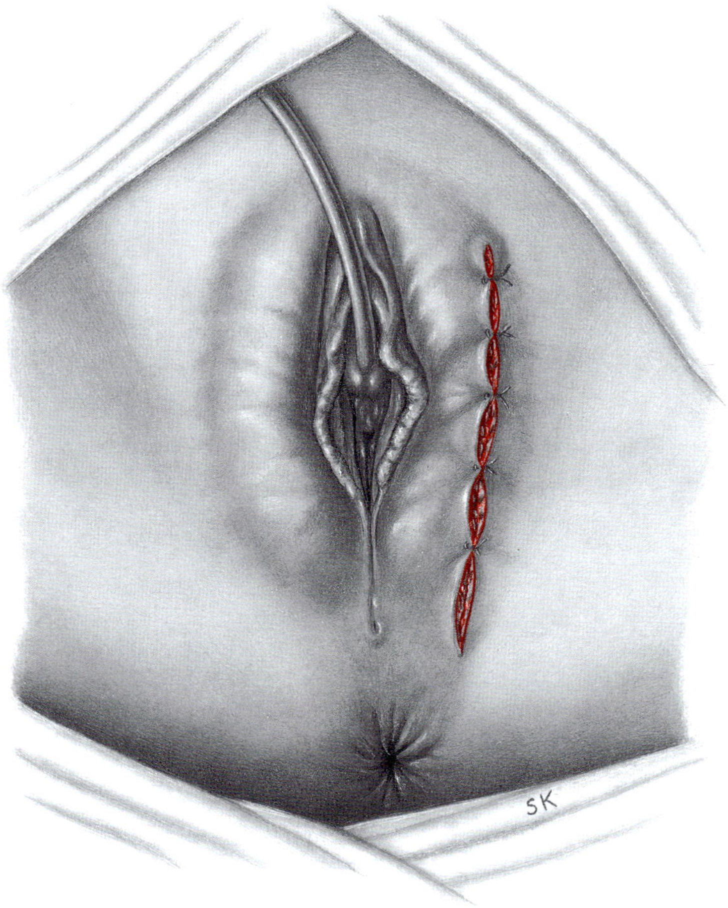

Figure 18.14. Symonds-Knapstein myocutaneous bulbocavernosus repair.

After careful hemostasis has been achieved, it will be easy to close the donor wound of the vulva with cutaneous interrupted sutures without tension (use size 000 to 0000 absorbable monofile suture). Subcutaneous sutures will not be needed. Two no. 12 Robinson drains will adequately drain the wound area for 3–4 days.

Latzko High Colpocleisis Fistula Repair

Technique

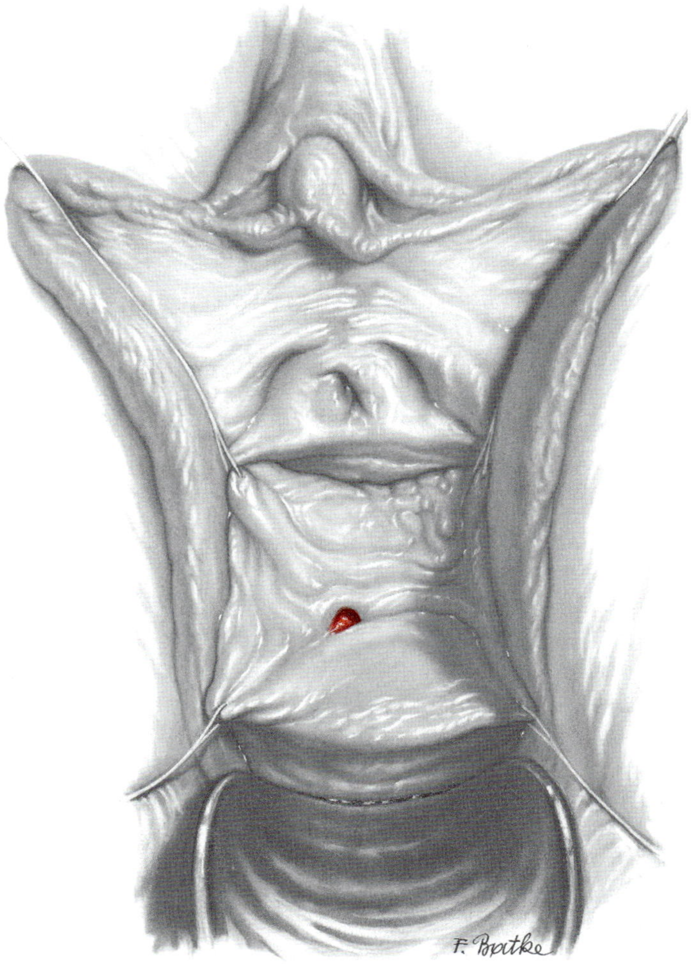

Figure 18.15. Latzko fistula repair. Exposing the fistula.

High in the vaginal vault, a small vesicovaginal fistula is pulled forward by four untied silk traction sutures placed symmetrically in the vaginal wall. The upper sutures are placed in the anterior vaginal wall, and the lower ones in the posterior vaginal wall.

If the fistula is fixed so that it cannot be pulled forward by the sutures alone, one may insert a thin Foley catheter through the fistulous tract into the bladder. When the balloon of the catheter is inflated, traction on the catheter will pull the fistula down and help place the vaginal wall on stretch in preparation for the vaginal wall circumcision.

When needed, access to the fistula can be further improved by a vaginoperineal incision.

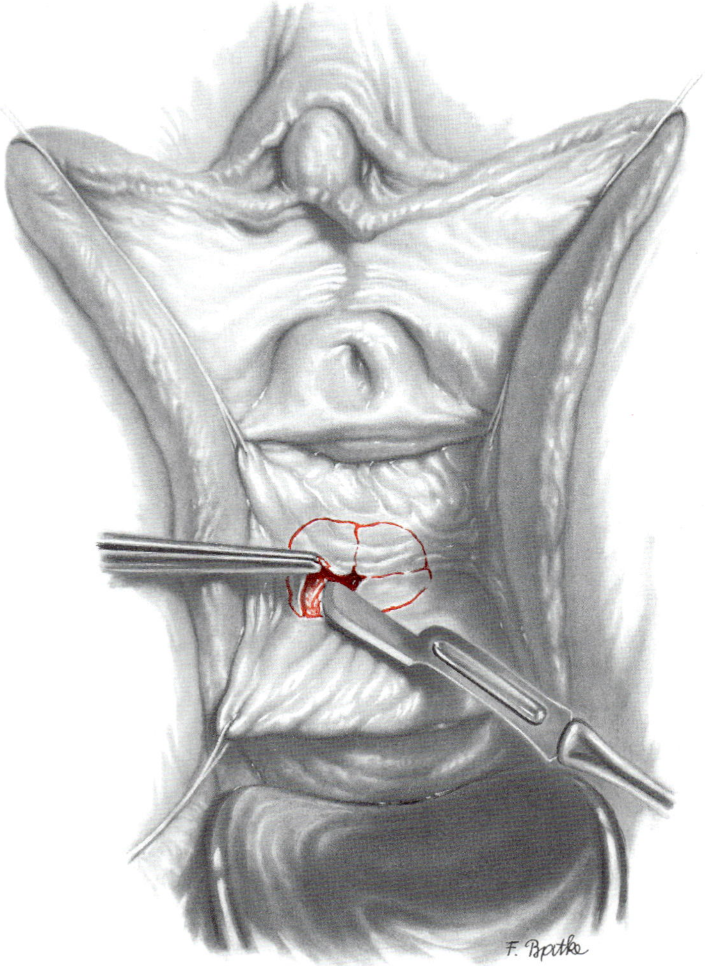

Figure 18.16. Latzko fistula repair. Dissecting the vaginal mucosa.

Traction on the silk sutures places the vaginal wall on stretch. The fistula is circumcised superficially with a long, delicate fistula knife at a distance of about 2 cm from the edge. Only vaginal mucosa is incised, and the vaginal fascia underlying the mucosa remains undisturbed. The area to be resected is divided into four quadrants with a cruciate incision.

The extent of the incision within this area, corresponding to the location of the fistula, usually encompasses tissues of anterior and posterior vaginal walls. Vaginal mucosa in this area is carefully dissected off sharply. Technically, this is performed most easily if one begins the dissection in the posterior quadrants. One removes the vaginal mucosa up to the edge of the fistula, thereby exposing the bladder mucosa. One does not construct a fistula collar.

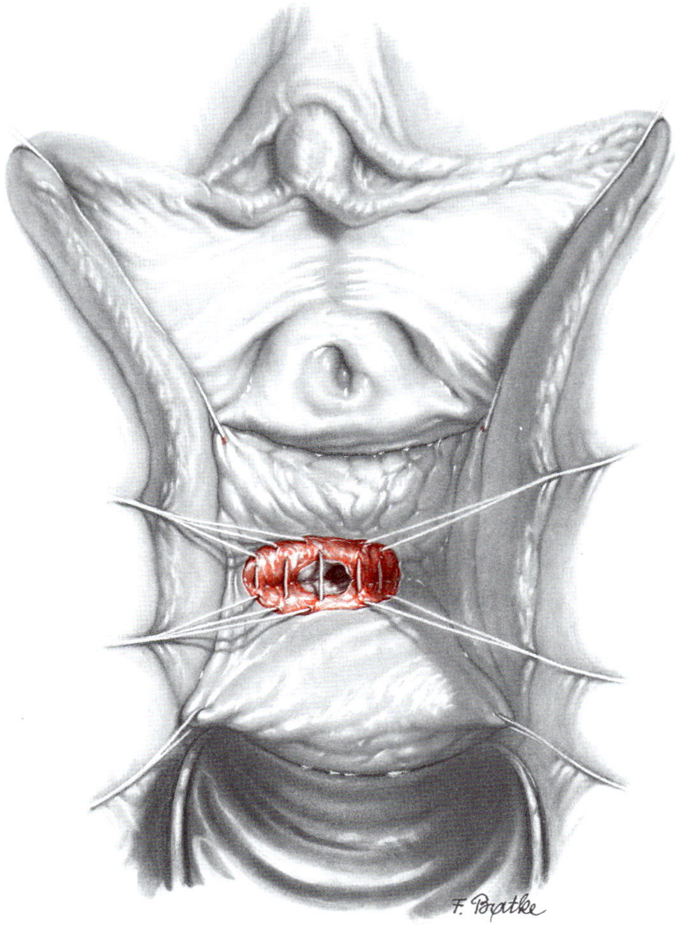

Figure 18.17. Latzko fistula repair. Closing the fistula.

The vaginal wound surfaces in this area are now apposed with a series of transversely placed atraumatic chromic catgut sutures (size 00 to 000) above the fistula. First, all sutures are laid in place, and then they are tied. There may be a second row of sutures needed, depending on the size of the incision area.

Technical Problems—Figures 18.15–18.18

1. During *circumcision* of the fistula, the *incision must not extend too deeply*, or it will accidentally sever the vaginal fascia up to the bladder fascia. The result of this error is extirpation of the full thickness of vaginal wall in the course of dissecting around the fistula, exposing the outer surfaces of the bladder and the rectum. When the fistula is later closed with a suture, the rectal and bladder walls will be approximated by mistake.
2. *Lateral dissection around the fistula should not be too limited.* When this happens, the lateral vaginal fascia sutures used to close the fistula will not cover enough tissue and, therefore, will provide an incomplete closure.

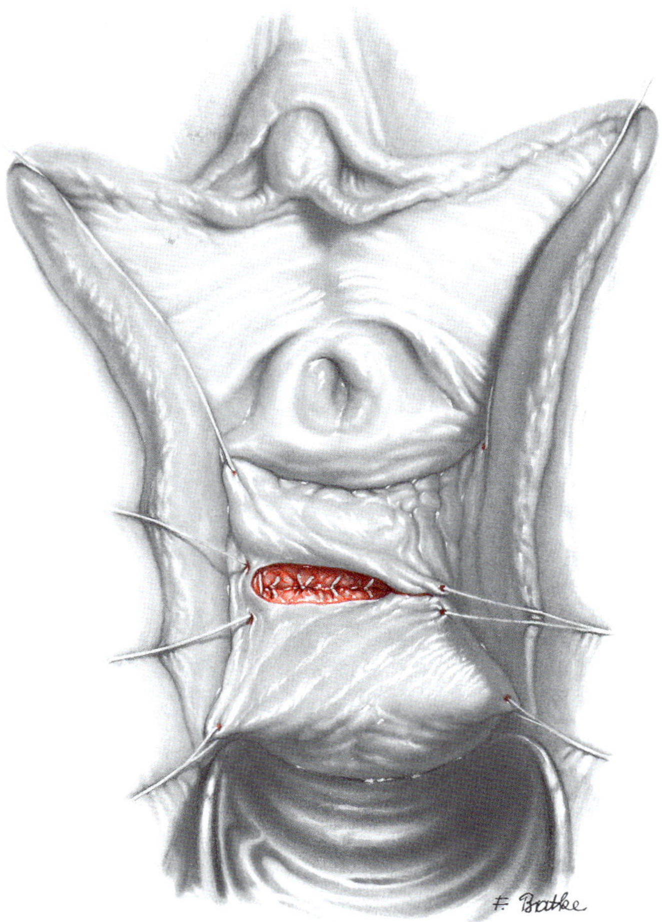

Figure 18.18. Latzko fistula repair. Closing the wound.

The fistula is closed by means of one or two rows of sutures.

The anterior and posterior vaginal wound edges are closed by means of a transverse row of chromic catgut sutures that include both vaginal mucosa and fascia.

The same practices suggested for postoperative care at the beginning of this chapter are recommended here. However, duration of the bladder catheterization and bed rest can be reduced to 1 week because the Latzko method does not put any tension on the bladder wall by virtue of the fact that only the vaginal wall, and not the bladder, was sutured.

Doederlein Rolled-Flap Fistula Repair

TECHNIQUE

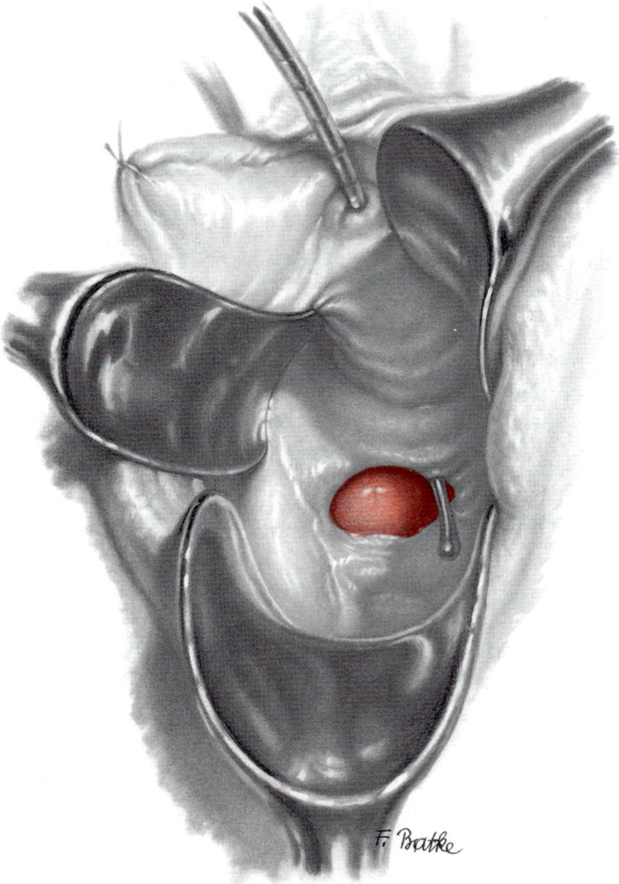

Figure 18.19. Doederlein rolled-flap fistula repair. Sounding the fistula.

Larger vesicovaginal fistulas often cannot be exposed in their entire extent by stretching the vagina with retractors. Therefore, one first inserts a knobbed uterine probe through the urethra into the bladder to trace the extent of the scarred and often retracted edges of the fistulous opening from inside.

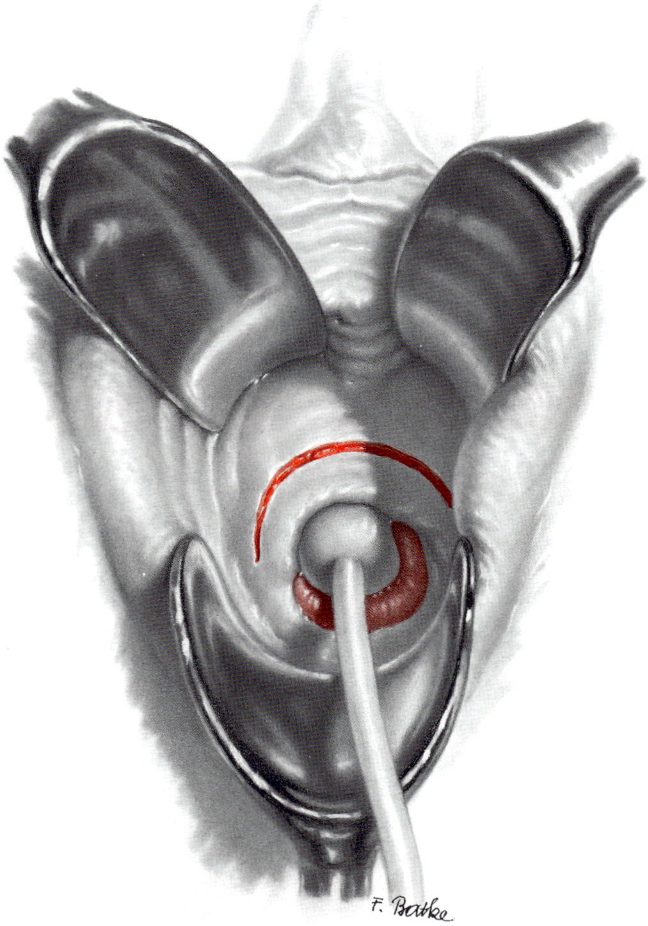

Figure 18.20. Doederlein rolled-flap fistula repair. Anterior circumcision.

The vaginal vault is exposed with three retractors. The fistula is pulled forward by the intravesical balloon of a Foley catheter.

It is imperative for the correct placement of the incision that the vaginal wall be placed on stretch in a very precise manner. The fistula is circumferentially incised anteriorly with a scalpel 1.5 cm distant from the edge.

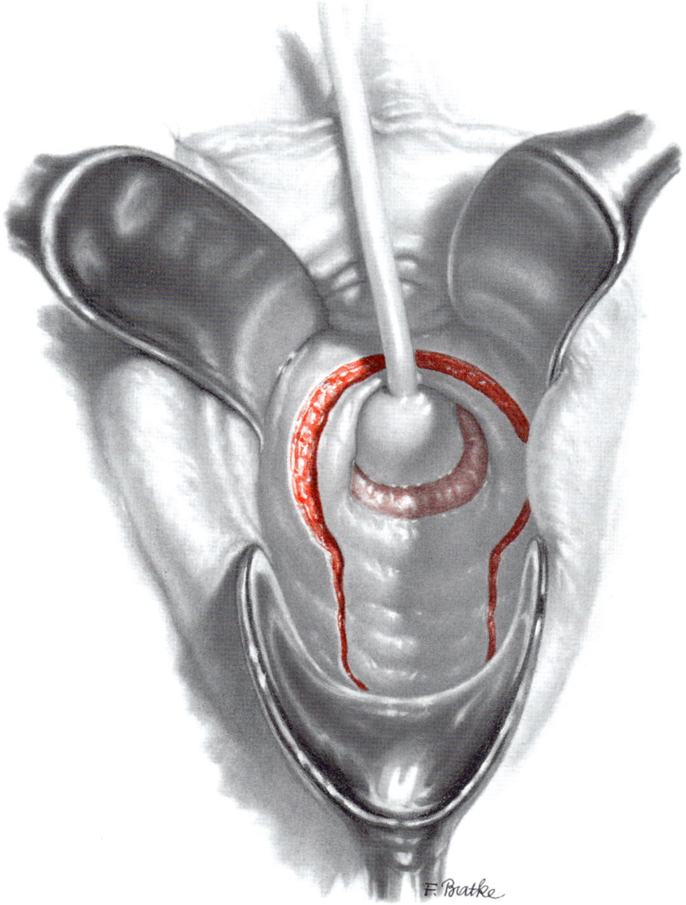

Figure 18.21. Doederlein rolled-flap fistula repair. Forming the vaginal flap.

The anterior and lateral circumferential incision has been made. The balloon catheter is pulled straight upward.

The lateral circumcision wounds are elongated dorsally along the posterior vaginal wall, outlining a 7-cm rectangular flap for excision. Note that the posterior edge of the fistula is not circumcised because the rectangular flap will be pedunculated at this site.

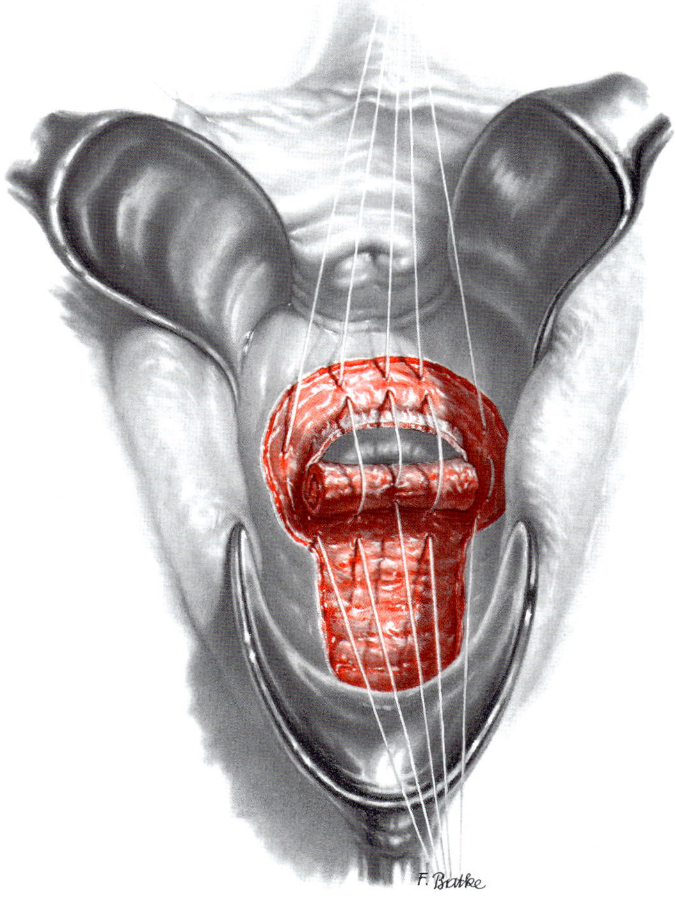

Figure 18.22. Doederlein rolled-flap fistula repair. Forming the roll.

Next, an anterior fistula is constructed by dissecting the vaginal mucosa, just as in the Füth procedure, by mobilizing it from the bladder.

The rectangular flap, dissected free from the posterior vaginal wall, is rolled, stuffed into the fistula, and fixed medially with a suture to the anterior bladder wound surface. (The suture is not yet tied to provide better visualization.) The flap remains attached as a pedicle at the posterior edge of the fistula.

Above the roll, the bladder tissue is approximated broadly by a first transverse suture to seal the fistula. Observe how far laterally the bladder sutures are placed.

At this point, the bladder is tested slowly with 100 ml irrigation fluid to ensure that it is watertight.

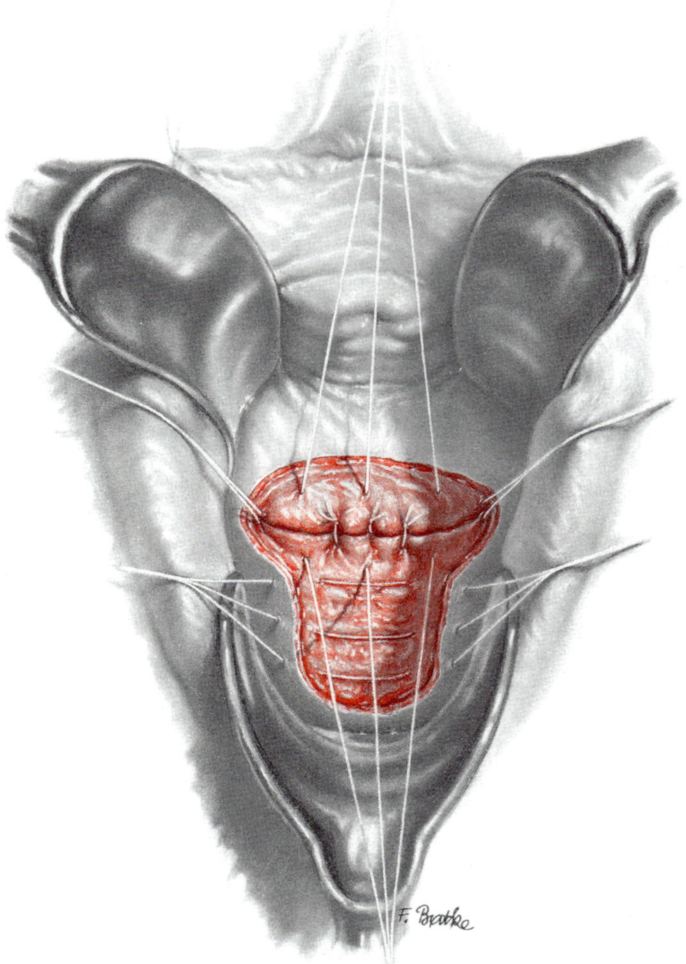

Figure 18.23. Doederlein rolled-flap fistula repair. Second suture row.

The bladder tissue has been joined by a tier of transverse sutures placed above the roll. The angle sutures of the first row have been left long and are used for traction.

The second row of sutures in the bladder wall covers and secures the first row; three sutures are in place.

The vaginal wound edges of the posterior rectangular wound are then closed by a vertical tier of chromic catgut sutures.

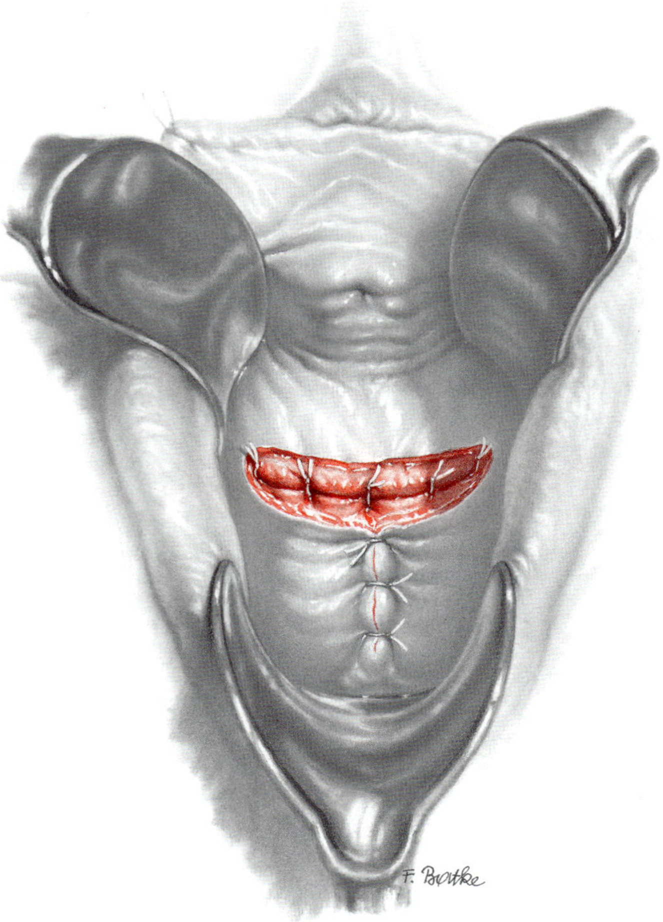

Figure 18.24. Doederlein rolled-flap fistula repair. Closing the wound.

The fistula has been occluded by use of the rolled flap and a two-layered bladder suture; the posterior vaginal wound edges were closed by vertical mattress sutures.

The anterior vaginal wound is now closed with transverse sutures.

TECHNICAL PROBLEMS—FIGURES 18.19–18.24

1. The *flap* formed from the posterior vaginal wall *must not be made too narrow*. To do so would yield a roll that could not adequately stop the ''leak.'' The roll must be wide enough to overlap the fistula laterally.
2. The *flap should not be dissected too thinly*, because it will tear off at the fistula edge. It should consist of both vaginal mucosa and fascia.
3. If the *flap is inadequately fixed* when it is rolled, it may unroll. Then it would no longer occlude the fistula opening completely. The needle must penetrate the entire roll when fixing the flap in place.
4. *Technical problems* listed under ''Füth Plastic Repair of Fistula'' also apply here.

19/ Surgical Treatment of Rectovaginal Fistulas

Indications

The transvaginal correction of a rectovaginal fistula remains a classical gynecological surgical procedure. In most cases, the fistula emerges postoperatively after inadequate repair of a third degree perineal laceration, after a levator perineal plasty, or even after a hysterectomy. Surgical treatment of a transvaginal postoperative fistula that is easily accessible at the lower or middle third region of the vagina is discussed in Chapter 19.

Larger *postirradiation* fistulas require a special perioperative management and also in most cases a vaginoabdominal approach, preferably in cooperation with a specialist. Vaginal perforations caused by *inflammatory intestinal diseases* such as Crohn's disease or diverticulitis should be handled by a gastroenterologist and surgeon; these perforations should never be treated exclusively by a gynecologist. Necrotic fistulas *caused by tumors* that are, depending on their size, still operable require a pelvic exenteration.

The transvaginal correction requires the same *timetable* as does the vesicovaginal fistula: one should wait at least 2–3 months after surgery until all inflammation has subsided. One might even expect a spontaneous recovery within that time. Postirradiation rectovaginal fistulas should not be treated surgically until 18–24 months have passed.

Perioperative management has a critical impact on successful treatment. With smaller, postoperatively developed fistulas one may decide not to perform a diverting colostomy before the correction: it presents a considerable strain for the patient, yet it is of medicolegal significance for the surgeon in charge.

Before surgical therapy of the rectovaginal fistula the entire bowel must be thoroughly cleansed. By using a duodenal probe, the intestines are perfused with approximately 10–12 liters saline solution enriched by calcium chloride of a specific electrolyte composition (a so-called colostomy trunk) 48 hours before surgery. The rectum is irrigated once more with a high cleansing enema 24 hours before surgery. The antibiotic prophylaxis (e.g., 2 × 2 g Cephalosporin per/day) that is begun 12 hours before surgery and continued for 8 days is important. To prevent premature evacuation of the bowels that might lead to infection of the wound region, the patient follows a bland astronaut (free of roughage) diet for 6 postoperative days. In addition, the bowel is put to rest during this time with tincture of opium.

To secure surgical success with larger postirradiation fistulas, it is impossible to avoid the diverting colostomy that is conducted 6 weeks before the correction.

Surgical Technique for Rectovaginal Fistula

Figures 19.1–19.7 illustrate the transvaginal closure of a fistula at the lower vaginal region—above the anal sphincter—as it may develop after inadequate repair of a third degree perineal laceration or after a levator perineal repair. Figures 19.8–19.11 demonstrate how the result of the operation is improved significantly by means of an additional transposition flap plasty.

After the suprasphincteral fistulous tract has been elevated with a thin knobbed probe, all tissue layers above the probe are dissected sharply with a scalpel. Also dissected are the skin, with the connective tissue of the perineum, and the vagina, all fibers of the external sphincter ani muscle, and finally the rectal mucosa down into the fistulous tract. Each end of the sphincter muscle is ligated with a thin monofilament suture (Figs. 19.1–19.3). To avoid a recurrence, the entire epithelialized lining membrane of the fistulous tract must be carefully resected to the healthy rectal mucosa (Fig. 19.4). One has thus created a clean wound comparable with that of a fresh third degree perineal tear, allowing a two-tiered closure of the rectal mucosa (Figs. 19.5 and 19.6). Above these first two suture rows the ends of the anal sphincter may now be approximated (Fig. 19.7), as described under repair of a fresh third degree perineal laceration (Figs. 17.9 and 17.10).

With this, the rectovaginal fistula is removed, and the skin of the vagina, introitus, and perineum can be closed again with a primary continuous subcutaneous suture.

However, there is risk that scar tissue stenosis of the introitus might develop, resulting in severe dyspareunia. For that reason, we repair the vaginal introitus after each suprasphincteral rectovaginal fistula operation with a transposition flap plasty, as illustrated in Figures 19.8–19.11.

Transposition Flap Repair Technique

With this method, an elongated, basilar pedunculated skin flap is mobilized from the wider region surrounding a defect and placed by means of transposition onto the wound in the area immediately neighboring it. The flap itself remains without tension; traction on the sutures is transferred onto the healthy donor site. For this purpose, the flap outline is drawn onto the vulvar skin of the thigh; a surface of 2 × 5 cm is generally enough (Fig. 19.8). The transposition flap is circumcised to its base, while the tissue (consisting of the labium majus and minus) is mobilized toward the defect in one motion (Fig. 19.9). After that, the skin flap can be exchanged—*transpositioned*—with the simultaneously mobilized pointed flap and placed onto the wound above the anal sphincter (Fig. 19.10). There it may be attached without tension by means of interrupted mattress sutures, while the actual traction on the tissue is carried over to the sutures of the donor site (Fig. 19.11). Advantages of this approach are that the fistula closure is secured with two additional healthy and well-perfused tissue layers (which aids the primary and recurrence-free healing process), that a tension-free wound closure is achieved, and that scar tissue stenosis of the introitus is avoided.

Technique

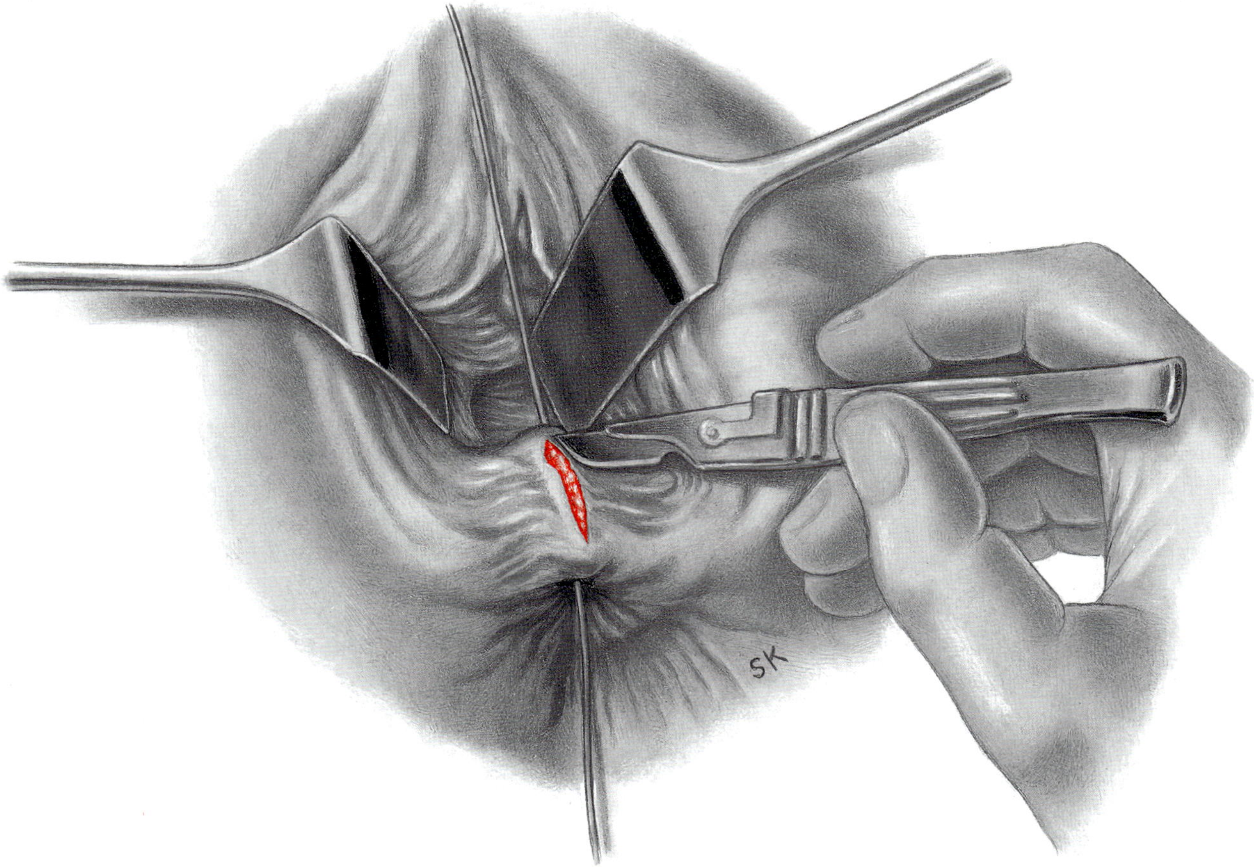

Figure 19.1. Surgical treatment of a suprasphincteral rectovaginal fistula.

A thin knobbed probe elevates the tissue layers in the fistulous tract; the skin of the perineum, introitus, and lower vagina are incised with a scalpel.

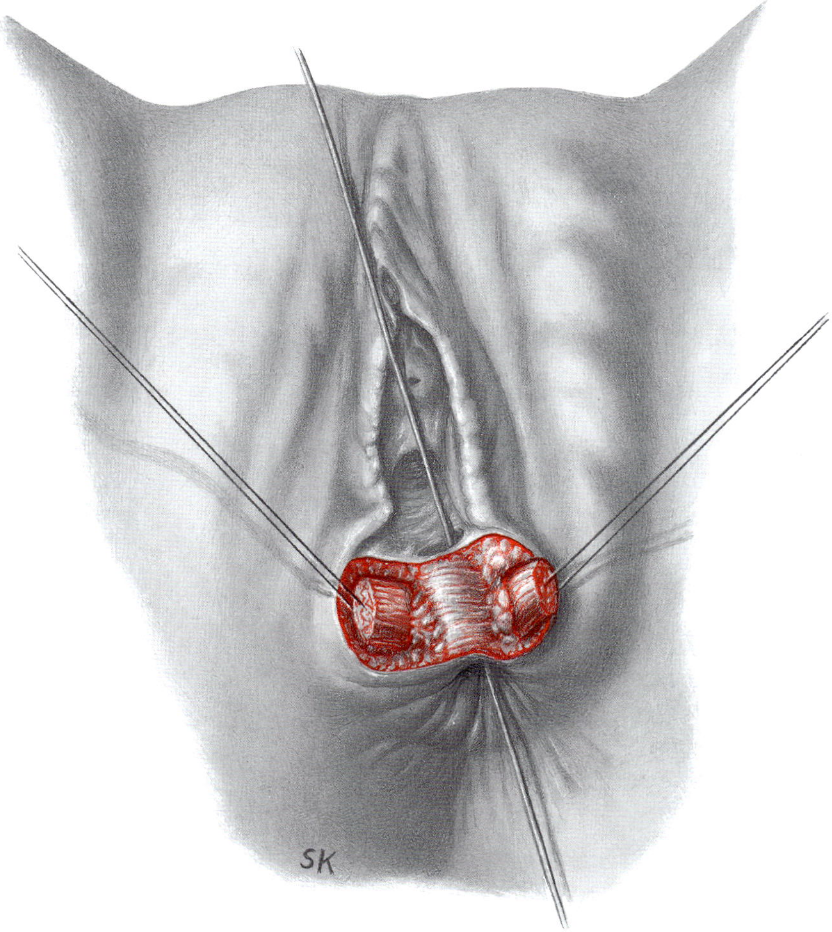

Figure 19.2. Surgical treatment of a suprasphincteral rectovaginal fistula.

Fibers of the external sphincter ani muscle are also sharply dissected down to the rectal mucosa, and each of its ends are ligated with a thin suture thread (size 0000 absorbable monofilament suture).

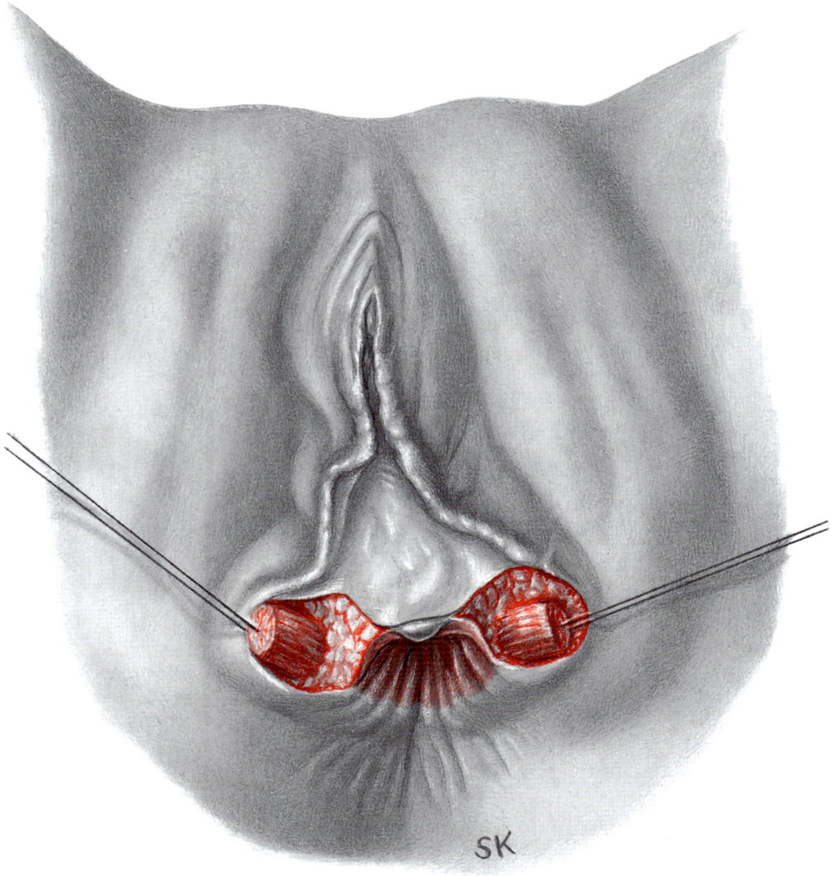

Figure 19.3. Surgical treatment of a suprasphincteral rectovaginal fistula.

After the mucosa of the anus and the lower rectum has been incised, the fistulous tract lies folded open.

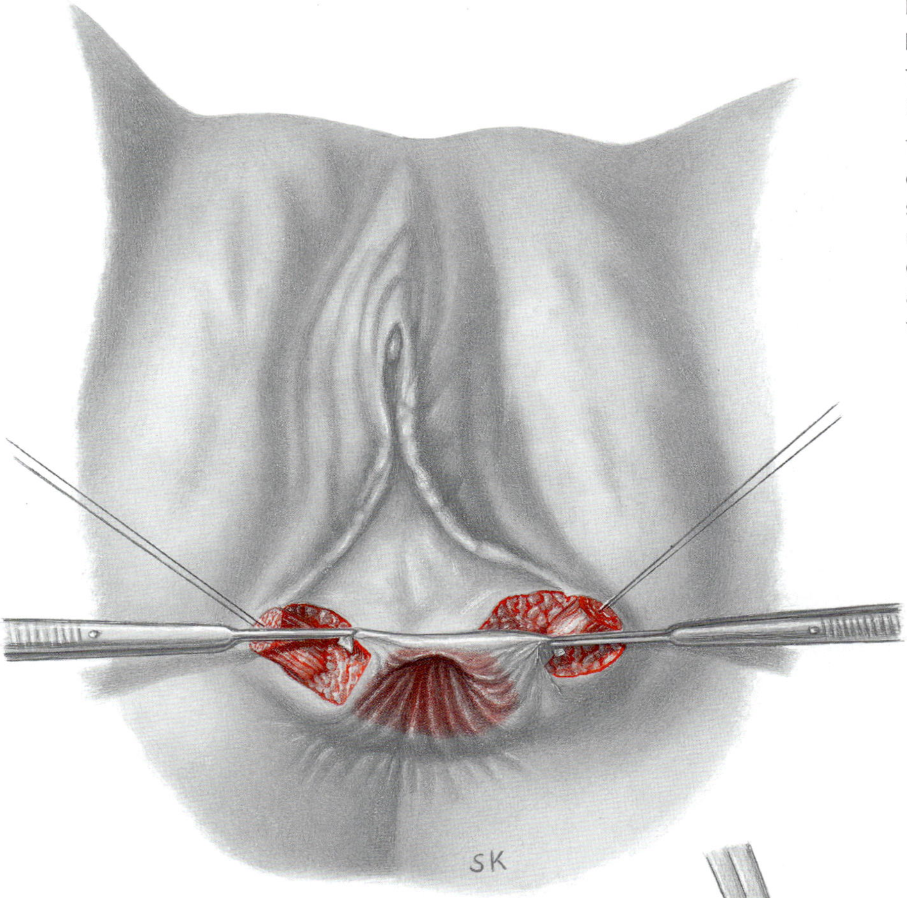

Figure 19.4. Surgical treatment of a suprasphincteral rectovaginal fistula.

The opened fistulous tract is grasped with two delicate, sharp tissue forceps and lifted upward.

The entire epithelial lining membrane must be carefully resected with a scalpel, or pointed scissors, until the normal mucosa of the rectum is reached. Care must be taken to create smooth edges during the resection process. In this manner, a wound is created comparable with that of a fresh third degree perineal laceration.

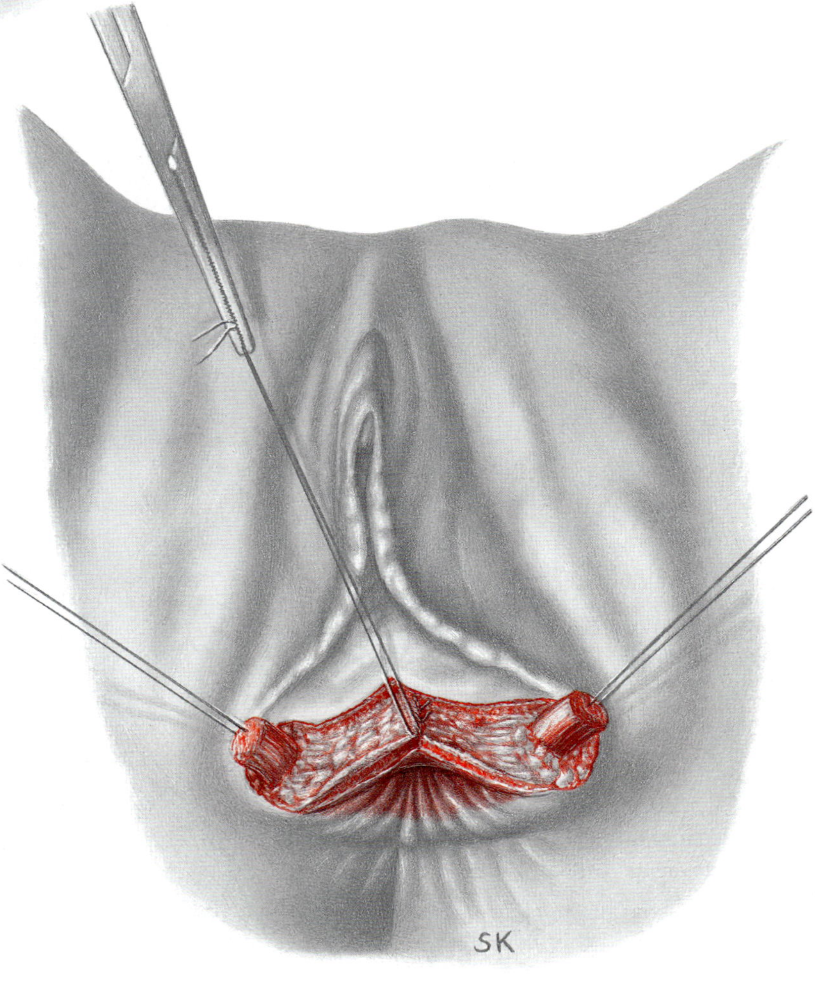

Figure 19.5. Surgical treatment of a suprasphincteral rectovaginal fistula.

The tissue layers of the anterior rectal wall are far enough mobilized from the surrounding scar tissue to allow a two-tiered wound closure free of traction with interrupted mattress sutures (use size 0000 absorbable monofilament suture). For the first suture row, the atraumatic needle punctures the muscular rectal wall immediately above the mucosa so that the wound edges are juxtaposed "layer by layer" onto each other. The mucosa itself is not punctured (in contrast to the multilayered suture of the bowel). The uppermost mattress suture is located above the highest wound angle of the rectum in the area of the excised fistula; the lowest one closes the anal mucosa at the perineum.

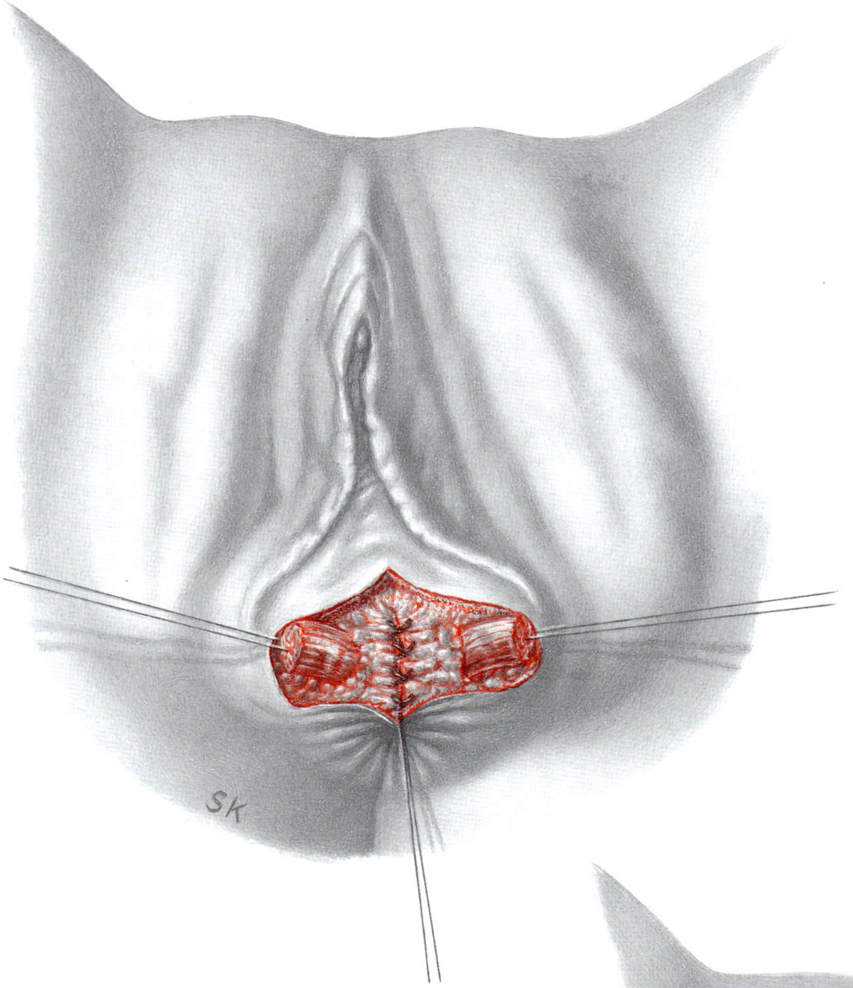

Figure 19.6. Surgical treatment of a suprasphincteral rectovaginal fistula.

A second suture row secures the first one in its entire length and covers it under the still severed sphincter ani muscle.

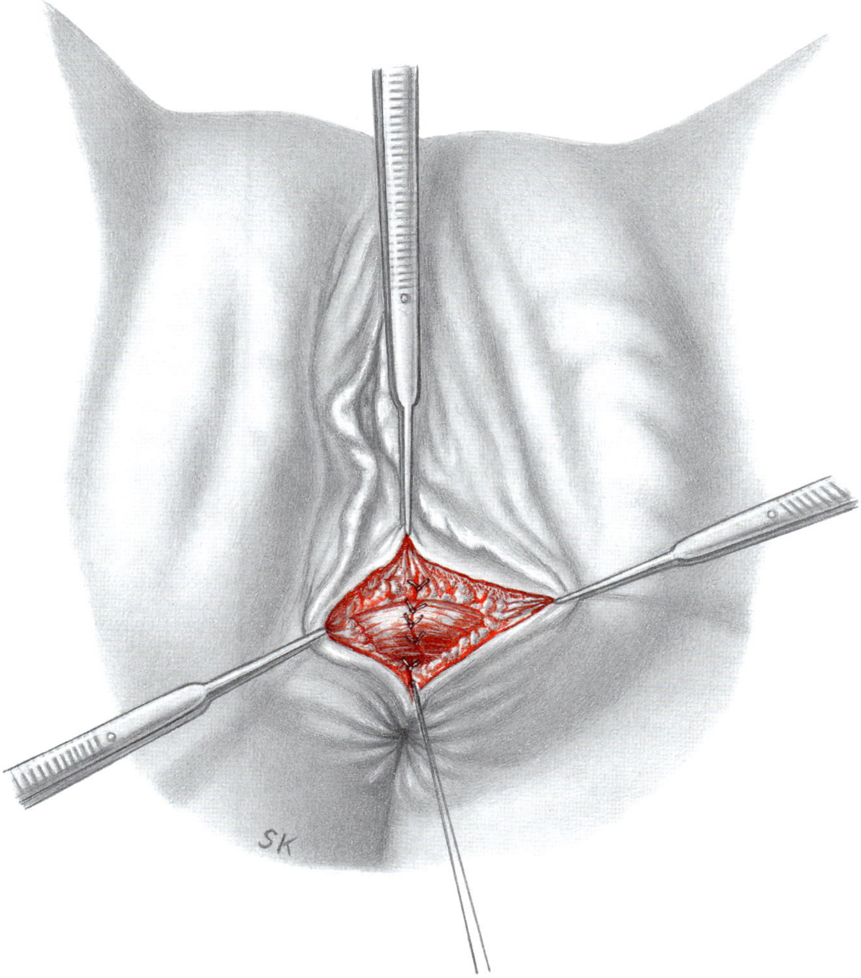

Figure 19.7. Surgical treatment of a suprasphincteral rectovaginal fistula.

Above the second suture row of the bowel closure the sphincter ani muscle is now reconstructed in its circumference. The technique for this procedure is illustrated Figures 17.9 and 17.10.

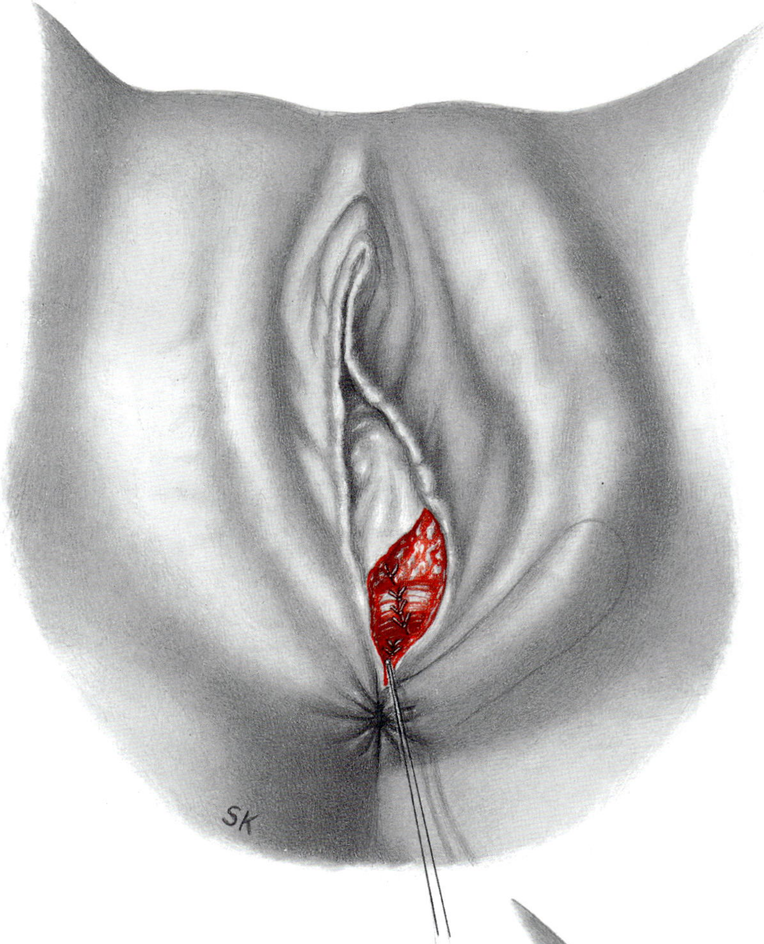

Figure 19.8. Surgical treatment of a suprasphincteral rectovaginal fistula. Transposition flap repair; transposition flap at the vaginal introitus. Circumcision incision for the flap in the vulvar skin area at the transition to the thigh.

The approximately 2 × 5 cm large flap is supposed to close the wound at the introitus without causing stenosis.

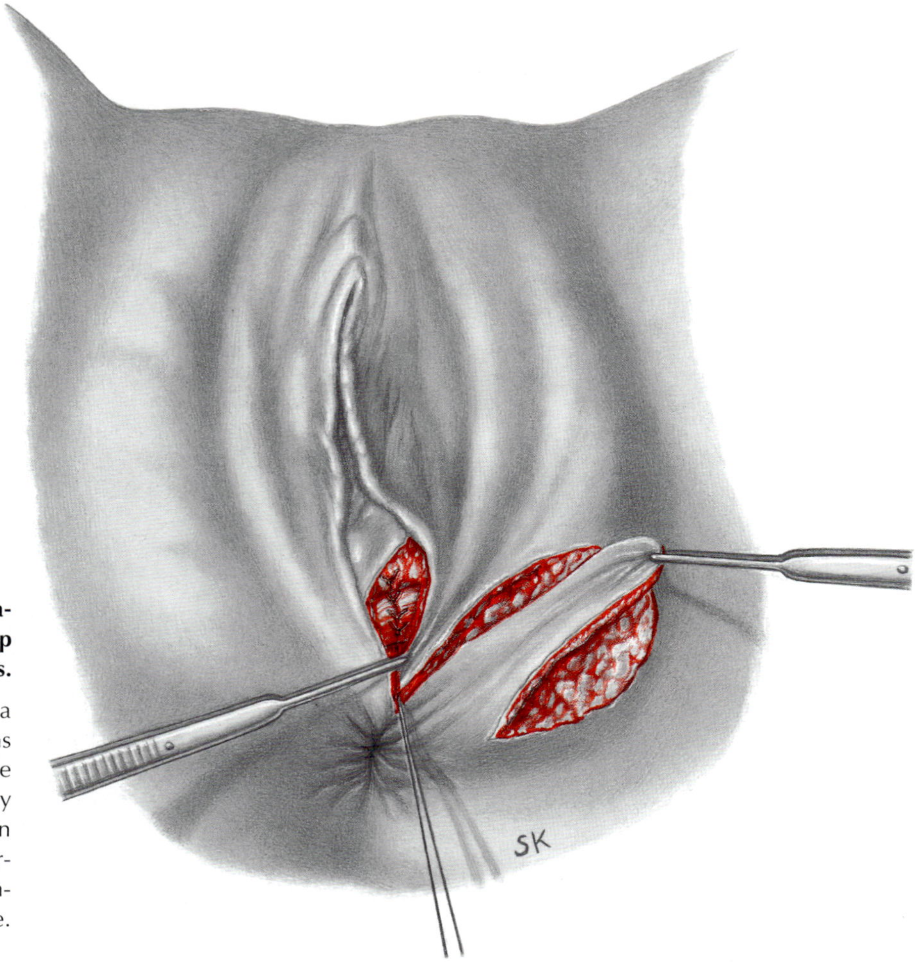

Figure 19.9. Surgical treatment of a suprasphincteral rectovaginal fistula. Transposition flap repair; transposition flap at the vaginal introitus.

The skin flap is circumcised to its base, while a 1.5- to 2-cm thick layer of adipose tissue remains beneath the skin. One must take care to leave the vessels coursing from the internal pudendal artery at the base of the flap intact; they are useful in providing blood supply. At the same time, the dorsal parts of the labium majus and minus are undermined between the introitus and the donor site. This will create a second pointed flap.

Figure 19.10. Surgical treatment of a suprasphincteral rectovaginal fistula. Transposition flap repair; transposition flap at the vaginal introitus.

By means of an exchange—which is the actual transposition—the skin flap is moved onto the wound at the introitus.

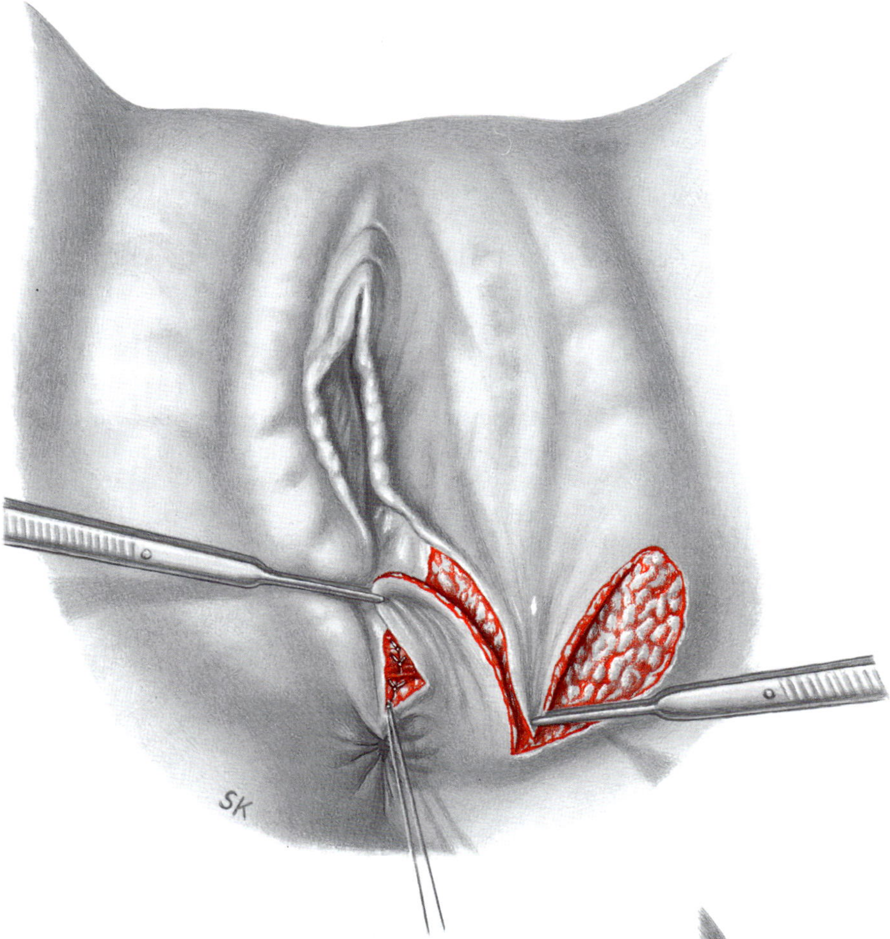

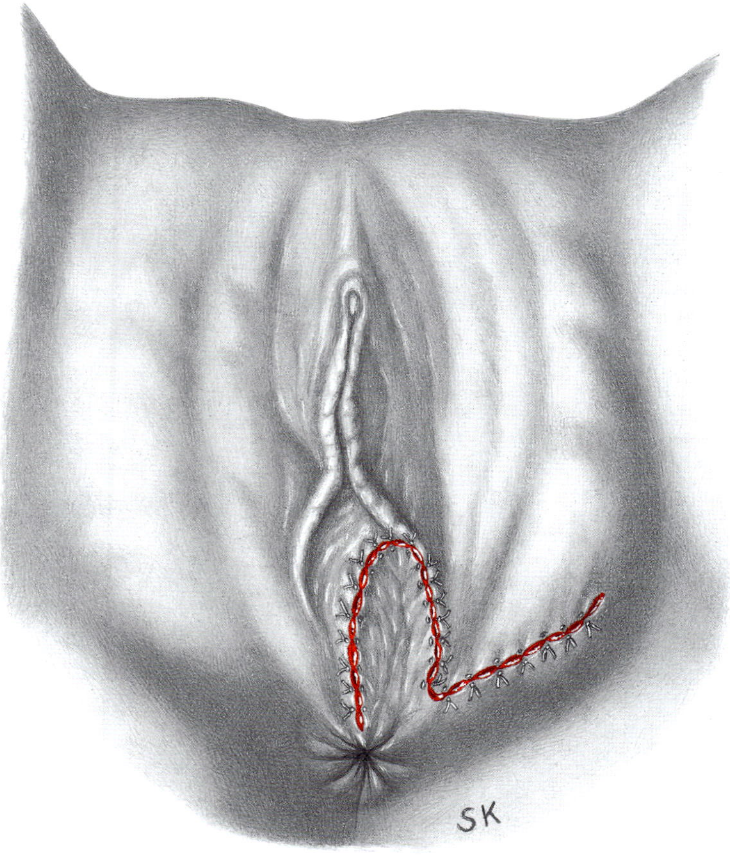

Figure 19.11. Surgical treatment of a suprasphincteral rectovaginal fistula. Transposition flap repair; transposition flap at the vaginal introitus.

The transposition flap is fixed to the wound edge of the vagina, or of the introitus, with interrupted mattress sutures (use size 0000 monofilament absorbable suture). This ensures that the fistula closure is performed without traction and that no stenosis occurs. After mobilization of the surrounding skin and careful hemostasis, the donor site is easily closed.

Technical Problems

For surgical treatment of a rectovaginal fistula in the lower vaginal region that is planned to be performed without a diverting colostomy, perioperative management is critical. A bowel perfusion by means of a duodenal probe with a 10- to 12-liter colostomy trunk, a high cleansing enema, antibiotic prophylaxis, astronaut diet, and additional resting of the bowel induced by tincture of opium are just as much part of the therapy concept as are refined surgical technique and the choice of the right suture material. Among our own patient pool composed of 35 women, we experienced two failures in the beginning. They happened when, because of omissions, bowel movements occurred on the second postoperative day, with resulting infection of the wound region and abscess formation. During the procedure itself, one must take special care to perform a complete resection of the epithelial lining of the fistula and an adequate mobilization of the mucosa and the anterior rectal wall. This will allow a two-tiered closure without tension. In every case, the additional transposition flap repair offers better healing results.

Treatment of a High Rectovaginal Fistula

Rectovaginal fistulas that develop postoperatively in the middle or upper third region of the vagina may be successfully repaired transvaginally as long as they are not too large. Exposure and complete excision of the fistulous tract may be performed without severing the sphincter ani muscle. In this case as well, the anterior rectal wall must be mobilized far enough to allow a two-tiered closure without tension. In every case, the two suture rows must be covered with an additional flap, making sure that no stenosis develops within the vagina. The myocutaneous bulbocavernosus repair, described in detail in Chapter 18 (Figs. 18.9–18.14), is particularly well suited for this purpose. Larger or postirradiation fistulas require a diverting colostomy and a vaginoabdominal approach that includes interposition of a greater omentum flap. This is best performed in cooperation with a general surgeon.

20/ Surgical Treatment of Vaginal Agenesis

Indications

Complete vaginal agenesis often coincides with agenesis of the uterus. This calls for laparoscopic evaluation to define the status of the inner genital organs before surgery. A chromosomal examination is also recommended preoperatively (Mayer-Rokitansky-Küster syndrome). Urologic malformations may frequently also be present (renal anomalies, unilateral kidneys, and ureteral duplications). These require precise urologic evaluation before deciding to proceed with the surgical construction of an artificial vagina. In most cases the procedure is done at a time in a patient's life when she wishes to be capable of sexual intercourse.

If a uterus is present, early construction of a vaginal lumen shortly after puberty is indicated to prevent the occurrence of a hematometrium. The decision to perform this operation should not be postponed; at the latest it should be made when the patient becomes aware of the anomaly. Otherwise, psychological damage may occur.

Construction of an Artificial Vagina

Technique

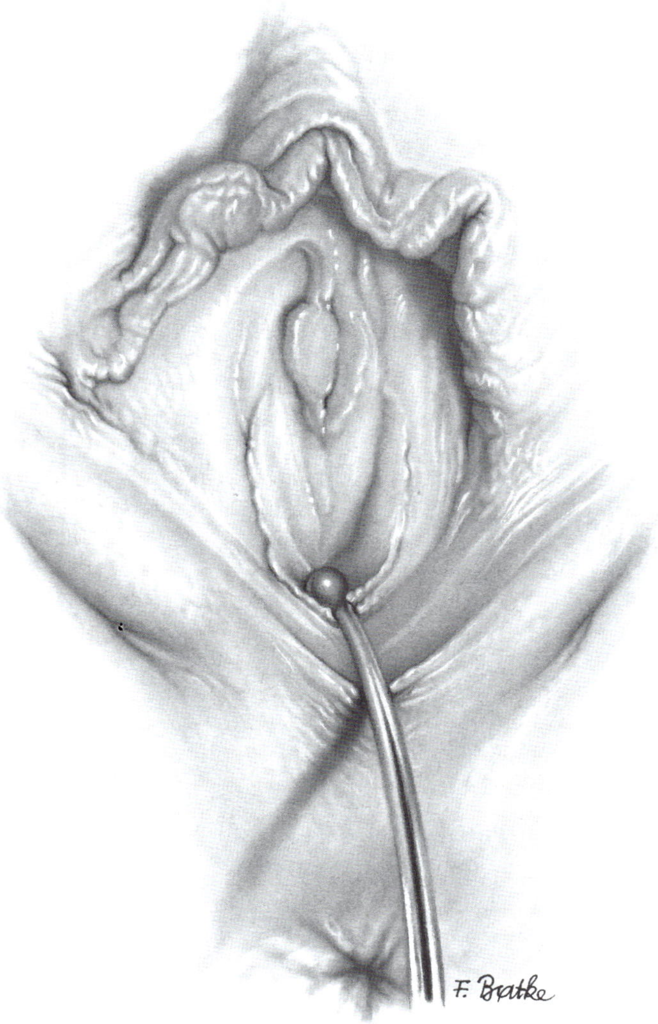

Figure 20.1. Artificial vagina. View of external genitalia.

The labia and clitoris are normally developed. One can see the external urethral meatus, the normally situated hymen, and the fossa navicularis, which is pushed posteriorly with a knobbed probe. Instead of the vaginal introitus, a tissue bridge reaches from the urethral meatus to the posterior commissure.

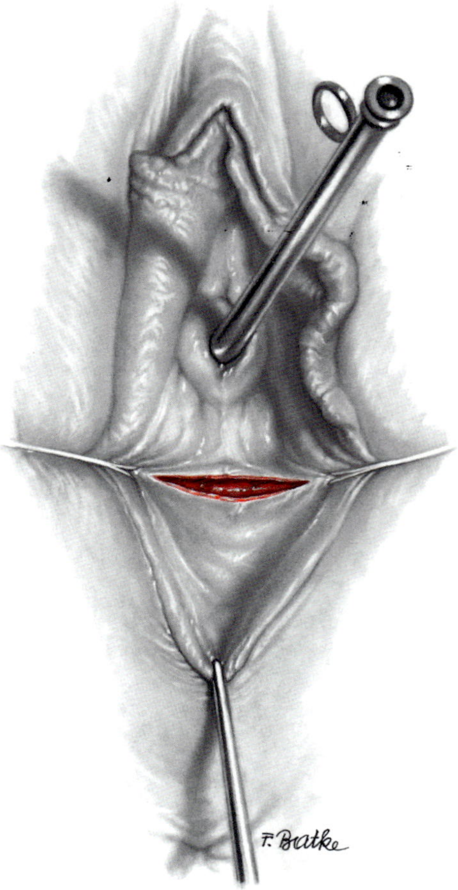

Figure 20.2. Artificial vagina. Splitting the skin bridge. Constructing a neovagina.

Two silk traction sutures are fastened laterally at the site of the future introitus. A clamp is placed at the posterior commissure and pulled downward.

The stretched skin of the closed vaginal introitus is transversely incised equidistant from the external urethral meatus and the posterior commissure.

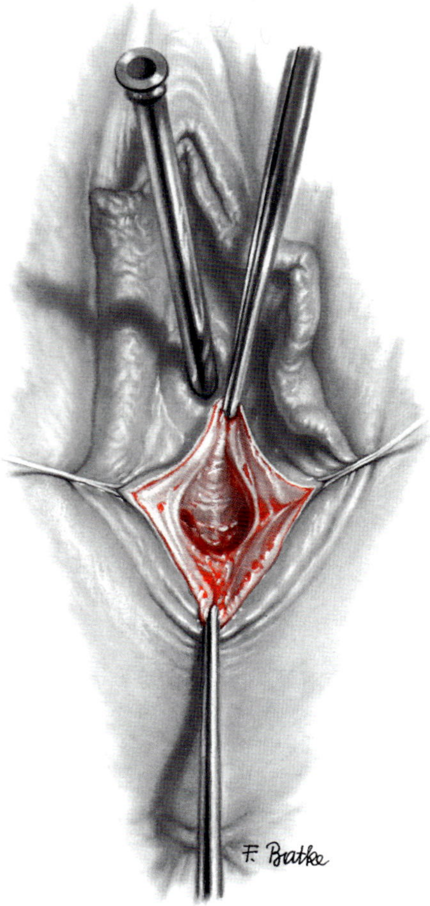

Figure 20.3. Artificial vagina. Separating the bladder and urethra from the rectum. Constructing a neovagina.

After the skin of the introitus has been incised, the cleft separating the urethra and the rectum is visible.

The cleft is deepened first in its lateral aspects by moving the dissection scissors with a fan-like motion; this creates umbilicated indentations. Since these pockets are filled with loose connective tissue, they are easily expanded cephalad up to the peritoneal reflection of the cul-de-sac of Douglas.

The thickened, denser connective tissue fibers (urethrorectal septum) are separated in midline with very small cuts of the scissors until the peritoneum is reached. Thus an artificial canal has been constructed that must be lined with epithelium.

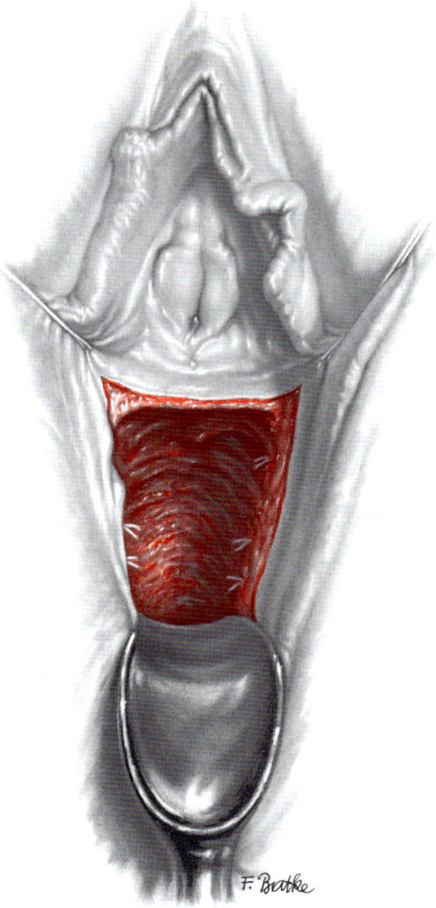

Figure 20.4. Artificial vagina. Constructing a neovagina.

The space between the urethra/bladder and the rectum has been opened further to the cul-de-sac of Douglas using sharp and blunt dissection.

This artificially constructed vaginal lumen is approximately 10–12 cm long and three fingerbreadths wide. The narrowest part is located just above the vaginal introitus where fibers of the urogenital diaphragm course laterally. These must be separated with the fingers, or severed with a scalpel, to ensure that this beginning part of the canal will be wide enough.

Precise hemostasis is required.

10 to 12 long
3 FB wide

Lining the Neovagina

We have successfully used three methods for *lining the artificial vagina*:

- Epidermal flap—Thiersch method;
- Meshgraft transplant;
- Peritoneal tissue—Davidov-Friedberg method.

Epidermal Flap—Thiersch Method

Special postoperative care. The prosthesis is held in place by a T-binder for additional support. An indwelling catheter is inserted into the bladder. Strict bedrest is recommended for 8 days. A fresh gauze strip impregnated with an antibiotic solution is inserted daily into the lumen of the glass prosthesis. This gauze strip also serves to aid drainage of wound secretions. On the 6th day after surgery the external sutures are removed from the vaginal introitus. On the same day, one begins to loosen the glass prosthesis gently by turning it slightly (no more than about 10°). On the 7th postoperative day, the glass prosthesis is loosened once again with a slight (10°) circular motion. During these last 2 days of strict bedrest the T-binder should be held in place tightly to prevent the prosthesis from moving any further.

The vaginal prosthesis is changed for the first time after 8 days. At this point, the skin flap will have grown almost completely onto the wound canal as long as the technique was applied correctly.

Should defects develop on the healing skin flap, a Sofratyl gauze strip is wound around the new prosthesis to expedite the healing process. After being discharged from the hospital the patient will wear a Plexiglas or wooden prosthesis overnight (to prevent injury, the prosthesis is lubricated with petroleum jelly). This nightly stretching of the vaginal cul-de-sac should be continued for at least 6 months after surgery. Removing the prosthesis too early leads to a poor end result because the skin flap in the artificial vagina has a tendency to shrink.

The site on the thigh from which the skin flap was removed is dressed with Sofratyl gauze; as a rule, the bandage is not changed until the 8th day (even in the presence of a foul odor). The wound in the thigh is redressed with Sofratyl. It usually dries completely after 3 weeks and will require no further care.

Technique

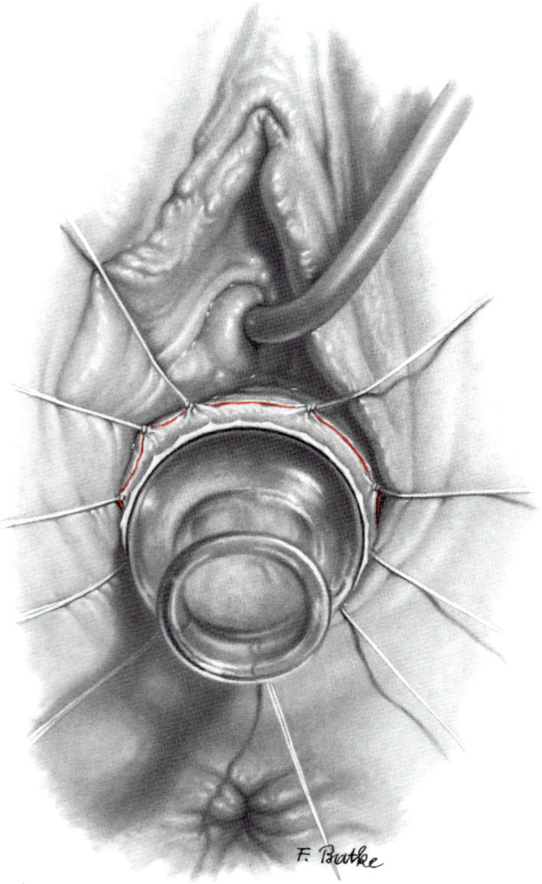

Figure 20.5. Artificial vagina. Constructing an epidermal flap.

Two Thiersch flaps 6 cm wide, 15 cm long, and 0.5 mm thick are removed from the thigh with a dermatome. They are placed on a sterile cork plate and stretched out next to one another with sterile tacks. The two flaps are then sutured together with atraumatic needles to form a single 12×15 cm flap. This dermatome flap is drawn onto a glass prosthesis—wound surface facing the outside—and the edges united radially with lateral sutures.

Where the skin flap stretches over several round holes in the prosthesis, it should be perforated with stitch incisions to ensure that accumulated postoperative secretions from the wound surface will flow into the lumen of the prosthesis.

The skin-covered prosthesis is now inserted into the artificially formed vaginal wound canal using a spiraling motion, whereby the two wound surfaces of the skin flap and the wound canal will lie face-to-face with one another.

The distal edge of the skin flap is fixed radially with fine silk sutures to the skin of the newly formed vaginal introitus.

Meshgraft Transplant

Indications

The original Thiersch flap approach may be improved by using it as a so-called meshgraft transplant. The surface of the free epidermal flap is enlarged by "mechanical fenestration," which allows for a proportionally smaller site of skin removal. In addition, drainage of wound secretions from the new neovagina and the healing process at the transplant site are aided. In our experience, the tendency of the neovagina to shrink was lowest when using a meshgraft skin flap among all methods discussed. For this reason it is our method of choice.

Technique

Two skin flaps are removed with an electrodermatome, each 5 × 10 cm large and 0.3–0.5 mm thick. The best sites for their removal are the inside of the thigh and/or its outside in the hip region. To transform the free skin flaps into meshgraft transplants, they are placed into a special device and perforated with an expansion factor of 1 to 3. This will transform the skin flaps into a tissue net three times larger. Thus prepared, the two flaps are united with fine catgut sutures to create one surface (Fig. 20.6). To aid the tissue net's insertion into the neovagina, a perforated glass or Teflon prosthesis is wrapped in Branolind gauze, and the meshgraft flap is drawn over this structure (Fig. 20.7). The epidermis has usually healed after 12 days, at which point the prosthesis may be carefully removed. Before the removal, the site is rinsed frequently with a sterile physiological saline solution to aid the separation of the gauze, which may remain within the neovagina for a few more days.

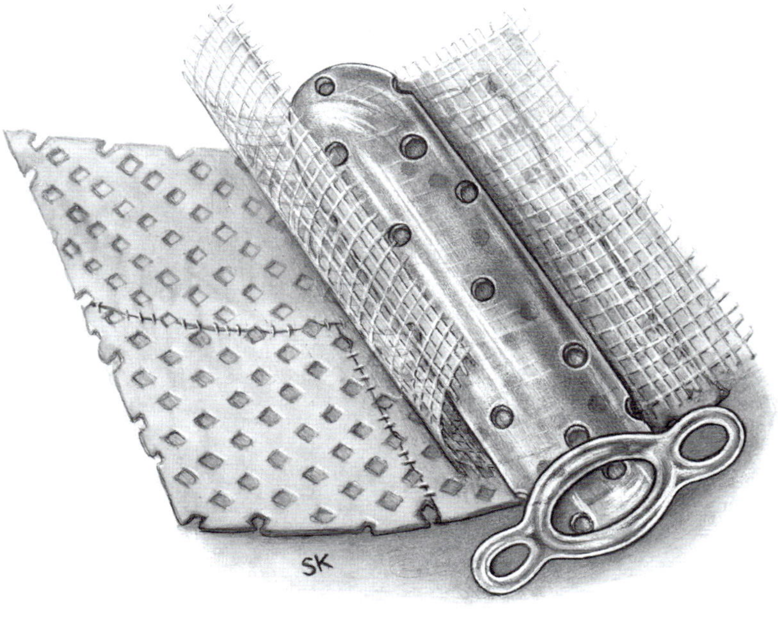

Figure 20.6. Artificial vagina. Preparing the prosthesis and the meshgraft transplant.

A perforated glass or Teflon (better) prosthesis is used, 12 cm long and 3 cm in diameter. The two epidermal flaps that had been mechanically transformed into a meshgraft network are united with thin catgut sutures (size 00) to form one surface. Adhesions are prevented by placing Branolind gauze between the transplant and the prosthesis surface. This will also aid the removal of the prosthesis at a later time. The surface of the skin faces the gauze strip, placing the skin removal site abreast with the wound surface of the neovagina.

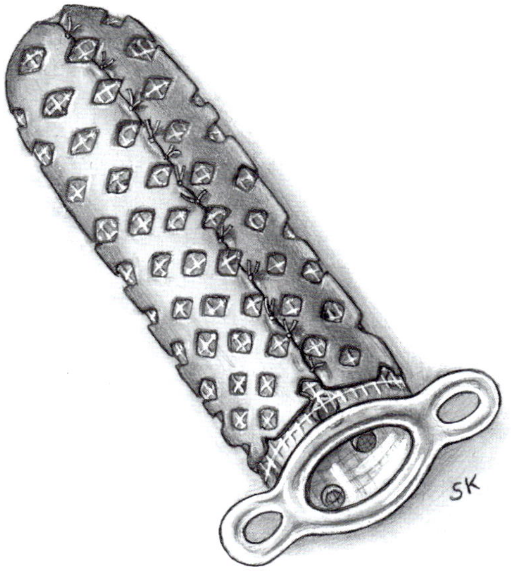

Figure 20.7. Artificial vagina. Meshgraft transplant pulled onto prosthesis, which may now be inserted into the neovagina.

Two loops serve to fixate the prosthesis onto the skin of the pelvic floor. The prosthesis interior is cleansed daily with a Nebacetin solution; it is removed on the 12th day after surgery. Frequent rinsing with physiological saline solution aids the separation of the Branolind gauze strip, which may be left in place for a few more days.

Peritoneal Tissue—Davidov-Friedberg Method

Indications

As mentioned previously, our experience leads us to favor the meshgraft method when constructing a neovagina. However, some surgeons prefer to use the peritoneal flap according to Davidov-Friedberg. Hence, this interesting approach is included in our methodologic discussion. Its advantage lies in the fact that there are no visible secondary scars at the donor sites used for creation of skin flaps. In Davidov's original method, the peritoneum used to line the neovagina is mobilized by means of a laparotomy. However, a skilled surgeon may be able to accomplish this transvaginally without using an additional laparotomy. Long-term results are acceptable, although not as good as those gained with the meshgraft method. This has convinced us to prefer the latter method.

Technique

In general, the peritoneum of the cul-de-sac of Douglas is mobilized, pulled downward through the neovagina, and fixed to the introitus. The peritoneal lining serves as a conducting surface for the squamous epithelial growth reaching from the skin of the introitus. As illustrated in Figures 20.1–20.4, the neovaginal cavity is opened to the peritoneal reflection of the cul-de-sac of Douglas. It can be dissected free from both the posterior bladder wall and the anterior rectal wall, partly bluntly by using a finger and partly sharply using scissors (Fig. 20.8). After the lower pole of the peritoneum is clearly visualized (Fig. 20.9), it is incised transversely, thus creating an anterior and a posterior flap, both of which are mobilized even more until they can be pulled all the way to the introitus without tension (Fig. 20.10). The peritoneal cavity is closed tightly with interrupted mattress sutures (Fig. 20.11). With the help of additional sutures a tube is constructed from the flaps (Fig. 20.12) that is apposed to the introitus (Fig. 20.13). Any remaining lateral gaps occurring during the neovaginal lining process may be covered by means of two additional transpositional flaps from the vulva (cf. Figs. 19.8–19.11). A prosthesis wrapped in Branolind gauze will prevent the peritoneal flap from forming premature adhesions during the first 12 days after surgery (Fig. 20.14). The patient should engage in intercourse very soon after the procedure. This will be crucial in a favorable long-term result. This must be made clear to the patient, preferably in her partner's presence.

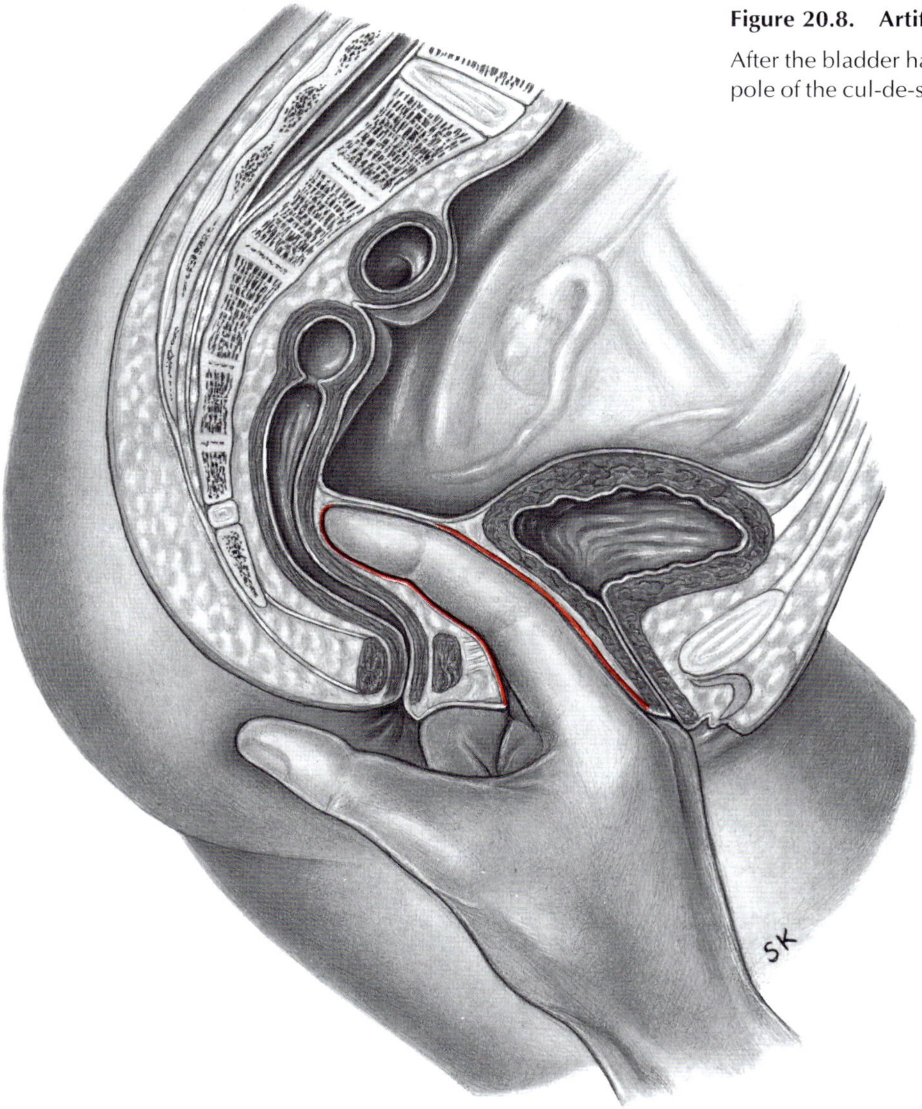

Figure 20.8. Artificial vagina. Lining with peritoneal tissue.

After the bladder has been dissected free from the rectum, the lower pole of the cul-de-sac peritoneum is mobilized bluntly with a finger.

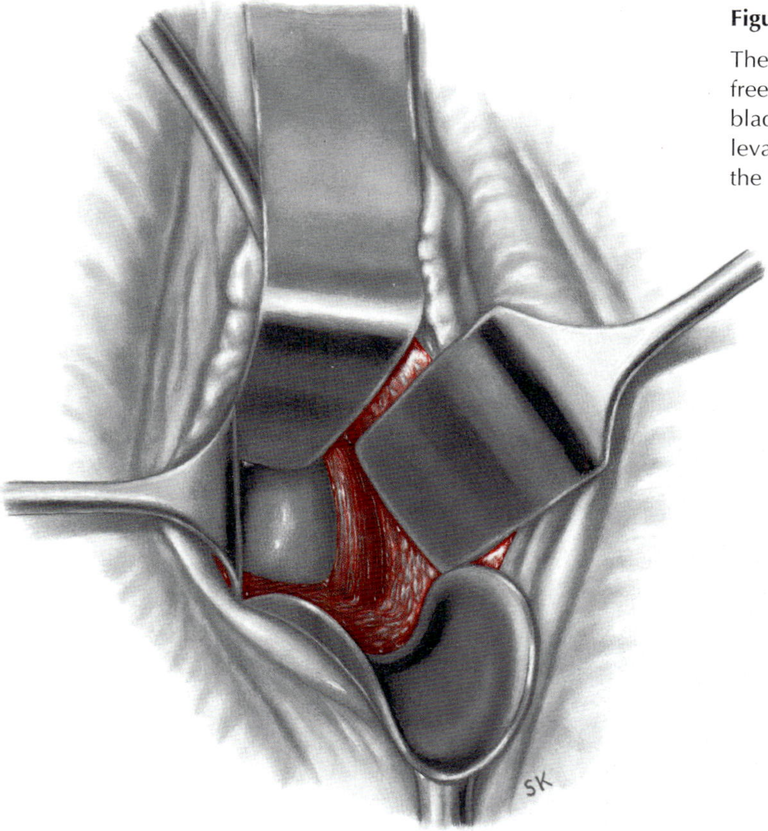

Figure 20.9. Artificial vagina. Lining with peritoneal tissue.

The lower pole of the cul-de-sac peritoneum has been dissected free. With scissors, it can be further sharply mobilized from the bladder, rectum, and lateral pelvic wall. The medial border of the levator ani muscle, shown on the left side, is a good marker for the topography of the true pelvis.

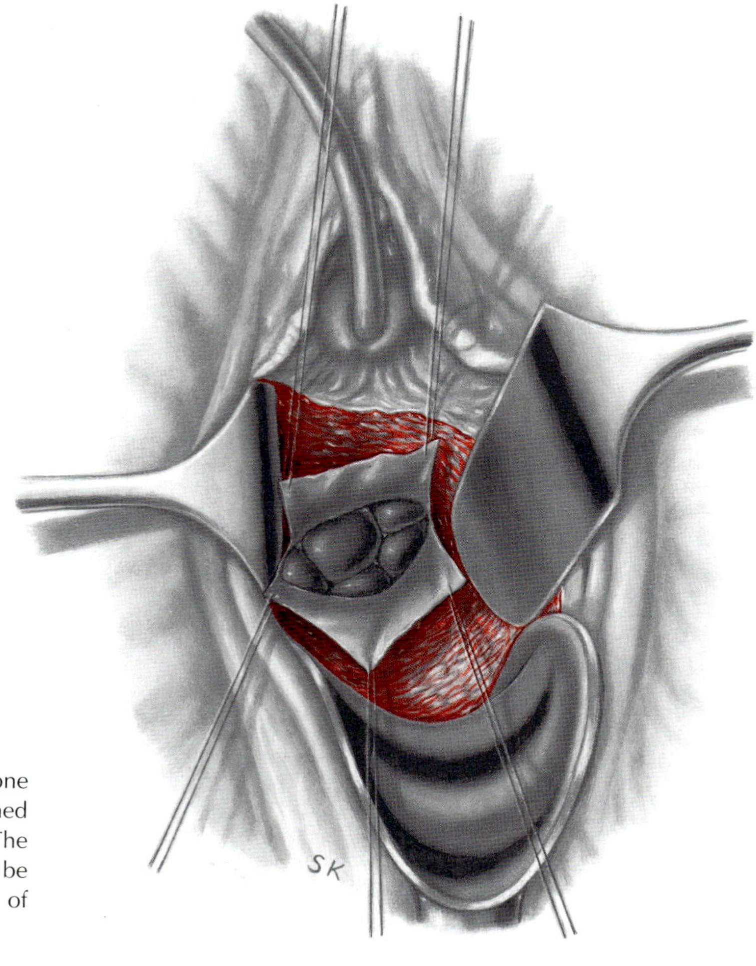

Figure 20.10. Artificial vagina. Lining with peritoneal tissue.

After the cul-de-sac peritoneum has been incised transversely, one can see the intestinal loops in the true pelvis (they should be pushed upward and out of the way with a long moist abdominal pack). The newly created peritoneal flaps are mobilized until they can be pulled back comfortably all the way to the introitus by means of traction sutures.

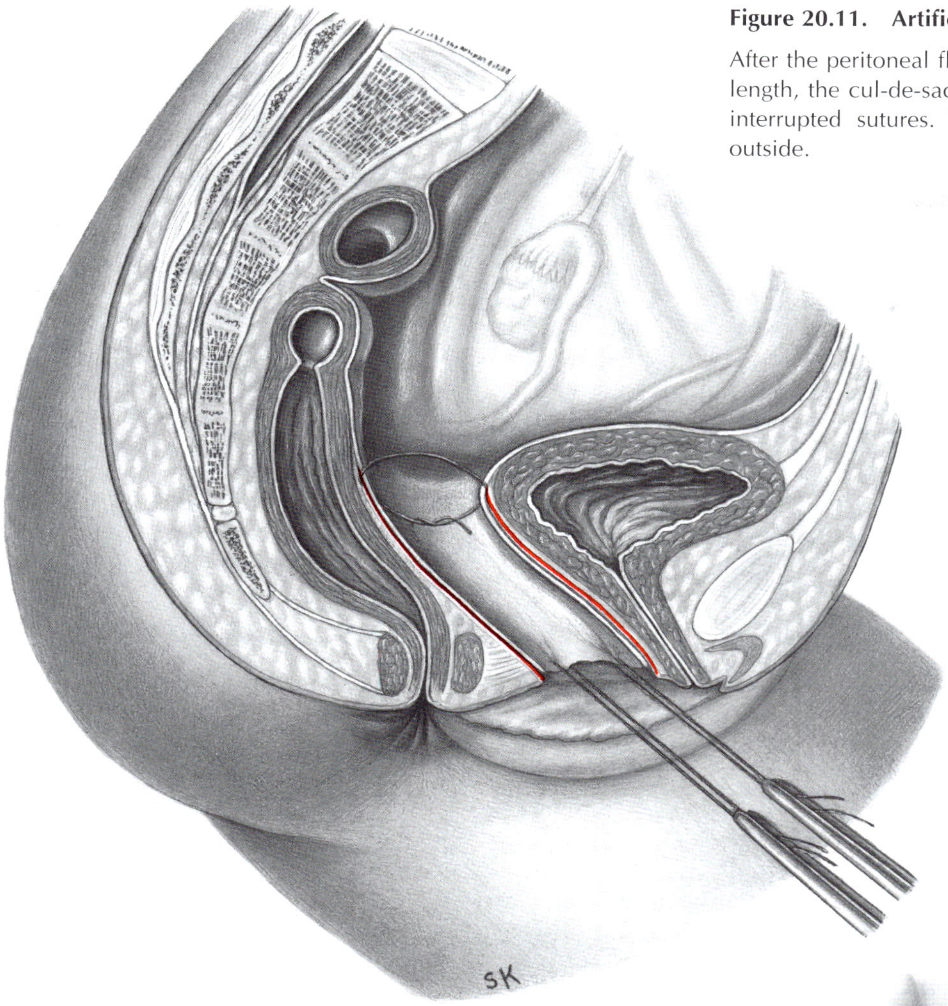

Figure 20.11. Artificial vagina. Lining with peritoneal tissue.

After the peritoneal flaps have been dissected free to an adequate length, the cul-de-sac of Douglas may be closed completely with interrupted sutures. The sutures are tied transvaginally to the outside.

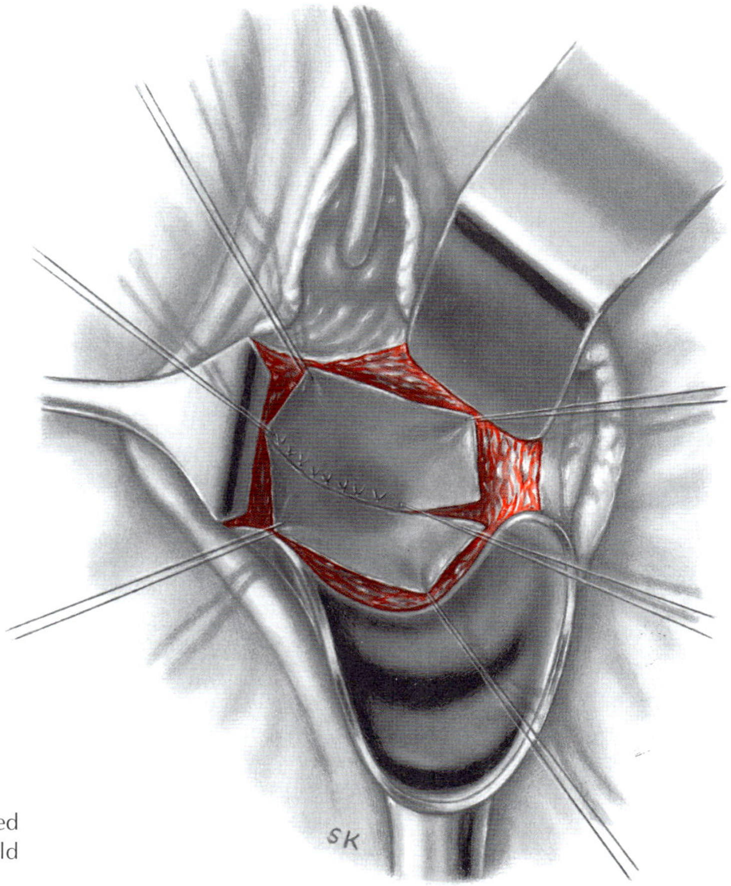

Figure 20.12. Artificial vagina. Lining with peritoneal tissue.

With additional interrupted mattress sutures a tube is constructed from the anterior and posterior peritoneal flaps. This tube should line the neovagina completely.

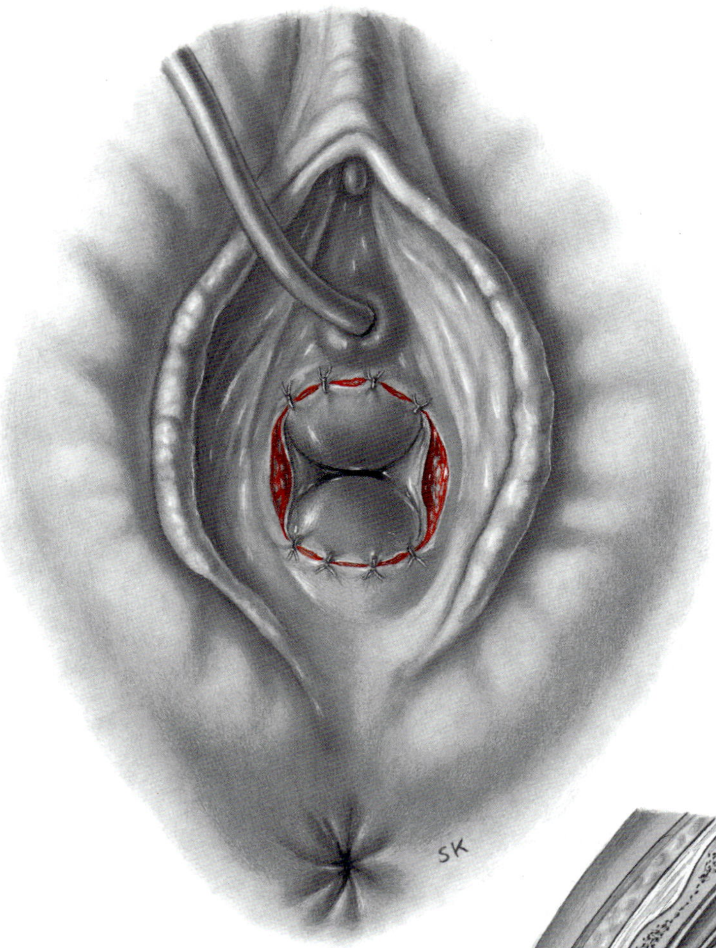

Figure 20.13. Artificial vagina. Lining with peritoneal tissue.

The flaps are fixed at the introitus with interrupted mattress sutures. Any remaining gaps may best be covered with transposition flaps from the perivulvar skin (cf. Figs. 19.8–19.11).

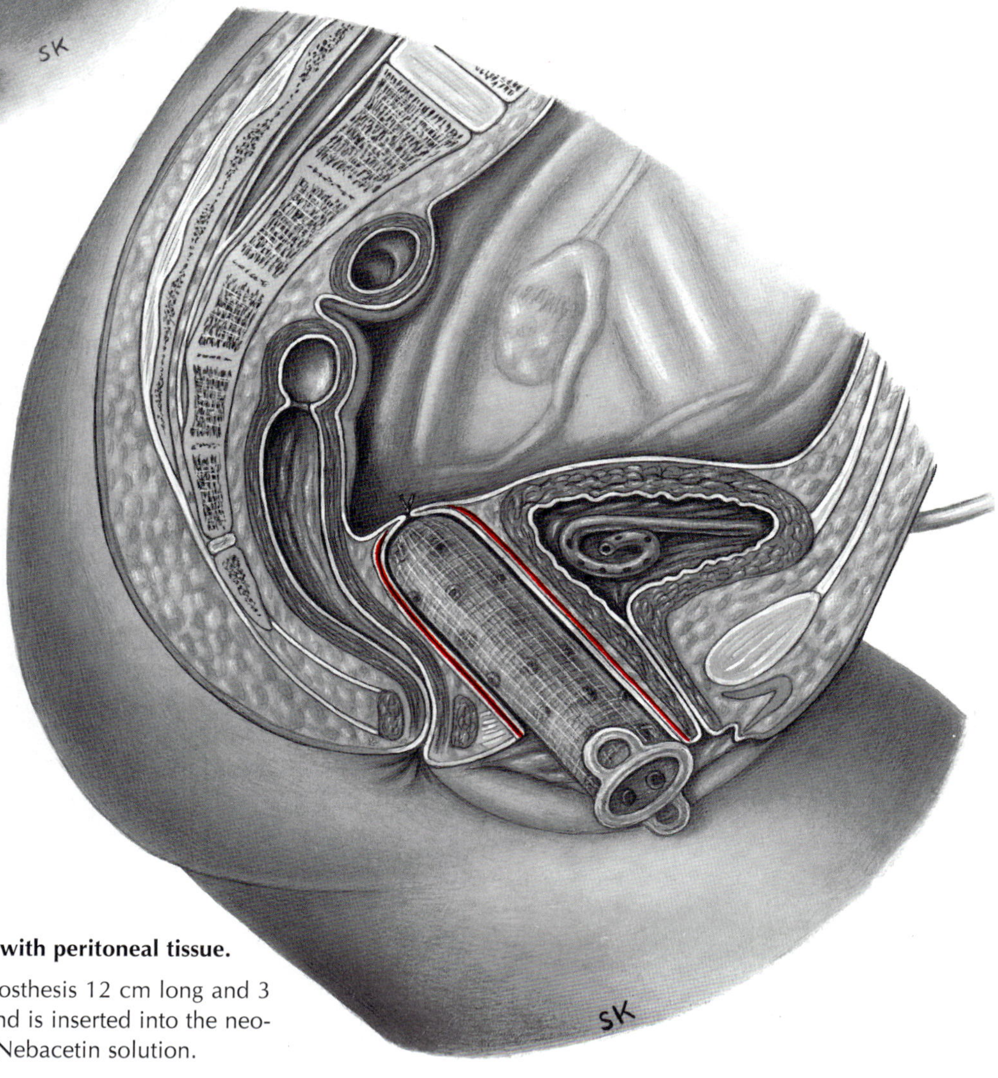

Figure 20.14. Artificial vagina. Lining with peritoneal tissue.

For the first 12 days a glass or Teflon prosthesis 12 cm long and 3 cm in diameter and wrapped in Branolind is inserted into the neovagina. It should be rinsed daily with a Nebacetin solution.

21/ Surgical Treatment of Vulvar Carcinoma

Radical Vulvectomy and Lymphadenectomy (''En-Bloc'' Resection)

Indications

Käser wrote in 1973,[a] ''In America, England, Ireland, Scandinavia radical vulvectomy for vulvar carcinoma is the therapy of choice. We are also of the opinion that the best results may be achieved with a one-sided en-bloc resection.'' In 1987 [b] F. di Re concluded that in the presence of a vulvar carcinoma, lymphadenectomy appears to be therapeutic as long as it is performed systematically and not selectively.

Within the past few years, however, the tendency toward selective surgical treatment of a vulvar carcinoma has been increasing.

1. With microinvasion, a wide local excision or a subtotal vulvectomy without lymphadenectomy suffices. With this approach one may expect an almost 100% cure rate.
2. Stromal invasion between 1 and 3 mm is treated with wide local excision or subtotal superficial vulvectomy.
3. A one-sided vulvar carcinoma may be treated with a one-sided lymphadenectomy as long as the lymph nodes are ''negative.''
4. Five-year cure rates with ''negative'' inguinal lymph nodes compare with those in cases exhibiting a single positive lymph node.
5. With a tumor larger than 2 cm in diameter, metastatic invasion of the lymph nodes increases considerably (in the presence of ''positive'' lymph nodes, the 5-year cure rate is lowered to 50%). Radical vulvectomy and bilateral inguinofemoral lymphadenectomy remain standard therapy for invasive vulvar carcinoma. The choice of a pelvic lymphadenectomy depends on positive results from a frozen section examination of the inguinofemoral lymph nodes.

The problematic nature of individualized vulvectomy suitable for various patients as well as for different stages of carcinoma, including plastic reconstruction, has been discussed exhaustively elsewhere[c]. We have chosen to concentrate on describing the extended radical ''en-bloc'' resection, because the restricted radical operations are easily derived from this method. Only the inguinal lymphadenectomy via triple incision is covered separately. For basic anatomical concepts, see ''Schauta vs. Wertheim'' in Chapter 22 and also the monograph by G. Reiffenstuhl[d].

For treatment of advanced vulvar carcinoma, one begins with an inguinal lymphadenectomy. The inguinal lymph nodes are removed ''en bloc'' in connection with the vulva.

---

[a]Käser O, Iklé FA, Hirsch HA. Atlas der gynäkologischen Operationen, 3rd ed. Stuttgart: Thieme, 1973:434.

[b]di Re F. Third International Symposium of Gynecological Oncology. Tokyo, October 1987.

[c]Knapstein PG, di Re F, di Saia P, Haller U, Serin B-U (eds). Malignancies of the vulva. New York: Thieme, 1991.

[d]Reiffenstuhl G. Das Lymphsystem des weiblichen Genitale. Munich: Urban & Schwarzenberg, 1957.

TECHNIQUE

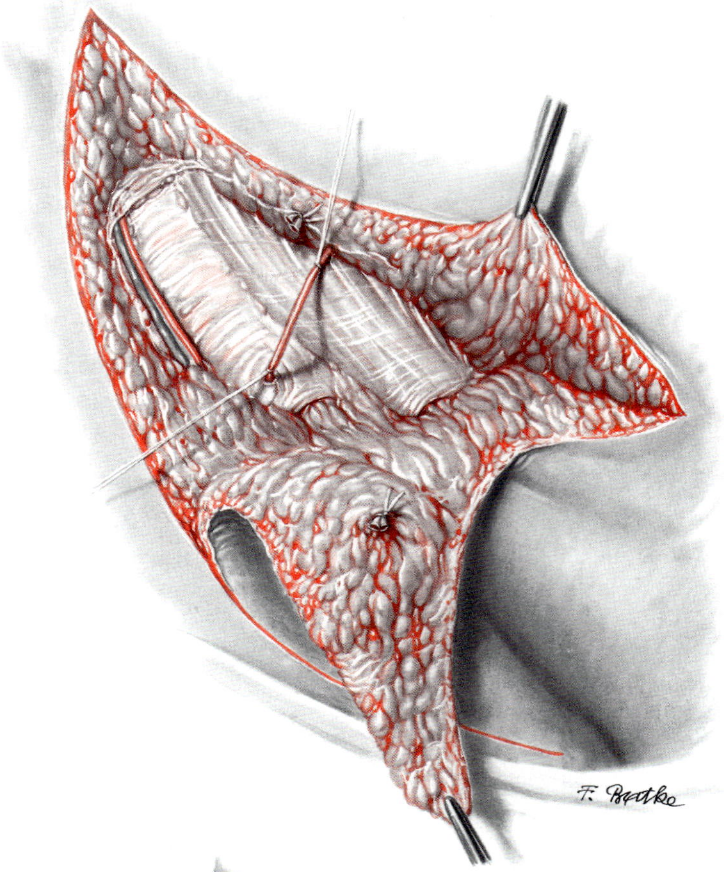

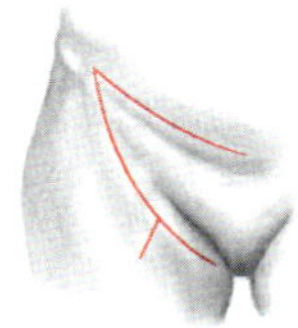

Figure 21.1. Right inguinal lymphadenectomy. Mobilizing the skin flap.

The skin incision (*detail*) begins at the anterior superior iliac spine and curves to the mons pubis. With a second incision, the skin of the inguinal crease is incised in a lancet shape: it begins laterally at the origin of the first incision, courses in a curve toward the thigh, and ends medially almost in the genitofemoral sulcus.

The subcutaneous adipose tissue of the inguinal region is divided by a delicate intervening connective tissue lamella into two strata, one above the other. The inguinal lymph nodes (horizontal tract) and the inguinal blood vessels lie in the deeper layer of the subcutaneous tissue. This makes it possible to incise the skin down to the intervening lamella without risk of injury to blood vessels.

One begins laterally with mobilizing the lancet-shaped skin flap. The intervening layer is divided with scissors. Deep down, the circumflex iliac artery and vein become visible. While continuing the dissection medially, the freed superficial epigastric arteries and veins (which are usually multiple in number) are ligated and severed.

After deepening the bow-shaped incision down to the fascia, the fatty lymph node bundle in the inguinal crease can be dissected relatively easily in toto in a medial direction. This step in the dissection is continued only until one can identify the proximal border of the fossa ovalis (cornu superius) and the round ligament where it exits from the inguinal canal medially.

The superficial epigastric artery is isolated from the adipose tissue and doubly ligated.

Detail. Right inguinal lymphadenectomy. Making the incision.

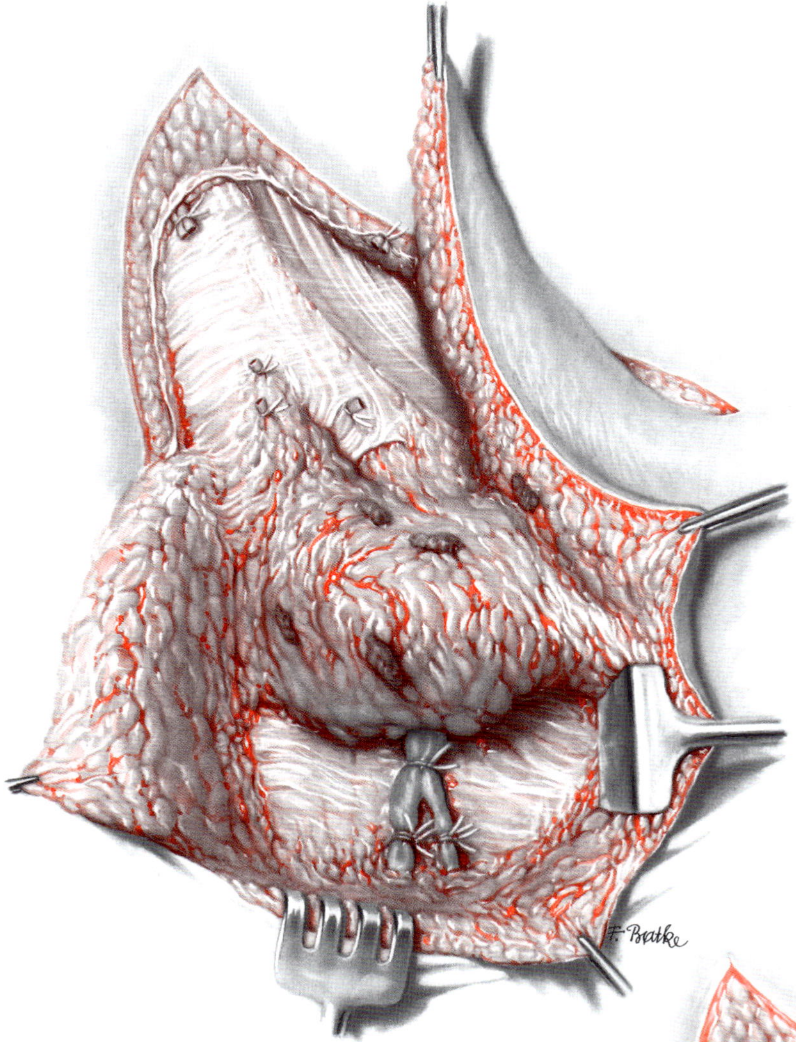

Figure 21.2. Right inguinal lymphadenectomy. Node removal and ligating the greater saphenous vein.

The lancet-shaped flap of fatty tissue has been dissected to the foramen ovale (saphenous hiatus) and retracted upward. The peripheral parts of the superficial circumflex iliac artery and vein and the superficial epigastric artery and vein are divided.

For the peripheral mobilization of the greater saphenous vein, a third skin incision is made perpendicularly to the second (Fig. 21.1, *detail*). It begins at the middle of the second skin incision and runs parallel to the femoral vessels along the thigh.

The tips of the femoral skin flaps are grasped with clamps and pulled downward. The lowermost wound angle is pulled caudally with a rake retractor. The greater saphenous vein and its accessory tributaries are mobilized and ligated.

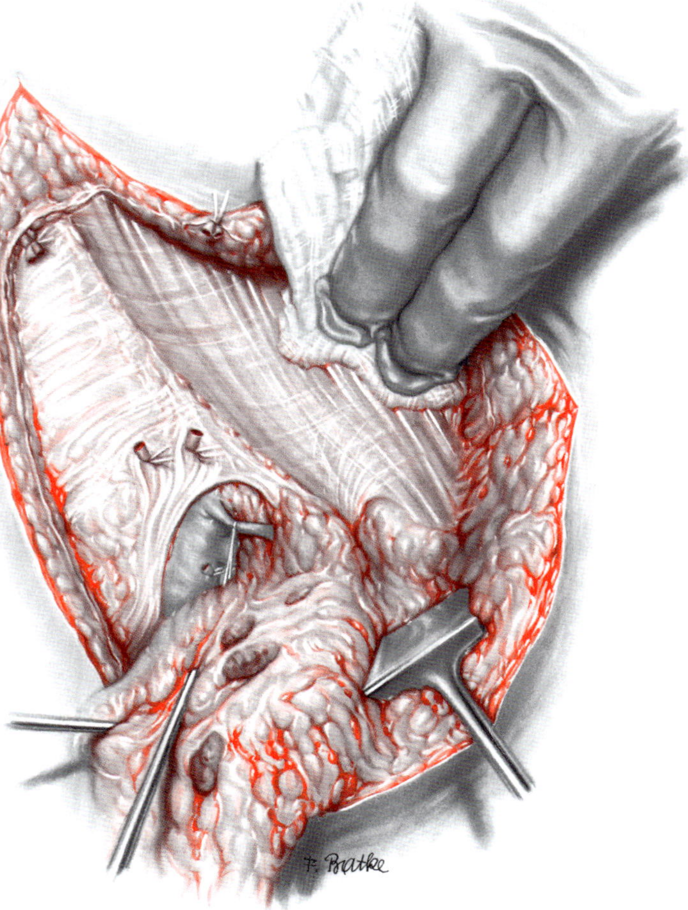

Figure 21.3. Right inguinal lymphadenectomy. Dissecting free the fossa ovalis.

The fatty tissue flap has been mobilized laterally from the fascia and pulled downward. Several lymph nodes of the horizontal tract can be seen in it.

The circumflex iliac and superficial epigastric vessels are divided peripherally. The round ligament is visible in the external inguinal ring (anulus inguinalis subcutaneus).

The fossa ovalis (saphenous hiatus) is dissected free from above and laterally; in its depth, the femoral vein is visible. The external pudendal vein is ligated near its entrance into the femoral vein.

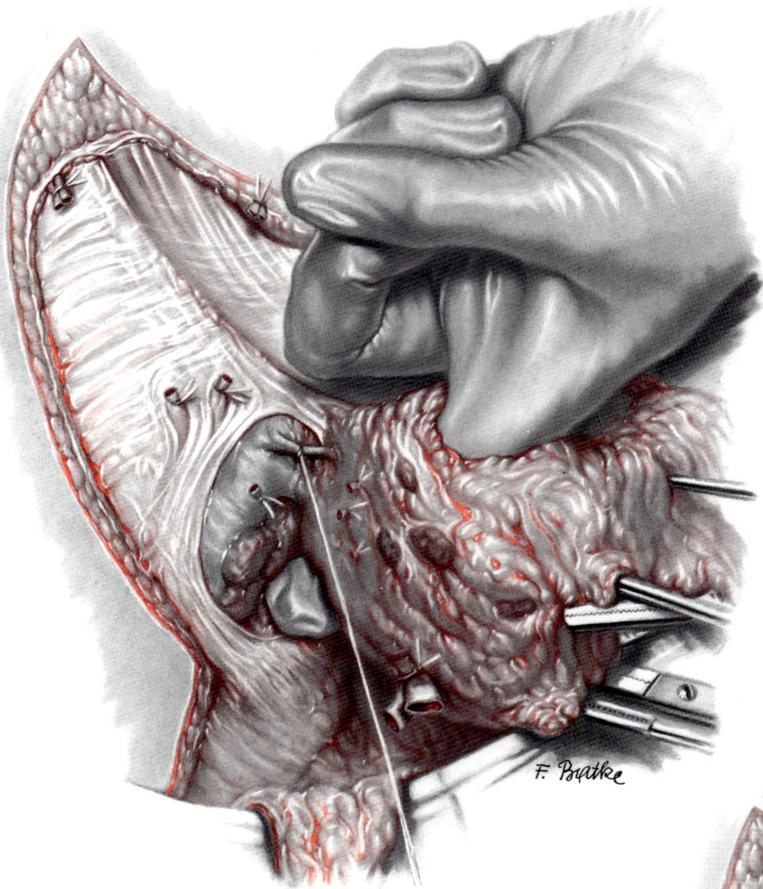

Figure 21.4. Right inguinal lymphadenectomy. Forming the lymph-bearing fatty pedicle.

The tissue flap is extensively mobilized at the side and is being retracted medially. The superior cornu, falciform margin, and inferior cornu of the fossa ovalis are all dissected free.

The femoral vein is visible in the saphenous hiatus. Underneath the ligated external pudendal vein is the central juncture of the greater saphenous vein into the femoral vein. Peripherally, the greater saphenous veins and accessory tributaries are ligated and divided; their stumps are recognizable at the lower border of the fatty lymph node flap.

The surgeon dissects the flap also medially to the fossa ovalis (saphenous hiatus) in the following manner: after the peripheral ligation and division of the external pudendal vein, the index finger is inserted medially to the external inguinal ring and is moved laterally toward the saphenous hiatus out to the fascia lata of the thigh, thus guiding it underneath the flap (the fingertip is visible in the fossa ovalis).

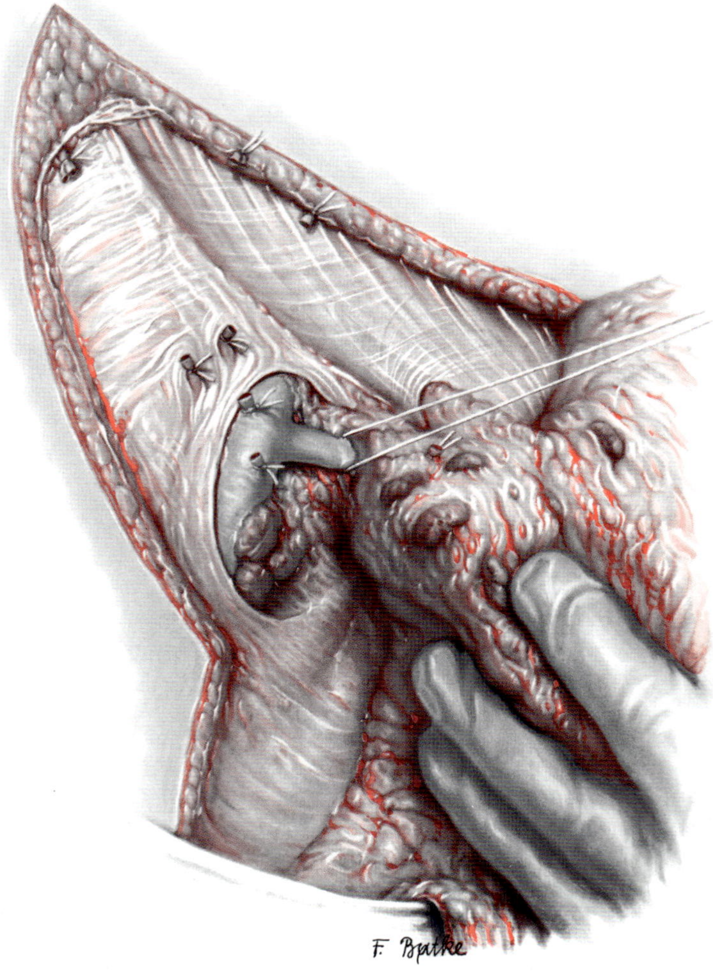

Figure 21.5. Right inguinal lymphadenectomy. Ligating the greater saphenous vein centrally.

The pedicle formation from the fatty lymph node flap is almost completed and the flap folded over medially. It is progressively narrowed by dissecting free the blood vessels located at its center. These vessels are severed and ligated close to their juncture with the femoral vein. The stumps of the external pudendal vein, the superficial circumflex iliac vein, and the superficial epigastric vein are visible.

The fossa ovalis is exposed at its proximal, lateral, and distal borders and partly at its medial margin also. On the medial side of the femoral vein two deep inguinal lymph nodes can be seen.

The greater saphenous vein is ligated at its entrance into the femoral vein.

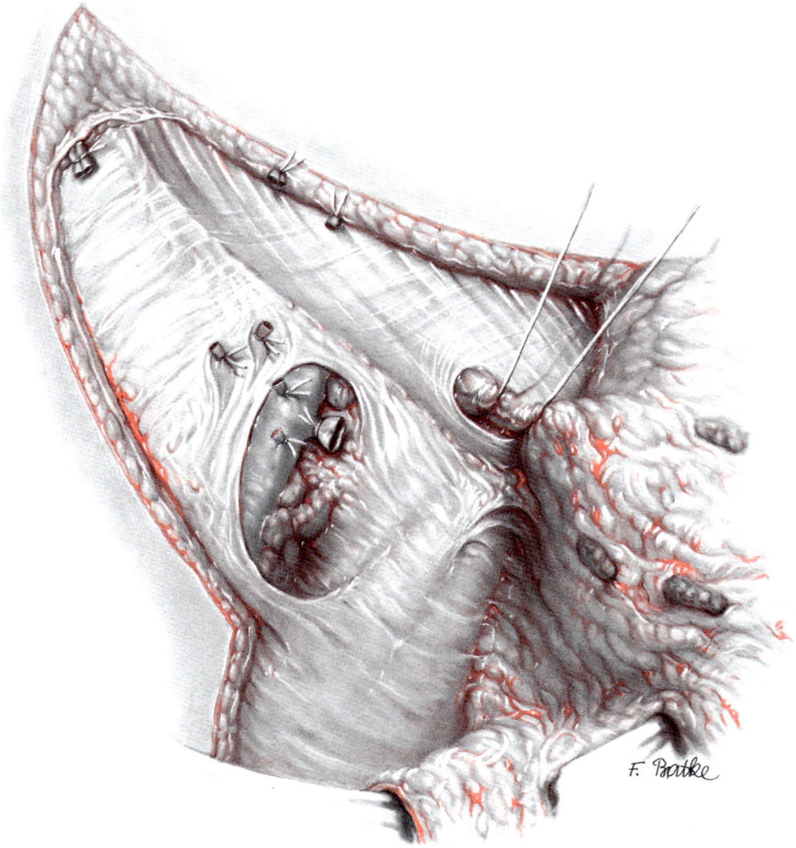

Figure 21.6. Right inguinal lymphadenectomy. Ligating the round ligament.

The fatty lymph node tissue has been removed (together with a lancet-shaped segment of skin from the inguinal region) down to the fascia of the external oblique abdominal muscle and to the fascia of the thigh. The fossa ovalis (saphenous hiatus) is dissected free. The veins are ligated and severed near their junctures with the femoral vein.

In the proximal part of the fossa ovalis at the medial side of the femoral vein, one can see Rosenmüller's node beneath the superior cornu.

The round ligament is doubly ligated and divided where it exits from the inguinal canal.

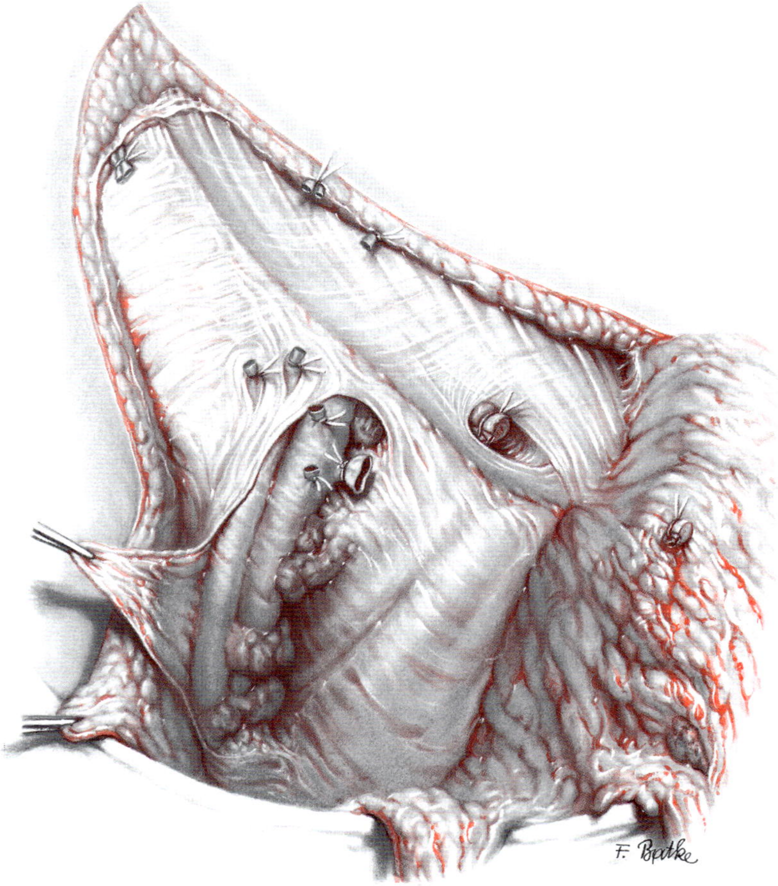

Figure 21.7. Right inguinal lymphadenectomy. Dissecting the deep inguinal lymph nodes.

The superficial inguinal lymph nodes have been dissected en bloc in conjunction with the surrounding adipose tissue and a skin flap and retracted in a medial direction.

To expose the deep inguinal lymph nodes, the fascia lata is split along the femoral vessels and retracted laterally. The fascial incision begins at the inferior cornu of the fossa ovalis and extends to the abductor canal.

The deep inguinal lymph nodes are visible at the medial side of the femoral vein and, more distally, are also seen lying on the vein. Lateral to the large femoral vein courses the femoral artery.

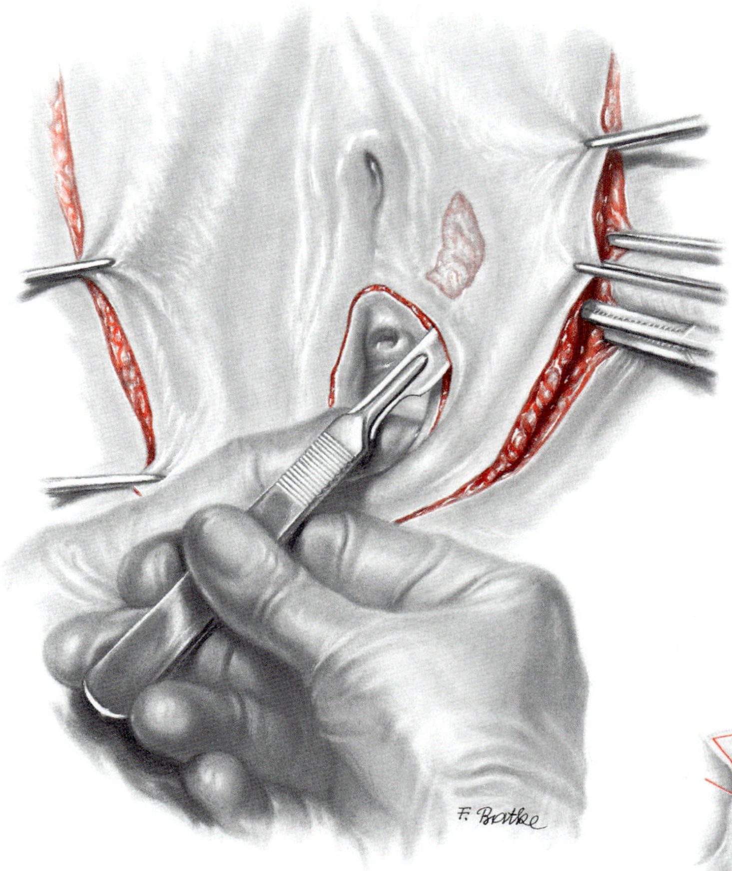

Figure 21.8. En bloc vulvectomy. Joining the inner with the outer circumcision wound.

The outer circumferential vulvar incision is placed laterally to the labia majora in the genitofemoral sulcus, curving caudally to encompass the greater part of the perineal skin. In the cephalad direction, it ends bilaterally in the inguinal skin incision.

The inner circumferential incision in the vaginal introitus begins above the urethral meatus and curves bilaterally along the hymenal edge, reaching the posterior commissure.

After partial dissection of the vulva from the anterior surface of the symphysis, the inner circumcision is joined to the outer wound area. This is done laterally from the exterior urethral meatus by advancing the scalpel diagonally outward from the inner circumcision edge until it meets the wound surface of the symphysis.

Detail. En bloc vulvectomy. Circumcising the vulva.

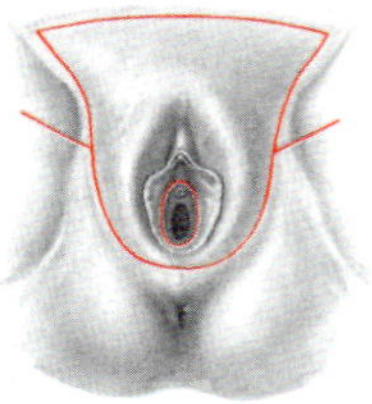

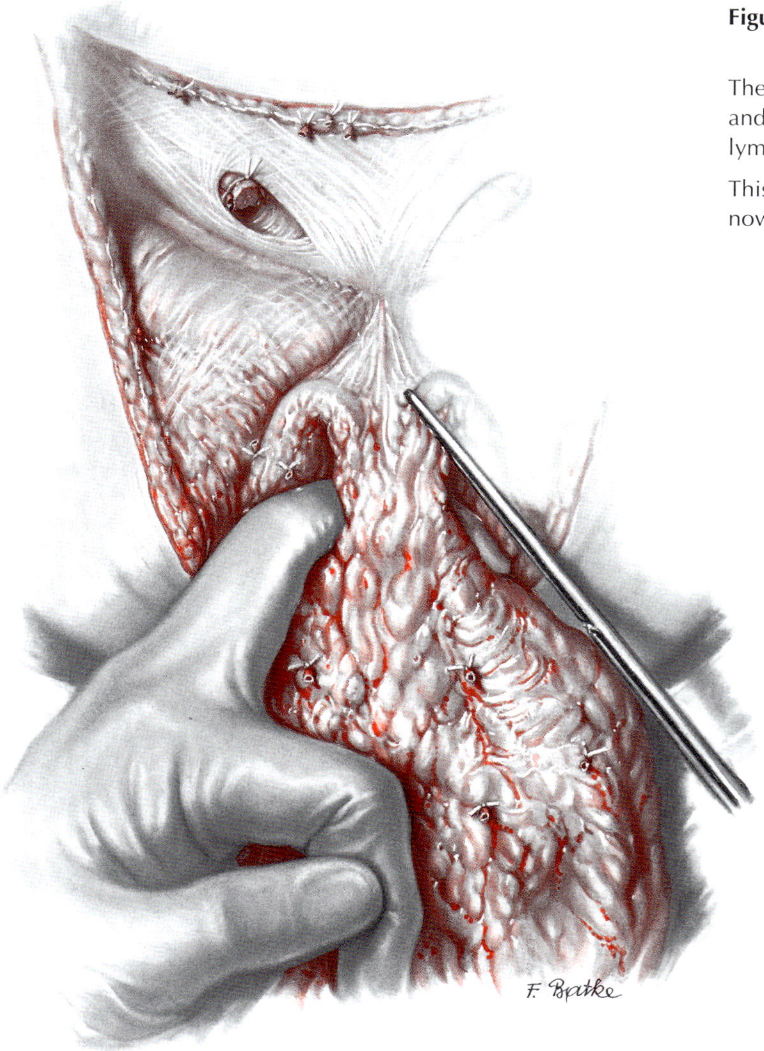

Figure 21.9. En bloc vulvectomy. Dissecting the clitoral crura.

The vulva is dissected from the anterior surface of the symphysis and retracted downward together with the entire block of fatty lymph node tissue of the inguinal region.

This tissue block is still attached to the crura clitoridis, which are now divided at the pubic arch by the clamp method.

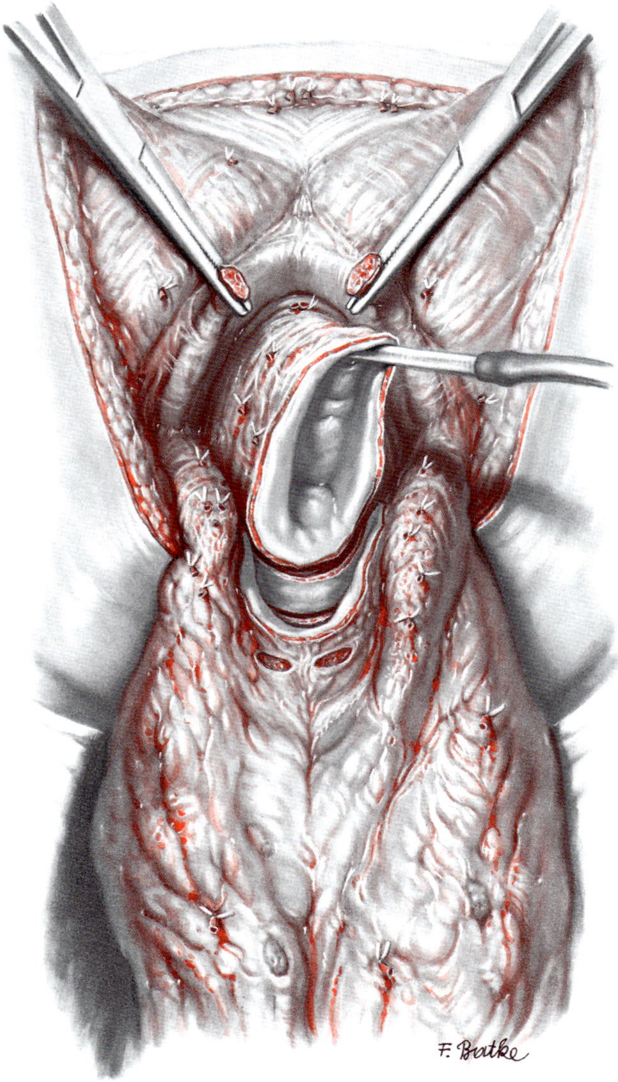

Figure 21.10. En bloc vulvectomy. Dissecting the vulva in conjunction with the regional lymph nodes.

The clitoral crura are clamped and severed. For orientation purposes, a catheter is temporarily inserted into the urethra.

The vulva is dissected from the vaginal canal and retracted downward; it remains fixed only by the perineal skin.

Note the radical removal of the tissue from the anterior surface of the symphysis and from the genitofemoral sulcus bilaterally.

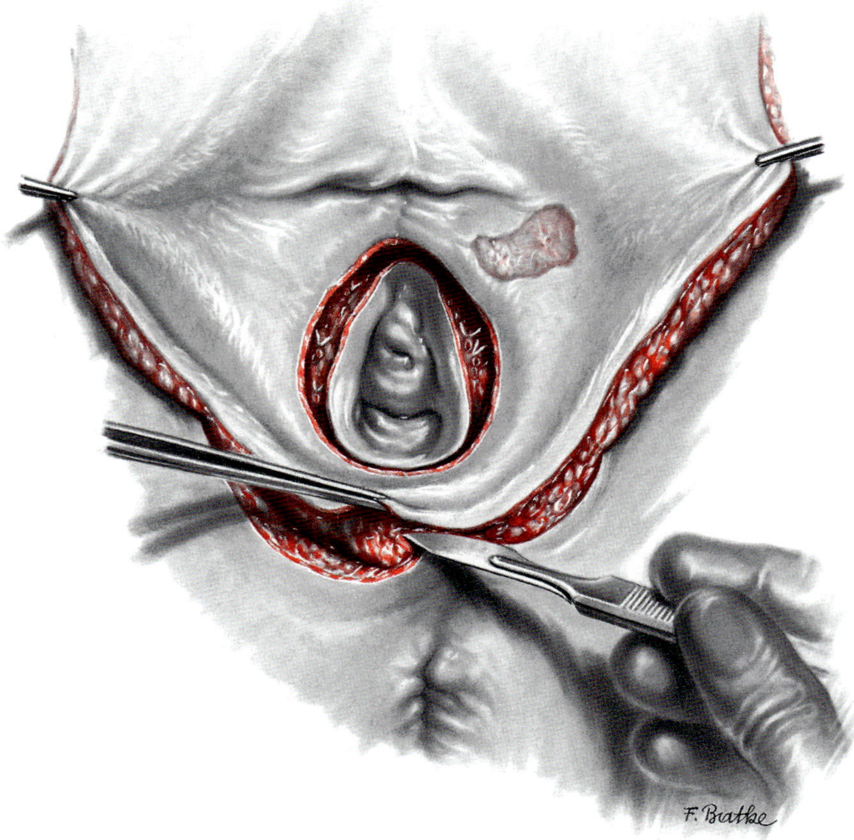

Figure 21.11. En bloc vulvectomy. Dissecting the perineal skin.

The vulva is almost completely dissected; the entire tissue block is held upward.

The perineal skin can be dissected sharply from caudal to cranial.

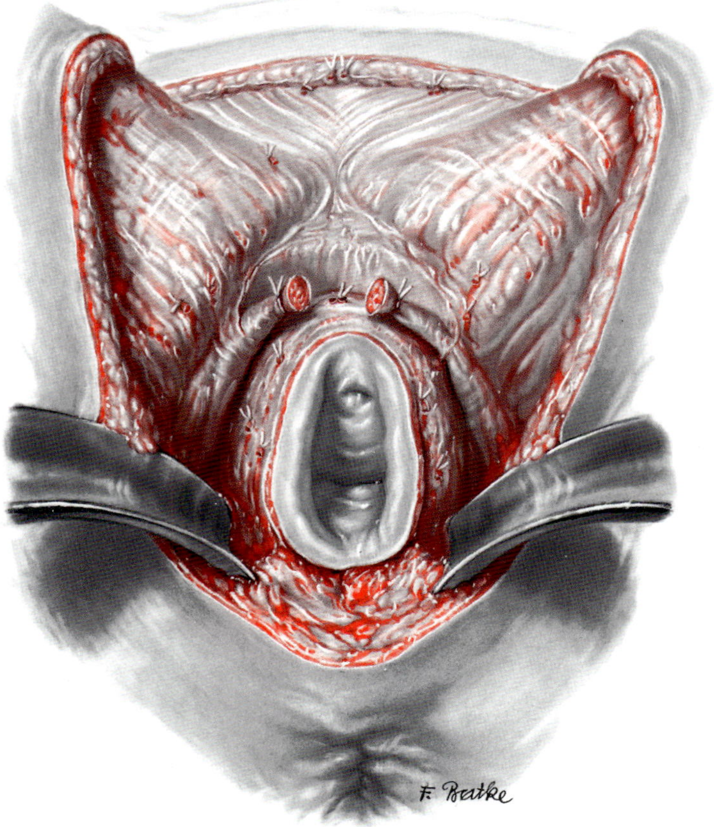

Figure 21.12. En bloc vulvectomy. View after vulvectomy and bilateral inguinal lymphadenectomy.

At the lower edge of the symphysis the severed clitoral crura and the stumps of the dorsal clitoral artery and vein are visible.

The fatty lymph node tissue was removed down to the fasciae of the abdominal wall and the thigh. The vulva was removed to the anterior surface of the symphysis and deep into the genitofemoral sulcus. Precise hemostasis is obtained.

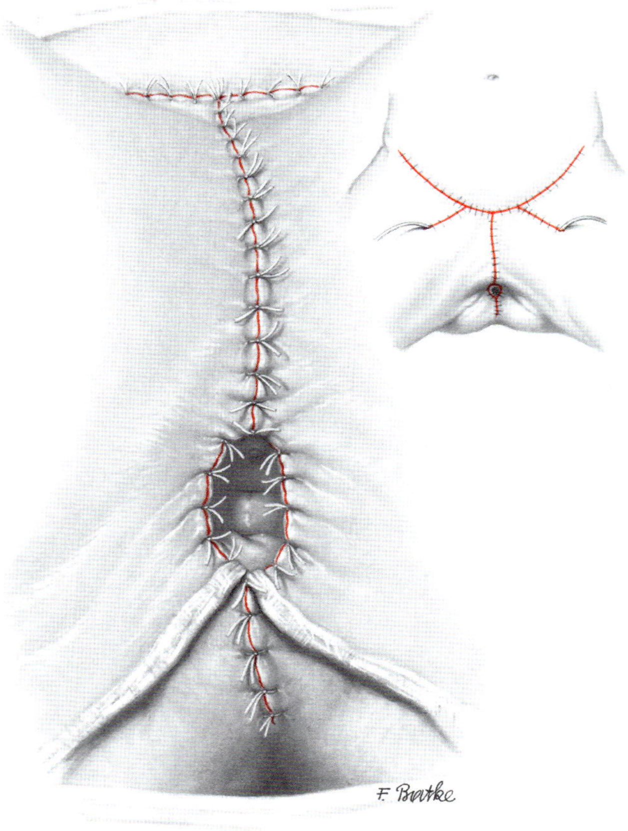

Figure 21.13. En bloc vulvectomy and inguinal lymphadenectomy. View after uniting the wound edges.

The skin edges at the inguinal region are joined at the thigh, at the anterior surface of the symphysis, at the vaginal introitus, and at the perineum with silk sutures.

The inguinal wound surfaces are cleansed with Redon drains that are brought out at the lowermost wound angles of the thigh. The genitofemoral sulcus is drained with Penrose drains.

Technical Problems—Figures 21.1–21.13

1. *Fatty lymph node removal* from the cranial border of the fossa ovalis *should not be continued in a caudal direction*. If this happens, the vessels coursing in the fossa ovalis just before emptying into the large vessels of the leg might be injured because the lower and lateral borders of the saphenous hiatus have not yet been exposed by dissection. It is preferable to discontinue any further dissection of the fatty lymph node tissue temporarily once the upper border of the fossa ovalis comes into view, continuing instead with the exposure of the saphenous vein. Only then should one mobilize the lower and lateral border of the fossa ovalis by caudal dissection.
2. In *locating and exposing the saphenous vein, it is possible to incise too deeply* and injure the fascia lata in the process. This can damage the femoral vein, particularly if one dissects deeply in the area lateral to the greater saphenous vein.
3. One *must not proceed too aggressively when dissecting the fossa ovalis*. In this stage of preparation, the tissue must be dissected carefully with tiny scissor cuts. Otherwise, the vessels coursing in the saphenous hiatus will be damaged.
4. Before dissecting the clitoris from the symphysis, the *inner circumcision wound above the urethral meatus must be deepened down to the pubic arch*. If this is not done, the urethra will not be well separated from the clitoris. As the clitoris is being dissected from the lower surface of the symphysis (which is always done in a craniocaudal direction), one might injure the urethra just below the pubic arch.
5. While covering the wound area, the *skin over the symphysis may be pulled together* caudally with too many interrupted transverse sutures. As a result, the external urethral meatus retracts into the depth of the wound and becomes accessible for catheterization only with difficulty. If one were to affix the vaginal wound edge above the urethral meatus to the skin located above it, the topography of the urethra will be maintained undisturbed.
6. *The skin and vaginal wound edges must not be united under tension*. If this is done, the sutures will cut through very soon, and the wound will dehisce. The same is true for joining the skin edges on the anterior surface of the symphysis. Complete closure should, therefore, not be forced to cover the large wound area, despite mobilization of the skin and the subcutaneous adipose tissue on the lower abdomen. Instead, one might perform a sliding flap plasty or cover the remaining wound surface in the presence of cleansed granulations about 6 weeks after the vulvectomy with a skin graft (Thiersch flap). The plastic vulva reconstruction is depicted in separate monographs[e,f].

[e] Knapstein PG, di Re F, di Saia P, Haller U, Serin B-U (eds). Malignancies of the vulva. New York: Thieme, 1991.

[f] Knapstein PG, Friedberg V. Plastische Chirurgie. Stuttgart: Thieme, 1987.

Superficial Inguinal Lymphadenectomy via a Triple Incision

TECHNIQUE

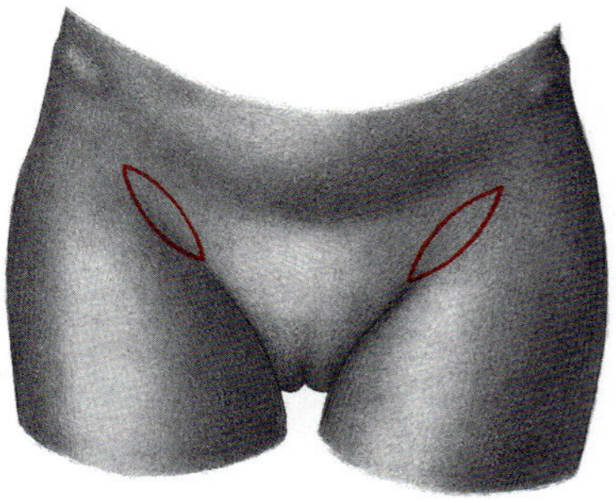

Figure 21.14. Superficial inguinal lymphadenectomy.

Outlining the spindle-shaped skin region in the groin.

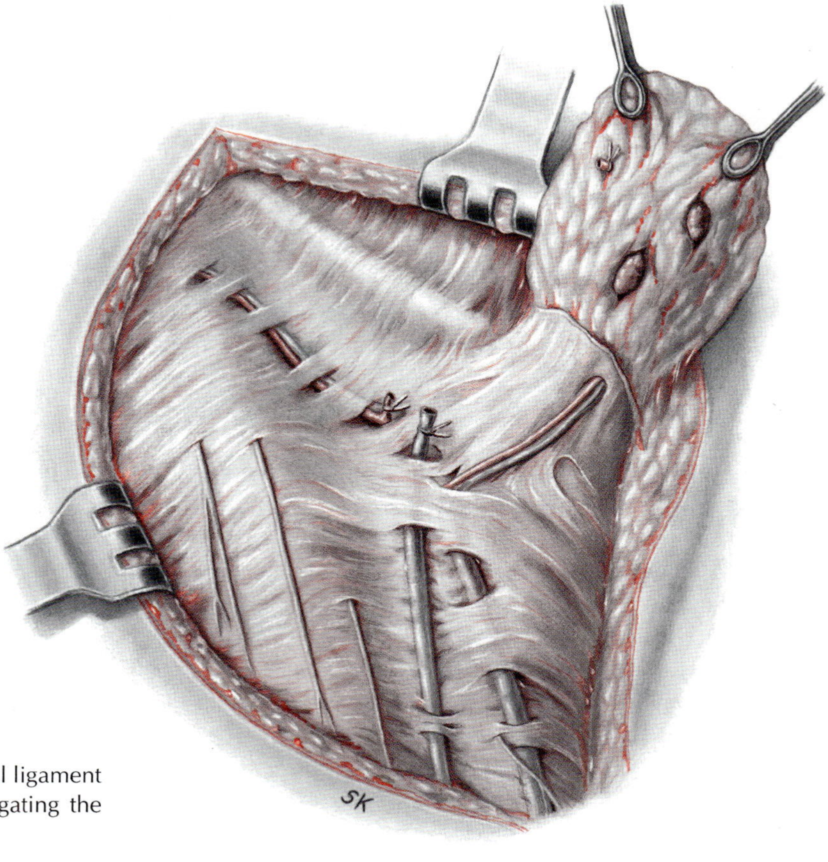

Figure 21.15. Superficial inguinal lymphadenectomy.

Dissecting the fatty node-bearing tissues from the inguinal ligament downward and from lateral to medial. Exposing and ligating the superficial vessels (cf. Fig. A.42).

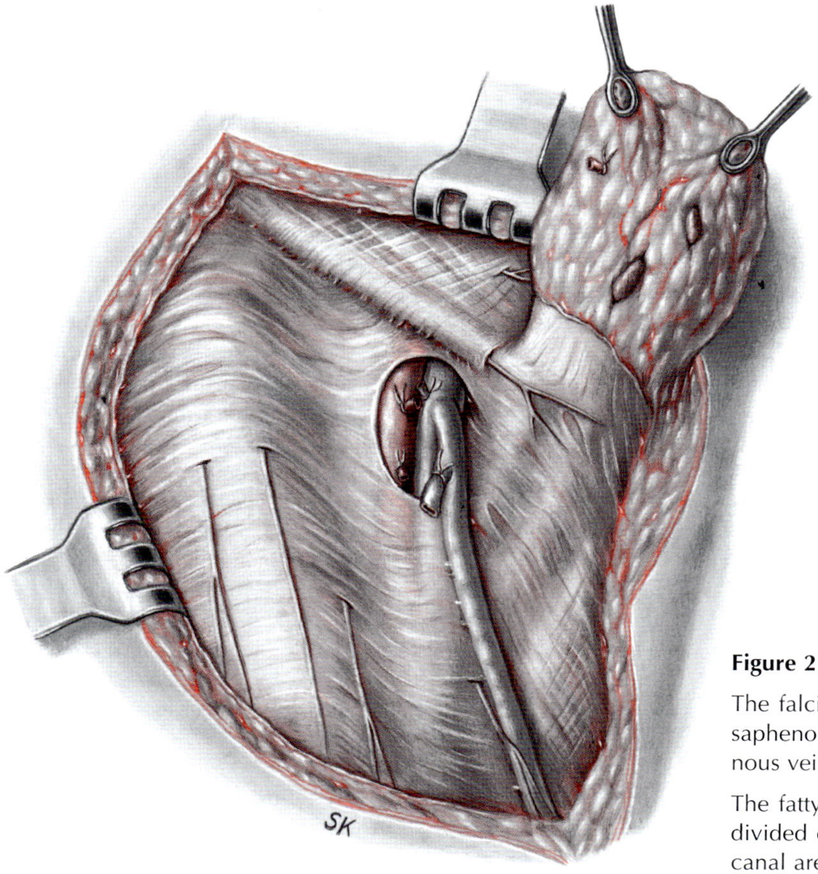

Figure 21.16. Superficial inguinal lymphadenectomy.

The falciform margin is exposed, as is the juncture of the greater saphenous vein with the femoral vein. The lateral accessory saphenous vein is ligated.

The fatty lymph node bundle, pediculated medially, can now be divided over a clamp. The deep lymph nodes within the femoral canal are left intact.

22/ Schauta-Amreich Radical Vaginal Hysterectomy

Indications

General Aspects

1. When treating carcinoma of uterine cervix stage 1b, a 5-year cure outlook of 87% is reached with a radical vaginal operation without lymphadenectomy.
2. Because the Schauta-Amreich procedure causes considerably less stress than the Wertheim method, it can be performed on women of advanced age.
3. The parametria may be resected at the same level vaginally as they are abdominally. Resection of the vagina as far as deemed necessary may be performed vaginally without difficulty.
4. Dissection of the ureter can be just as gentle with the Schauta-Amreich procedure as with the Wertheim.
5. General postoperative problems are almost nonexistent with the Schauta-Amreich procedure. We are continually surprised how quickly patients recuperate from the vaginal radical operation.

''Schauta'' vs. ''Wertheim''

Vienna is the cradle of the two procedures that typify surgical treatments of cervical carcinoma worldwide. Friedrich Schauta (University-Clinic for Women, Vienna) and Ernst Wertheim (University-Clinic for Women, Vienna) were neighbors. Their surgical procedures at first were in competition because each had a completely different approach to treatment of regional lymph nodes. Schauta (1904, 1908) refrained from removing the regional lymph nodes; he viewed the reduced surgical risk as one advantage of his method. Wertheim (1911), in contrast, at first always removed the lymph nodes during abdominal carcinoma surgery. But long-term results for women with cancerous lymph nodes were disappointing; despite the fact that their nodes were routinely removed, the primary mortality rate increased. Wertheim then substituted the obligatory lymph node removal with a node search where only enlarged lymph nodes were removed. However, this did not result in an improved cure rate.

The advance of radiation therapy during the subsequent years pushed the surgical approach to therapy for cervical carcinoma into the background. In 1913 Wertheim planned a definitive paper for the German Gynecology Congress in Halle an der Saale. In it he discussed a surgical method he had developed for treating carcinoma of the uterine cervix. However, Wertheim withdrew his paper after he heard about the extraordinary success rate of intracavitary thorium and radium. To make matters worse, A. Doederlein approached Wertheim at the congress and with a hearty pat on Wertheim's shoulders announced: ''My dear Wertheim, you are now a historic relic, your operation will no longer be performed!''

Scientific development, however, soon advanced in a different direction. Vaginal and abdominal operations returned because long-term effects of radiation therapy for positive lymph nodes were poor at the time. Moreover, technical improvements in anesthesiology and blood transfusions eventually allowed a more radical approach to surgery.

In case of carcinoma of the cervix, primary mortality rates and permanent results (5-year cure rate) were the sole deciding factors in the choice of a radical operation. In 1950 Amreich, a student under Schauta's direction, noted that Wertheim and Schauta in 1914 achieved identical results: the same percentage of 5-year survivals (36.6%). But he could not explain this surprising correlation. After all, one would expect far better results from the radical abdominal method, which included removal of metastasized lymph nodes, than from the radical vaginal method alone, where the regional pelvic lymph nodes were not considered. This led Amreich to conclude as late as 1950 that there must be previously unknown anatomical relationships in the regional lymphatic system of the pelvis.

In 1955 Navratil discovered that in cases of cervical carcinoma stage 1b, in which approximately 20% of the regional lymph node stations were affected, removal of the regional lymph nodes did not affect cure results significantly. Among 48 cases of cervical carcinoma stage 1b, on which he used primarily the Schauta-Amreich procedure, Navratil performed an abdominal extraperitoneal, preferably radical, pelvic lower para-aortic lymphadenectomy subsequent to the procedure and found that results did not improve. Consequently the use of an extraperitoneal lymphadenectomy as a supplemental procedure to a vaginal radical Schauta-Amreich operation was no longer used after this series.

Rauscher and Spurny from Antoine's clinic demonstrated in an often-quoted paper published in 1956 that only an insignificant difference exists in the 5-year cure rate regardless of whether the obligatory lymphadenectomy is used. This prompted Antoine to postulate that lymphadenectomy was overrated while the rest of the operation, especially the vaginal cuff and parametrium, was somewhat neglected. In 1961 Anselmino, a Schauta surgeon who excluded lymphadenectomies, claimed he could nearly duplicate the results of hospitals that preferred the Wertheim method (Meigs 1956; Antoine, Navratil 1957). Since then, innumerable papers have been published on this subject; they cannot be detailed here. Antoine believed that it must be a matter of luck in each case whether one could remove every carcinomatous node. This should not lead to a final judgment about the value of a lymphadenectomy, but it prompted Amreich in 1951 to advocate in-depth study of Reiffenstuhl's work on the anatomical conditions of the pelvic lymphatic system.

For anatomical representation of draining lymphatic pathways of the uterus, Reiffenstuhl used bodies of stillborn infants. A Paris blue celloidin solution was injected into the portion of the uterine vaginal cervix (portio vaginalis uteri) of 35 specimens, and their now clearly visible draining lymphatic pathways as well as regional lymph node stations were viewed under the microscope. (Using fully grown bodies for injection experiments was not recommended because then it was no longer possible to fully present the lymphatic uterine vessels and their

---

Sources of illustrations:

Figures 22.1–22.4. Reiffenstuhl G. The lymphatic system of the female genitalia. Munich: Urban & Schwarzenberg, 1957.

Figure 22.5. Reiffenstuhl G. The pelvic lymph nodes of a case of multiple myeloma. Zbl Gynecol 1956;78:79.

Figures 22.6–22.22. Reiffenstuhl G. The lymph node problem with carcinoma colli uteri. Munich: Urban & Schwarzenberg, 1967.

pathways connecting them to the regional lymph nodes. This may be explained with the changes that have already taken place in their connective tissue.) The results of these experiments were publicized extensively in 1957 (Reiffenstuhl G. The lymphatic system of the female genitalia. Munich: Urban & Schwarzenberg, 1957).

Draining lymphatics of the uterine cervix, with few exceptions, follow the course of the blood vessels flowing to the lymph nodes at the pelvic wall. Figure 22.1 depicts 10 lymph node groups combined, all of which are primary pathways from the uterine cervix. Pathways 8–10 (outlined in boldface on Fig. 21.1) lead to those lymph node groups that are most often reached by lymphatics of the uterine cervix.

Note that some of the inferior gluteal lymph nodes located near the ischial spine (collecting channel 10) are hidden behind large blood vessels—at the location where the inferior gluteal artery and the internal pudendal artery pass through the true pelvis via the sciatic foramen.

The detailed course of the cervical lymphatics and the hidden position of important regional nodes are illustrated in Figures 22.1–22.5.

Lymph node removal using the Wertheim method and its modifications (i.e., Wertheim-Meigs, Latzko, Okabayashi) is performed in different treatment centers to a variable extent, but all discuss a ''radical'' removal of the regional lymph nodes of the cervix. Even though generally only the hypogastric, obturator, external, and communal iliac lymph nodes are removed, some surgeons extend the lymphadenectomy to the aortic lymph nodes or at least parts of them. The superior gluteal and sacral lymph nodes are removed only in isolated cases, and then only partially; this is never performed routinely. *The inferior gluteal lymph nodes are left in place.* These nodes cannot be made visible at the pelvic wall even with lymphangiography using oil based iodine stains or with radioactive technetium.

As a general rule, inguinal nodes are divided into superficial and deep nodes (Figs. 21.2–21.7).

The *superficial* inguinal nodes (n = 8–10), lie immediately beneath the skin. They can be divided into two groups:

- An upper horizontal group, placed along Poupart's ligament; they communicate with lymphatic vessels from the vulva, clitoris, urethra, and skin of the perineum;
- A superficial group coursing in a vertical direction (n = 8–5) surrounding the termination of the great saphenous vein that predominantly receives superficial lymphatics of the lower extremities but also a few of those of the vulva and the anus.

The *deep* inguinal nodes (n = 5–8) lie in the femoral triangle (fossa ovalis) on the fascia of the iliopsoas muscle; they are separated from the superficial inguinal nodes by the fascia lata. The uppermost node of this lymph node chain lies deep in the femoral canal; this is known as Cloquet's or Rosenmüller's node.

Lymphatics of the superficial inguinal nodes perforate the fascia lata as well as the cribriform fascia and drain into the deep nodes. Subsequent drainage flows into the pelvic nodes.

In adult patients, superficial and deep inguinal nodes are dissected free by removing the subcutaneous inguinal fatty tissue as well as the cribriform fascia and bisecting the fascia lata laterally. *After applying a staining solution directly to the superficial inguinal lymph nodes (Reiffenstuhl), one can observe three drainage pathways* to the pelvic lymph nodes (Figs. 22.6–22.8).

- *First pathway:* numerous efferent vessels of the inguinal lymph nodes course *laterally from the femoral vein* through the lateral aspect of the lacuna vasorum into the pelvis (see 1 in Figs. 22.6–22.8), turn upward along the exterior and posterior side of iliac artery, and drain into the superficial and deep lateral external iliac nodes (see 16 in Fig. 22.8); from there, lymph flows to the common iliac nodes and after that to the aortic nodes.
- *Second pathway:* numerous efferent vessels of the inguinal nodes course *upward along the femoral vein*, reach the femoral ring nodes (see 11 in Fig. 22.8), and drain, in most cases, into the medial external iliac nodes (14); from there, numerous lymphatic vessels course to the obturator (4) and hypogastric (5) nodes and also to the like-named nodes located on the lateral side of the external iliac artery (16).
- *Third pathway:* numerous efferent vessels of the inguinal nodes turn upward *medially to the femoral vein* (see 3 in Figs. 22.6–22.8) and enter the pelvis at the most medial aspect of the lacuna vasorum; they course past the femoral ring nodes (see 11 in Fig. 22.8) and drain into the obturator and inferior gluteal nodes (7).

During lymphangiography using the Kinmonth method, the stain applied to the dorsum of the foot is first absorbed by the lymphatic vessels of the leg and then transported to the inguinal nodes. It drains into the nodes of the vertical tract and then flows along the path of least resistance (most of the efferent vessels of the vertical tract course to the lateral group of the horizontal tract of the inguinal nodes) *only on the first and second pathway* (Figs. 22.7 and 22.8) along the large blood vessels of the pelvic wall to the obturator, external iliac, communal iliac, and aortic lymph node groups. *The third pathway is not depicted from the dorsum of the foot.*

It is understandable after these studies that a preoperative marking of the lower gluteal lymph nodes is not possible with the often used Kinmonth method of lymphangiography. The following quote illuminates F. diRe's position on this subject: ''Even lymphangiography is not sufficiently accurate in determining the status of the inguinofemoral nodes on account of the difficulty in obtaining complete visualization of lymph nodes in the inguinal area. Only one to four superficial nodes can be detected well, although an accuracy of 85% should be achievable in detecting pelvic nodes.''

The inferior gluteal nodes can only be made visible before surgery by directly applying a contrast medium to a node in the medial group of the inguinal node's horizontal tract (method of Reiffenstuhl). Lymphangiographic examinations (Reiffenstuhl direct inguinal lymphangiography) supplement and confirm anatomical knowledge of inguinal lymphatic drainage (Figs. 22.9–22.20).

Success rates for lymphadenectomy performed along with the Wertheim radical operation are thus significantly lowered because the inferior gluteal nodes, which are often affected with carcinoma of the cervix, cannot be removed. To remove these lymph nodes (which lie alongside and partially behind the inferior gluteal artery, the internal pudendal artery, and their accompanying veins), one would have to resect the large blood vessels of the pelvic wall all the way to their exit from the true pelvis (see also Fig. 22.5). Even though it is technically possible to dissect free the large arteries all the way to the sciatic foramen, the presence of the thin-walled, easily injured veins does not allow this procedure on living patients without running a significant risk for hemorrhage. In fact, the inferior gluteal nodes are not visible to the surgeon during the entire abdominal radical operation and can therefore not be removed! In this regard, nothing has changed to this date.

One may begin with the assumption that the gluteopudendal nodes, which act as an important regional lymphatic station with carcinoma of the cervix, cannot be removed during the Wertheim operation without danger of a massive hemorrhage. Therefore carcinomatous lymph nodes remain in many cases, which might later clinically manifest themselves in this region as ''lymph node metastases.''

A scientific paper from 1962 confirms this fact. Figure 22.21 depicts the localities of lymph node metastases (i.e., positive lymph nodes) from 70 patients who underwent the Wertheim procedure with a radical lymphadenectomy. They were compared with ''recurrences'' (Fig. 22.22) among 35 patients whose carcinomatous nodes had been removed during the radical operation. These supposed recurrences were observed almost exclusively in the region of the inferior gluteal nodes (so-called pelvic wall recurrence), which already contained carcinomatous cells, almost certainly, at the time the Wertheim procedure was performed. That means the inferior gluteal nodes that had not been removed contained true lymph node metastases. These women died later from carcinoma metastases that existed (but had not been detected) before the operation was performed. This proves that the Wertheim procedure did not achieve surgical removal of all regional lymph nodes affected by carcinoma of the cervix!

Furthermore, in the abdominal radical operation of cervical carcinoma, suppose that one proceeds on the false premise that all regional lymph nodes of the cervix, including the lower gluteal nodes, may be removed. In that case, one should expect significantly better 5-year cure rates than those achieved with the radical vaginal procedure. The clinic reports the following on this subject.

In 1985 Noda reported a 5-year cure rate of 88.8%, among 30,000 cases of patients in stage 1b after undergoing the Wertheim-Okajashi procedure for carcinoma of the cervix. Glitsch (personal observations) achieved a 5-year cure rate of 87% using the Wertheim-Latzkosch radioisotope radical operation on patients suffering from carcinoma of the cervix stage 1b. We achieved a 5-year cure rate of 87% using the Schauta-Amreich procedure (Reiffenstuhl) while treating more than 300 cases of patients with cervical carcinoma stage 1b.

Schauta and Amreich asserted that the ''radical lymphadenectomy'' allows only partial, but not complete, removal of the regional lymph nodes of cervical carcinoma. That they were correct is confirmed by the three almost identical incidences of 5-year cures in stage 1b just cited. Additional evidence is provided by the fact that in cases of carcinomatous nodes removed during the Wertheim procedure the ''recurrence'' occurred predominantly in the region of the ischial spine (the region of the lower gluteal nodes). The conditions and cure results described here have been confirmed by numerous European, American, and Japanese publications up to 1994.

These data justify the choice of the vaginal approach in cases of stage 1b cervical carcinoma after careful preoperative histological confirmation of lack of metastases to these areas.

The clinic teaches that the incidence of pelvic wall failure can be reduced only marginally by the abdominal radical operation even though consensus has not been reached in the medical community—the anatomy is the reason. The value of a laparoscopic pelvic and lower aortic lymphadenectomy in connection with the Schauta-Amreich procedure remains to be seen. This applies also to an extraperitoneal lymphadenectomy performed with a Purandase incision. We reach this conclusion after carefully examining the anatomical illustrations depicting the location of regional lymph node stations of the cervix. Some are found behind the blood vessels of the false pelvis and cannot be removed without danger, even by laparotomy (Wertheim procedure).

The Schauta-Amreich procedure is considerably less traumatic for the patient than the Wertheim method and may be performed at an advanced age (the oldest patient undergoing the Schauta-Amreich procedure was 86; she survived the procedure without any complications). This method allows a more radical removal of the vaginal cuff in addition to an at least equal extensive resection of the parametria. Furthermore, there are fewer severe postoperative complications than are observed with the abdominal approach. Of course, up to a certain degree this result depends on the surgeon's skill.

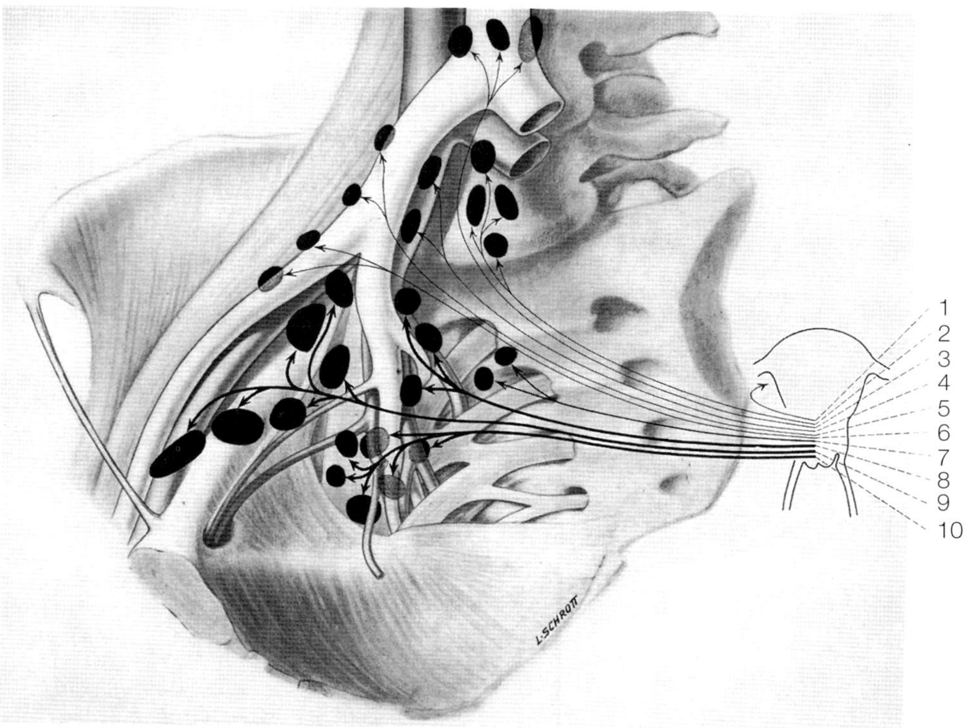

Figure 22.1. The regional lymph node groups of the uterine cervix.

Pathways 8–10 are boldface because they lead to those regional lymph nodes that are used most often by the lymphatics of the cervix. Despite that fact, we must also consider that carcinoma cells may reach the lymphatics of the pelvis via tracts 1–7, unless there has been prior interruption.

1 to pararectal nodes
2 to subaortic (promontori) lymph nodes
3 to aortic lymph nodes
4 to medial common iliac lymph nodes
5 to lateral common iliac lymph nodes
6 to lateral external iliac lymph nodes
7 to sacral lymph nodes
8 to superior gluteal lymph nodes
9 to internal iliac lymph nodes (hypogastric and obturator)
10 to inferior gluteal lymph nodes

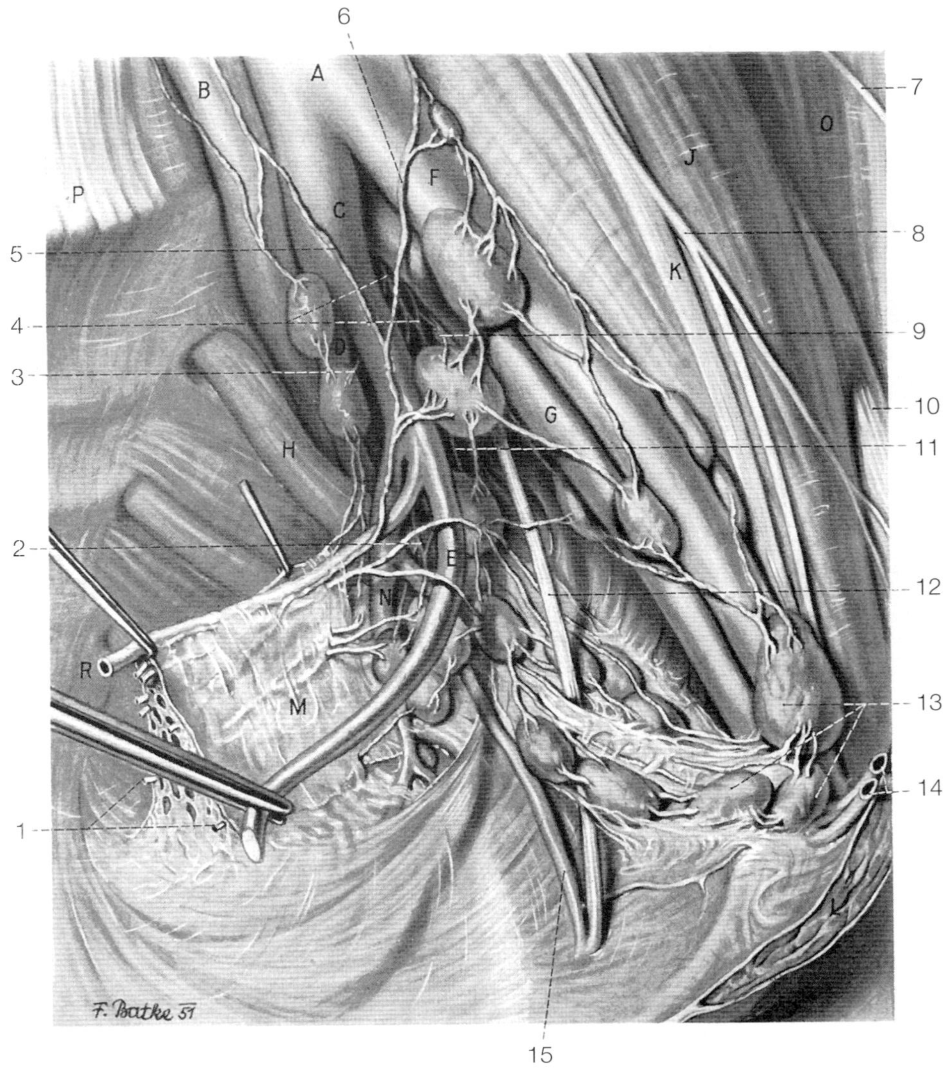

A common iliac artery
B common iliac vein
C internal iliac artery
D superior gluteal artery
E lateral umbilical ligament
F external iliac artery
G external iliac vein
H sacral nerve I
J psoas major muscle
K psoas minor muscle (tendon)
L abdominal internal and transverse oblique muscles
M Mackenrodt's ligament
N inferior gluteal artery
O iliac muscle
P promontory
R uterine artery
1 cervical lymphatic vessels
2 efferent lymphatic vessels
3 efferent lymphatic vessel
4 efferent lymphatic vessels
5 cervical lymphatic vessel
6 cervical lymphatic vessel
7 lateral femoral cutaneous nerve
8 genitofemoral nerve
9 lateral deep external iliac lymph node
10 femoral nerve
11 efferent vessel
12 obturator nerve
13 femoral ring lymph nodes
14 inferior epigastric vessels
15 obturator artery

Figure 22.2. Lymph drainage of uterine cervix.

View of the anterior surface of the Mackenrodt's ligament (M) previously separated from the uterus.

The triangular incision surface of the Mackenrodt's ligament demonstrates that its base is wider and that it is bordered by the uterine artery (R) on its upper edge. The ureter has been removed; the lateral umbilical ligament (E) was pulled medially; and the obturator nerve (12) remained in situ.

Numerous lymphatic vessels accompany the uterine artery and join the internal iliac nodes. Individual lymphatics of the cervix course past the internal iliac nodes, turn medially (5), and finally reach the medial side of the common iliac artery (A). Other lymphatic pathways of the cervix (6) cross the external iliac artery (F) without interruption and then reach the nodes located on the lateral surface of the common iliac artery. Additional lymphatic vessels of the cervix course alongside the uterine artery (they were pulled from behind with a small hook) to the pelvic wall and drain into the superior gluteal nodes where the like-named artery (D) branches from the internal iliac artery (C).

In the deeper sections of Mackenrodt's ligament, lymphatics of the cervix (1) course to the inferior gluteal nodes that occupy the sides of the pelvic wall caudally to the obturator artery (15). These nodes are partially obstructed by the lateral umbilical ligament, and some have not yet been removed from the base of the Mackenrodt's ligament.

The femoral ring nodes (13) connect with the nodes in the obturator fossa (they surround the like-named nerve from medial and lateral) as well as with the nodes located along the external iliac artery and vein. Note the deep drainage canals (2, 11, 4) that come from the inferior gluteal and internal iliac nodes, cross under the parietal blood vessels, and reach this group's deep nodes from behind the common iliac vessels.

A rectum
B uterus (intestinal surface)
C Mackenrodt's ligament (medial part)
D sacral nerve I
E piriform muscle
F internal iliac artery
G external iliac artery
H external iliac vein
J psoas muscle
K promontory
L Mackenrodt's ligament (posterior fascia)
1 cervical lymphatic vessels
2 rectouterine ligament
3 cervical lymphatic vessels
4 cervical lymphatic vessels
5 sacral lymph nodes
6 rectum
7 subaortic (promontory) lymph nodes
8 medial common iliac lymph node
9 cervical lymphatic vessels
10 efferent vessels
11 superior gluteal lymph nodes
12 efferent vessels
13 efferent vessels
14 ureter
15 lateral umbilical ligament
16 obturator nerve
17 uterine artery
18 obturator artery

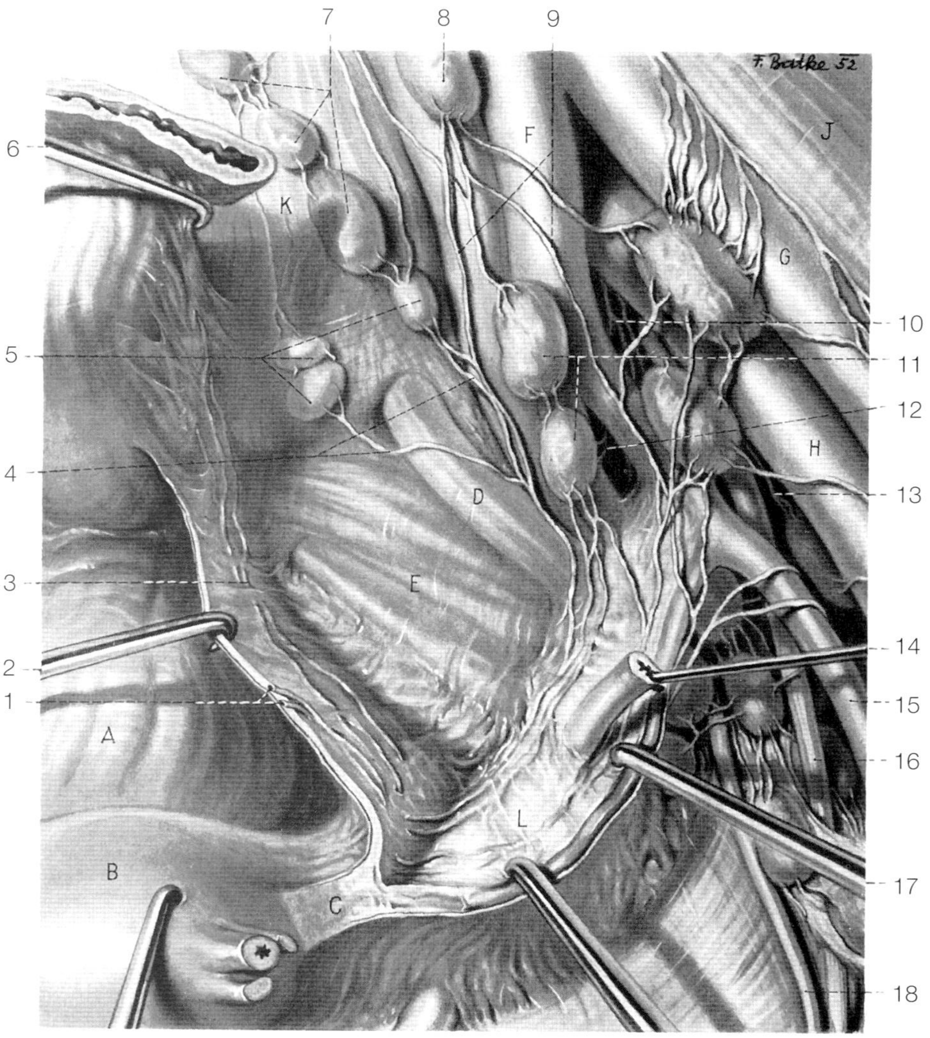

Figure 22.3. Lymph drainage of the uterine cervix to the rectum and pelvic wall.

The uterus (B) and uterine artery (17) are pulled forward. View of the posterior surface of the Mackenrodt's ligament (L). Ureter has been severed.

The sagittal rectal pillar (2) has been separated from the pelvic wall and pulled aside with hooks. Its surface originates from the posterior area of Mackenrodt's ligament.

Several lymphatics of the cervix (3) course to the rectum through the sagittal rectal pillar (2) and drain into the nodes behind it (superior rectal nodes). Some (1) move upward into the ureter leaf.

Those among the lymphatics of the cervix that drain into the superior gluteal nodes (11) course ventrally in the Mackenrodt's ligament (L) and dorsally upward from the ureter (14). Some of these lymphatics (4) turn toward the sacrum at the level where the superior gluteal artery takes off medially and reach the sacral nodes (5) as regional nodes. Other lymphatics of the cervix (9) course past the superior gluteal nodes and are interrupted for the first time by a medial common iliac node (8).

Note especially the deep drainage canals (12, then 10) coming from the superior gluteal and internal iliac nodes that course upward behind the parietal blood vessels to finally drain into the lateral deep common iliac nodes.

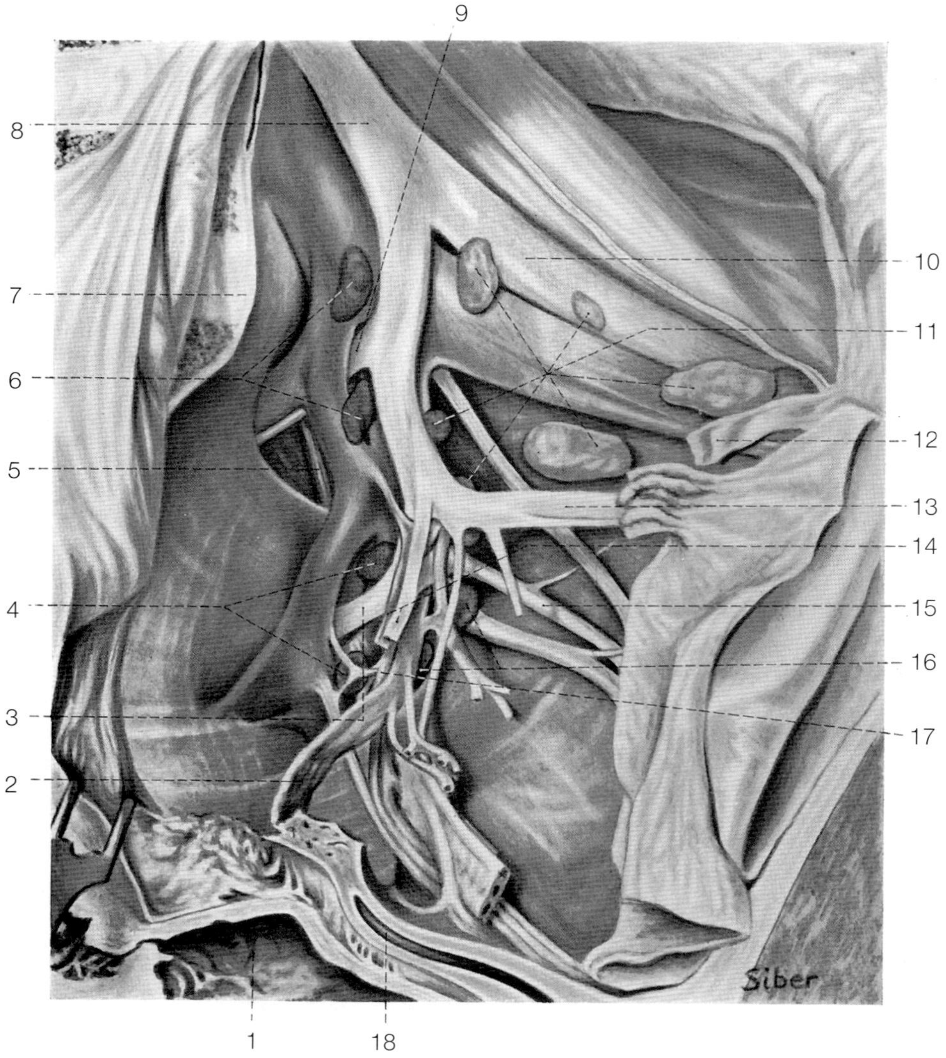

Figure 22.4. Position of caudal pelvic lymph nodes in relationship to parietal blood vessels.

Medial view of the left half of the pelvis split sagittally. The visceral pelvic blood vessels have been severed close to their exit from the vessels of the false pelvic wall. The wound surface of the rectum (1) and the vagina (18) are visible.

The superior gluteal nodes (6) are grouped around the beginning portion of the superior gluteal artery (9). A few of the internal iliac nodes (11) are found in the space between the large iliac blood vessels all the way back to the obturator artery (15).

The inferior gluteal nodes (4, 16) are particularly distinguished by their locations; they are partially hidden behind the blood vessels and reach down to the sciatic foramen. There they lie medial and lateral to the point where the internal pudendal artery exits from the true pelvis (17), close to the ischial spine.

1 rectum
2 Mackenrodt's ligament (inferior part) (hypogastric and obturator)
3 inferior gluteal artery
4 inferior gluteal lymph nodes
5 sacral nerve I
6 superior gluteal lymph nodes
7 promontory
8 common iliac artery
9 superior gluteal artery
10 external iliac artery
11 internal iliac lymph nodes
12 round ligament
13 lateral umbilical ligament
14 uterine artery and vein
15 obturator artery
16 inferior gluteal lymph nodes
17 internal pudendal artery
18 vagina

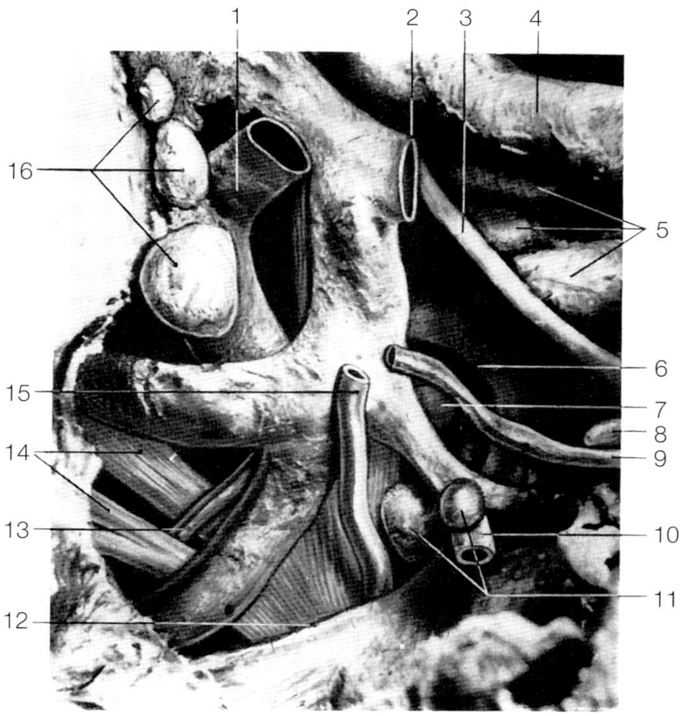

Figure 22.5. Medial view of the left pelvic wall of an adult. Cause of death was lymphoma.

The stem of the hypogastric artery (internal iliac) and the external iliac vein have been resected. In addition, numerous drainage veins of the uterovaginal plexus were removed. The piriform muscle has been removed to allow clearer orientation and a better view of the sacral nerves.

On this preparation, the inferior gluteal artery originates from the superior gluteal artery. Two nodes (11) occupy the place where the internal pudendal artery exit; an additional node (7) is found more cranially in the greater sciatic foramen. Three nodes (16) can be seen by the superior gluteal artery; several internal iliac (hypogastric) nodes are grouped around the obturator node (5,8) and reach cranially to beneath the external iliac artery and vein.

1 superior gluteal artery
2 external iliac vein (incision edge)
3 obturator nerve
4 external iliac artery
5 internal iliac (obturator) lymph nodes
6 sciatic notch
7 inferior gluteal lymph node
8 obturator lymph node
9 obturator artery
10 branch of uterovaginal venous plexus
11 inferior gluteal lymph nodes
12 sacrospinal ligament
13 inferior gluteal artery
14 sacral nerves I and II
15 internal pudendal artery
16 superior gluteal lymph nodes

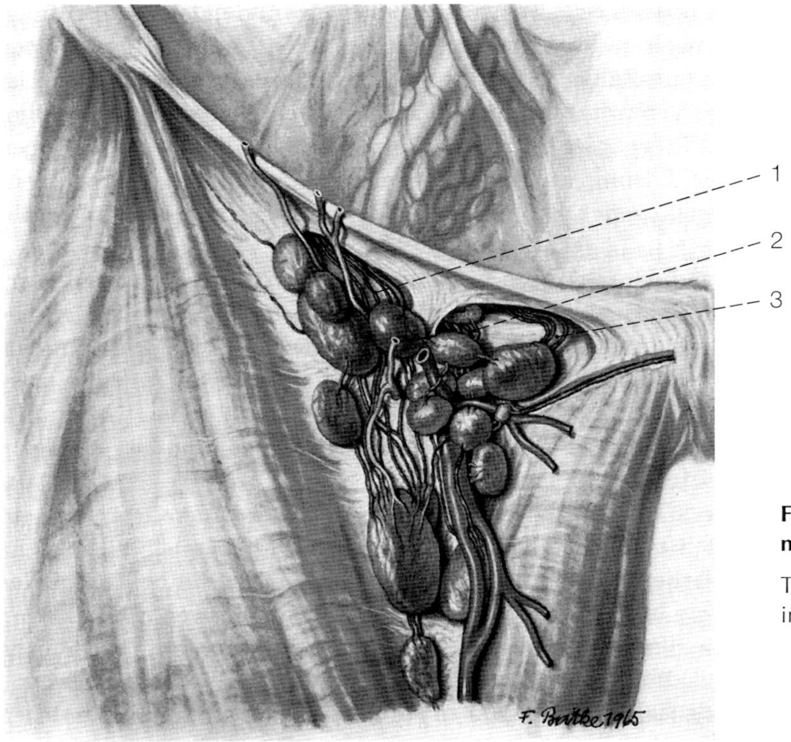

Figure 22.6. Inguinal lymph drainage over right inguinal nodes.

Three major pathways drain the lymph from the inguinal nodes into the pelvis:

1 lymph drainage to lateral external iliac nodes
2 lymph drainage to median external iliac nodes
3 lymph drainage to obturator and gluteal nodes.

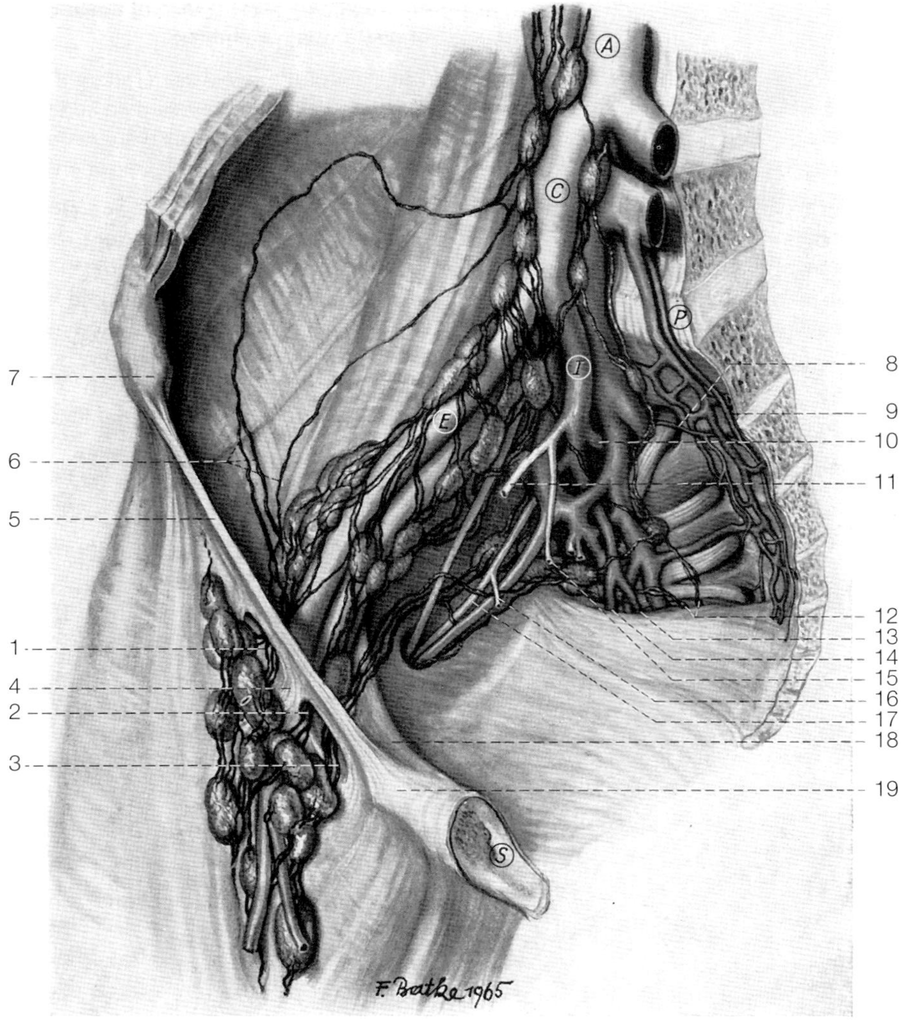

Figure 22.7. Connecting pathways between inguinal lymph nodes and pelvic lymph nodes (1, 2, 3).

A aorta
C common iliac artery
E external iliac artery
I internal iliac artery
P promontory
S symphysis

1 lateral path to lateral external iliac nodes and common iliac nodes
2 medial path to medial external iliac and hypogastric nodes
3 medial path to obturator and inferior gluteal nodes
4 pathways of adventitia to the fascia
5 inguinal ligament
6 circumventing pathways from inguinal, or external iliac, to the common iliac lymph nodes
7 superior anterior iliac spine
8 lateral sacral artery
9 medial sacral artery
10 superior gluteal artery
11 lateral umbilical ligament
12 lymphatic pathways to gluteal region
13 inferior gluteal artery
14 internal pudendal artery
15 uterine artery
16 inferior vesical artery
17 obturator artery
18 superior ramus of the os pubis
19 pubic tubercle

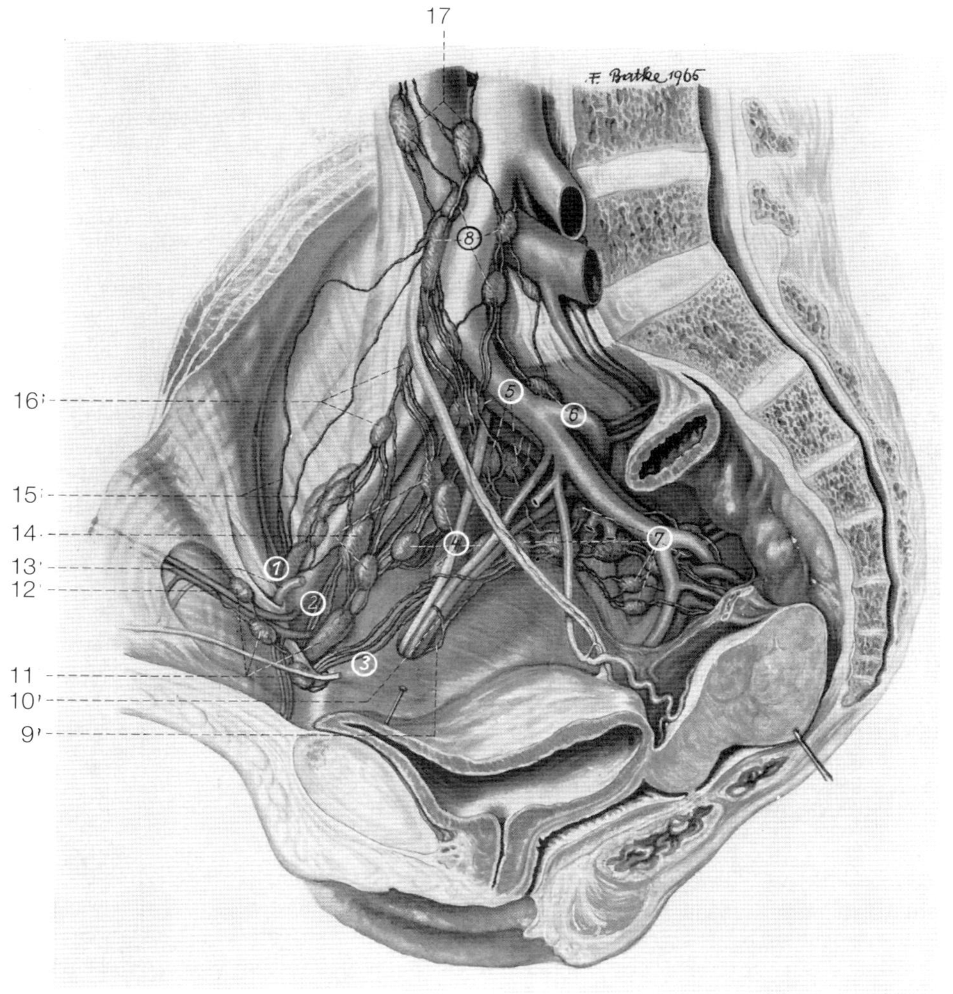

Figure 22.8. Inguinal lymph drainage in humans. Median-sagittal section of the pelvis.

View of right half of the pelvis. The efferent vessels of the inguinal nodes enter the pelvis via three major pathways (1, 2, 3).

1 lymph drainage to lateral external iliac nodes
2 lymph drainage to medial external iliac nodes
3 lymph drainage to obturator nodes and inferior gluteal nodes
4 obturator nodes
5 hypogastric nodes
6 superior gluteal nodes
7 inferior gluteal nodes
8 medial and lateral common iliac nodes
9 lymphatics through obturator foramen
10 connecting lymphatic pathway
11 femoral ring nodes
12 inferior epigastric artery and vein
13 round ligament
14 medial external iliac nodes
15 circumventing lymphatic pathways from the inguinal (or lateral external iliac) nodes to the lateral common iliac nodes (or aortic nodes)
16 lateral external iliac nodes (superficial)
17 aortic nodes

Case 1.

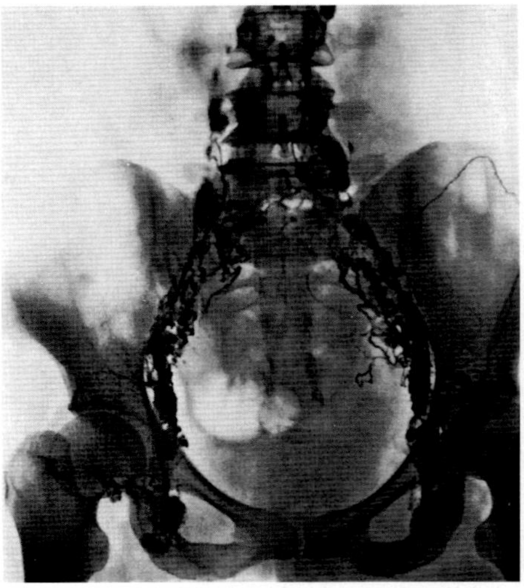

Figure 22.9. Lymphangiography (Reiffenstuhl method), case 1. Lymphangiogram, anteroposterior view.

30-year old woman; cervical cancer IIb; 10 ml oily contrast medium have been injected bilaterally into the medial inguinal nodes of the horizontal group (Figs. 22.9 and 22.10).

The pelvic lymphatic nodes are for the most part projected on top of each other. A dilated lymphatic vessel can be recognized on the left pelvic bone next to the filled pelvic lymphatics; it connects the *distal external iliac with the common iliac nodes.*

Results. Pelvic lymphatics are completely filled by injecting the contrast medium into a medial inguinal node. The pelvic nodes are partially projected on top of one another in anteroposterior radiographs; their true size can only be highlighted by taking radiographs from a lateral angle. A dilated vessel is found between the external iliac and common iliac nodes that courses laterally along the pelvic bone.

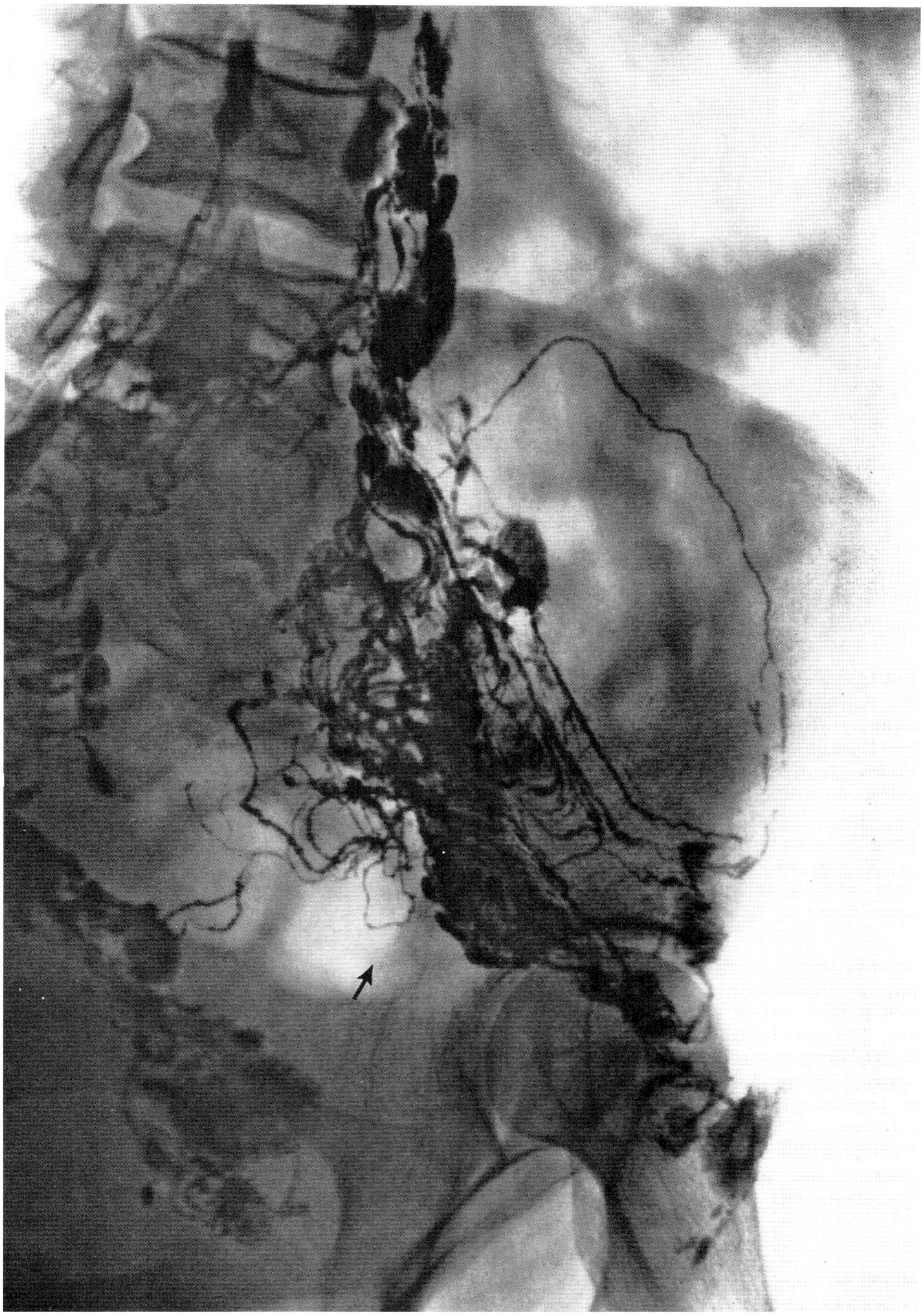

Figure 22.10. Case 1. Lymphangiogram, lateral view.

View of left pelvic wall. Lymphatic network situated along the pelvic blood vessels is particularly well depicted. Note dilated lymphatic vessels overlying the pelvic bone, lymphatic pathways alongside the external iliac vessel, dense lymphatic network in the obturator fossa, lymphatic pathways reaching to the sciatic foramen, and sacrum. *Arrow*, ischial spine.

Only the lateral radiographic view allows us to recognize the true topographic location of the pelvic lymphatic pathways and nodes. We could demonstrate all these pathways by injecting contrast medium into a left medial inguinal node on the horizontal tract.

Case 2.

42-year old woman, vaginal cancer, very obese; 8 ml Lipiodol ultrafluid have been injected bilaterally into a medial inguinal node on the horizontal tract (Figs. 22.11–22.13).

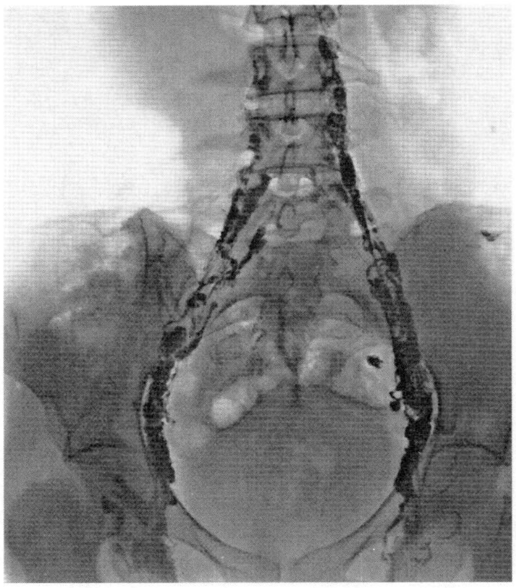

Figure 22.11. Case 2. Lymphangiogram. Filling phase. Anteroposterior view. Lymphatics have been filled to L2.

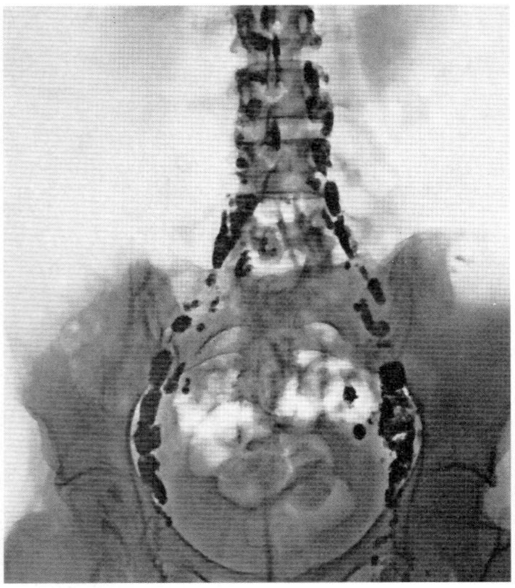

Figure 22.12. Case 2. Lymphangiogram. Nodal phase. Anteroposterior view.

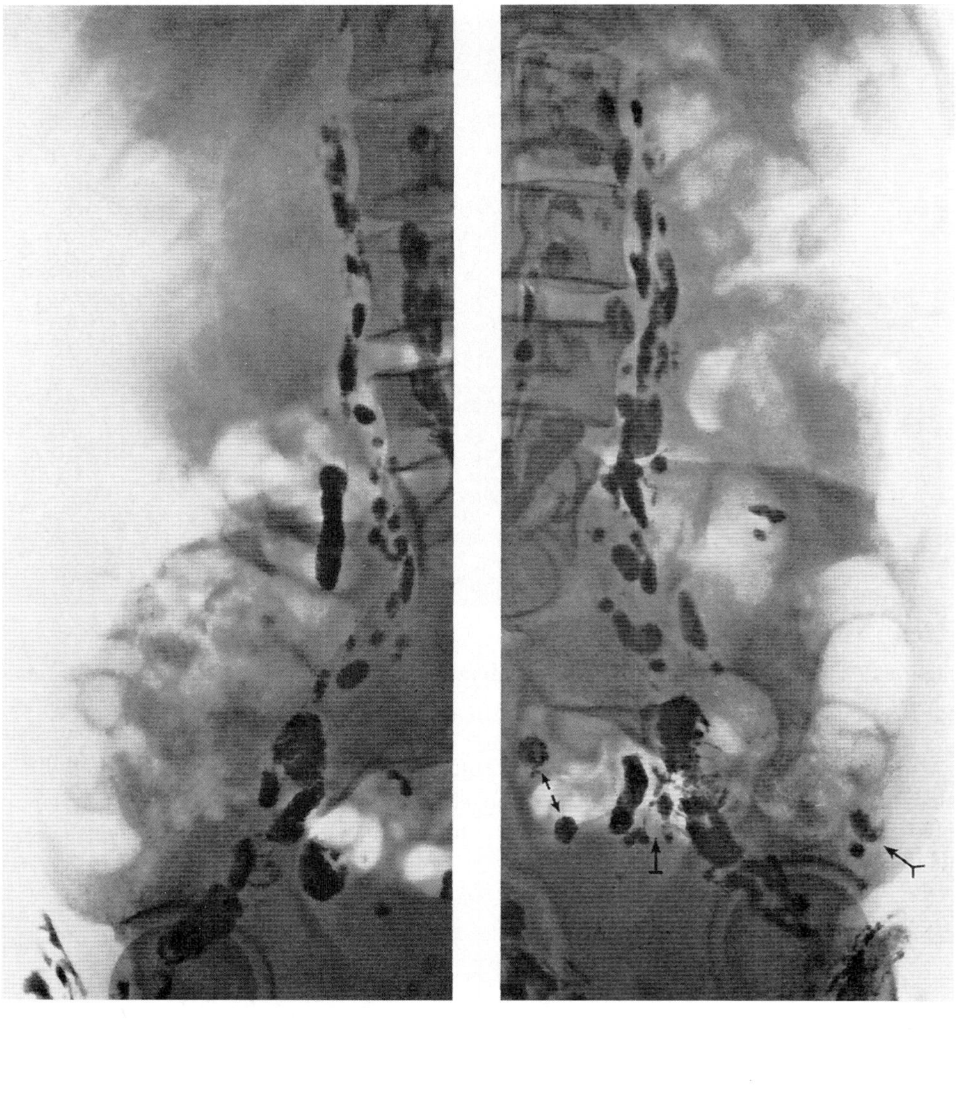

Figure 22.13. Case 2. Lymphangiograms, nodal phase, lateral view, showing right (*left*) and left (*right*) pelvic wall.

Right, note location of gluteal (↕), obturator (↑), and external iliac (↖) nodes on left pelvic side wall.

Case 3.

44-year old woman, cervical cancer 1b, obstruction of the lymphatics; 10 ml oily contrast medium have been injected into a right lateral superficial inguinal node on the horizontal tract (Figs. 22.14 and 22.15).

Results. The lateral, as well as medial, drainage pathway from the inguinal node is brought into view by injecting contrast medium into a lateral node. The anteroposterior radiographic view projects the inguinal lymphatic drainage pathways and the obturator, external iliac, and gluteal lymphatic areas partially resting on top of each other (Fig. 22.14). Only the lateral radiographic view (Fig. 22.15) allows recognition of their true topographic location.

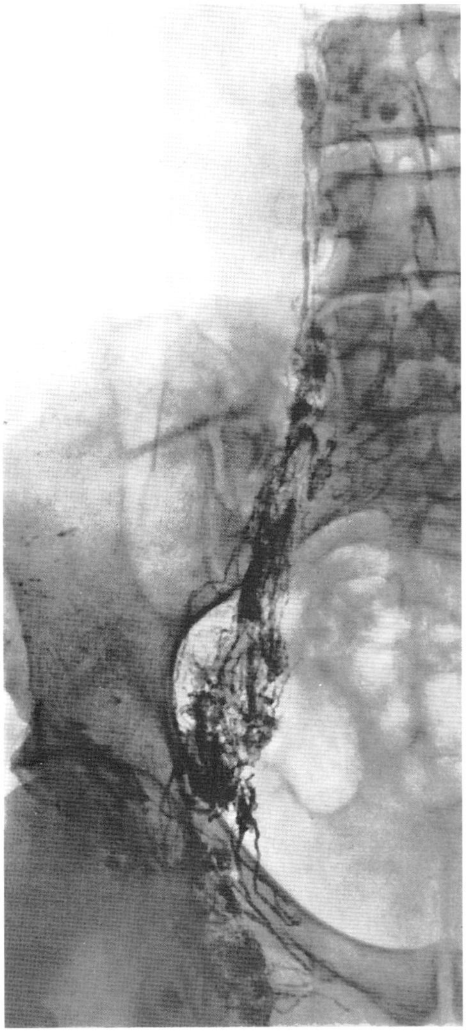

Figure 22.14. Case 3. Lymphangiogram, filling phase, anteroposterior view, right pelvic wall.

Numerous inguinal dilated vessels of the lymphatics are present. Lymphatic drainage from the inguinal region appears to be coursing predominantly into the obturator fossa.

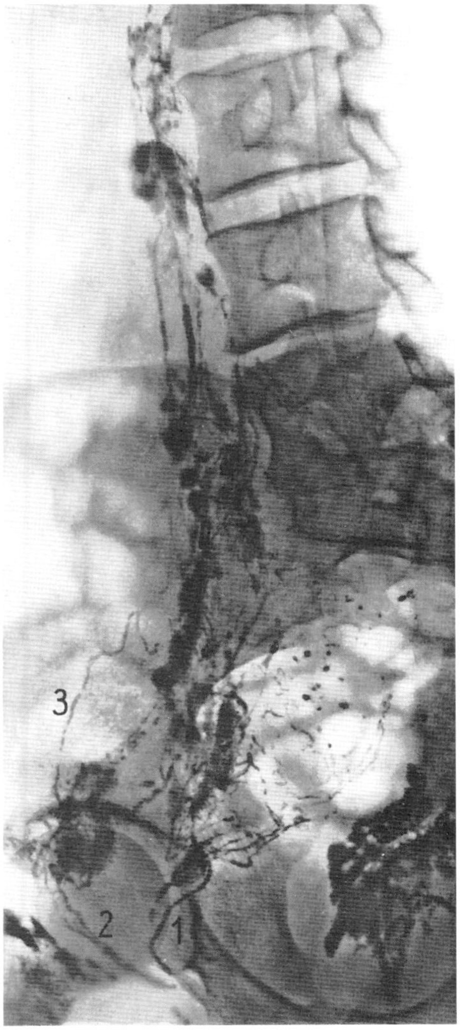

Figure 22.15. Case 3. Lymphangiogram, filling phase, lateral view, right pelvic wall.

Note lymph drainage from inguinal medially (1) to the obturator and then the gluteal nodes and sacrum and also the lateral drainage pathway (2) to the external iliac nodes.

A dilated lymph vessel (3) courses in a bow-like curve in lateral direction upward to the common iliac nodes. This lymph vessel originates from a node that is located laterally to the external iliac artery and is also the most distal.

Case 4.

Lymphangiography on a cadaver.

35-year old woman, status posthemorrhage at cesarean section; 26 hours after death, 2 ml oily contrast medium were injected into each *medial inguinal node* (radiographs, filling phase).

The medial lymph nodes on the horizontal tract of the inguinal lymphatics had deliberately been injected with a very small amount of contrast medium so that the lymphatic drainage from the medial inguinal nodes can be studied separately. The pelvis has been removed from the body, and x-rays were taken from different directions. The pelvis was then placed in a deep freeze and split sagittally.

Results (obtained from anatomical x-ray examinations).

Looking at an anteroposterior radiograph of the pelvis (Figs. 22.16 and 22.17), one may mistakenly assume that lymphatic drainage from the inguinal nodes occurs only upward along the external iliac artery. Only the lateral views demonstrate that lymph drainage occurs predominantly from the medial inguinal nodes into the obturator fossa and to the branches of the internal iliac artery. We could show this by marking the blood vessels of the pelvic wall with ureteral catheters (Fig. 22.18) and designating points of orientation using small lead plates (Figs. 22.19 and 22.20). The obturator nodes, inferior gluteal nodes, and superior gluteal nodes can be demonstrated by injecting contrast medium into a medial inguinal node. The lateral view shows clearly how lymphatics of the pelvis are filled to the sciatic foramen.

By injecting only 2 ml (a relatively small amount) of contrast medium into a medial inguinal node, the medial lymphatic drainage passage of the inguinal node was predominantly highlighted. Should one inject a larger amount of contrast medium into a medial inguinal node, one can fill the entire lymphatics of the pelvic wall from there. This has been demonstrated by means of lymphangiograms performed on live patients, as shown in Figures 22.9–22.15.

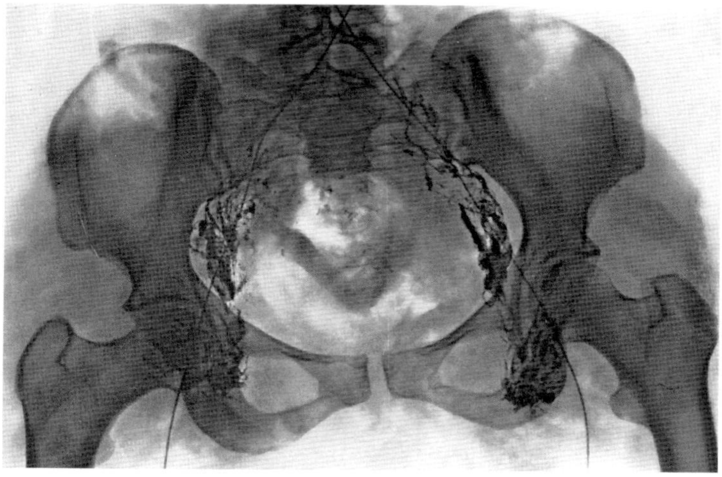

Figure 22.16. Case 4. Pelvis is slightly tilted forward. Anteroposterior view.

Ureteral catheters are located bilaterally from the aorta to the femoral artery. Medial to the linea terminalis one can see a network of lymphatic vessels and nodes that appears to stretch along the external iliac vessels and that is demonstrated on the left along the common iliac vessels, reaching to the level of the promontory.

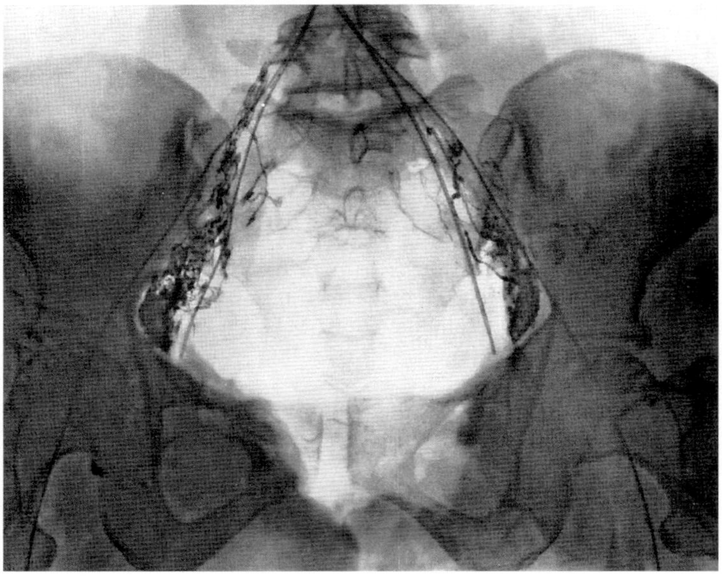

Figure 22.17. Case 4. Anteroposterior view of pelvis.

Ureteral catheters have been inserted bilaterally from the aorta along the common and external iliac arteries as well as along the common iliac and internal iliac arteries to the sciatic foramen. The anteroposterior radiograph depicts the radiographically illuminated lymphatic system of the pelvis mainly between the inserted ureteral catheters.

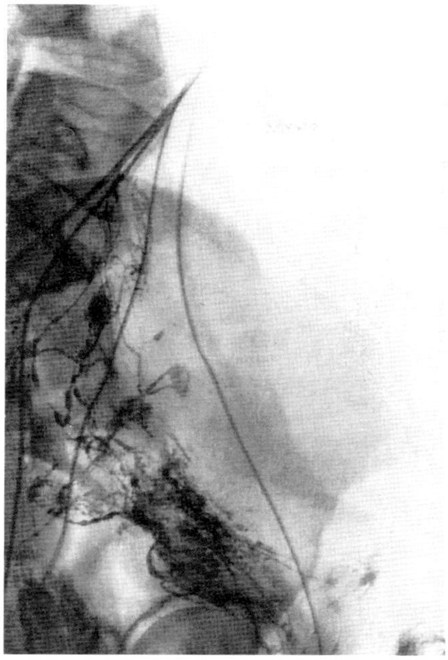

Figure 22.18. Case 4. Medial view of left pelvic wall.

The ureteral catheters have been inserted in a manner analogous to that shown in Figure 22.17. One ureteral catheter marks the common and the left external iliac arteries; the other is inserted into the common and internal iliac arteries.

This lateral radiographic view demonstrates the important fact that lymph from the medial inguinal nodes does not drain upward alongside the left external iliac artery but rather empties into the obturator fossa and flows to the peripheral branches of the internal iliac artery and then flows all the way to the sciatic foramen. The obturator, inferior gluteal, and superior gluteal nodes were reached from the medial inguinal nodes.

Note that there is a tendency for drainage to occur from the medial inguinal nodes to the obturator fossa.

By injecting only small amounts of oily contrast medium into a medial inguinal node, lymphatic pathways and nodes coursing along the ureteral catheter that had been inserted into the external and common iliac arteries were not highlighted.

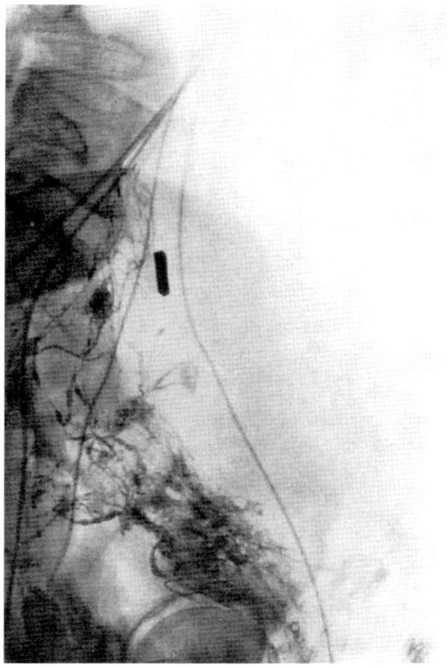

Figure 22.19. Case 4. View from medial to left pelvic wall.

The left hypogastric angle (internal iliac artery) has been marked with a small lead plate.

The radiographically illuminated lymph drainage of the medial inguinal nodes resembles that shown in Figure 22.18. In this case as well the contrast medium flows from the medial inguinal nodes to the obturator and gluteal nodes. The lymphatics coursing alongside the external and left common iliac arteries are not shown.

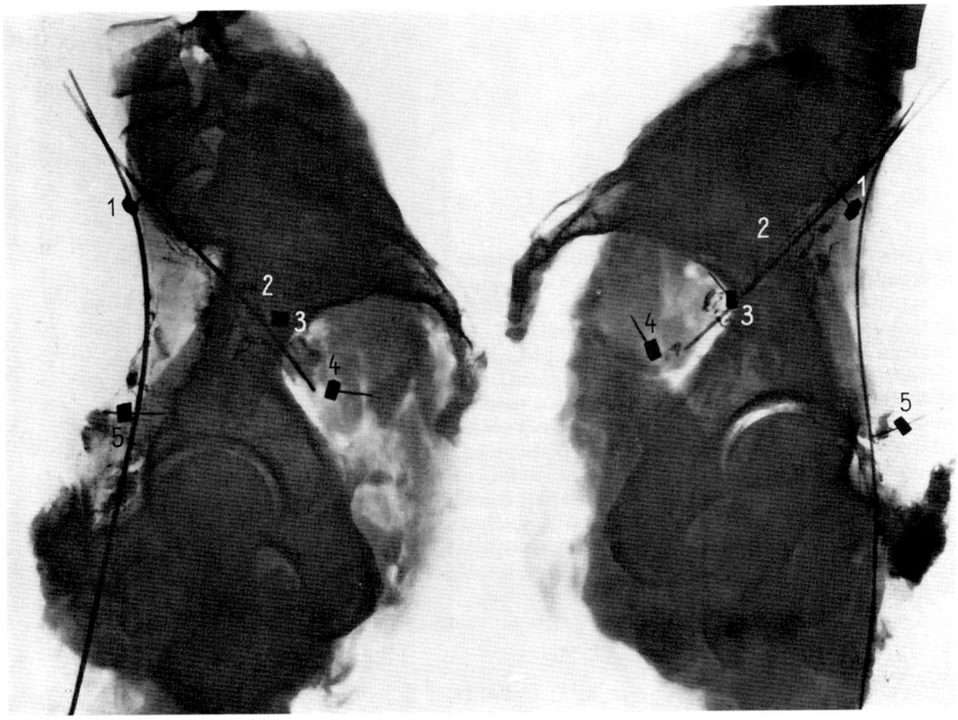

Figure 22.20. Case 4. Pelvis split in midline. Medial views to the right and left pelvic wall.

For anatomical orientation, additional small lead plates have been used to designate points of interest:

1 hypogastric angle (internal iliac artery)
2 point where the superior gluteal and internal iliac arteries branch off
3 point where the inferior gluteal and internal iliac arteries branch off
4 point of exit of the pelvic blood vessels from the sciatic foramen
5 point of exit of the external iliac artery from the pelvis

On the left, one can see lymphatic vessels and nodes in the sciatic foramen very close to mark 4, to the exit point of the inferior gluteal artery (mark 3), and along the primary stem of the internal iliac artery (mark 2). Injection of contrast medium into a medial inguinal node made this possible.

In the left external iliac artery, lymphatic vessels and nodes cannot be seen along the ureteral catheter. However, on the right side, along the external iliac artery, one can recognize scattered lymphatic vessels and nodes filled with contrast media. Observe on the left the considerable distance from the inferior gluteal node (mark 4 on the sciatic foramen and mark 3 on the branching point of the inferior gluteal artery) to the hypogastric angle (mark 1).

Summary.

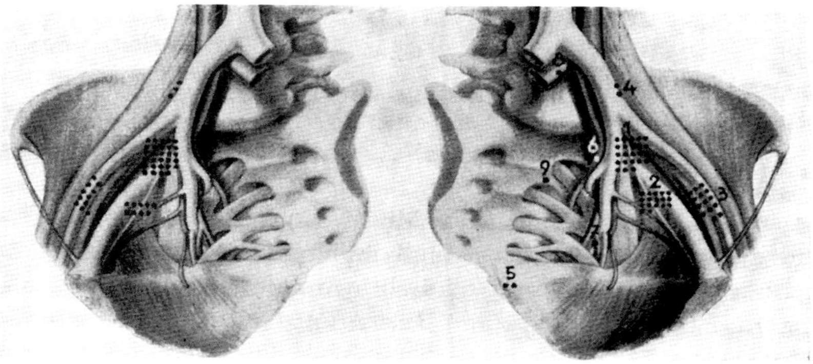

Figure 22.21. Summary of location of lymph node metastases.

Subjects were 70 patients who underwent the Wertheim-Meigs procedure and who had as radical a lymph node dissection as possible.

Each point designates an affected lymph node group but not the number of affected nodes in each group. Note that this overview does not demonstrate lymph node metastases in the area of the inferior gluteal nodes. This may be explained by the fact that the nodes were not removed from this region during the "radical operation."

1 hypogastric nodes
2 obturator nodes
3 external iliac nodes
4 common iliac nodes
5 parametrial lymph nodes
6 superior gluteal nodes
7 inferior gluteal nodes
8 subaortic nodes
9 pararectal nodes

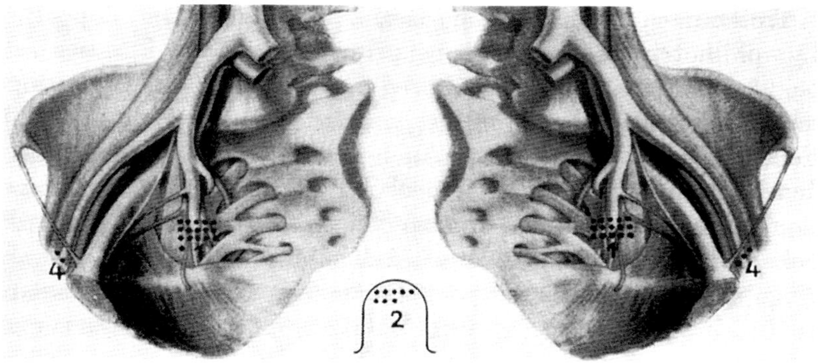

Figure 22.22. Summary of "relapse" locations.

Among the 70 patients whose positive lymph nodes had been removed during a radical operation, 35 died of recurrent carcinoma.

Observe the clear evidence of "lymph node recurrence" predominant on those locations on the pelvic wall that correspond to locations of the inferior gluteal nodes that had not been removed. This demonstrates that these recurrences are not true recurrences but are really lymph node metastases that had already been present when the Wertheim radical operation was performed but that had either not been detected or were technically too difficult to remove.

1 pelvic wall recurrence
2 localized recurrence
3 inguinal recurrence

Technique

Schuchardt Incision (Vaginal-Perineal-Levator Incision)

A sufficiently large opening to the operative field is achieved by means of a left-sided Schuchardt incision that opens the left pararectal and paravesical space. Correct dissection of the so-called ''paraspaces'' is imperative for successful execution of the radical vaginal operation. One can reach these spaces safely if one first infiltrates the tissues with fluid (physiologic saline solution plus five units vasopressin/100 ml).

Figure 22.23. Schauta-Amreich procedure. Infiltration of the left-sided Schuchardt incision.

The surgeon's left index finger is inserted into the vagina to palpate the ischial tuberosity.

A long needle is used to perform perineal tissue infiltration of a fan-shaped area with 20 ml fluid. The needle is inserted about 3 cm laterally to the left of the anus and advanced close to the ischial tuberosity while the fluid is injected simultaneously.

Detail. Fan-shaped fluid injection (*red*).

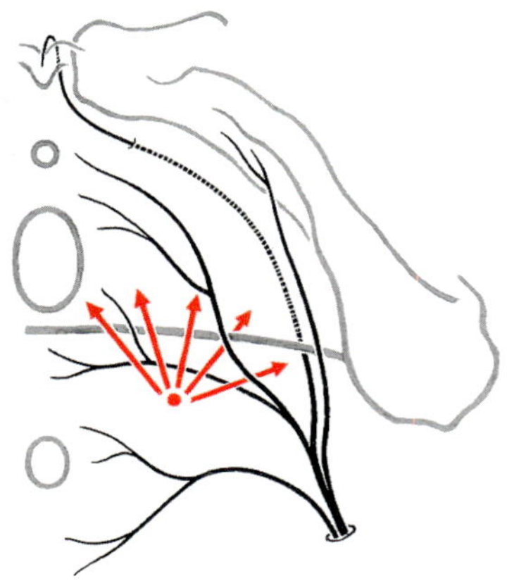

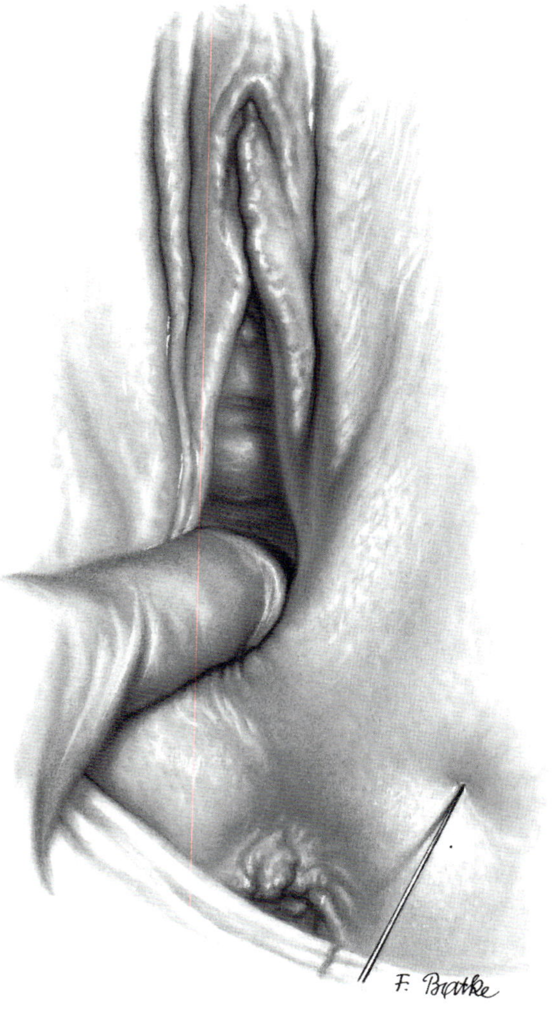

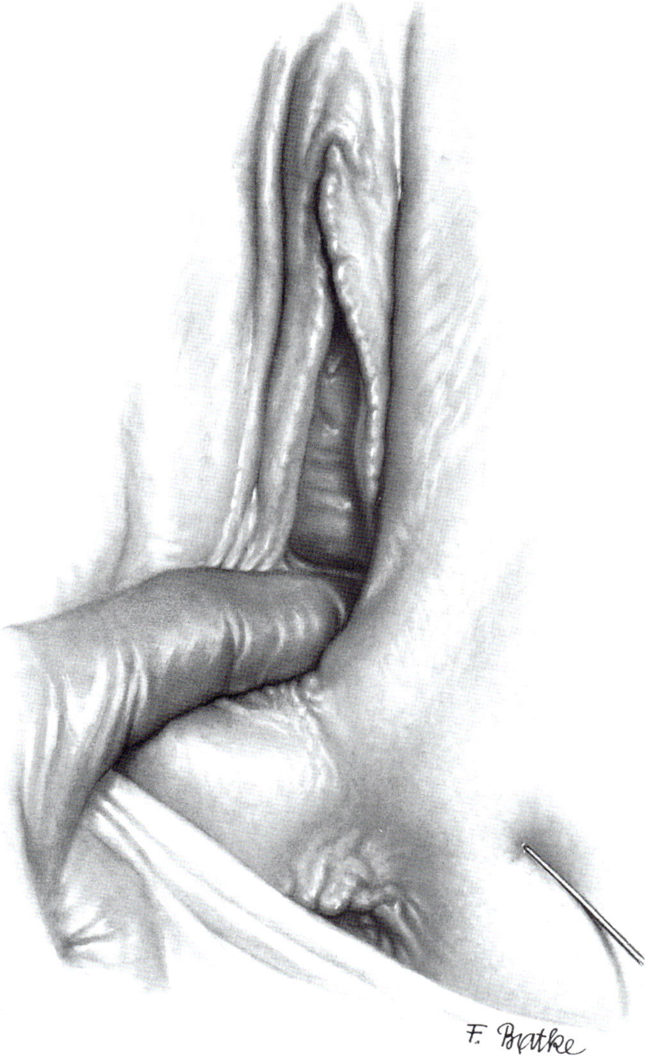

Figure 22.24. Schauta-Amreich procedure. Infiltration of the left-sided Schuchardt incision.

At the end of the fan-shaped perineal infiltration the needle is advanced subcutaneously up to the posterior commissure, and the left lateral vaginal wall is then infiltrated.

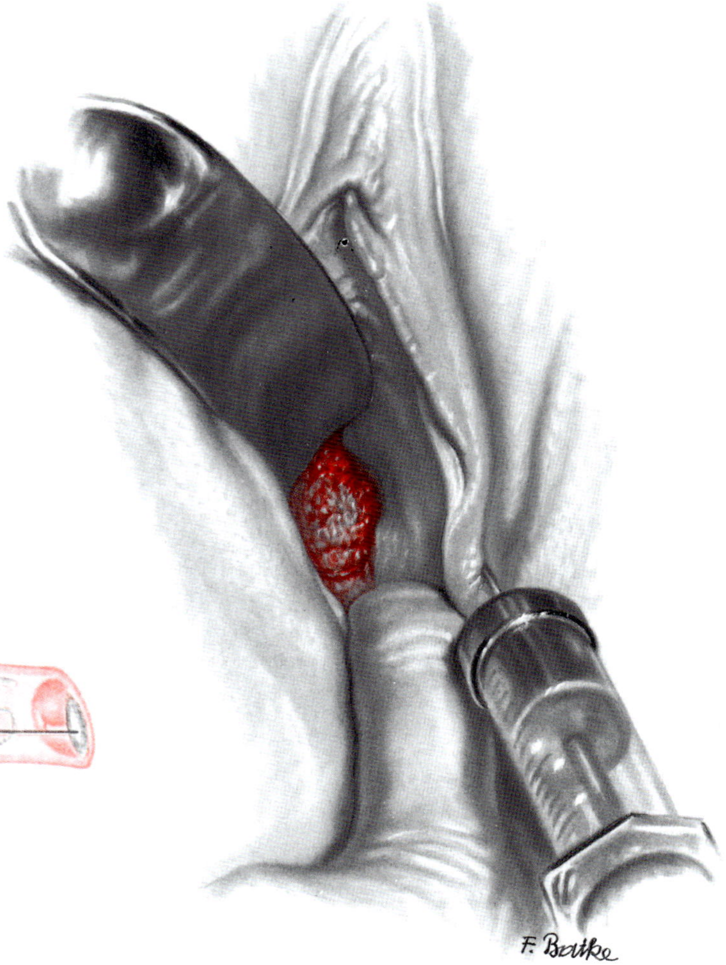

Figure 22.25. Schauta-Amreich procedure. Infiltration of the left-sided Schuchardt incision in the left vaginal wall region.

The surgeon inserts the index finger deeply into the vagina and pushes the left posterior vaginal wall downward; the assistant retracts the anterior vaginal upward to the right with a spatula.

The needle is inserted at the posterior commissure, and the left lateral wall is infiltrated up to the lateral fornix with 20 ml fluid.

Detail. The vagina is stretched, and the needle is advanced subfascially along the left vaginal wall up to the level of the left fornix (*gray*).

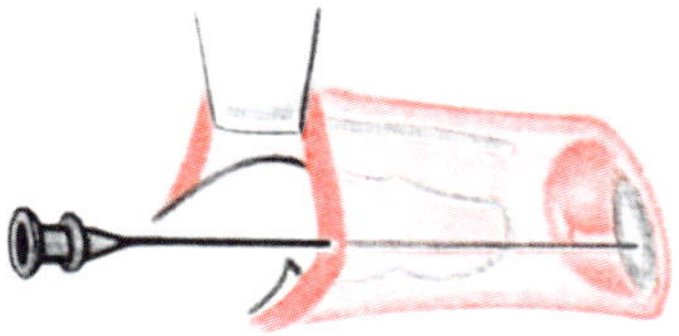

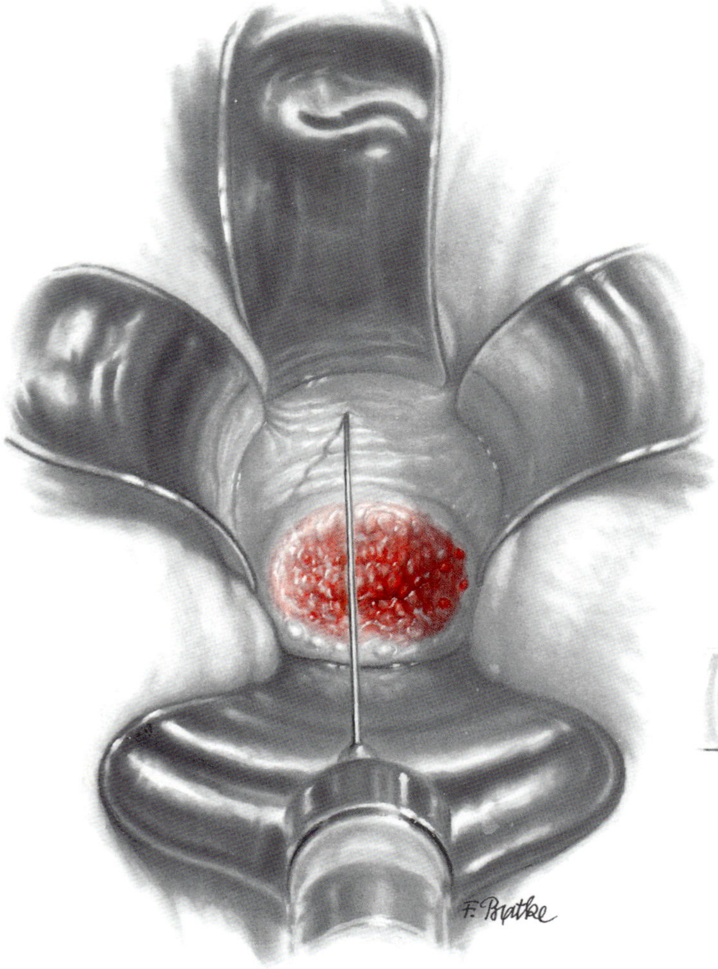

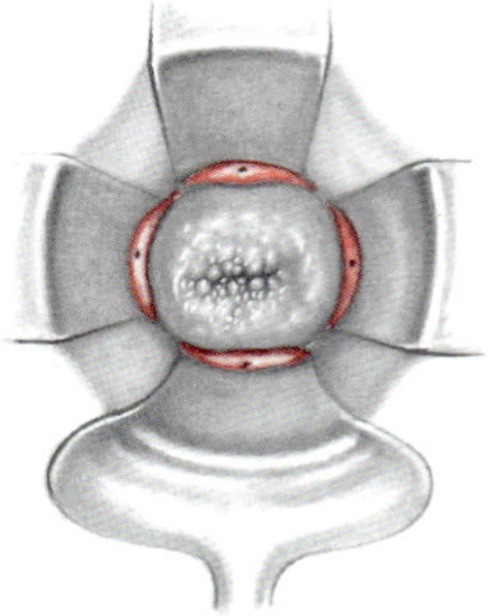

Figure 22.26. Schauta-Amreich procedure. Infiltration of the site of the vaginal circumcision.

The needle is inserted at 12 o'clock in the anterior vaginal fornix. Selecting the distance of the puncture site from the portio depends on the size of the carcinoma. Infiltration of the vaginal wall should be 3–4 cm distal from the edge of the carcinoma tissue because it is essential to perform the vaginal circumcision in an area of macroscopically healthy vaginal tissue.

Detail. Infiltration of the site of the vaginal circumcision through injection of 20 ml fluid at 12, 6, 9, and 3 o'clock in the anterior, posterior, and two lateral fornices (*red*).

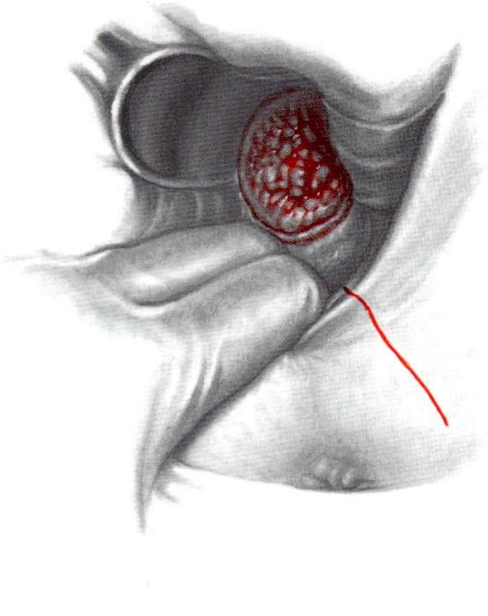

Figure 22.27. Schauta-Amreich procedure. Left-sided placement of the Schuchardt incision. Dividing the perineal skin.

The vagina is distended by an anterior retractor (held by the right assistant), by the left assistant's right index finger deeply inserted into the vaginal canal, and by the second and third fingers of the surgeon's left hand.

The incision begins at the posterior commissure three finger breadths to the left of the midline and curves to the left to reach the level of the anus. Customarily, the incision is performed using an electrocautery knife.

Figure 22.28. Schauta-Amreich procedure. Left-sided placement of the Schuchardt incision. Incision of the lateral vaginal wall.

The left assistant retracts the left lateral vaginal wall firmly upward with the index finger. The surgeon's index finger retracts the posterior vaginal wall and also the rectum downward.

The perineal skin is divided, and the left vaginal wall is incised up to the left fornix.

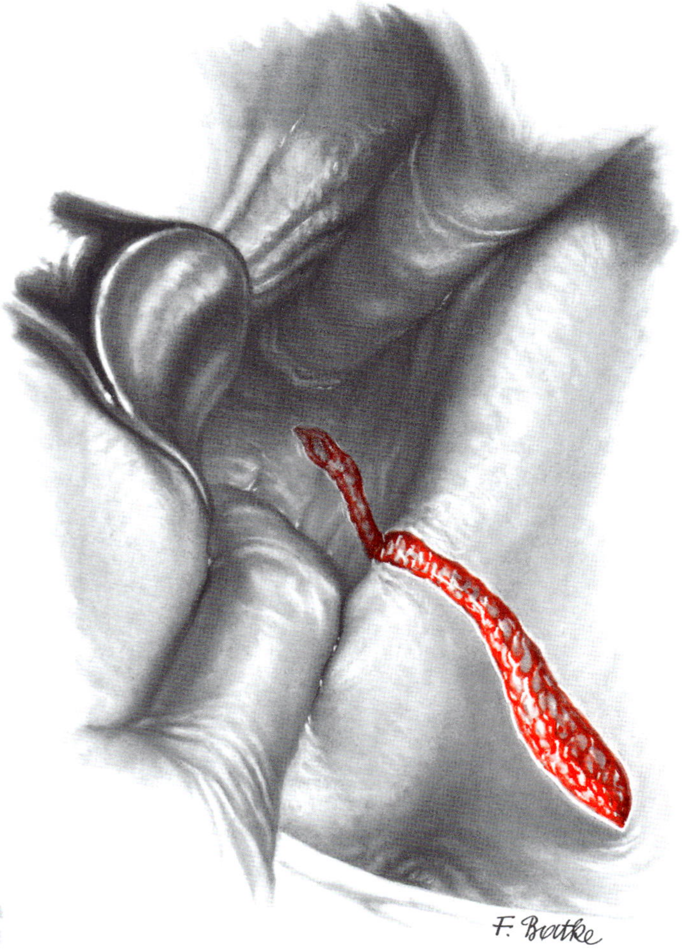

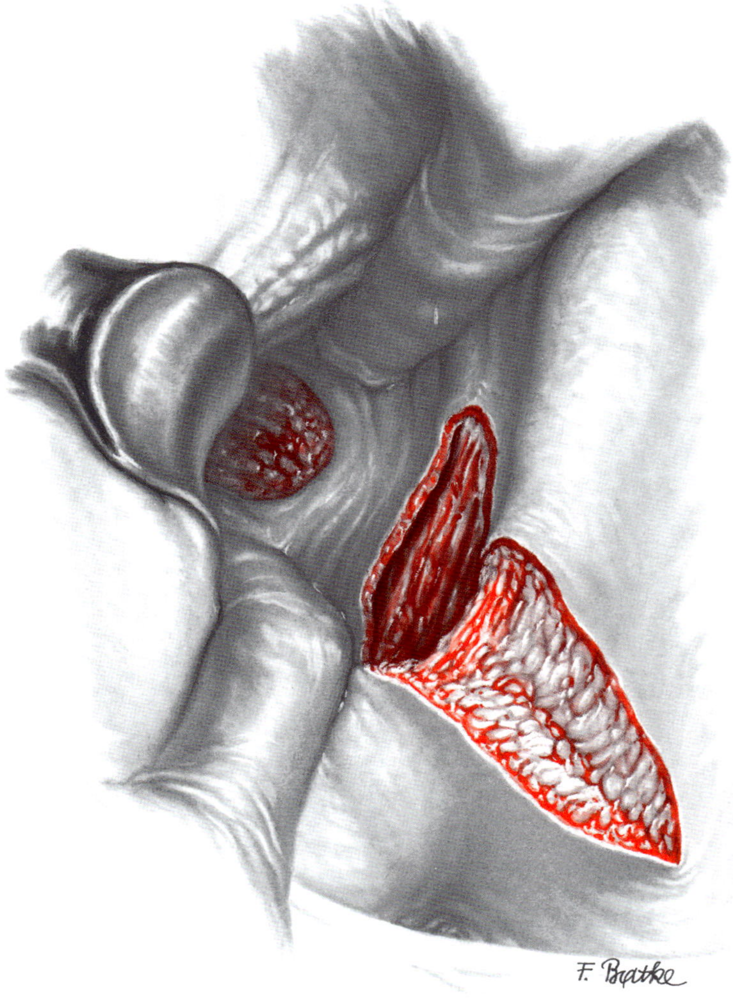

Figure 22.29. Schauta-Amreich procedure. Left-sided placement of the Schuchardt incision. Extending the perineal incision and opening the pararectal space.

The wound is gaping through pressure applied by both fingers after the vaginal wall has been incised; the levator fibers can then be seen cephalad.

Medial to the uppermost levator muscle fibers, the left pararectal space was opened bluntly with the blunt edge of the scalpel that had been advanced between the vaginal incision edge and the levator muscle.

The puborectal levator fibers are then sharply divided again using an electrocautery knife.

Figure 22.30. Schauta-Amreich procedure. Exposure of the para-spaces.

The levator muscle is almost completely severed so that the pararectal fossa is opened widely (a partial indentation of the levator muscle is often sufficient to allow enough access to the operating field). Deep down the rectum is visible.

The surgeon advances the index finger cephalad from the pararectal space between the rectum and the levator muscle, and thus advances into the paravesical space.

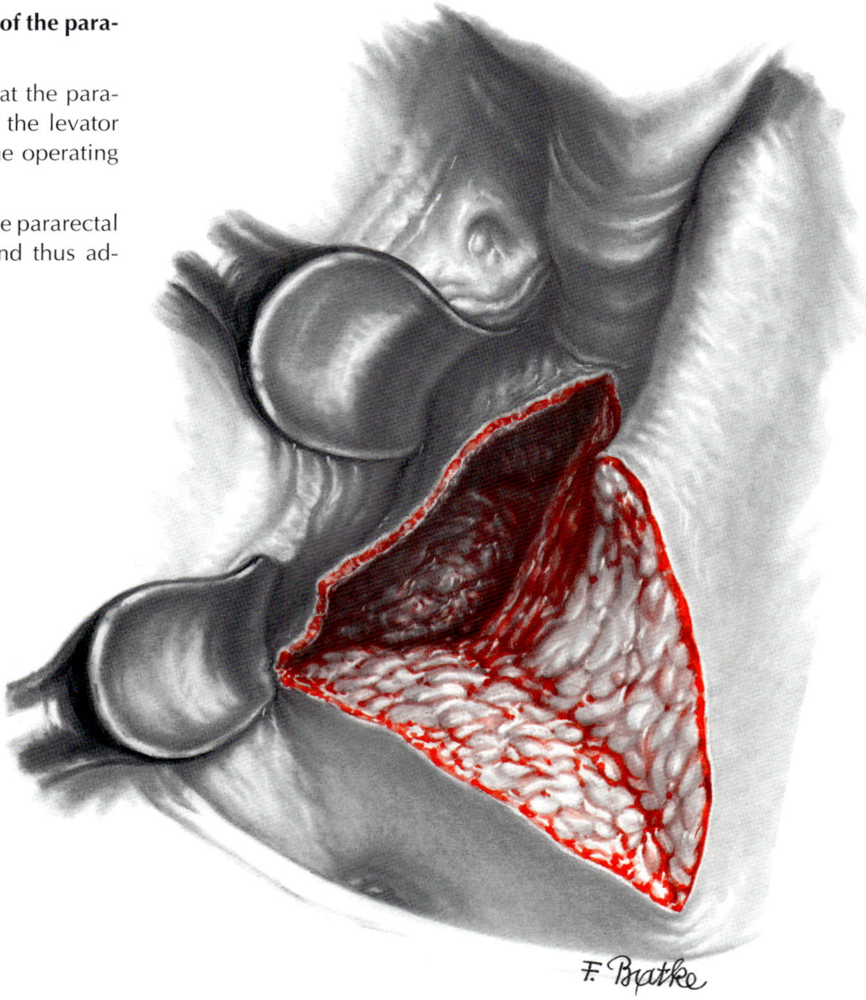

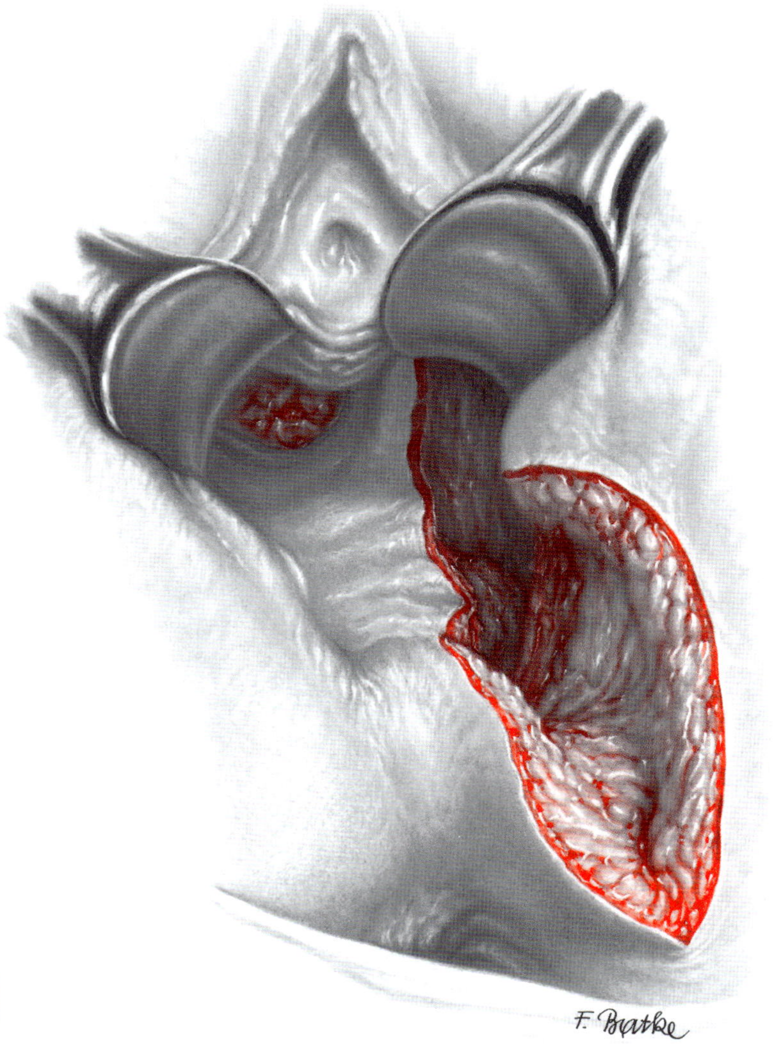

Figure 22.31. Schauta-Amreich procedure. Uniting the paraspaces.

The right assistant retracts the right vaginal wall to the right with a retractor. The left assistant inserts a retractor in the exposed left paravesical space and pushes the bladder upward.

The pararectal and paravesical spaces have been widely opened and joined. The bladder is visible anteriorly in the depths of the vaginal incision, and the rectum is seen posteriorly. Hemostasis has been accomplished in the region of the Schuchardt incision.

The Schuchardt incision is draped with a gauze pad that is secured at the lateral wound edges with several silk sutures.

Technical Problems—Figures 22.23–22.31

1. The rectum can be injured during the lateral vaginal incision *if the pressure exerted by the* left assistant's *index finger* (retracting the vaginal wall anteriorly and to the left) and by the surgeon's finger (pulling downward and to the right) *are inadequate* to distend the left vaginal wall sufficiently.
2. Opening the pararectal and the paravesical spaces is made more difficult if *only lateral fibers of the levator muscles are divided* during the electrocautery scoring of the levator ani muscles, leaving the medial puborectal fibers intact. In addition, when dissection of the paravesical space is extended too far caudally, the intact upper puborectal fibers of the levator adhere to the bladder pillar, making this structure unduly thick. This will complicate matters when the ureter is dissected free at a later stage.
3. If the left vaginal wall *incision is made too far medially*, one can injure the rectum or the larger pararectal veins. Should the incision be placed *too far laterally*, it may lacerate the larger veins of the bulbocavernous plexus (however, hemostasis is easy to accomplish).

Circumcision of the Vaginal Canal

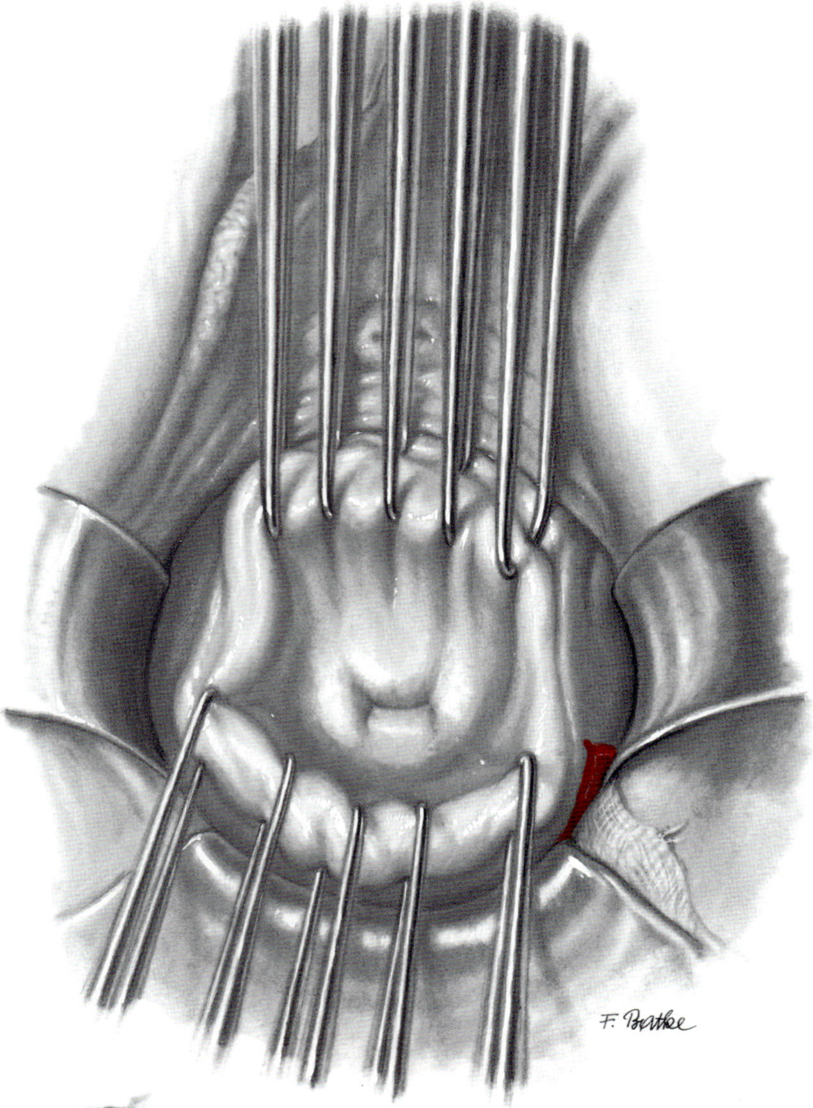

Figure 22.32. Schauta-Amreich procedure. Circumcision of the vaginal canal. Attaching the tenacula.

The vagina is distended by two lateral retractors and a self-retaining posterior retractor; the Schuchardt incision has been draped with a gauze pad.

The vaginal canal is grasped with several single-toothed tenacula at the preselected 4 cm distance from the portio first anteriorly, then posteriorly, in a circular manner. The uppermost wound angle of the vaginal longitudinal incision can be seen in the left fornix; it reaches to the level at which the vaginal circumcision will be conducted.

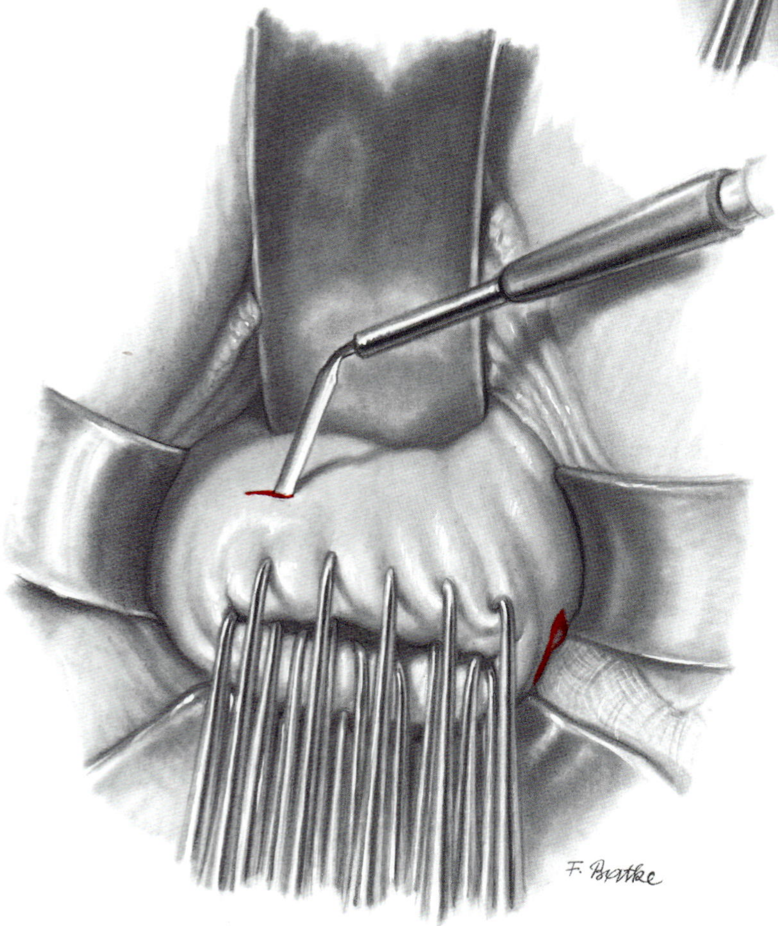

Figure 22.33. Schauta-Amreich procedure. Circumcision of the vaginal canal. Anterior circumcision.

The right assistant pushes the anterior vaginal wall vigorously upward with an anterior retractor; the surgeon pulls the attached tenacula down.

The surgeon applies the angulated tip of the electrocautery knife perpendicularly to the stretched vaginal wall and cuts it in a semicircle close above the tenacula. Both the vaginal mucosa and fascia are separated; one can recognize when the correct depth is reached by the wide gaping of the wound caused by retractor pressure.

Figure 22.34. Schauta-Amreich procedure. Circumcision of the vaginal canal. Posterior circumcision.

The right assistant pulls the tenacula upward. The surgeon stretches the posterior vaginal wall downward with tissue forceps and cuts in a semicircle just caudad to the tenacula. The vaginal circumcision is correctly accomplished when it meets the uppermost angle of the left vaginal incision wound.

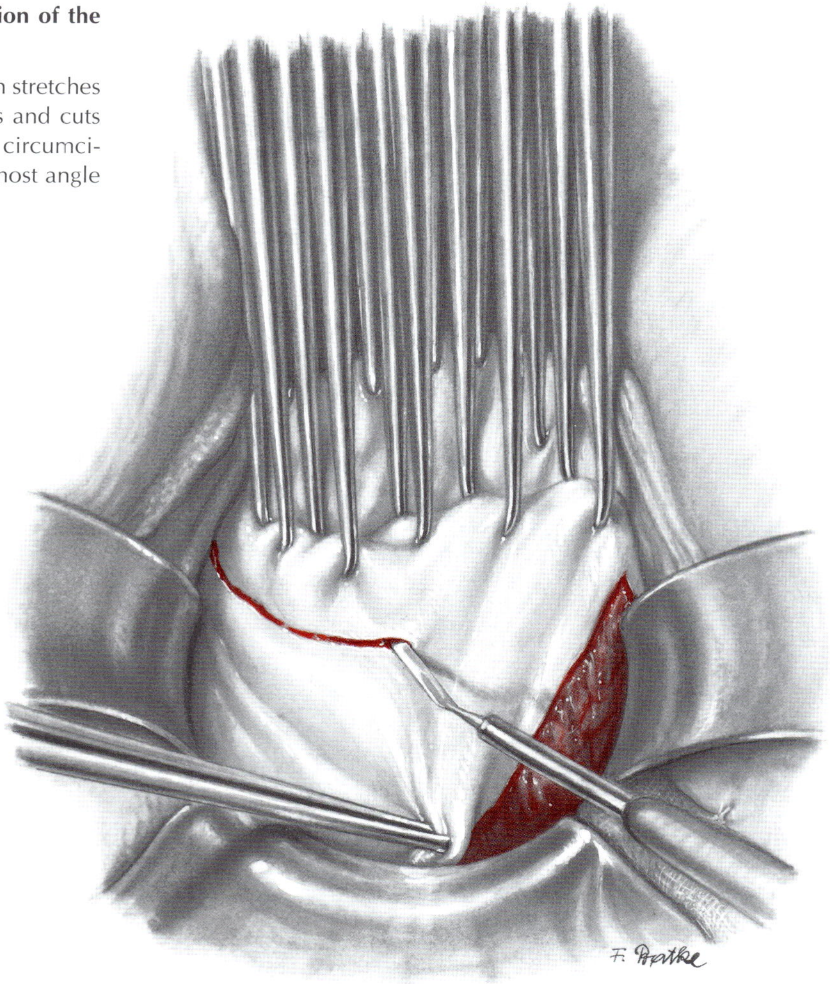

Technical Problems—Figures 22.32–22.34

1. The downward pull of the tenacula that are placed on the anterior wall does *not stretch the anterior mucosa uniformly* so that it may undulate lengthwise. This is particularly noticed in cases when the vaginal canal is very wide and many tenacula had to be used. Under these circumstances, the right half of the tenacula should be pulled down and to the right by the surgeon's left hand, and the other half pulled down and to the left with the free left hand of the left assistant. The anterior inverted vaginal wall is thus stretched flat without folds.
2. If the circular *incision is made too deeply in front* during vaginal circumcision, the vaginal cuff may be perforated at the anterior fornix.
3. The assistant on the right might *not lift the anterior vaginal wall upward with sufficient strength* during the anterior circumcision with the electrocautery. In such a case, the vaginal wall will not gape adequately, and consequently the bladder (which had been pushed upward) may be endangered by any further vaginal wall separation.
4. If the vaginal canal has *not been divided precisely at its lateral margin*, later dissection of the bladder pillar will be more difficult.

Formation of Vaginal Cuff

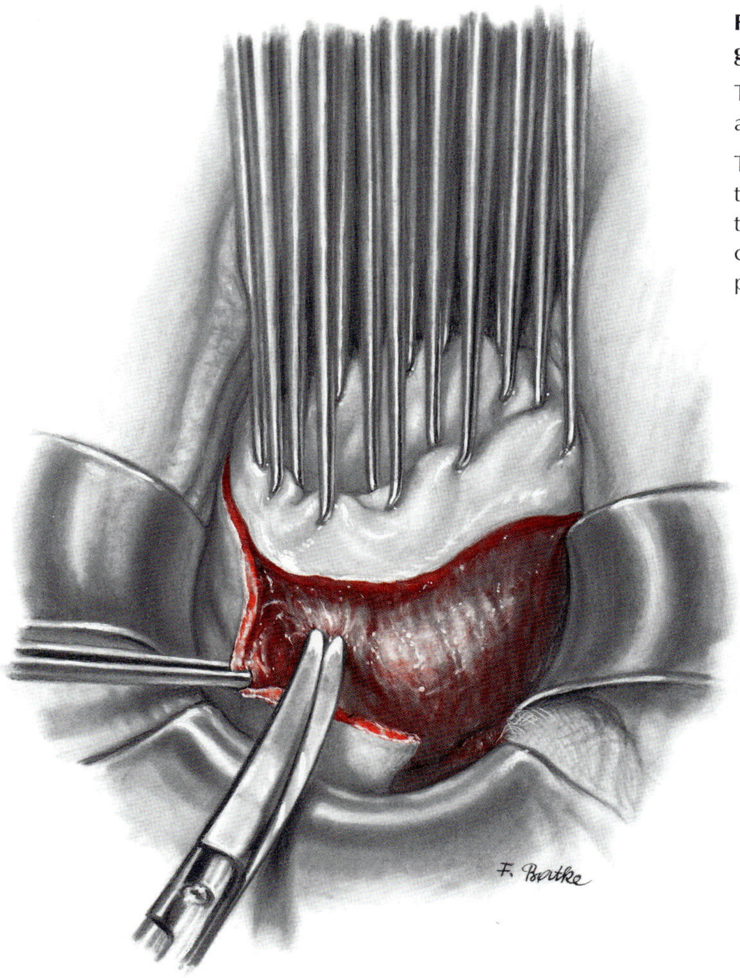

Figure 22.35. Schauta-Amreich procedure. Developing the vaginal cuff. Dissecting the rectum.

The vagina is placed on stretch with three retractors, the tenacula are raised up.

The surgeon pulls the posterior vaginal wound edge, together with the attached rectum, caudally with the toothed forceps. At the same time, above it, the taut retrocervical connective tissue is pushed caudally with slightly opened dissecting scissors, curved tips pointed upward. This maneuver moves the rectum away.

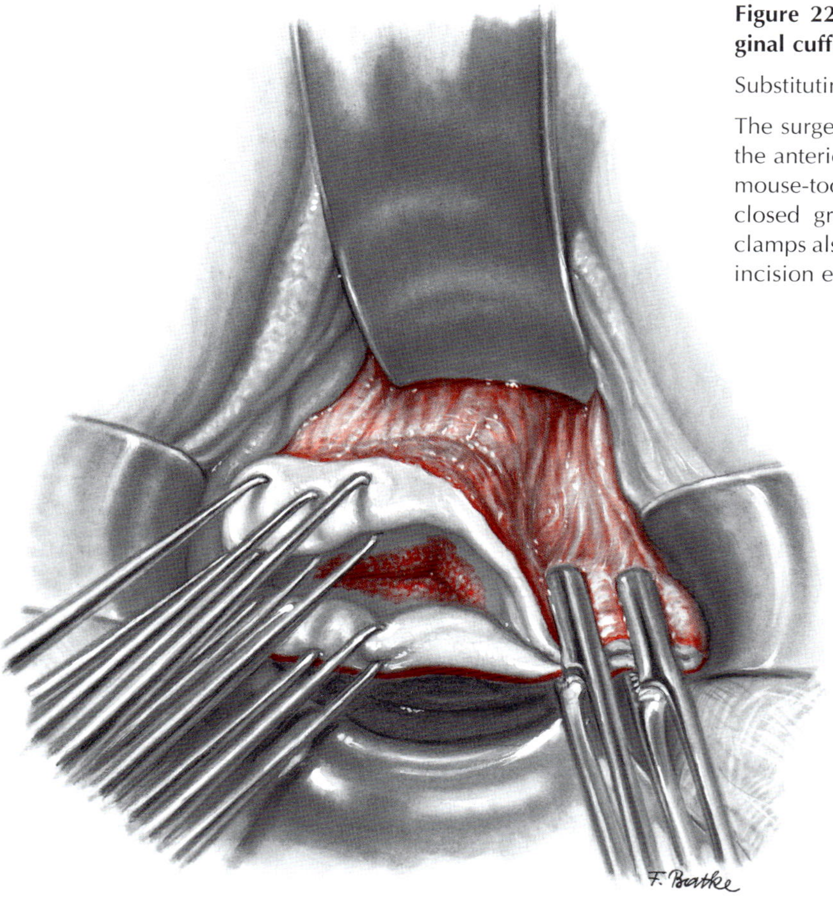

Figure 22.36. Schauta-Amreich procedure. Developing the vaginal cuff.

Substituting mouse-toothed clamps for the tenacula.

The surgeon removes the tenacula in a stepwise fashion and joins the anterior and posterior incision edges of the vaginal stump with mouse-toothed clamps. With this procedure the vaginal canal is closed gradually, completely covering the cervical tumor. The clamps also achieve effective hemostasis in the region of the vaginal incision edges.

TECHNICAL PROBLEMS—FIGURES 22.35 and 22.36

1. If the mouse-toothed clamps are attached too high anteriorly on a short vaginal cuff, the bladder may be caught up by them, particularly if it has not yet been dissected free.
2. Using heavy silk sutures instead of mouse-toothed clamps when suturing the vaginal stump has not been shown to be particularly advantageous. Mouse-toothed clamps can be held parallel to each other and therefore can be directed more exactly, which allows one to move the closed vaginal cuff like a broad band. In addition, the use of the clamps stretches both anterior and posterior vaginal walls flatly, presenting it in full breath. As a result, it is easier for the lower pole of the urinary bladder and the rectum to be dissected. A circular closure of the vaginal stump with silk sutures elevates the vaginal wall and makes it appear bumpy.

Dissection of Supravaginal Septum

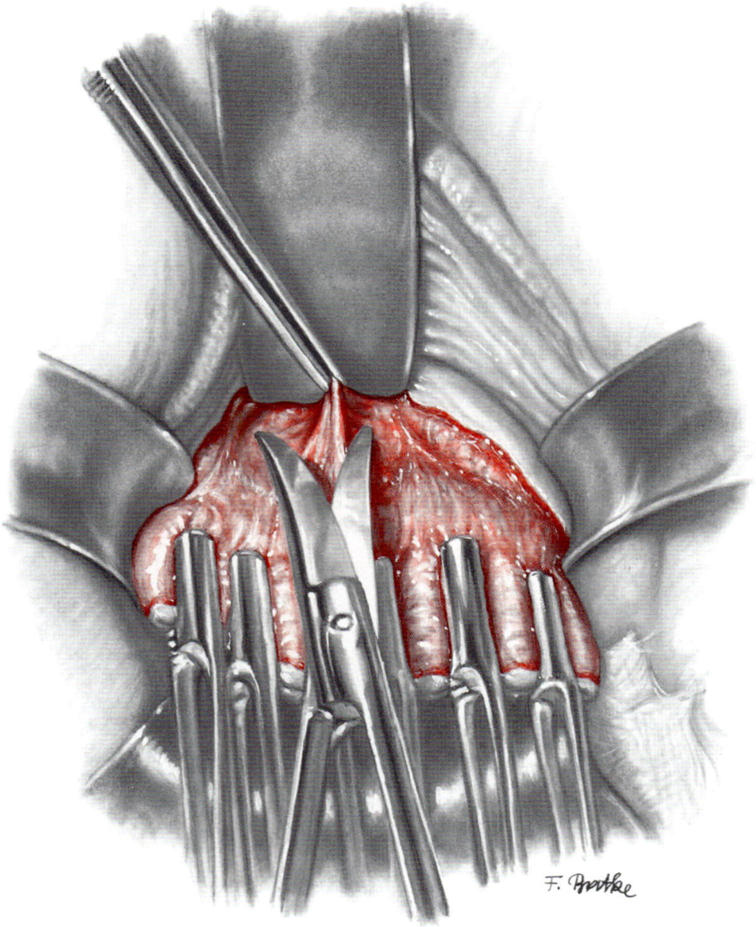

Figure 22.37. Schauta-Amreich procedure. Opening the vesicocervical space.

The left assistant pulls the vaginal cuff down with the mouse-toothed clamps.

The surgeon grasps the lower bladder pole somewhat with curved tissue forceps and lifts it somewhat to stretch the fibers of the supravaginal septum in a sagittal direction. The fibers are dissected with a pair of scissors directed toward the cervix and placed very close to the anterior wall of the cervix. In this way the vesicocervical space is opened. The lower pole of the bladder can then be easily mobilized upward with the index finger to the level above the peritoneal fold.

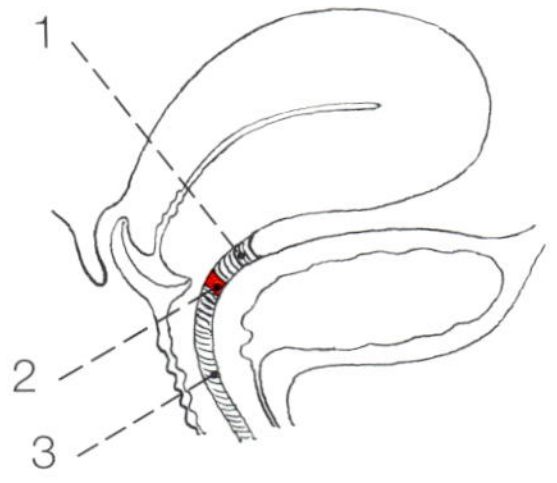

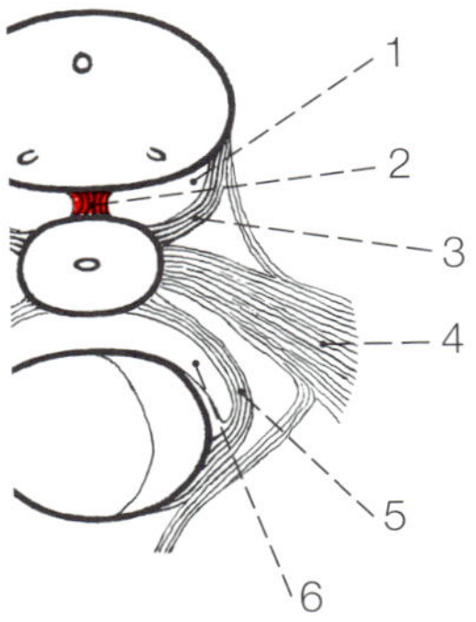

Left detail. Supravaginal septum and space: median sagittal view.

1 loose connective tissue in the vesicocervical space between uterus and urinary bladder
2 supravaginal septum
3 loose connective tissue between vaginal and vesical fascia and between vaginal and urethral fascia in the vesicovaginal and urethrovaginal spaces, respectively

Right detail. Supravaginal septum and spatia: cross-section.

1 vesicouterine space
2 supravaginal septum
3 vesicouterine ligament
4 cardinal ligament
5 rectouterine ligament
6 rectouterine space

Technical Problems—Figure 22.37

1. If the *anterior retractor pushes the vaginal wall too far upward,* the surgeon will not be able to elevate the lower pole of the bladder enough, and the fibers of the supravaginal septum will no longer be visibly stretched.
2. The supravaginal septum might be dissected too close to the bladder, and this could result in injury to the bladder.
3. The supravaginal septum might be divided *too close to the cervix*. This is one of the most frequently made mistakes of the inexperienced surgeon, who tends to dissect too close to the cervix for fear of injuring the bladder. The surgeon will cut into the anterior cervical wall, note erroneously that the ''layers are very poorly defined,'' and then experience the utmost difficulty when dissecting the bladder because the dissection is in the wrong layer. If one mistakenly advances into the anterior cervical wall, it will not be possible to open the vesicocervical space and mobilize the lower pole of the bladder to the level above the peritoneal fold. To avoid this, the surgeon must localize the lower bladder pole by inserting a uterine sound through the urethra into the bladder. It will then be clear that the dissection was too close to the cervix.

Dissection of Ureter on the Left

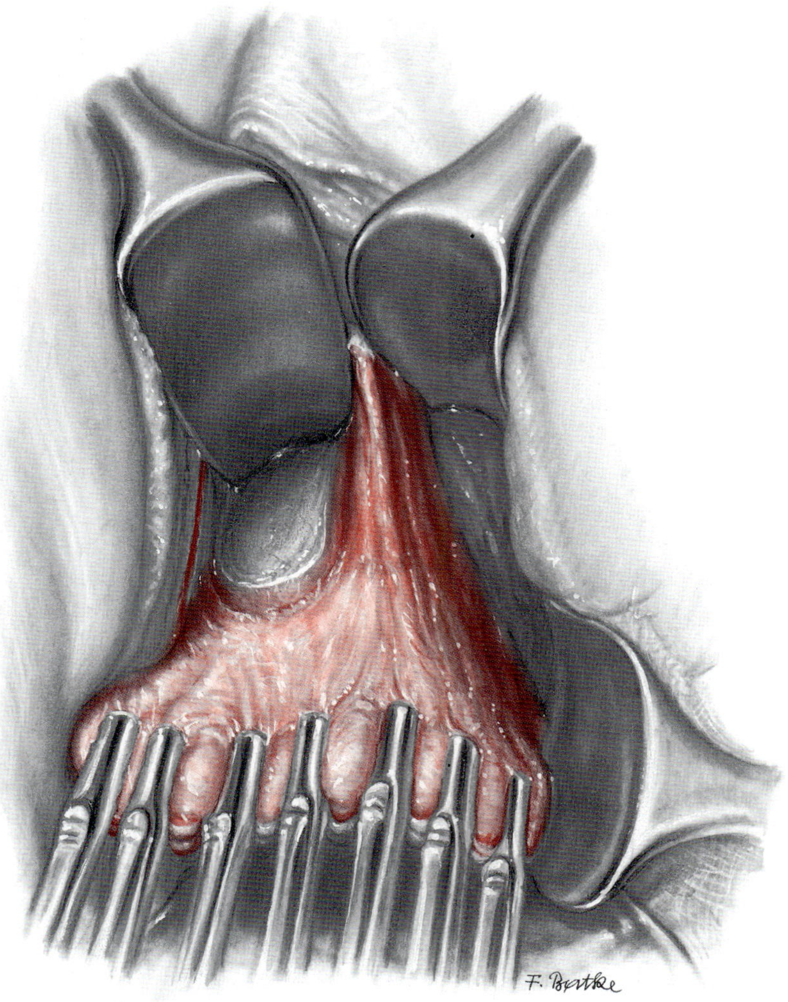

Figure 22.38. Schauta-Amreich procedure. Ureteral dissection on the left. Locating the ureter.

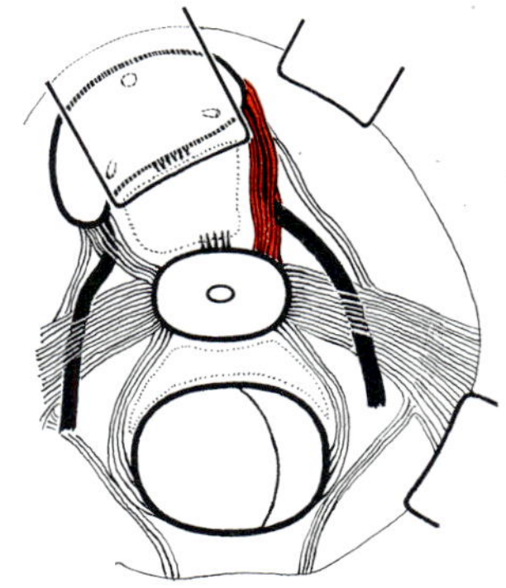

The supravaginal septum is divided and the vesicocervical space opened. The bladder is dissected upward to above the peritoneal reflection.

The right assistant pulls the vaginal cuff down to the right and pushes the bladder up with a retractor already in place in the vesicocervical space. The retractor is then tilted somewhat, which causes the left connective tissue pillar (through which the ureter courses) to be stretched. The left assistant inserts a narrow retractor laterally from the left bladder pillar into the paravesical space and tilts it as well, which further stretches the bladder pillar. By using the posterior retractor, the rectum is depressed to the left.

Detail. Correct pressure by the retractor causes the bladder pillar (vesicouterine ligament) to be stretched so that it is positioned as a sagittal tissue plane in which the ureter courses.

Figure 22.39. Schauta-Amreich procedure. Palpating the left ureteral knee in the bladder pillar.

The surgeon palpates the stretched bladder pillar with a scissor-like grasp of the second and third fingers. Letting the bladder pillar glide through the fingers, he or she can identify the ureteral knee coursing in it as a coarse cylindrical cord. If the bladder pillar is not too thick, and with correct palpation, the ureteral knee may spring audibly across the fingertips.

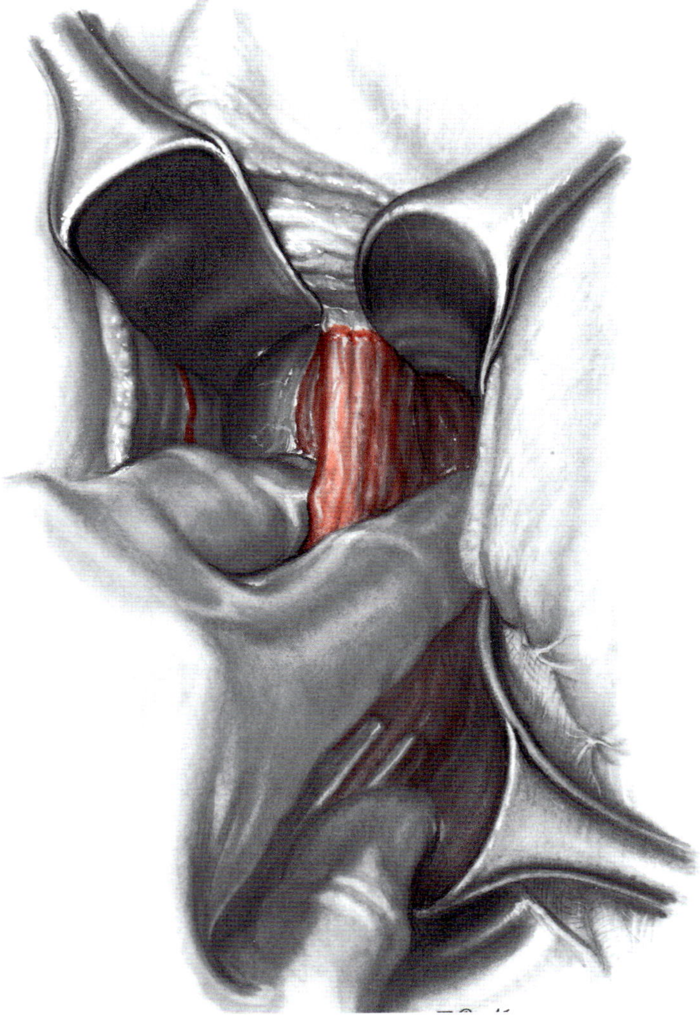

Figure 22.40. Schauta-Amreich procedure. Mobilizing the left ureter. Step-wise separation of the bladder pillar from the cervix.

The anterior retractors stretch the bladder pillar by applying upward pressure while they are somewhat tilted. One can recognize the tongue-like peritoneal reflection reaching down on the anterior surface of the uterus that has not yet been opened. The surgeon pushes the anterior cervical wall caudally with the middle finger; this stretches the bladder pillar even more, exposing its juncture at the edge of the cervix.

Fibers of the bladder pillar are separated in stepwise fashion close to the cervix anteriorly with several small scissor cuts. The tips of the scissors should point toward the cervix.

After separation of the caudal aspects of the bladder pillar, one approaches the ureteral knee coursing in the cephalad portion of the bladder pillar. One refrains therefore for the moment from further separating the bladder pillar from the cervix and ligates the uterine vascular bundle that now slowly comes into view.

Detail. Direction of ureter coursing in the bladder pillar.

1 vesicouterine ligament
2 lateral portion of the bladder pillar
3 cervix
4 cardinal ligament of Mackenrodt

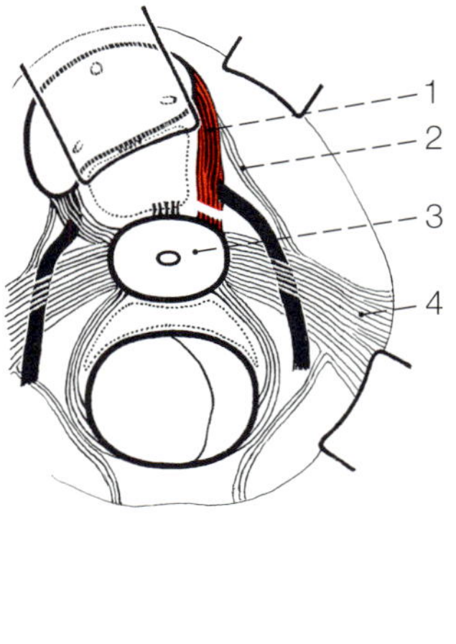

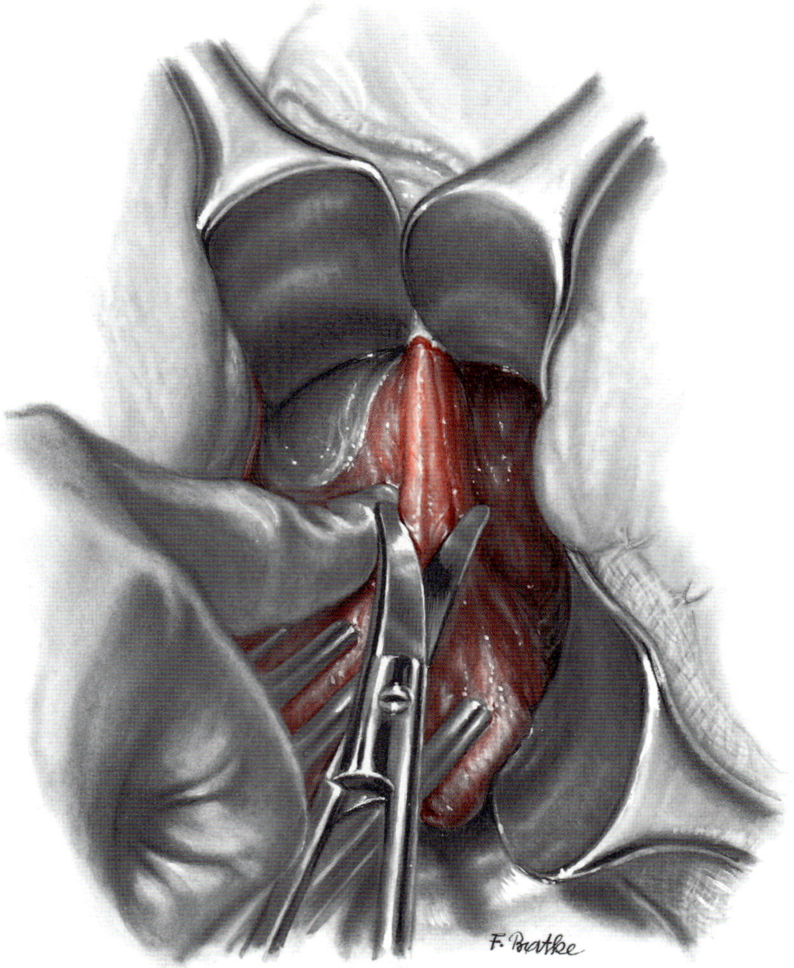

Figure 22.41. Schauta-Amreich procedure. Mobilizing the left ureter. Ligature of the uterine arteries and veins.

The caudal portions of the bladder pillar have been dissected from the cervix. The anterior retractors stretch the remaining part of the bladder pillar. With proper dissection, the uterine vascular bundle (uterine arteries and veins) appears medially from the bladder pillar. Vessels are ligated here with a silk Deschamps suture. The ligature is left long and pulled down to the right.

Because the uterine artery crosses over the ureteral knee (see *details*), downward traction on this vessel will displace the ureteral knee caudally (*right inset*) to make it more accessible for further dissection.

Details. Relationships of the uterine artery and the ureteral artery in situ (*left*) and after lateral and caudal displacement of the ureter (*right*).

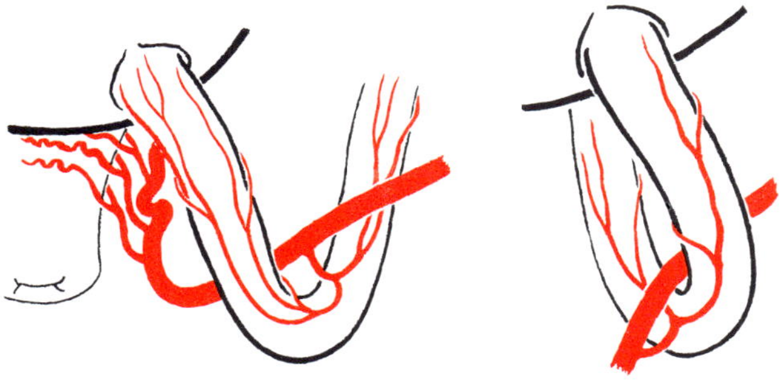

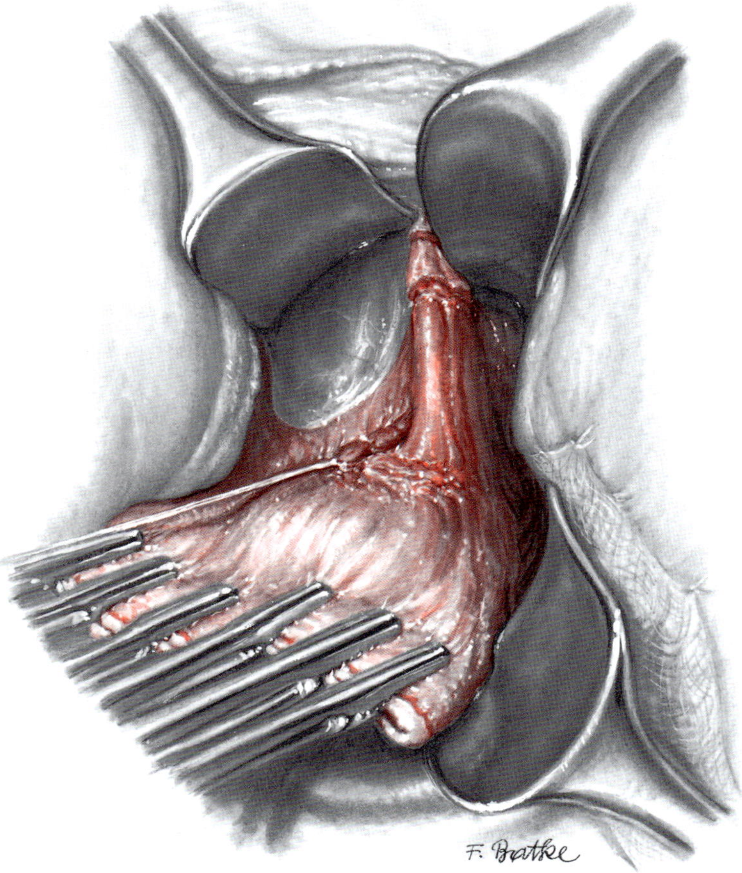

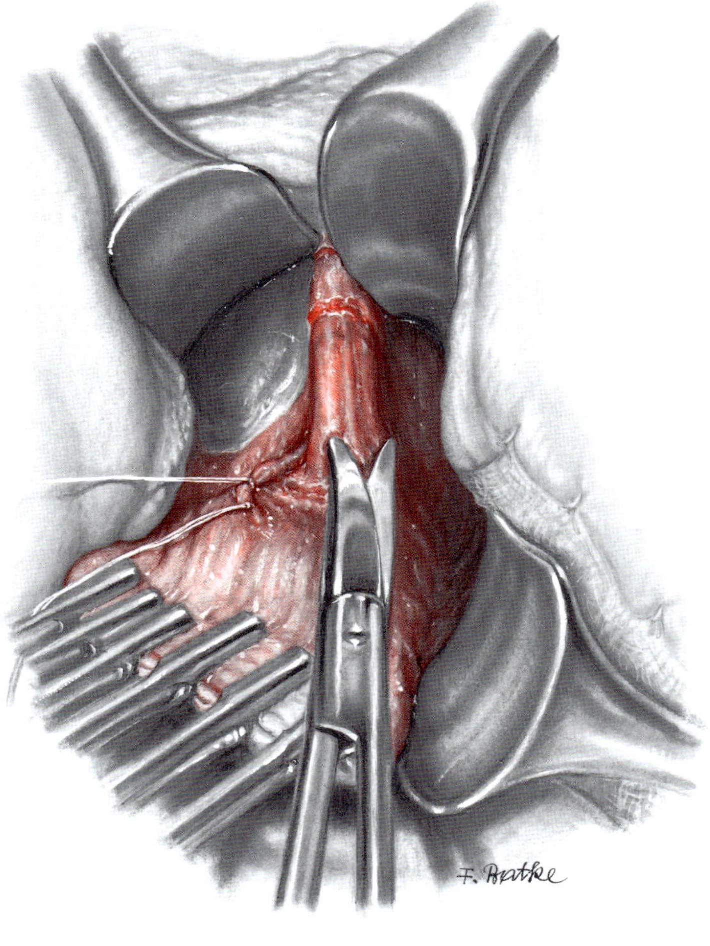

Figure 22.42. Schauta-Amreich procedure. Mobilizing the left ureteral knee. Further separation of the bladder pillar.

By tilting the anterior retractor up, the remaining part of the bladder pillar is stretched.

The uterine vascular bundle has been relegated proximal to the first suture, the end is left long, to be used as a new marker. This will further displace the ureteral knee caudally where it can be easily located through renewed palpation.

The surgeon carefully renews the division of the bladder pillar fibers with small scissor incisions near the cervix.

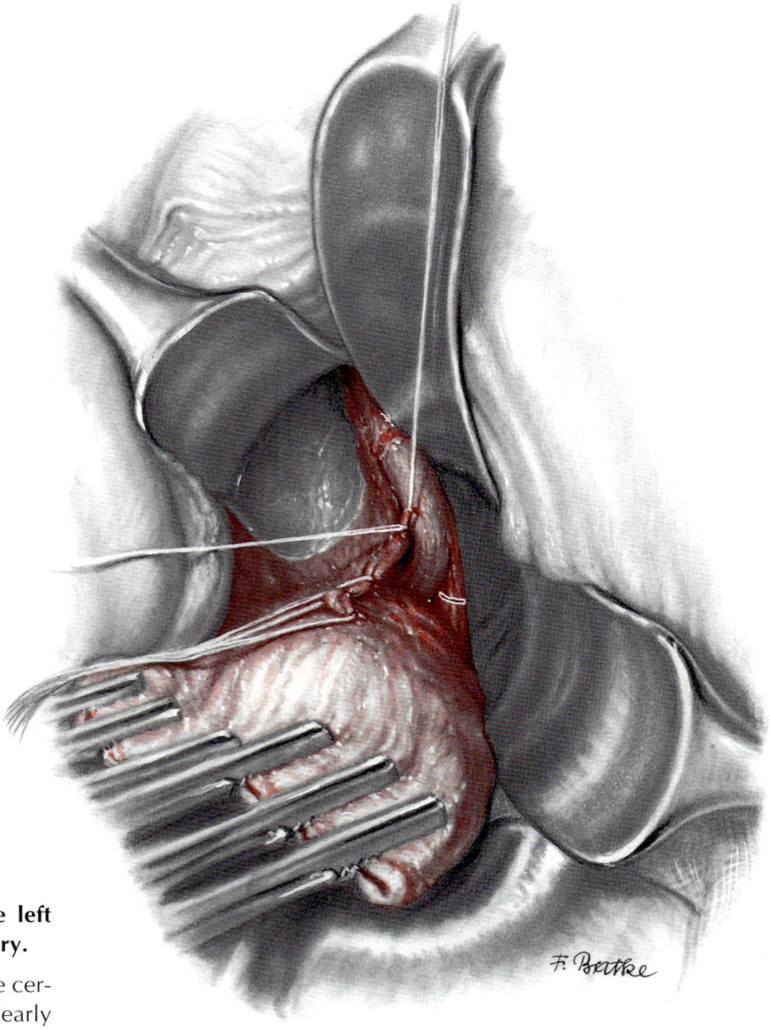

Figure 22.43. Schauta-Amreich procedure. Mobilizing the left ureter. Opening the ureteral canal. Ligating the ureteral artery.

The medial aspects of the bladder pillar are separated from the cervix. The ureteral canal is opened and the ureteral knee is clearly visible.

The uterine vascular bundle is triply ligated medially to the ureteral knee. The ureteral artery, originating from the uterine artery, is doubly ligated and divided.

When the bladder pillar is especially thickened, it is necessary to ligate its lateral aspects (*black line*). Only then can the ureteral knee easily be pushed upward with closed dissecting scissors.

Details. Uterine vascular bundle and ureteral artery.

1 traction on vascular bundle pulled to the ureter
2 uterine vascular bundle
3 ureter
4 ureteral artery
5 uterine artery

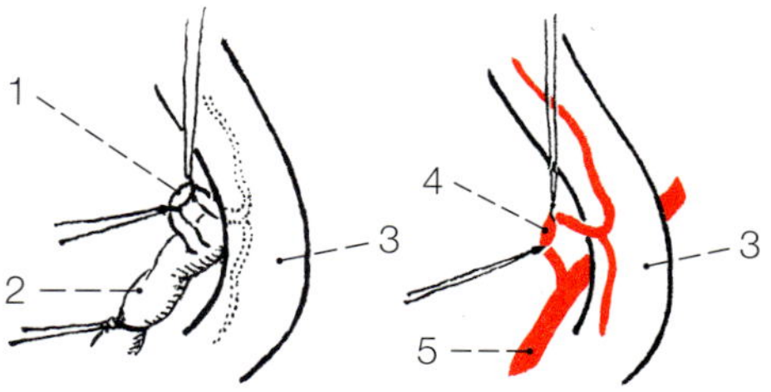

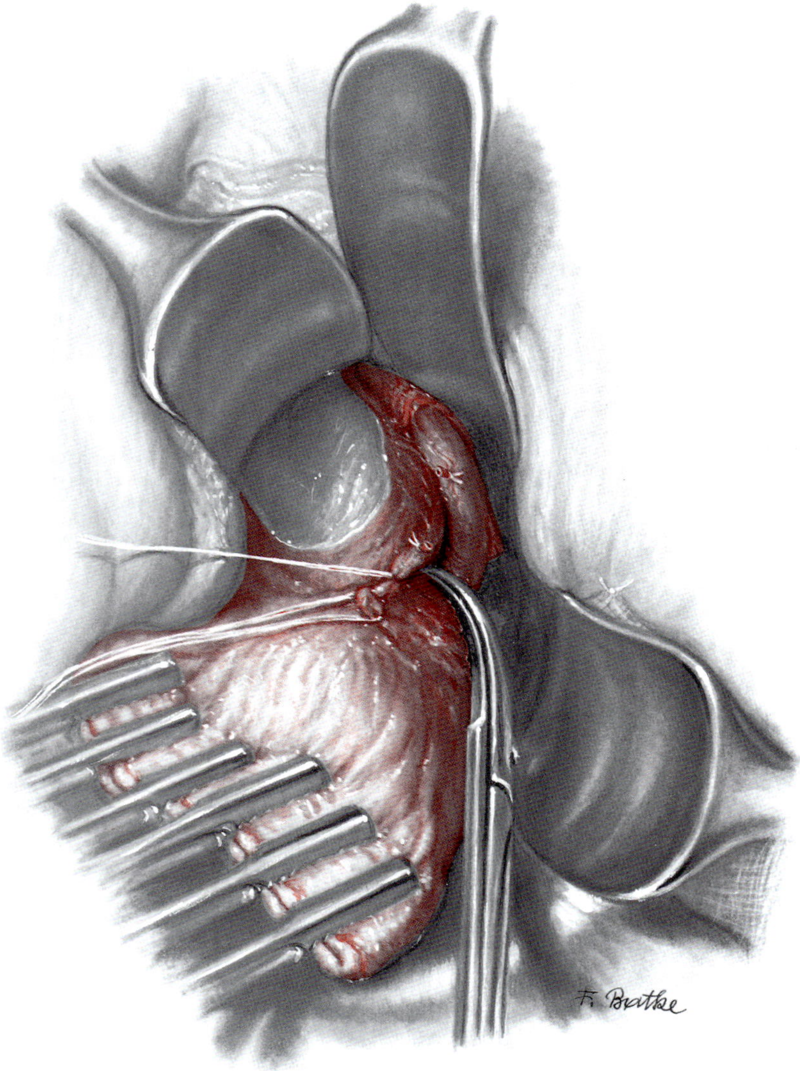

Figure 22.44. Schauta-Amreich procedure. Mobilizing the left ureter. Displacing the ureteral knee.

The uterine vessel bundle has been ligated several times; the ureteral artery has been divided.

The mobilized ureteral knee is pushed further upward with closed dissecting scissors that can now be ligated still higher. The higher the uterine vascular bundle is ligated, the better the lateral parametrium can later be resected.

Details. Relationship of the uterine vascular bundle (*left*) and uterine artery (*right*) to the ureter.

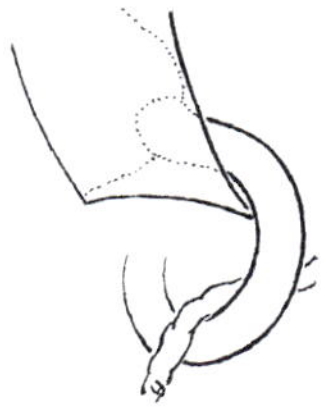

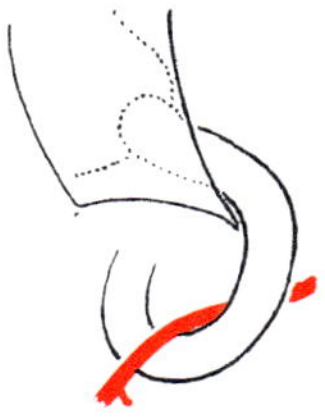

Figure 22.45. Schauta-Amreich procedure. Mobilizing the left ureter. Final cephalad ligation of the uterine vessels.

The left ureter is mobilized far up and laterally and pushed cephalad with the anterior retractor held by the left assistant. The anterior retractor of the right assistant elevates the bladder.

Once again, the uterine vascular bundle is doubly ligated up high.

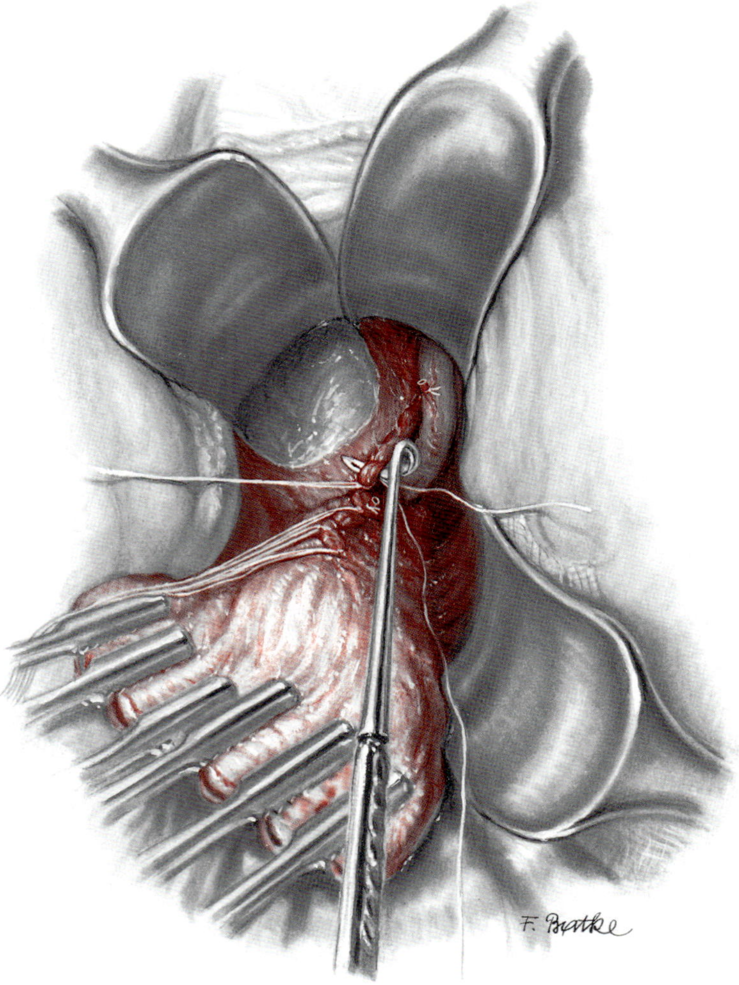

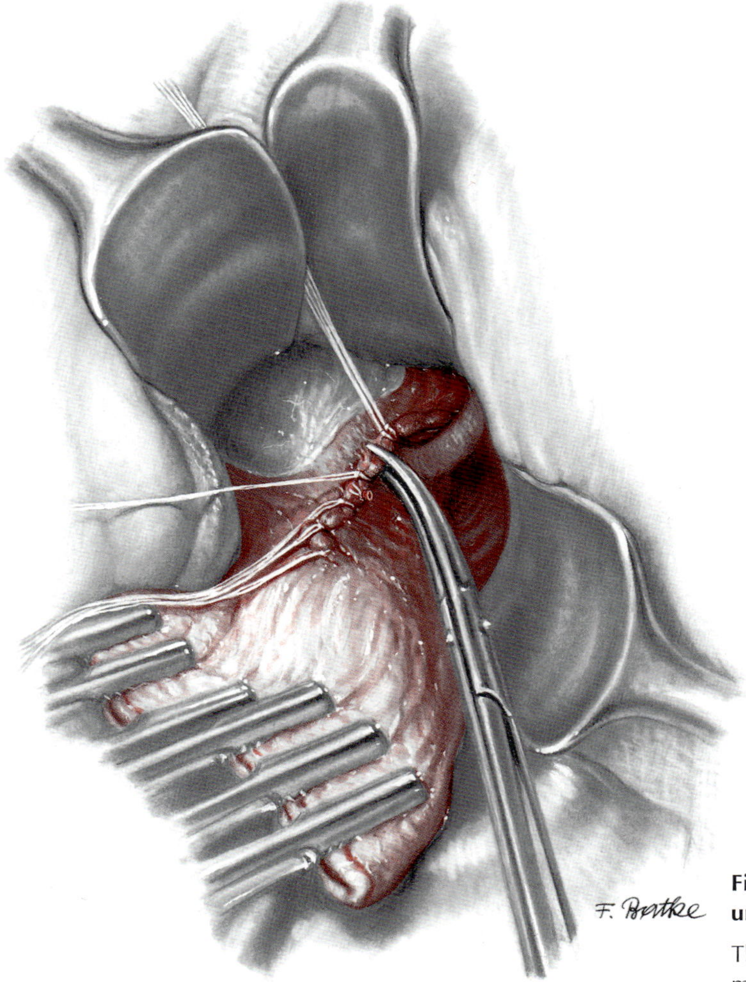

Figure 22.46. Schauta-Amreich procedure. Mobilizing the left ureter.

The uterine vascular bundles are divided distally to the two uppermost ligatures.

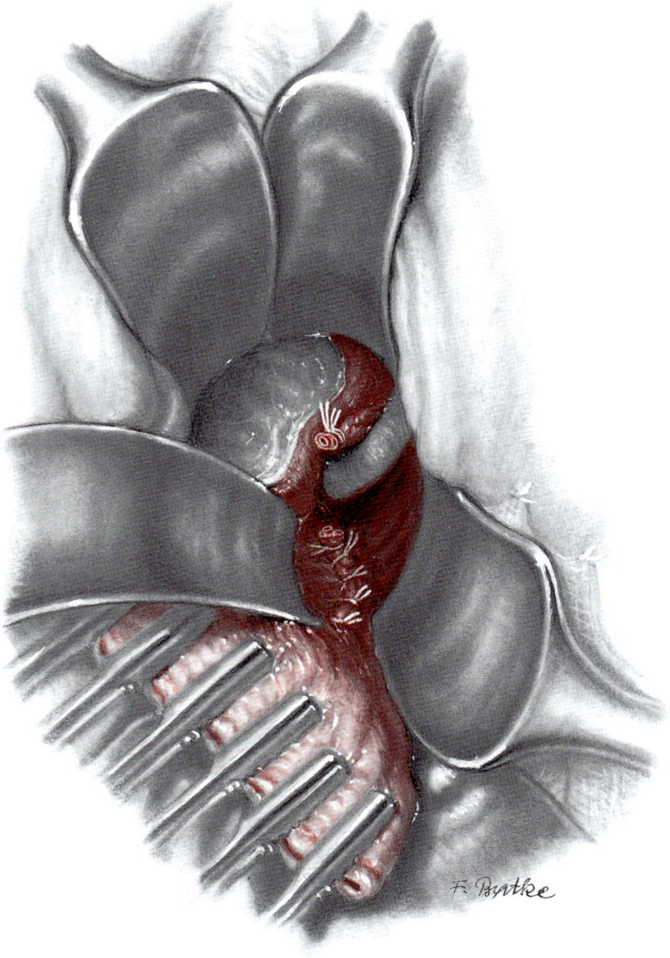

Figure 22.47. Schauta-Amreich procedure. The left ureter is freed. View of operative site.

The five uterine ligatures tied in stepwise fashion are visible at the edge of the cervix. The uterine vascular bundle has been divided; the cephalad portion of the vascular pedicle can be seen medially from the ureteral knee.

Along a short section, the ureter has been completely mobilized gently and can be displaced upward, which is important later in the surgical procedure.

Technical Problems—Figures 22.38–22.47

1. If the *bladder pillar is insufficiently stretched* because the retraction is insufficient, palpation of the ureteral knee is made more difficult, and it becomes possible to injure the ureter during dissection of the caudal part of the bladder pillar.
2. When the fibers of the bladder pillar are dissected *too close to the bladder*, there may be danger to the ureter as well.
3. Should the bladder pillar be divided *too close to the cervix*, massive hemorrhage from the uterine vessels may ensue.
4. In the event of *insufficient dissection of the bladder pillar*, freeing the ureteral knee becomes very difficult.
5. When a cystocele exists, the *bladder* may extend *far down* between the bladder pillars. It must first be carefully separated from the cervix and advanced before the uterine vessel bundle can be ligated higher up. Otherwise, bladder tissue may be incorporated in the uterine ligature.
6. In the course of the sharp division of the bladder pillar from the cervix, the assistants must be sure to hold the vaginal retractors very still because *every positional change produces a change in the location of the ureter* within the bladder pillar.
7. If the assistant on the right side *does not apply sufficient continuous traction to the right and downward* on the uppermost *uterine vascular ligature*, the ureteral knee in the bladder pillar is inadequately displaced caudally. This means that the ureteral knee remains high up out of reach and is therefore more difficult to mobilize.
8. During very high ligation of the uterine vascular bundle, especially if some bleeding occurs from it, the *juxtavesical segment of the ureter may be drawn into the ligature.*
9. The assistant on the left side can inadvertently tear veins located at the pelvic wall by *excessive pressure* applied to the *retractors* in the paravesical and pararectal spaces. Tying these veins can create great difficulties.

Preparation of Right Paraspaces

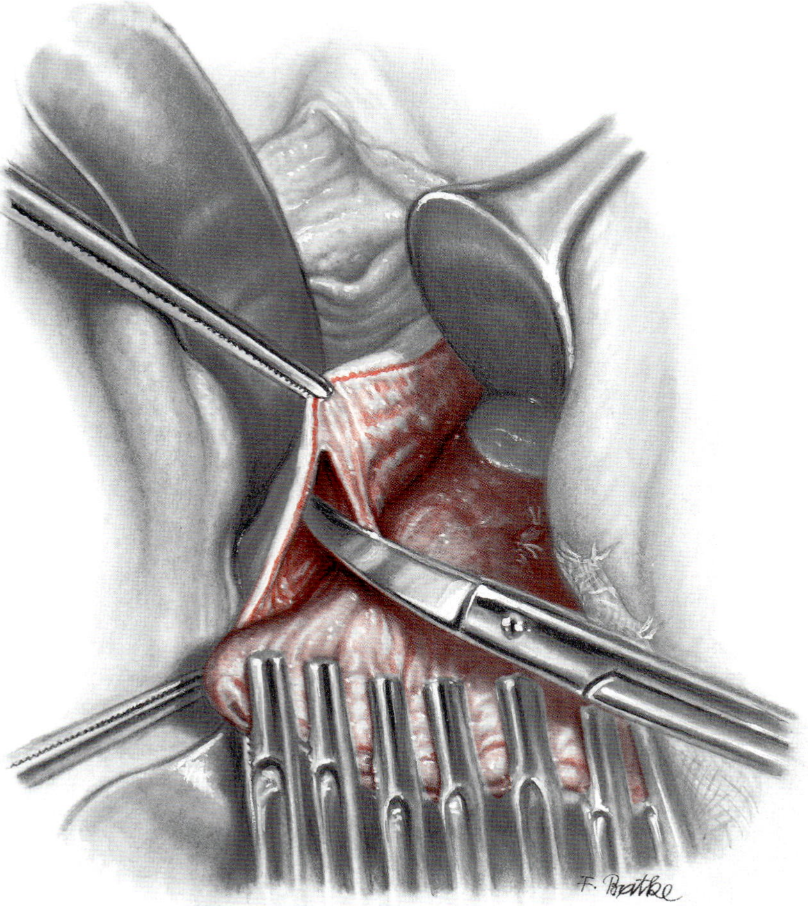

Figure 22.48. Schauta-Amreich procedure. Opening the right paravescical space.

The paravesical space must first be dissected to reach the lateral side of the right bladder pillar, which can now be seen as a sagittally reaching connective tissue plane in which the ureter courses. The surgeon places two toothed clamps at the lateral vaginal circumcision wound edge, one at the level of the paravesical space and the other further down at the pararectal space. The upper clamp is then pulled toward the surgeon. The right labia and the bladder are pushed downward with retractors.

The surgeon then opens the right paravesical space with a pair of curved dissecting scissors by incising just medial to the vaginal wound edge. This opening is enlarged somewhat by widening the scissor blades, which allows the surgeon to insert the finger and expose the entire paravesical space.

Correct and complete exposure of the right paravesical space is sometimes more difficult than mobilization of the ureters.

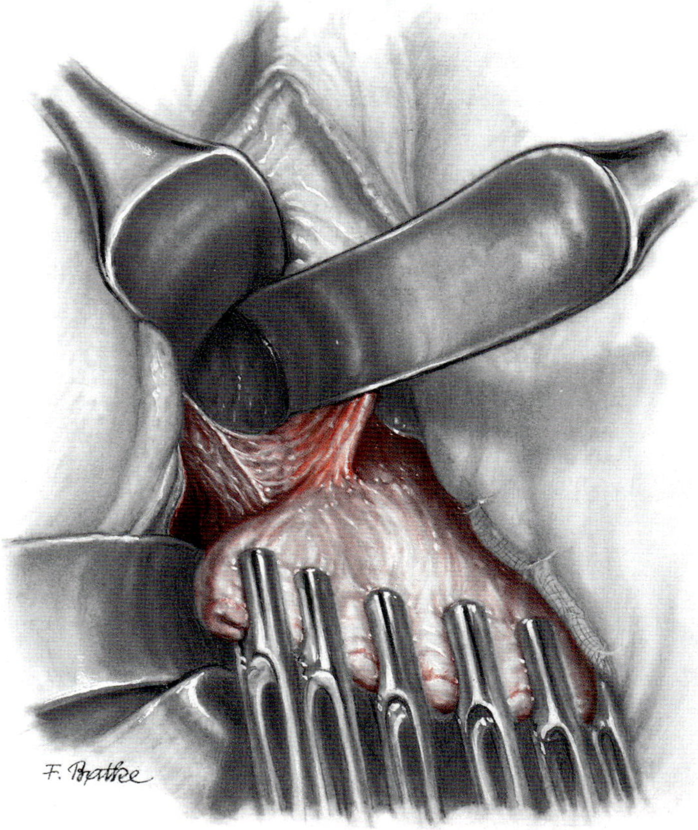

Figure 22.49. Schauta-Amreich procedure. Presentation of the right horizontal pelvic fascia.

The assistant on the right retracts the vaginal wall upward and to the right with a retractor inserted into the paravesical space, while holding back the protruding rectum with a lateral retractor placed in the pararectal space. The toothed clamps on the lateral side are removed from the vaginal incision edge. The assistant on the left side inserts a long narrow retractor into the right paravesical space and pushes the right bladder pillar toward the midline.

The horizontal pelvic fascia (dense connective tissue) may be seen as an intervening layer between the paravesical and pararectal space.

Figure 22.50. Schauta-Amreich procedure. Uniting the right paraspaces (paravesical with pararectal space).

The horizontal fascia is exposed with appropriate retraction. It is grasped with two long, straight clamps and divided between them. In this way the spaces lateral to the right bladder pillar and the rectum are completely united.

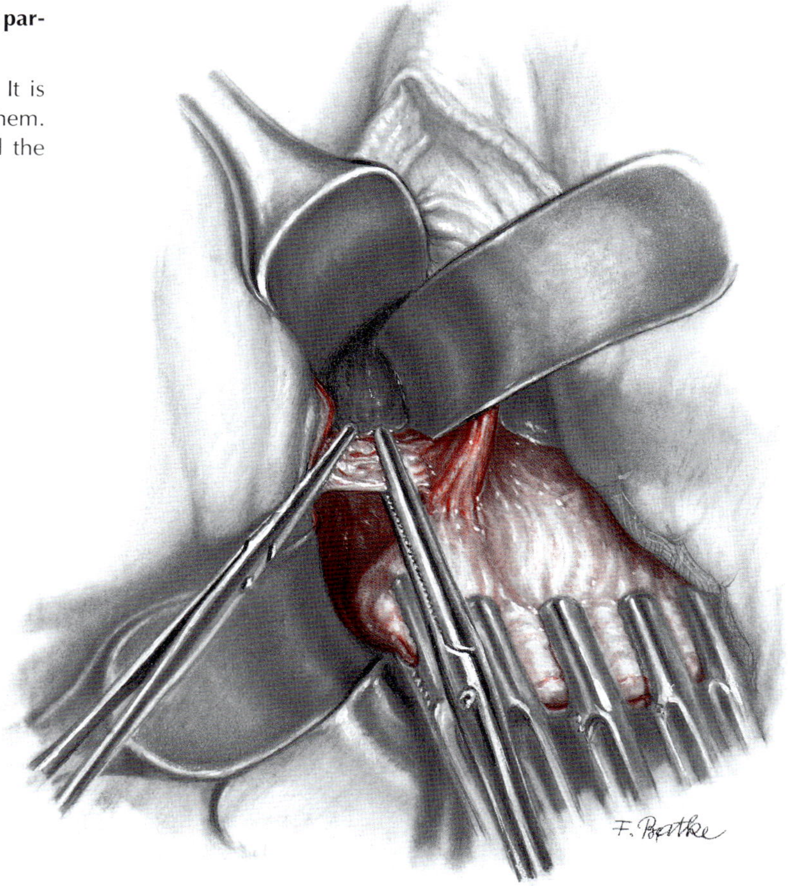

Technical Problems—Figures 22.48–22.50

1. The *sharp dissection* required for opening the paravesical space must be performed just under the vaginal fascia. If one incises somewhat more medially, bladder injury may occur.
2. The *scissors may be directed incorrectly* into the space. If the vaginal circumcision had been done relatively close to the cervix so that only a small amount of vagina was circumcised for later removal, the closed tip of the scissors for opening the paravesical space must be directed laterally to be certain that it will proceed laterally to the right bladder pillar. Conversely, if plenty of vaginal mucosa was removed (i.e., the circumcision was performed far from the cervix), the tip of the dissecting scissors should proceed directly upward into the paravesical space and parallel to the pelvic wall but not in a lateral direction because this might cause it to reach the obturator fascia and damage the pelvic wall veins.
3. After the paravesical wall has been opened, if *the scissors tip is advanced too far* into the space, the veins at the pelvic wall or the bladder can be damaged. Complete exposure of the opened paravesical space is best done bluntly with a finger.
4. If the paravesical space *has not been opened widely enough*, it will not be possible to expose the outer surface of the right bladder pillar completely. This will make later dissection of the ureter more difficult.
5. If *the clamps* are *applied too high* up the pelvic wall on the horizontal pelvic fascia, the blood vessels on the pelvic wall can be injured by the lateral clamp, and the ureter coursing in the bladder pillar can be injured by the medial clamp.
6. When the correctly placed medial clamp is replaced by sutures, one must not insert the needle *too deeply* into the bladder pillar because the ureter might be caught in the suture as well.
7. *Incomplete union* of the right paravesical space with the pararectal space will risk later problems because one will still find thickened tissue lateral to the mobilized right ureter while attempting to dissect the right ureteral knee free. This tissue courses in a cranial-caudal direction and may be part of the descended bladder or the levator. Because any connective tissue found lateral to the ureteral knee must be moved aside or divided to achieve complete mobilization, injury to the bladder is possible.

Dissection of Ureter on the Right

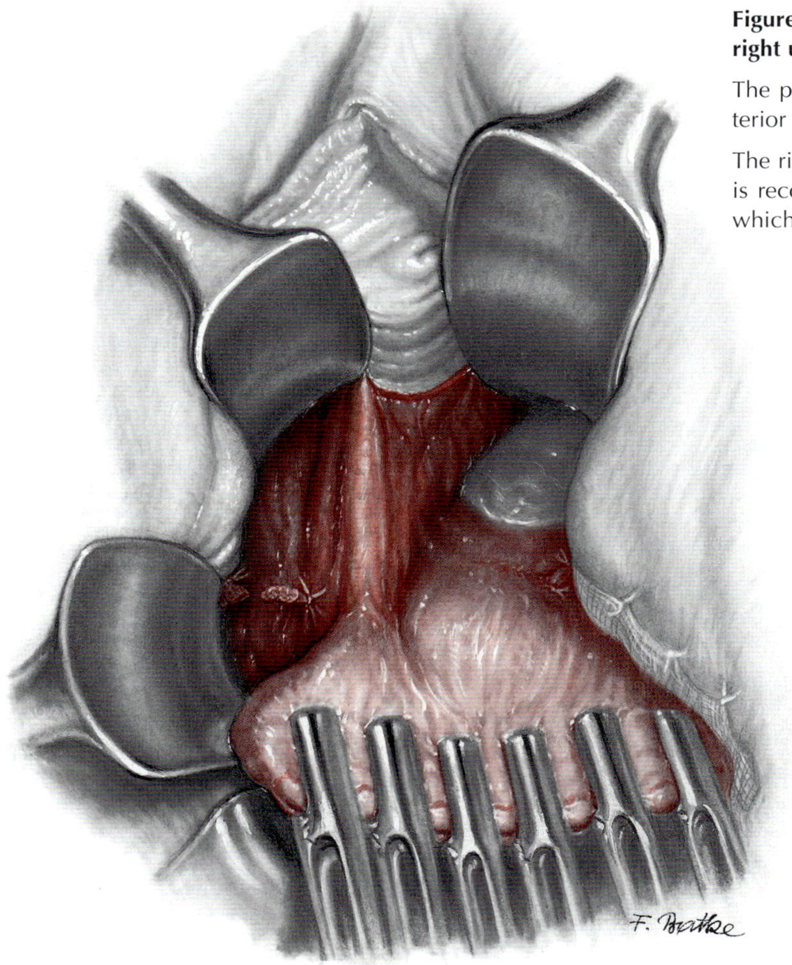

Figure 22.51. Schauta-Amreich procedure. Dissecting free the right ureter. Visualization of the right bladder pillar.

The paravesical and pararectal spaces have been united. The anterior peritoneal fold is visible on the anterior uterine wall.

The right bladder pillar is exposed with appropriate retraction and is recognizable as a connective tissue layer in a sagittal plane in which the ureter courses.

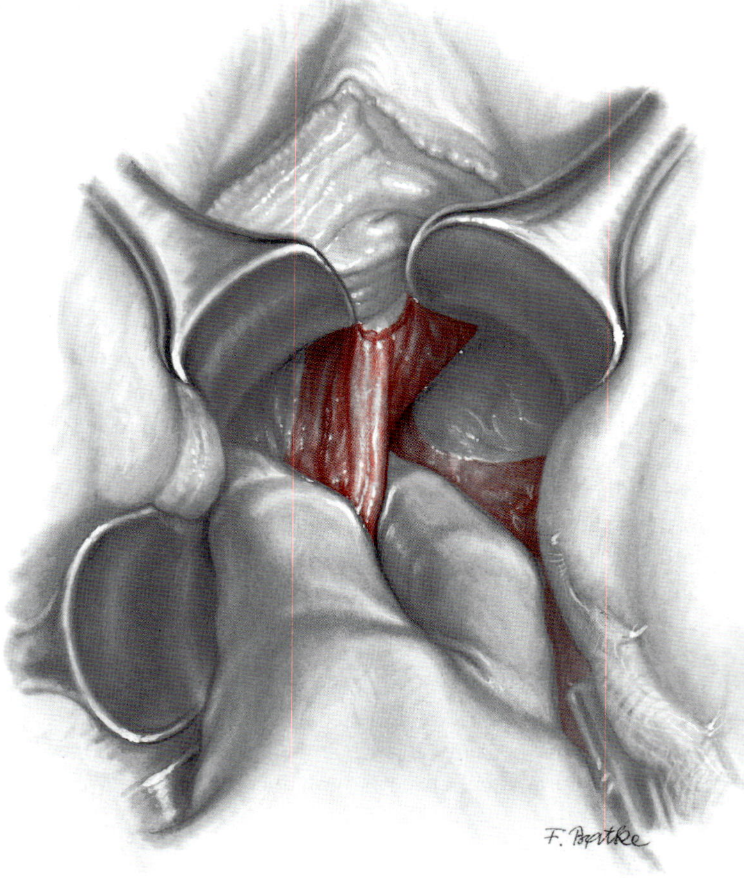

Figure 22.52. Schauta-Amreich procedure. Dissecting free the right ureter. Palpating the ureter in the bladder pillar.

The anterior retractors are tilted, which stretches the right bladder pillar noticeably.

The surgeon locates the ureteral knee by palpation with the second and third fingers by taking hold of the bladder pillar in a scissor-like grip.

Detail. The left vesical ligament (left bladder pillar) is divided from the cervix; the right vesical ligament [right bladder pillar (*red*)] is stretched.

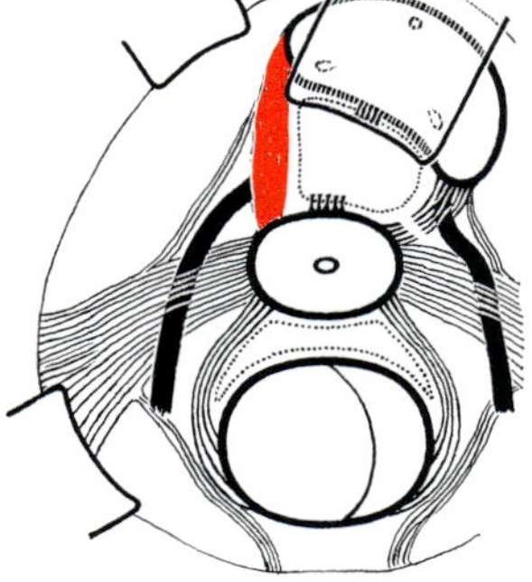

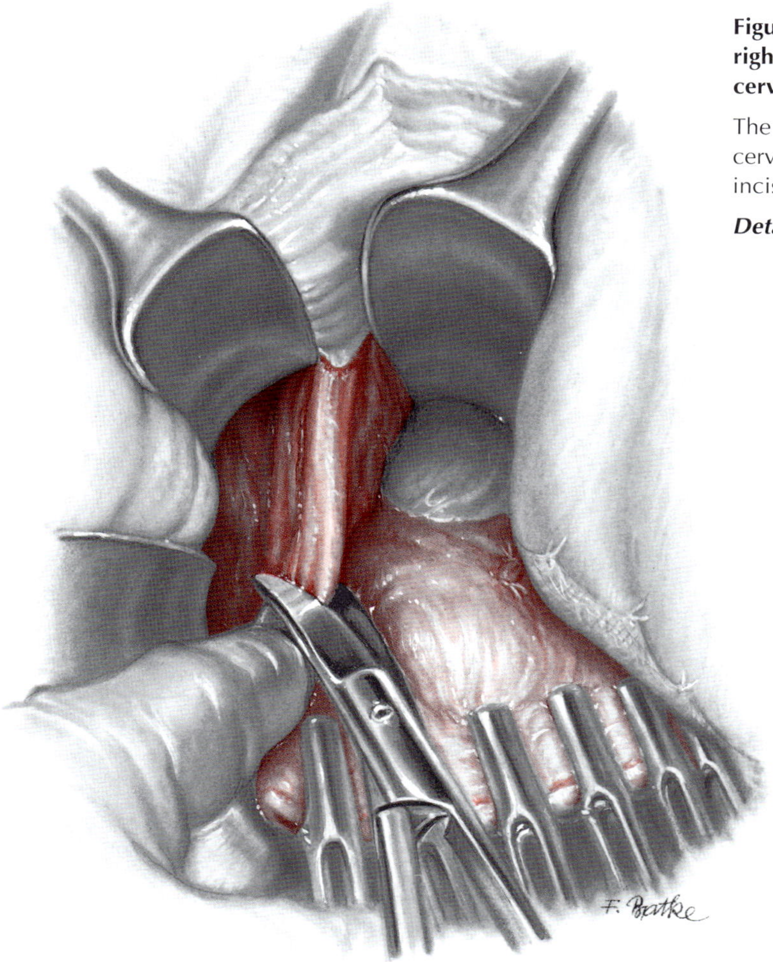

Figure 22.53. Schauta-Amreich procedure. Dissecting free the right ureter. Step-wise division of the right bladder pillar at the cervix.

The assistants stretch the bladder pillar. The surgeon depresses the cervix with the left index finger and, with short snips of the scissors, incises the bladder pillar at its base close to the edge of the cervix.

Detail. Both bladder pillars are divided from the cervix.

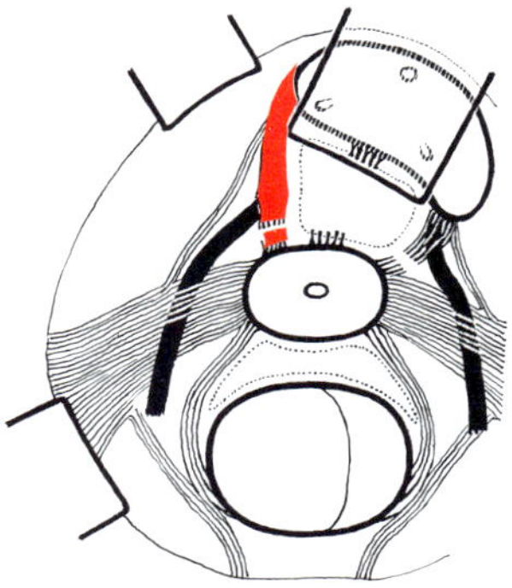

Figure 22.54. Schauta-Amreich procedure. Dissecting free the right ureter. Separating the right bladder pillar.

The uterine vascular bundle is ligated once; the right bladder pillar has only been partially separated from the cervix. In cases where there is much vaginal or bladder descensus the bladder edge must be dissected off the ureteral knee both laterally and medially and advanced upward. To accomplish this, the bladder base is elevated and pushed vigorously toward the symphysis with an anterior retractor.

The surgeon raises the descended bladder edge with toothed forceps medially to the exposed ureter. The bladder pole can now be divided with scissors close to the cervix.

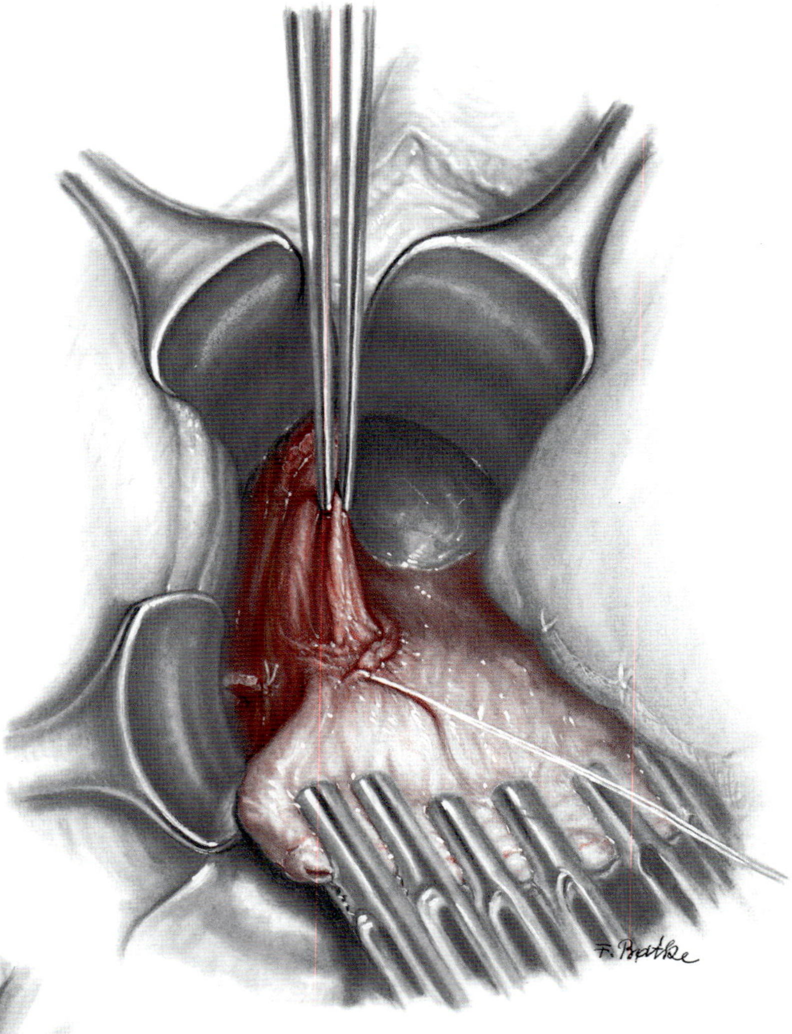

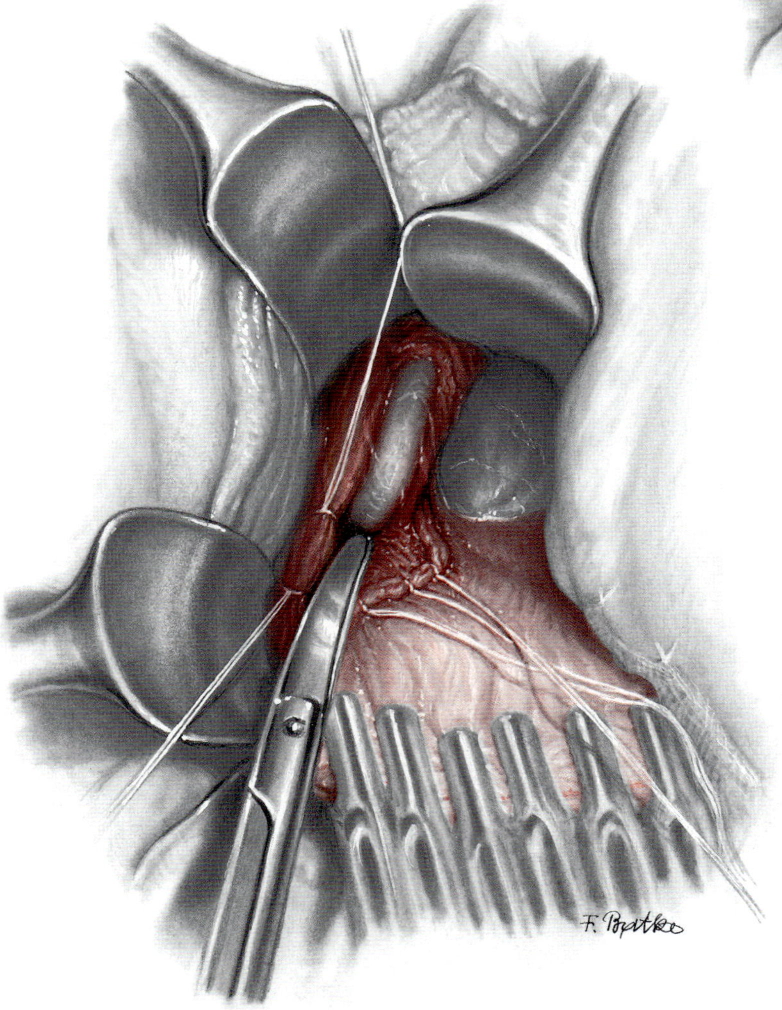

Figure 22.55. Schauta-Amreich procedure. Dissecting free the right ureter. Ligating and dividing the lateral aspects of the thickened bladder pillar.

The ureteral knee has been extensively mobilized anteriorly, and on its medial side the uterine muscular bundle has already been ligated three times.

The fibers of the bladder pillar stretching lateral to the ureter are doubly ligated. The points of the closed scissors are in the opened ureteral canal; they push the ureteral knee upward to move it out of the line of incision.

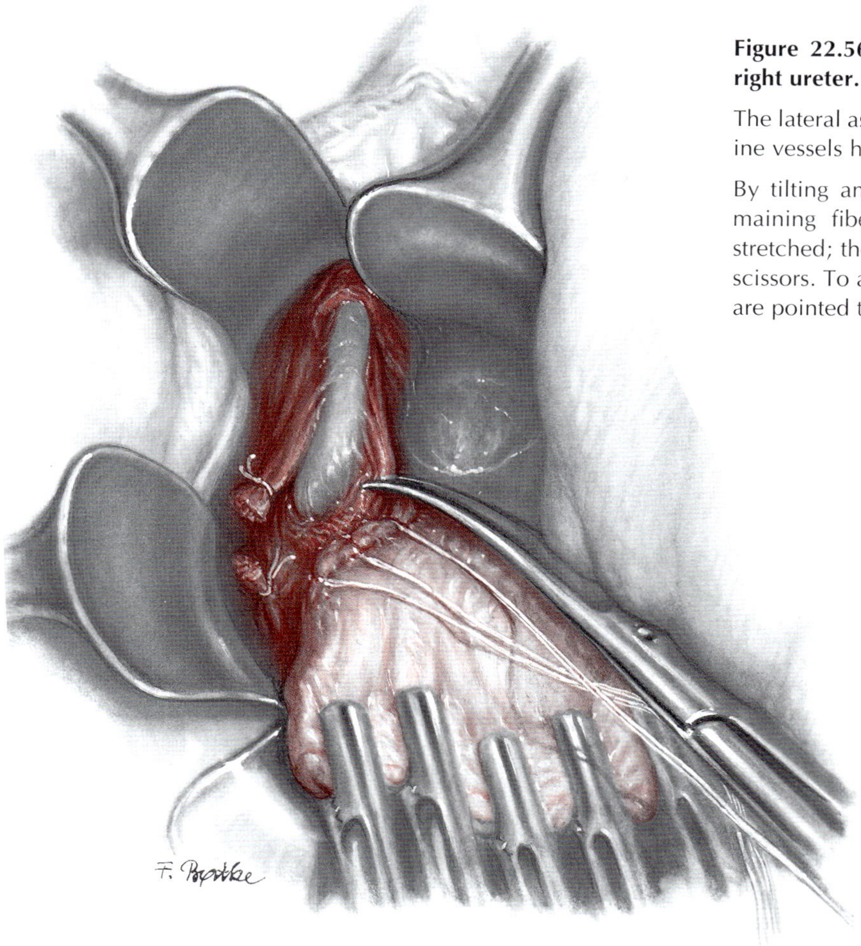

Figure 22.56. Schauta-Amreich procedure. Dissecting free the right ureter. Further separating the bladder pillar from the cervix.

The lateral aspects of the bladder pillar have been divided; the uterine vessels have been ligated three times.

By tilting and forcefully elevating the anterior retractors, the remaining fibers of the bladder pillar medial to the ureter are stretched; they are dissected or pushed back with slightly opened scissors. To avoid injuring the ureter, the curved tips of the scissors are pointed toward the cervix.

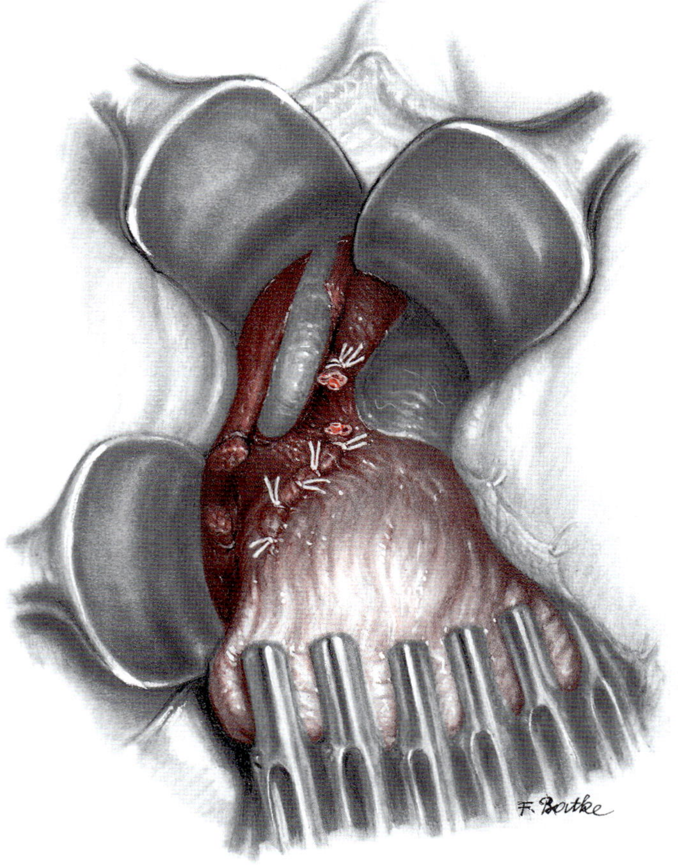

Figure 22.57. Schauta-Amreich procedure. Dissecting free the right ureter. Status after division of the uterine vascular bundle.

The right ureteral knee has been extensively mobilized. It can be lifted upward and laterally with a retractor after the uterine vascular bundle has been once more ligated and divided high up.

Opening Cul-de-Sac of Douglas

Figure 22.58. Schauta-Amreich procedure. Opening the cul-de-sac of Douglas.

The assistants pull the vaginal cuff with its attached mouse-toothed clamps toward the symphysis. The rectum, which is at times ballooning forward, is retracted aside with two lateral retractors. The surgeon pulls the peritoneal edge out with toothed tissue forceps in midline and divides it with a single cut of scissors whose curved tips are pointed upward.

Details. Opening the cul-de-sac of Douglas in a median-sagittal incision (*left*) and from below (*right*).

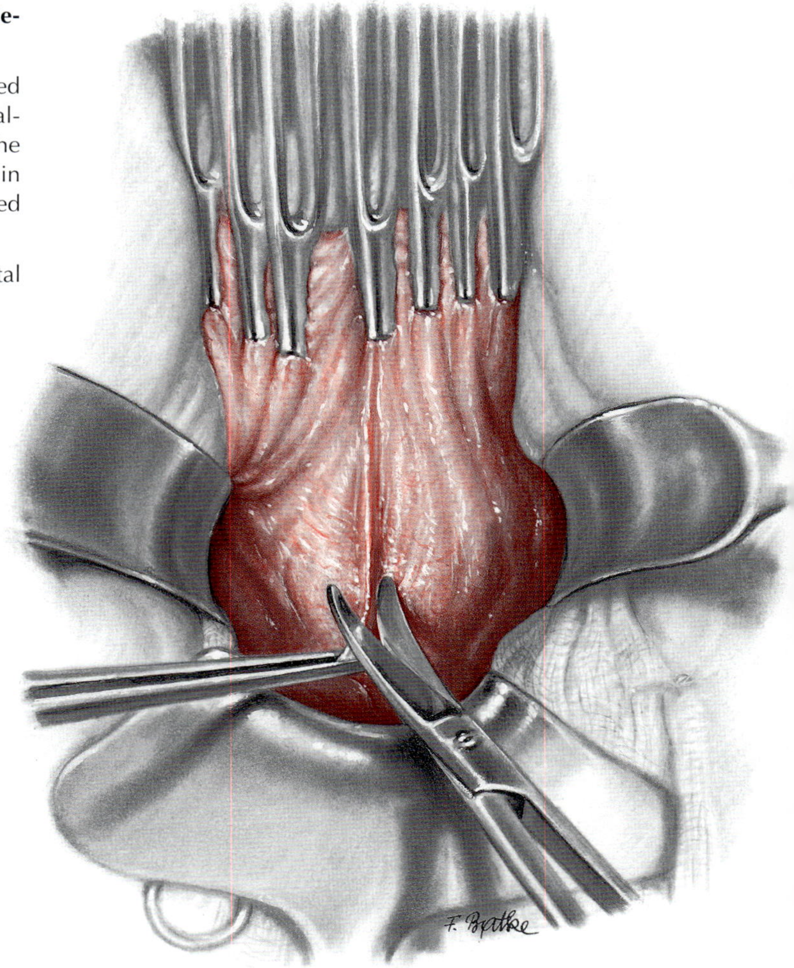

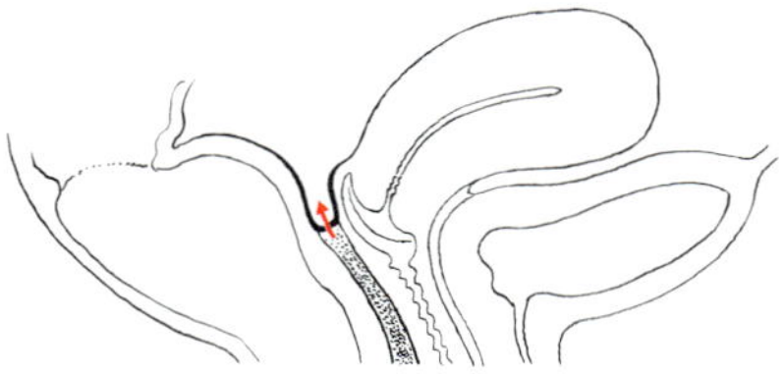

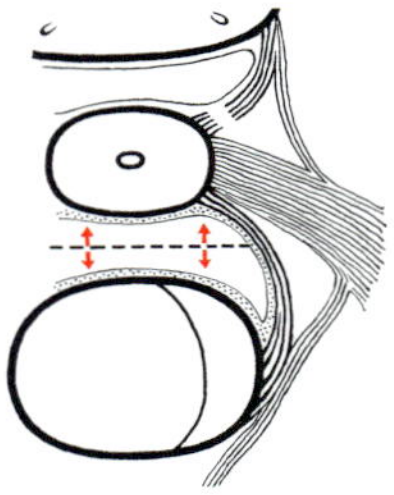

Technical Problems—Figure 22.58

1. Before the cul-de-sac of Douglas has been opened, the rectum has been retracted caudally in the midline of the posterior cervical wall, and the *stretched tissue fibers at the sides* are divided. These fibers are part of the rectal pillar and constitute the uterosacral ligaments that should not be dissected close to the posterior cervix at this time but, instead, close to the rectum later in the procedure.
2. While trying to avoid injury to the rectum, *the peritoneal cul-de-sac reflection might be sought too near the cervix.* This will cause the surgeon to dissect the posterior peritoneal pouch further from the posterior wall of the cervix or uterus. He or she will be working in a ''poor plane'' and will therefore not be able to reach the abdominal cavity. In such a case it is advisable to pull the incorrectly dissected tissues upward with a toothed clamp and to incise posterior to the clamp. Now the posterior peritoneal reflection can be opened without risk, provided there are no adhesions in the cul-de-sac.
3. It is sometimes not feasible to *expose* the *peritoneal reflection* clearly, if at all, but the surgeon might try to open the cul-de-sac with a single incision. Such a procedure is dangerous and should be avoided because the rectum or intestinal loops might be opened mistakenly. Ordinarily, dissection in the correct layer will permit clear definition of the cul-de-sac and make it easy to open. One should assume that adhesions are present if the peritoneum cannot be readily found; here it is better not to try to open the cul-de-sac but to await a better view of the situation in the cul-de-sac space later, after the vesicouterine fold has been opened and the uterus has been rolled anteriorly.

Division of Rectal Pillars (Rectouterine Ligaments)

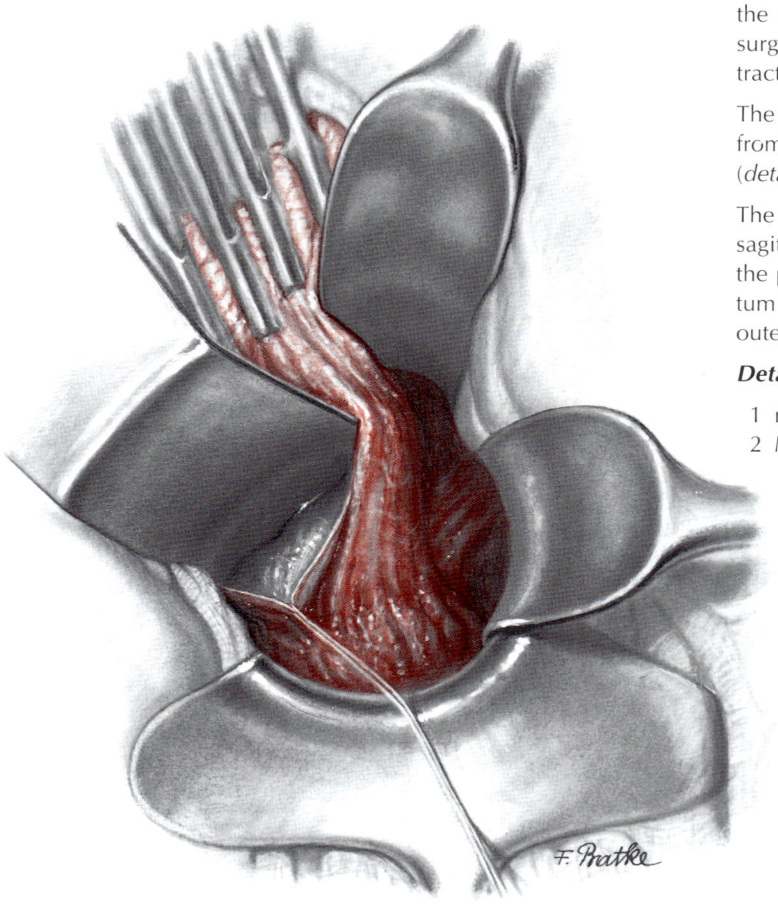

Figure 22.59. Schauta-Amreich procedure. Dividing the left rectal pillar. Preparing the operative field.

A long gauze strip is inserted into the widely opened cul-de-sac of Douglas and pushed toward the symphysis using a broad right-angled retractor; this will retract the intestinal loops upward. The left assistant lifts the well-mobilized left ureter (extraperitoneally in the paravescical fossa) with an anterolateral retractor and pushes back the rectum with a posterolateral retractor. At the same time, the surgeon should visually check that the ureter has actually been retracted well out of the way.

The left rectal pillar is thereby stretched so that it courses upward from the left lateral edge of the rectum to Mackenrodt's ligament (*detail*).

The medial surface of this tissue structure, which is now located sagittally, is covered by peritoneum. A traction suture is placed on the posterior peritoneal wound edge. The forward ballooning rectum must be dissected somewhat more from its attachments to the outer aspects of the rectal pillar.

Detail. Course of the rectal pillar.

1 rectal pillar
2 Mackenrodt's ligament

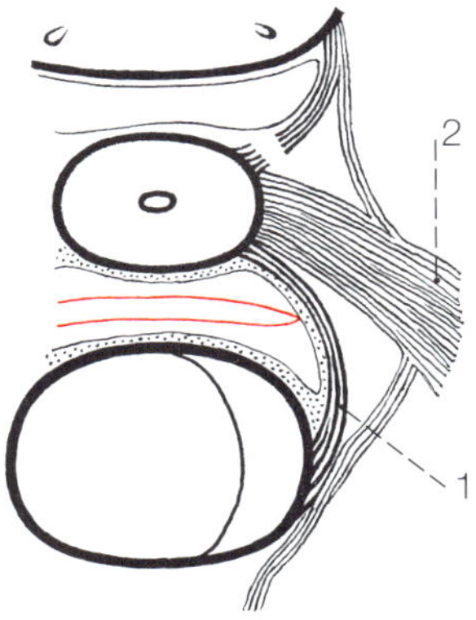

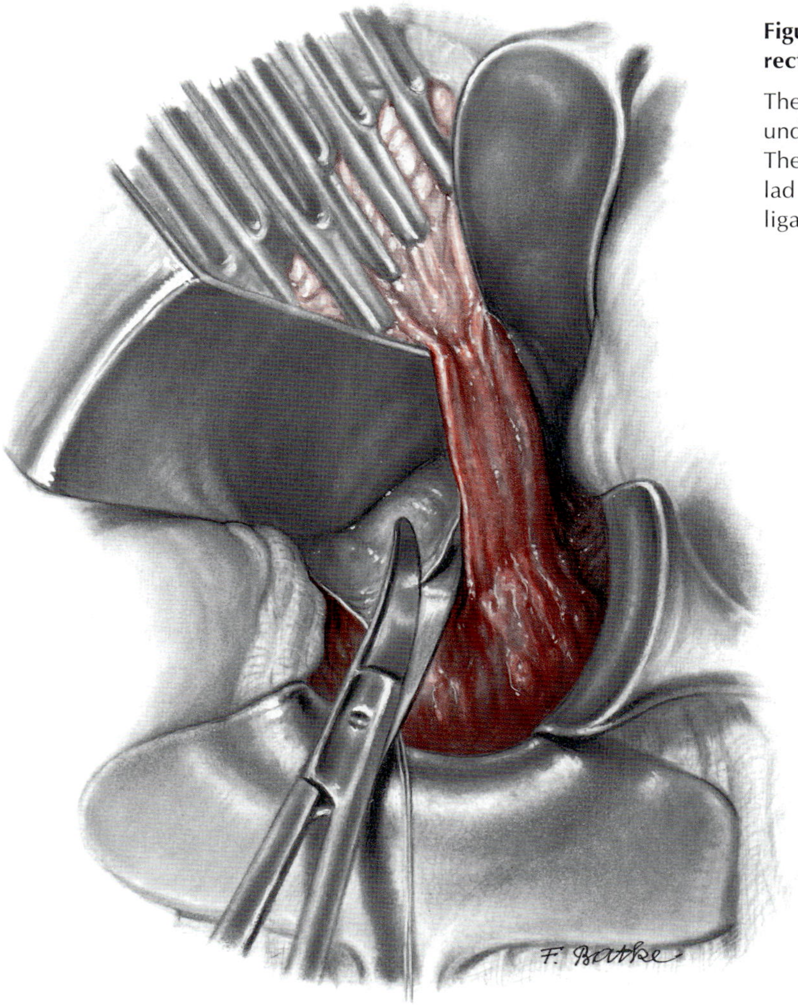

Figure 22.60. Schauta-Amreich procedure. Dividing the left rectal pillar. Incision of the peritoneum at the rectal pillar.

The peritoneum at the median side of the rectal pillar has been undermined with closed scissors and incised at the pillar's base. The peritoneal incision is now extended until it reaches cephalad to the entrance of the rectal pillar into the Mackenrodt's ligament.

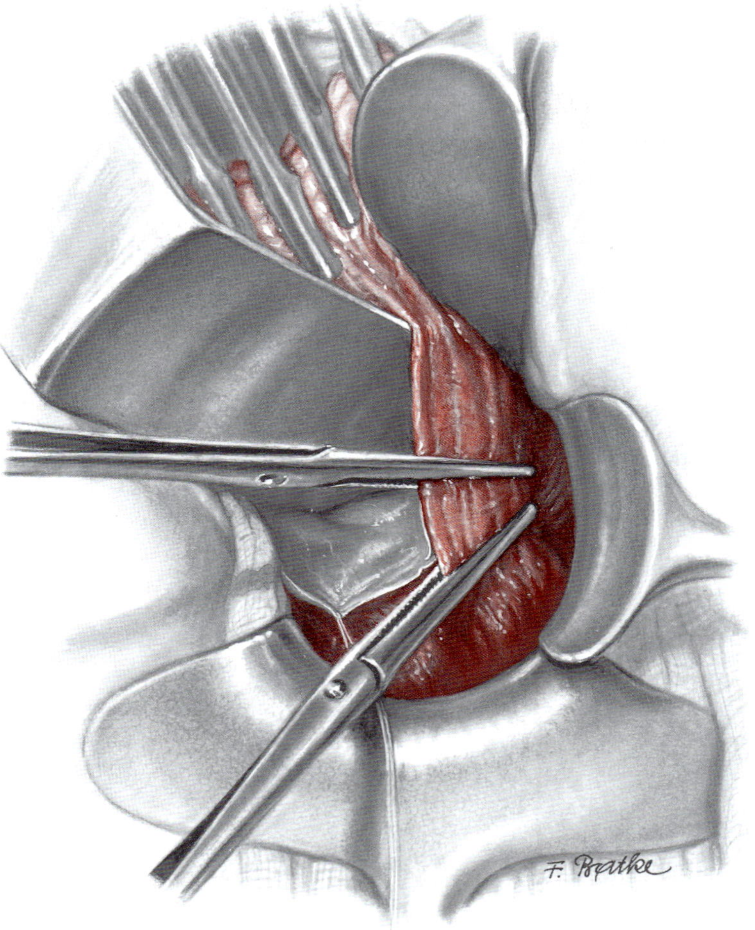

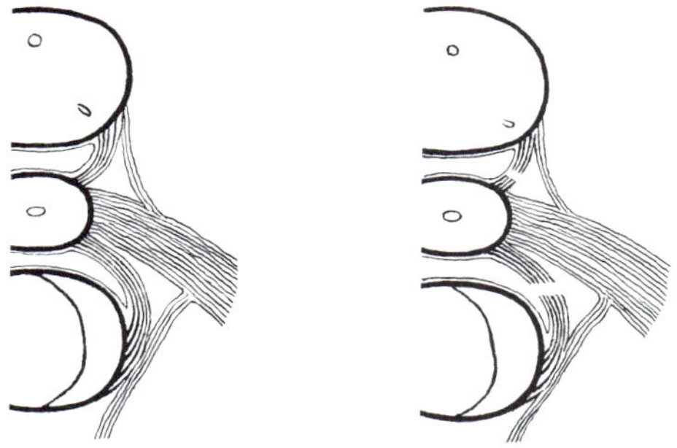

Figure 22.61. Schauta-Amreich procedure. Dividing the left rectal pillar.

Continuing retractor pressure applied on the rectal pillar will stretch the pillar in the sagittal plane.

The rectal pillar has been exposed medially from its peritoneal covering. Two long clamps are applied close to the rectum, and the pillar is divided between them.

Details. Connective tissues in situ (*left*) and location of division of the vesicouterine and rectouterine ligaments (*right*).

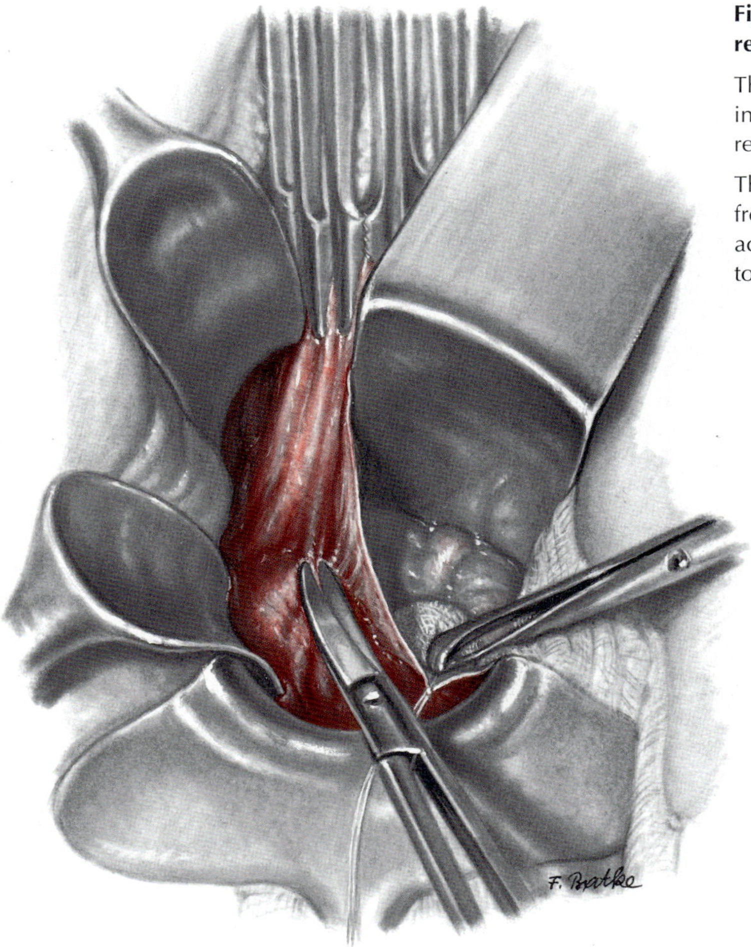

Figure 22.62. Schauta-Amreich procedure. Dividing the right rectal pillar. Additional dissection of the rectum.

The right assistant pushes the ureter upward with a retractor inserted into the paravesical space and applies downward pressure on the rectum with a retractor placed in the pararectal space.

The forward-ballooning rectum must be dissected somewhat more from its attachments to the outer aspects of the rectal pillar. To accomplish this, sponge forceps inserted intraperitoneally are used to depress the anterior rectal wall.

Technical Problems—Figures 22.59–22.62

1. During the process of dividing the rectal pillar, injury to the rectum is possible if the forward-ballooning rectum has not been sufficiently displaced caudally.
2. The *rectal pillar may be divided too far cephalad*, which will cause bleeding from the lateral parametrium.
3. If the entire rectal pillar is *divided freely* without clamping, bleeding from the medial rectal artery might ensue.

Opening the Vesicouterine Fold

Figure 22.63. Schauta-Amreich procedure. Opening the anterior peritoneum.

The vesicouterine fold is easily recognized at the anterior surface of the uterus as a tongue of shiny whitish membrane. It is lifted slightly off the anterior uterine wall with tissue forceps and is opened with one cut of the scissors.

A delicate silk ligature fixed to the peritoneal wound edge serves for traction. A second long tamponade strip is inserted anteriorly into the wide-open peritoneal cavity, which prevents intestinal loops from prolapsing.

Detail. Opening the vesicouterine peritoneal space.

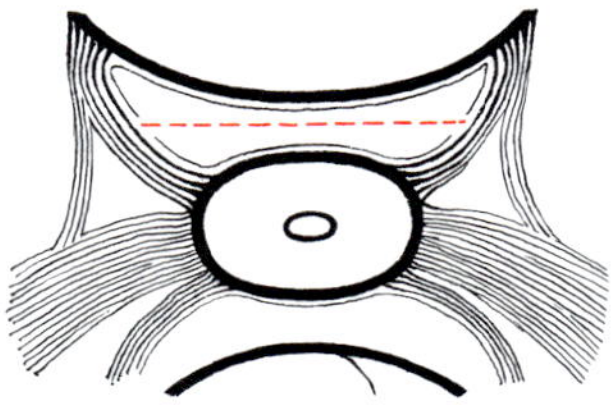

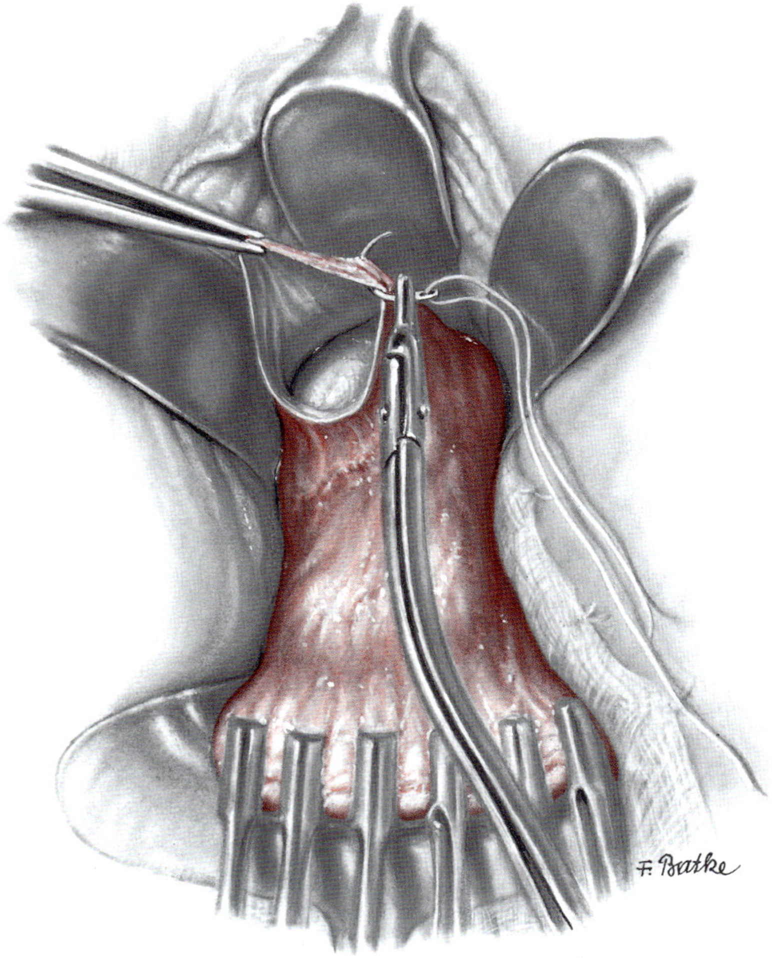

Technical Problems—Figure 22.63

1. If the *silk* used as a ligature at the anterior peritoneal wound edge *is too heavy*, the peritoneum may tear at the slightest pull.
2. If the *needle* used to suture the anterior peritoneal wound edge *is too large*, the peritoneum will tear during manipulation of the needle in the limited area of the vesicouterine space. As a consequence, the suture may pull out and cause the peritoneal edge to retract.
3. While tamponading the bowel, an anterior retractor must be inserted intraperitoneally to lift and support the anterior peritoneal wound edge. If the *gauze pad is inserted into the peritoneal cavity without the protection of the retractor*, the silk traction suture at the anterior peritoneal edge will tear out or the peritoneum will tear laterally and far upward. This type of peritoneal laceration may be difficult to repair.

Resection of Adnexa in Conjunction with Uterus

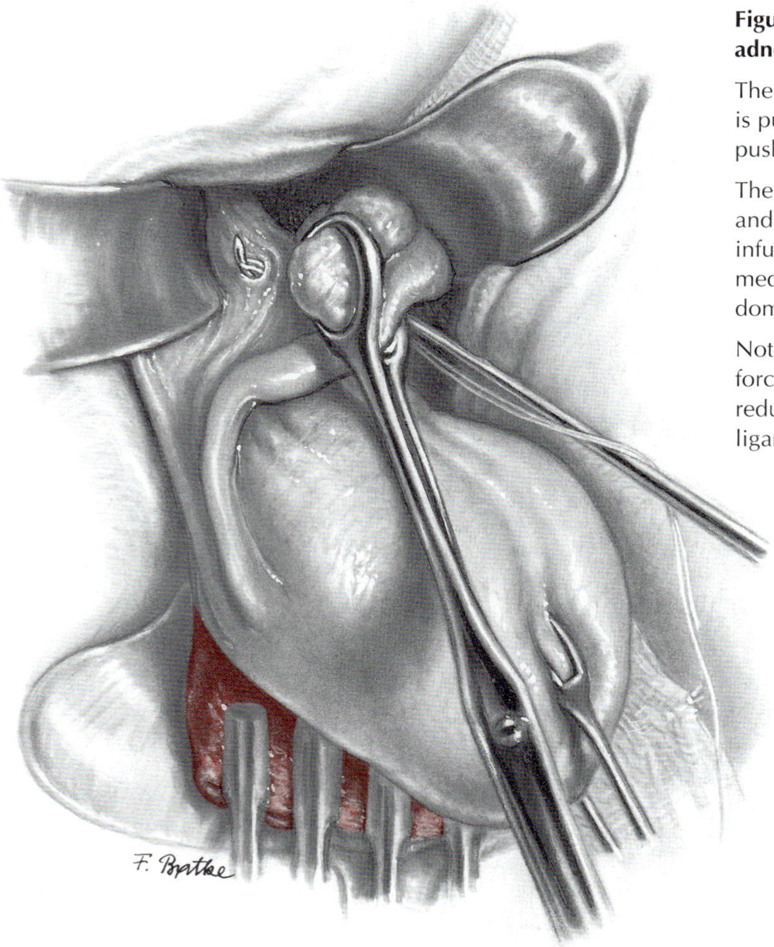

Figure 22.64. Schauta-Amreich procedure. Resecting the right adnexa. First ligation of the infundibulopelvic ligament.

The uterus has been tilted forward out of the abdominal cavity and is pulled downward with a claw tenaculum. The round ligament is pushed laterally with a lateral retractor.

The surgeon has grasped the tube and the ovary with ring forceps and lifted them somewhat away from the posterior uterine wall. The infundibulopelvic ligament is now clearly visible and is ligated from medial to lateral using a Deschamps needle 1–2 cm above the abdominal end of the ovary.

Note that during the infundibulopelvic ligation, the ovarian ring forceps lifts the adnexa somewhat away from the pelvic wall. This reduces the risk of damaging the ureter, which courses behind the ligament along the pelvic wall.

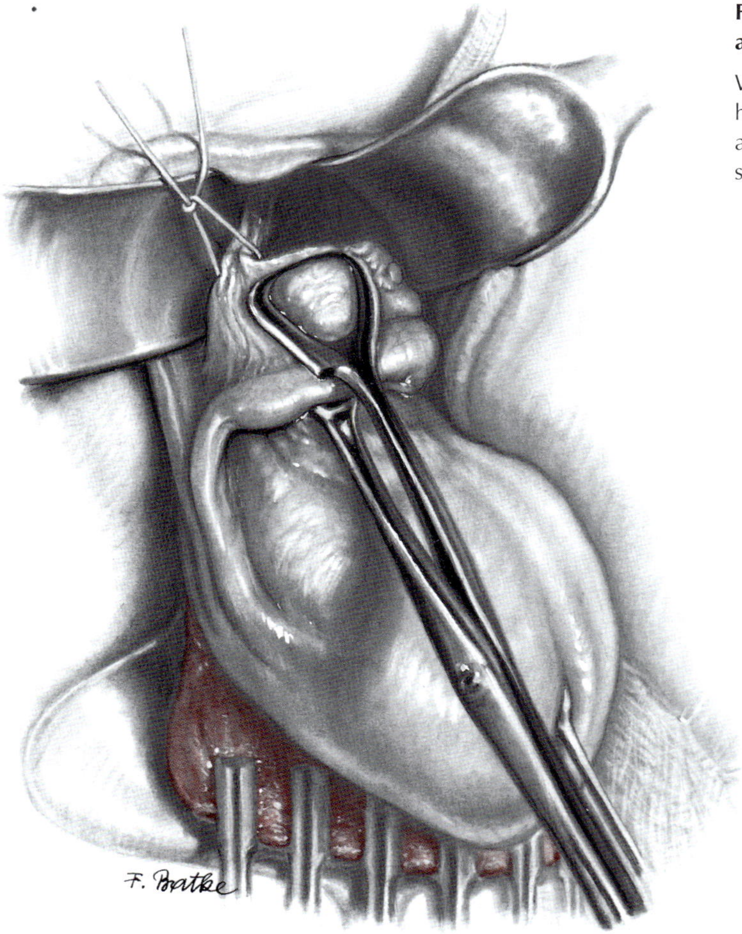

Figure 22.65. Schauta-Amreich procedure. Resecting the right adnexa. First ligation of the infundibulopelvic ligament.

When the infundibulopelvic ligature is tied, the ovarian forceps are held horizontally by the left assistant's left hand and placed flat against the posterior uterine wall. Thus the surgeon increases the space available for tying the ligature high up in the operative field.

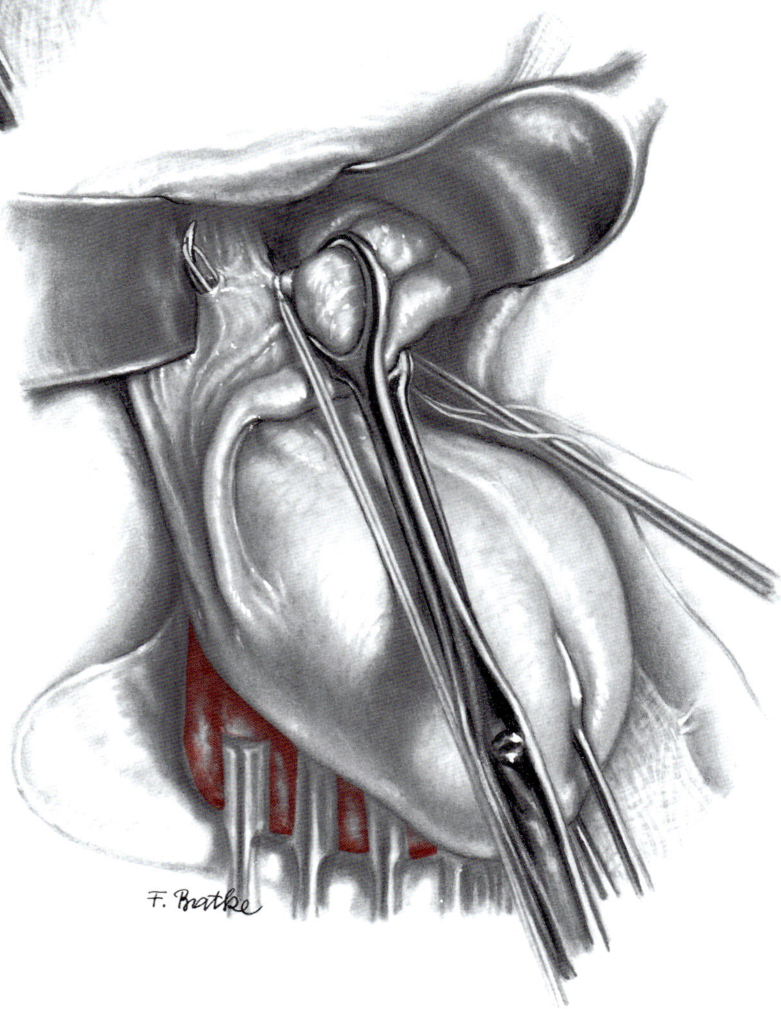

Figure 22.66. Schauta-Amreich procedure. Resecting the right adnexa. Second ligation of the infundibulopelvic ligament.

While pushing the infundibulopelvic ligament higher up, the surgeon once more grasps the right adnexa with ring forceps sagittally and lifts it somewhat away from the pelvic wall to avoid also ligating the ureter.

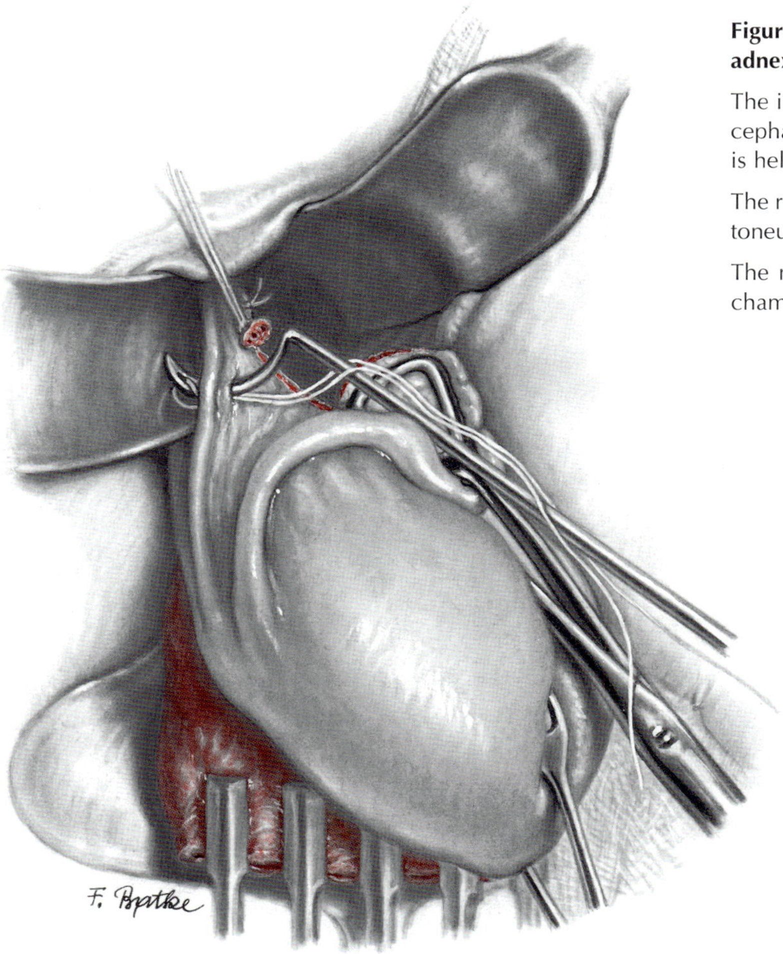

Figure 22.67. Schauta-Amreich procedure. Resecting the right adnexa. Ligating the round ligament.

The infundibulopelvic ligament is doubly ligated and divided. The cephalad ligature is cut short, and the long end of the caudal suture is held upward.

The right assistant releases the round ligament and retracts the peritoneum located laterally to the round ligament instead.

The round ligament is ligated from medial to lateral with a Deschamps needle.

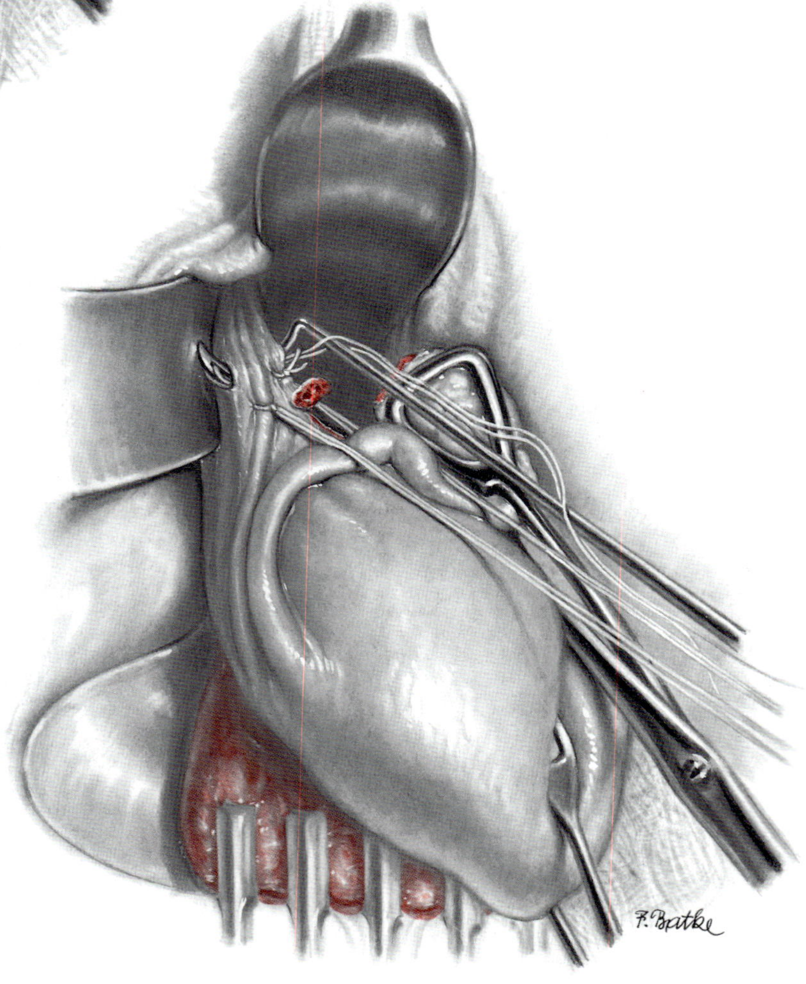

Figure 22.68. Schauta-Amreich procedure. Resecting the right adnexa. Ligating the round and infundibulopelvic ligaments conjointly.

The long ends of the sutures at the infundibulopelvic stump and the round ligament are pulled down to the left, and both ligaments are jointly ligated once more cephalad to all previously placed sutures with a Deschamps needle.

Figure 22.69. Schauta-Amreich procedure. Resecting the right adnexa. Dividing the round ligament.

The long ends of the ligament sutures are pulled upward. Laterally to the round ligament, the peritoneal leaf (the anterior leaf of the broad ligament) is pushed to the side, and the ligated round ligament can then be divided.

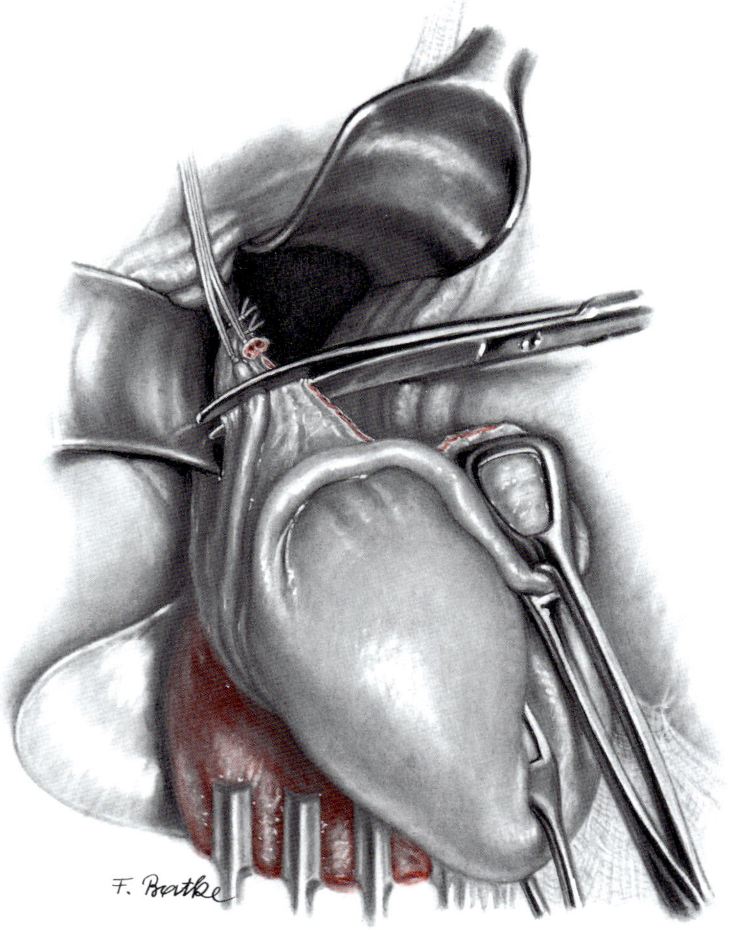

Technical Problems—Figures 22.64–22.69

1. Technical difficulties *may make it impossible to place a second tie on the infundibulopelvic ligament* proximal to the first one. A second safety ligature is always to be preferred, even if it has to be affixed close above the first one. If only one ligature has been placed, and it comes off because of a strong pull or poor purchase, massive hemorrhage will occur from the ovarian artery and vein. These severed vessels retract immediately upward into the infundibulopelvic ligament when a ligature comes off, and it is then difficult and even dangerous to grasp them again with a clamp because of the close proximity of the ureter to the cephalad portion of the ligament. To staunch the bleeding from these retracted vessels, laparotomy may be necessary. (However, in a series of more than 800 Schauta-Amreich radical procedures, this complication was never encountered because it was always possible to place the second infundibulopelvic ligature).

2. The infundibulopelvic and round ligaments can also be divided *between clamps.* However, we advise against this practice because it might become necessary to clamp the ligaments high. In such a case, the likelihood of injury to the closely underlying ureter by the clamp is much more pronounced than when ligating with a Deschamps needle.

Resection of Lateral Parametria (Cardinal Ligaments)

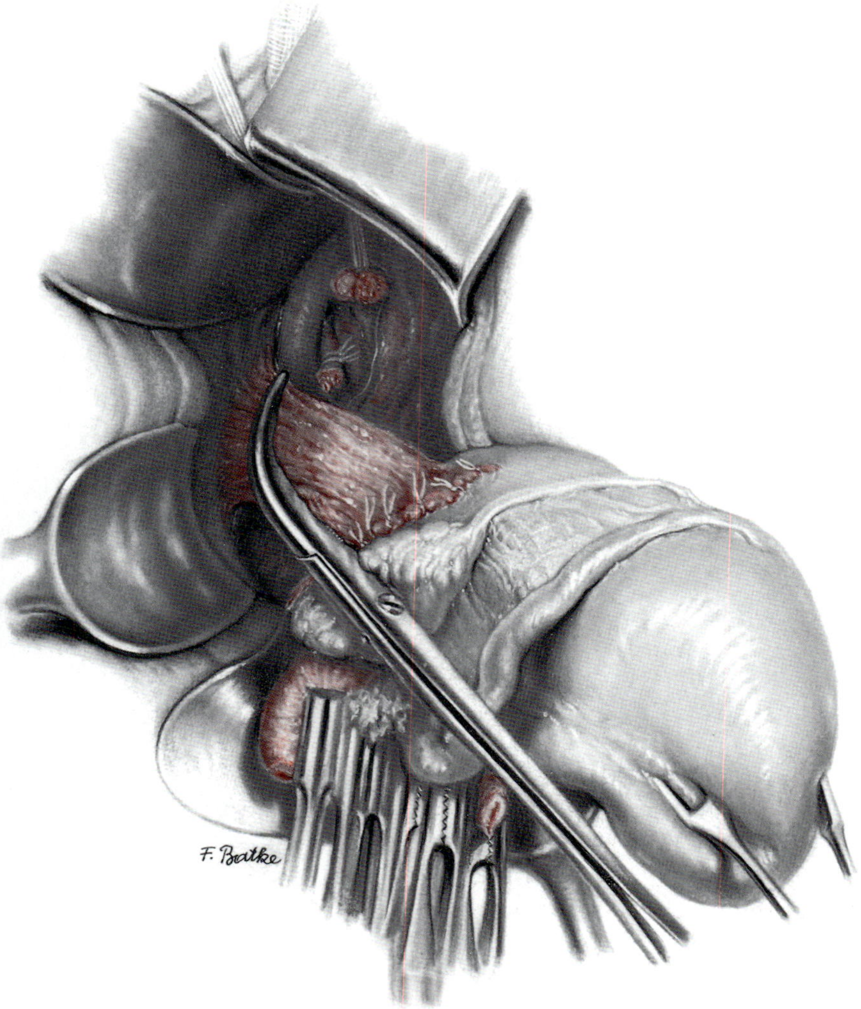

Figure 22.70. Schauta-Amreich procedure. Resecting the right lateral parametrium.

After separating the bladder pillar from the cervix, the rectal pillar from the rectum, and the adnexa from the pelvic wall, the uterus is left connected to the pelvic wall only by the lateral parametrium and is therefore rather mobile.

The surgeon visually checks to ensure that the right ureter is retracted well out of the way with appropriate retractor pressure before the parametrium is resected close to the pelvic wall. With an additional lateral retractor the forward-ballooning rectum is depressed toward the sacrum. The lateral parametrium is then clearly exposed as a wide tissue layer coursing diagonally upward from the edge of the cervix and laterally to the pelvic wall. One or more curved parametrial clamps can be placed close to the pelvic wall and the parametrium resected.

Details. Dividing the lateral parametrium in schematic cross-section. *Left,* connective tissue pillars, ureter and uterine vascular bundle in situ; *center,* view after division of the vesicouterine and rectouterine ligaments and the uterine vascular bundle; *right,* view after division of the cardinal ligament.

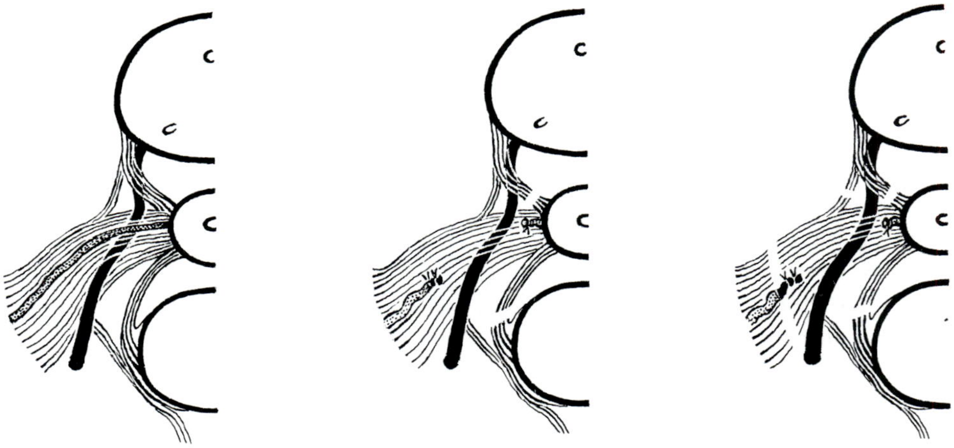

Technical Problems—Figure 22.70

The *parametrial clamps must not be placed too high* on the pelvic wall because large blood vessels in this area may be injured.

Closure of Peritoneal Cavity

A precise closure of the peritoneal cavity and extraperitonealization of the stumps is the best prophylaxis against infection and adhesion.

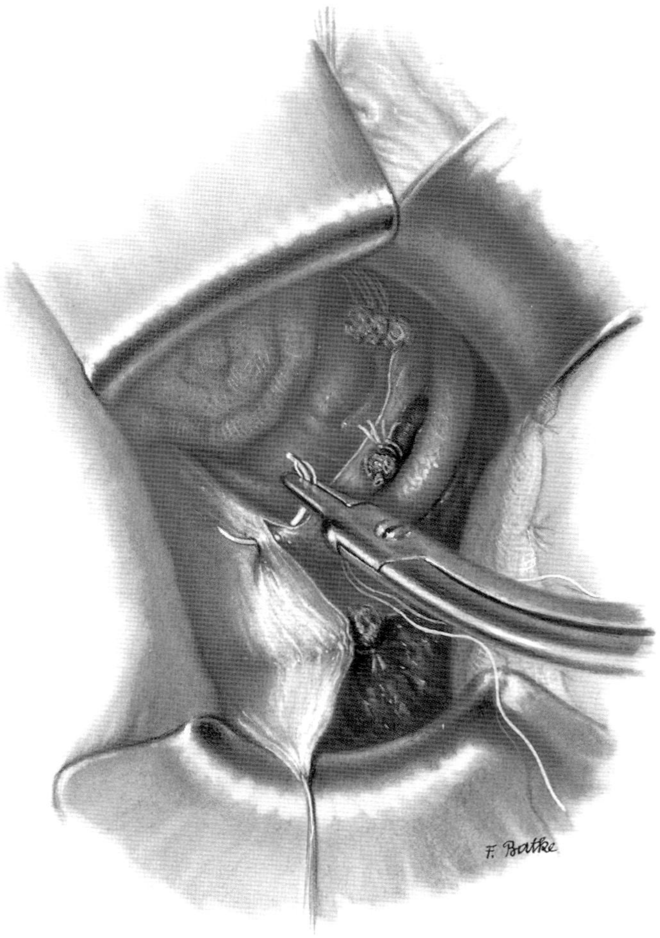

Figure 22.71. Schauta-Amreich procedure. Closing the peritoneal cavity. Placing the left angle suture.

The right assistant holds back the bowel with a gauze pack that is retracted upward with a wide right-angled retractor inserted intraperitoneally. The left assistant pushes the freed ureteral knee extraperitoneally upward and to the left with a retractor.

The uterine stump is seen medial to the ureteral knee; cephalad the pedicles of the infundibulopelvic and round ligaments are pulled upward, and caudally the pedicle of the rectal pillar is adherent to the rectal peritoneum (the lateral parametrial pedicle is not visible).

The surgeon grasps the uppermost angle of the peritoneal wound edge in the needle.

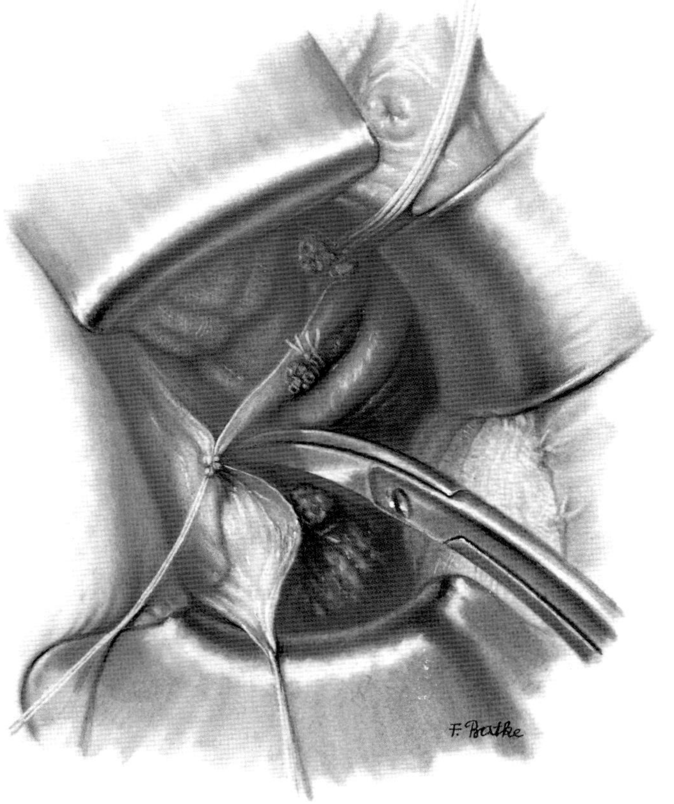

Figure 22.72. Schauta-Amreich procedure. Displacing the ureteral knee during closure of the peritoneal cavity. The angle suture is tied.

The closely adherent ureteral knee is pushed upward with the closed scissors and mobilized once more.

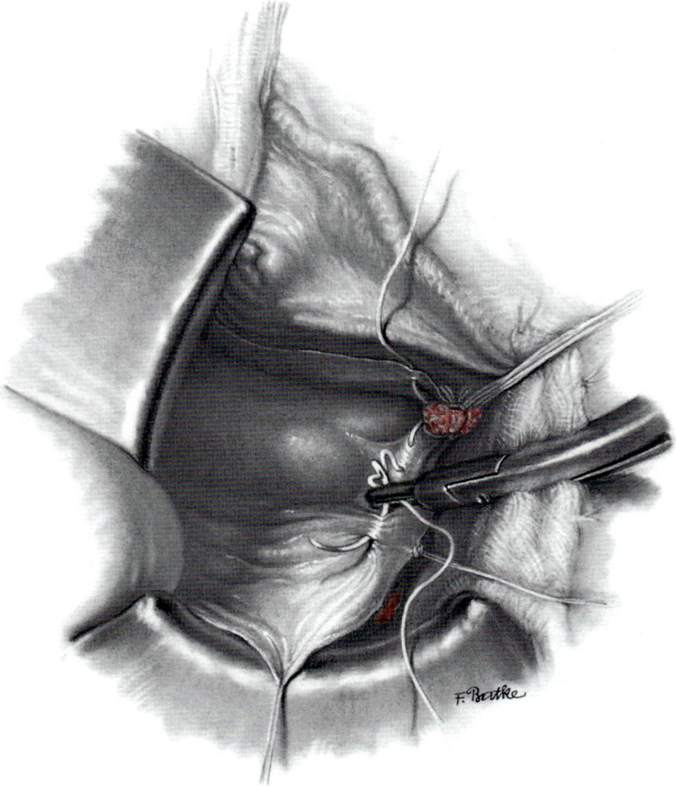

Figure 22.73. Schauta-Amreich procedure. Closing the peritoneal cavity. Left angle suture as half purse-string suture.

The assistant pulls the sutures on the round and infundibulopelvic pedicles up and to the left; at the same time he or she pulls down on the pseudoangle suture.

The peritoneal angle suture, begun anteriorly, is continued around to include the peritoneum medially to the infundibulopelvic and the round ligament pedicle and then medially to the pseudoangle suture.

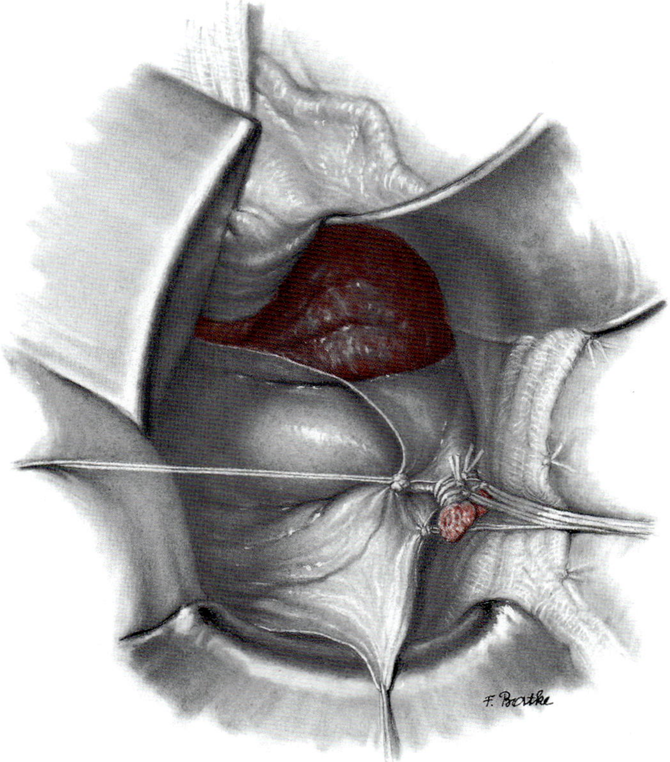

Figure 22.74. Schauta-Amreich procedure. Closing the peritoneal cavity.

The left half purse-string suture is tied; it lies somewhat cephalad and medial to the angle suture. The pedicles are thereby precisely extraperitonealized.

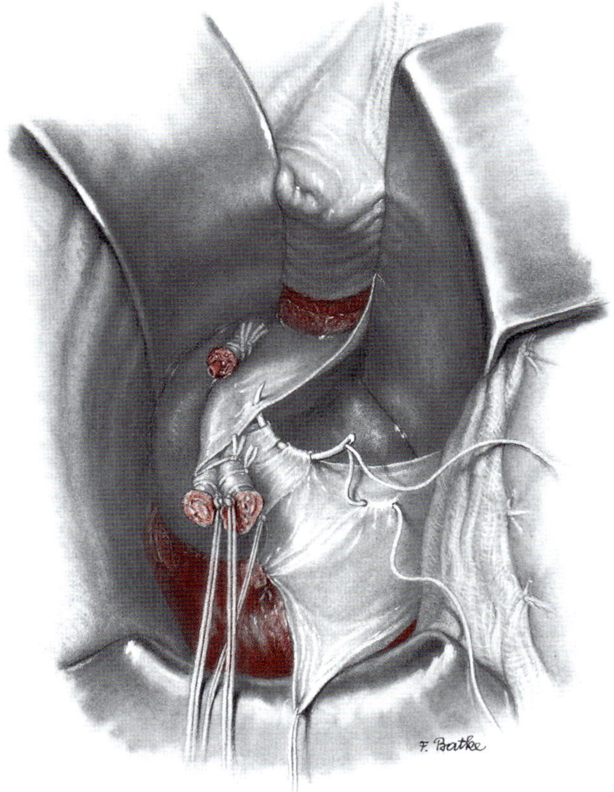

Figure 22.75. Schauta-Amreich procedure. Closing the peritoneal cavity. Placing the right peritoneal angle suture.

The left assistant takes over the large intraperitoneal right-angled retractor. With an extraperitoneal retractor, the right assistant pushes the ureter, the uterine pedicle, and the bladder upward, while pulling the sutures of the infundibulopelvic and the round ligaments downward.

The surgeon begins the peritoneal suture deep on the rectal peritoneum and continues upward by grasping the peritoneum in several places until the tip of the needle punctures the anterior peritoneal wound edge.

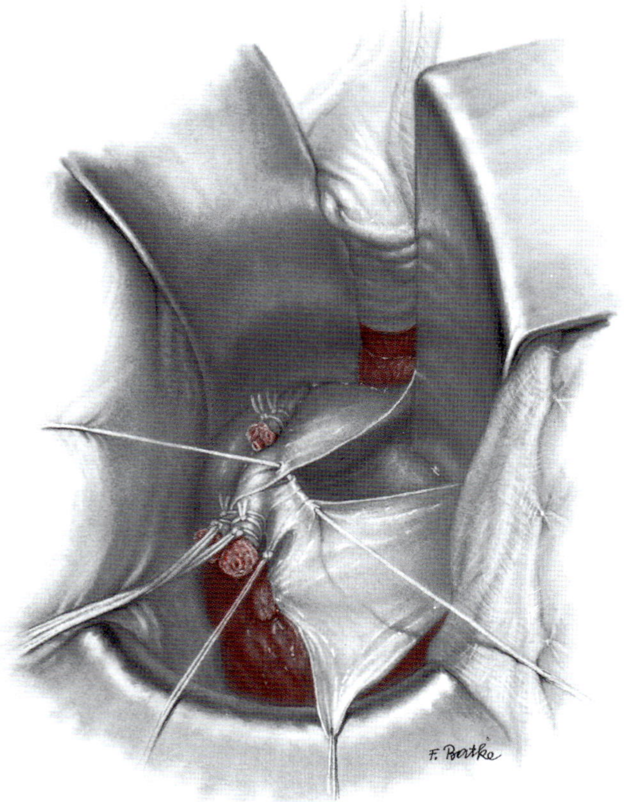

Figure 22.76. Schauta-Amreich procedure. Closing the peritoneal cavity. Tying the right peritoneal angle suture.

The ureteral knee is well visible; it is located at a safe distance from the suture. The pedicles are precisely extraperitonealized.

Figure 22.77. Schauta-Amreich procedure. Plicating the bladder.

The peritoneal cavity is closed; the bladder is noticeably descended after it had been extensively separated from the pelvic wall during the procedure. It must now be plicated with several catgut sutures, fixing it to the anterior vaginal circumcision wound edge.

The first bladder plication suture has already been tied on the left side; an additional suture is placed at several sites in the bladder wall, fixing it to the anterior vaginal wound edge.

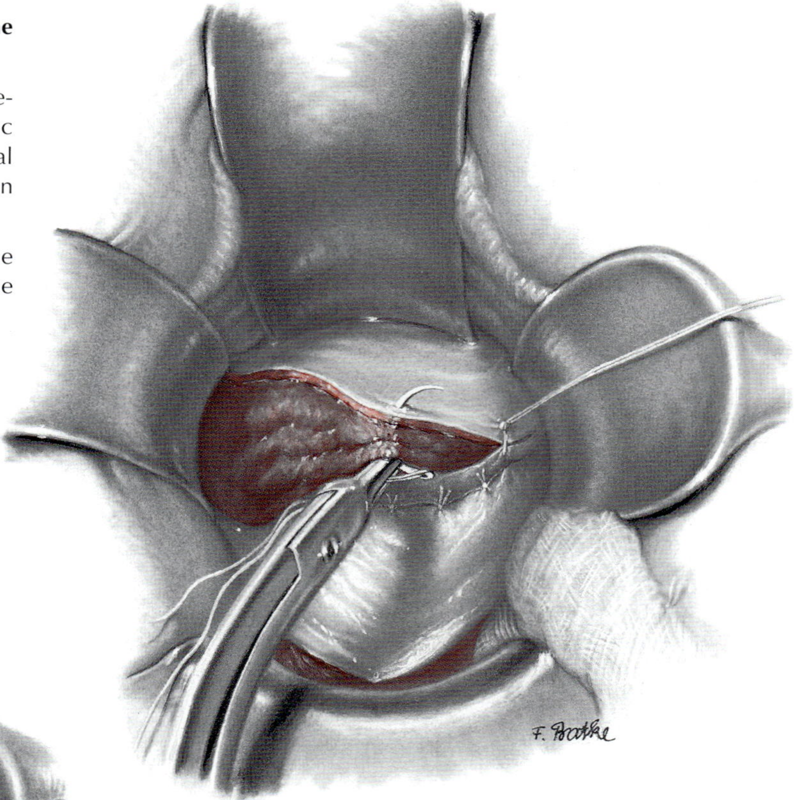

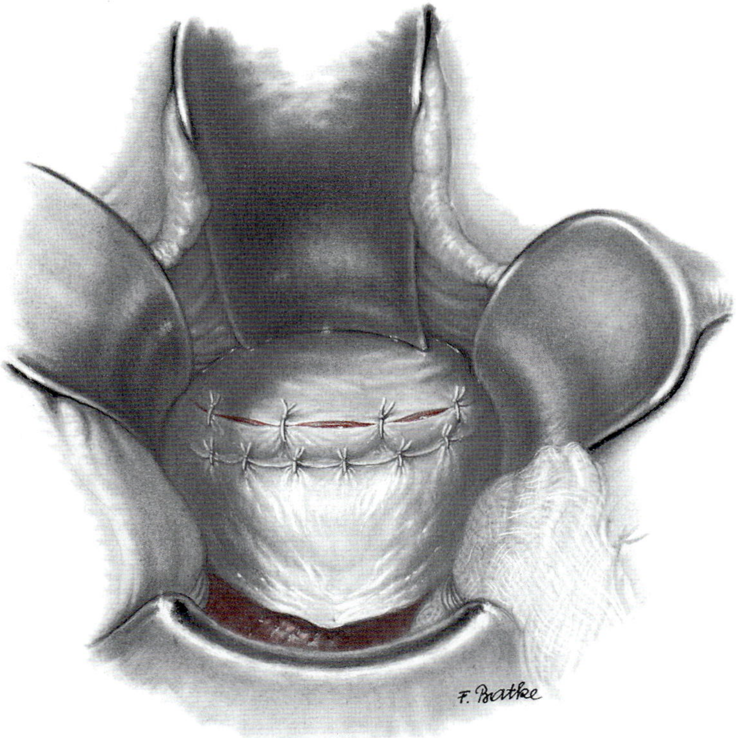

Figure 22.78. Schauta-Amreich procedure. Appearance of the field at the peritoneal closing, plicating the bladder.

Two transverse sutures are seen: the lower corresponds to the peritoneal closing sutures and the upper to the bladder plication.

Inspection and tamponade of the wound cavity follow. Retractors are placed in appropriate locations. The surgeon visually checks the course of the ureters to make certain that they are mobile. In addition, the pelvic wall is palpated to determine if the lymph nodes are pathologically enlarged. He or she also makes sure that any oozing of blood is controlled; this is easily done because there is good exposure and access to the pelvic wall once the internal genitalia and parametria have been removed. The large retroperitoneal cavities are tamponaded with gauze packings (two each) folded four times that are 4 m long and 6 cm wide and have been soaked in a Baneocin solution. Beginning with the 3rd postoperative day, the gauze packs are to be shortened daily and will be completely removed on the 5th day.

Technical Problems—Figures 22.71–22.78

1. When the pseudoangle suture is being placed, the ureter can be included if the needle is placed too deeply. The same may happen while the half purse-string suture is being placed, if too much peritoneal tissue is loaded on the needle medial to the uterine vascular pedicle.
2. Sometimes, after the peritoneal angle suture has been tied, the *ureter* appears to be *pulled up toward the ligature* and kinked. If that happens, it must be pushed away once more to make sure that urinary obstruction will not result.
3. If the sagittal *bladder plication sutures are performed too far laterally*, the needle may come too close to the uterovesical junction, causing the ureter to be injured.

Closing the Schuchardt Incision

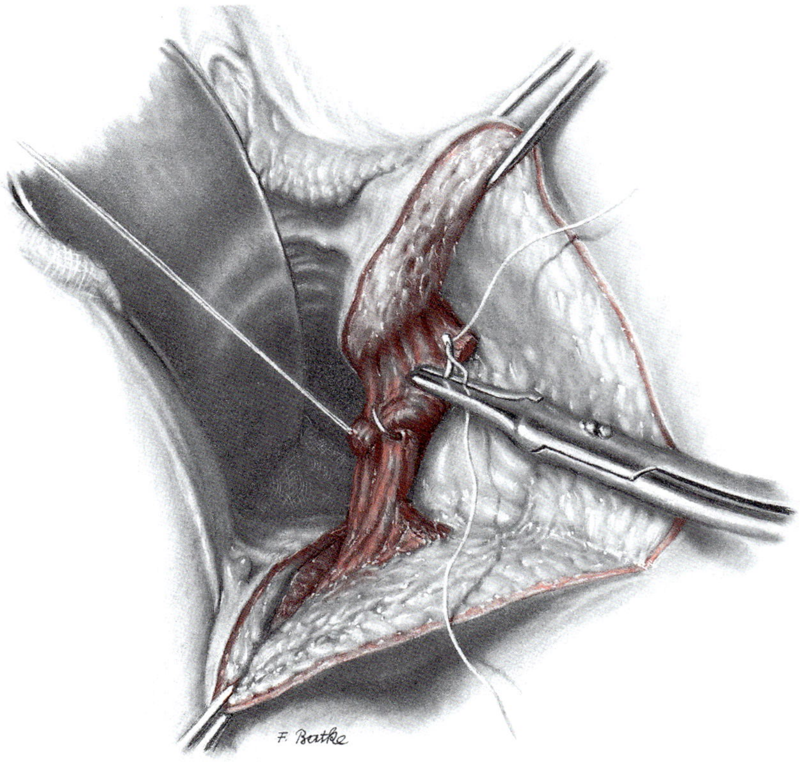

Figure 22.79. Schauta-Amreich Procedure. Closing the Schuchardt incision. Closing the levator muscle.

The Schuchardt incision is exposed with two single-toothed tenacula placed on either side of the posterior commissure.

The levator wound edges are approximated by several interrupted sutures.

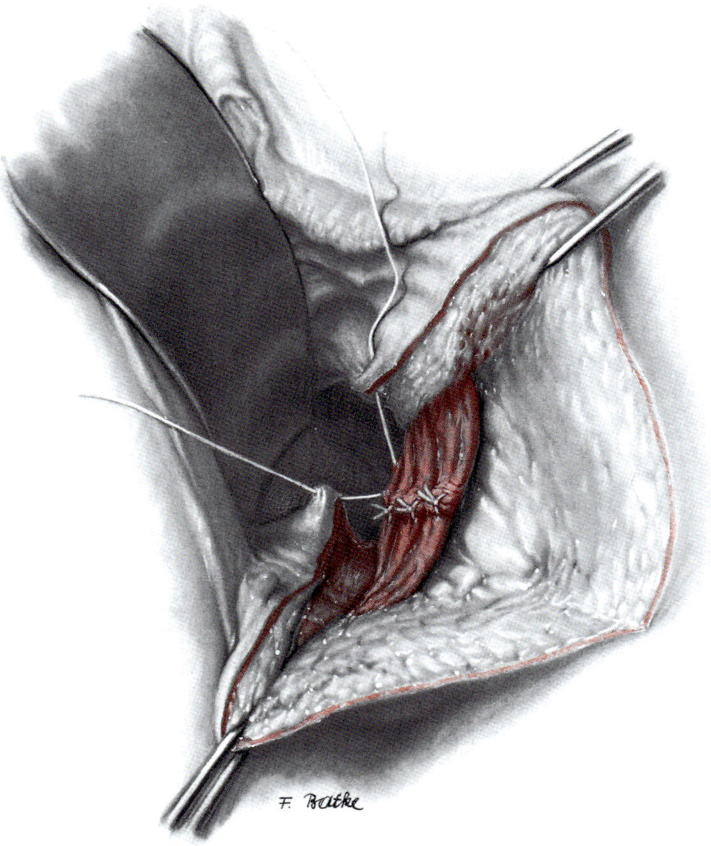

Figure 22.80. Schauta-Amreich procedure. Closing the Schuchardt incision. Apposing the vaginal wound edge.

The levator muscle is sewn. In closing the vaginal mucosa edges, one begins at the uppermost angle of the wound where the longitudinal vaginal incision meets the circumferential incision.

It is important that the levator muscle in the depth be included in the topmost suture of the vaginal cuff to prevent subperitoneal serous secretions from flowing down into the Schuchardt incision. This could result in dehiscence of the wound.

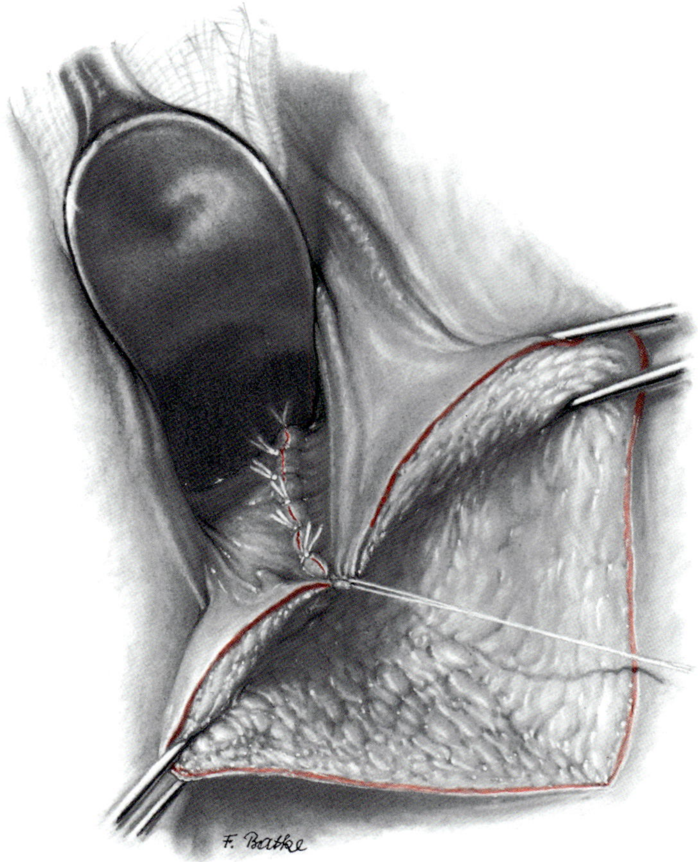

Figure 22.81. Schauta-Amreich procedure. Closing the Schuchardt incision. Suturing the vaginal wound edges.

The vaginal wall is closed with interrupted catgut sutures down to the posterior commissure. The ends of the last suture are left long for traction.

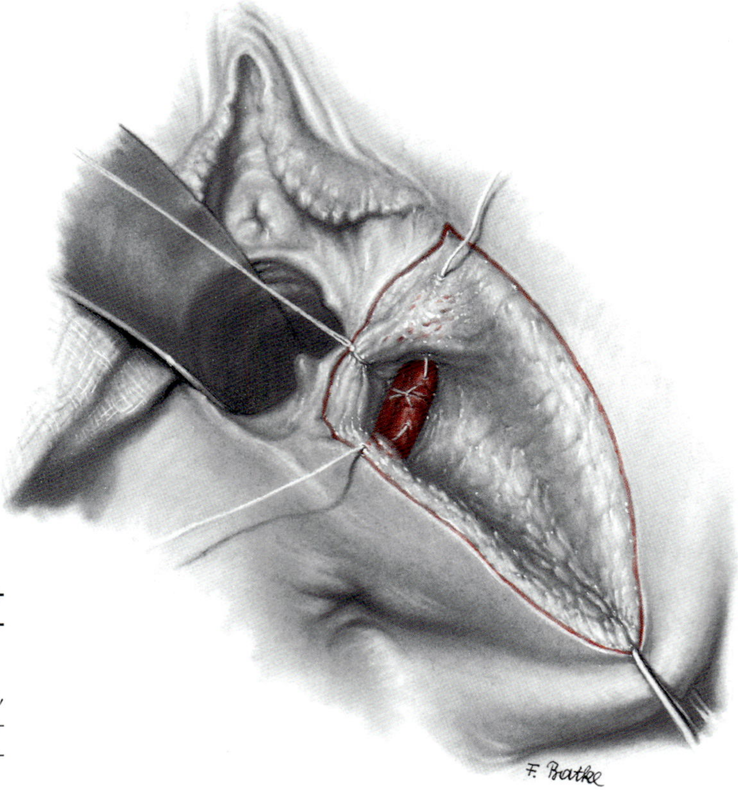

Figure 22.82. Schauta-Amreich procedure. Closing the Schuchardt incision. Suturing the bulbocavernosus muscle and the urogenital diaphragm.

To avoid leaving dead space while reconstructing the pelvic floor, the levator muscle deep down and the severed fibers of the urogenital diaphragm medially should be incorporated into the bulbocavernosus suture.

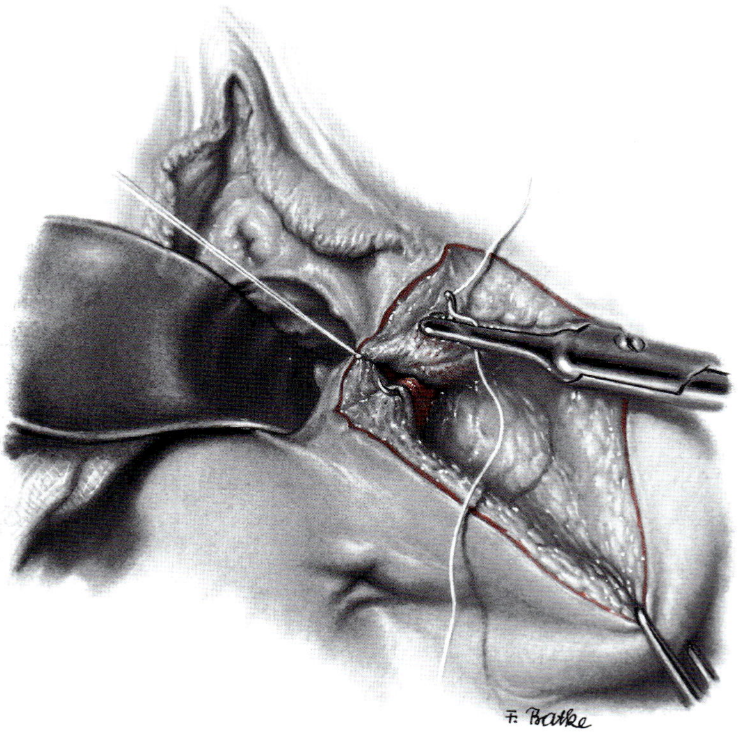

Figure 22.83. Schauta-Amreich procedure. Closing the Schuchardt incision. Closing the perineum in layers.

The deep tissues of the perineal incision are joined with interrupted sutures.

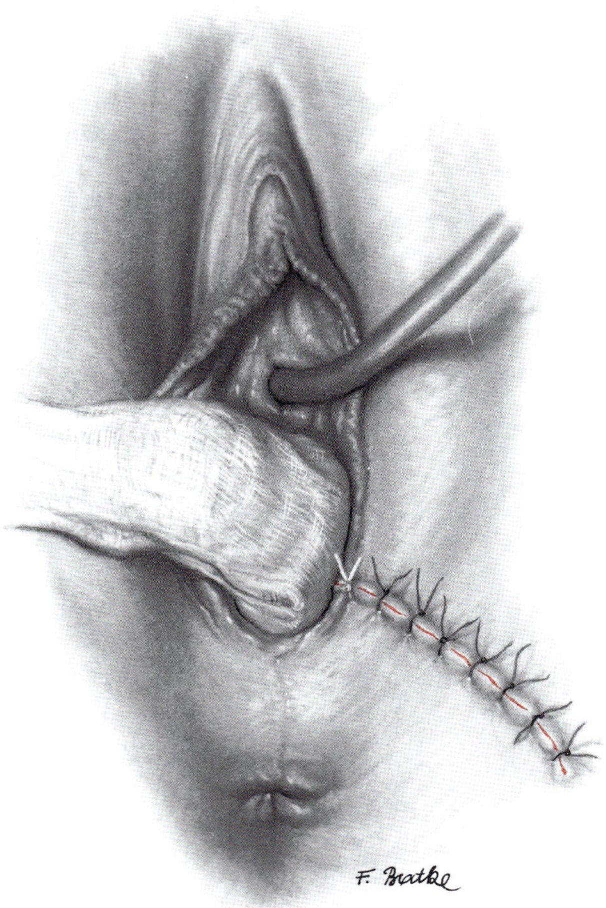

Figure 22.84. Schauta-Amreich procedure. Closing the Schuchardt incision. Approximating the skin wound edges. End view.

The perineal skin edges are joined with silk sutures. At the posterior commissure the last vaginal catgut suture can be seen. An indwelling catheter is inserted into the bladder (and the balloon inflated). In addition, the vaginal cuff has been loosely tamponaded with two gauze packings.

Technical Problems—Figures 22.79–22.84

1. When bringing the severed edges of the levator muscle together, one can grasp more tissue laterally than medially without any problem. In the *immediate vicinity of the medial levator stump is the rectum; one must proceed with care here, grasping only a small amount of muscle tissue to avoid damaging the easily punctured rectum.* The more caudal one gets in the layered closure of the Schuchardt incision, the less likely it is for the rectum to be damaged.
2. The uppermost vaginal suture must include the levator so that *no communication will remain between the retroperitoneal cavity and the levator incision.*
3. The perineal skin must be apposed precisely. Therefore, *closure of the perineal skin must be from the bottom up and not the reverse.* (An exact apposition of the vaginal wound edges is cosmetically not of great significance because the vagina possesses a good granulation capability.)

At the conclusion of the procedure, the vaginal cuff is tamponaded with the same two gauze pads, which had already been partially introduced into the retroperitoneal wound cavity.

Index